AF709126

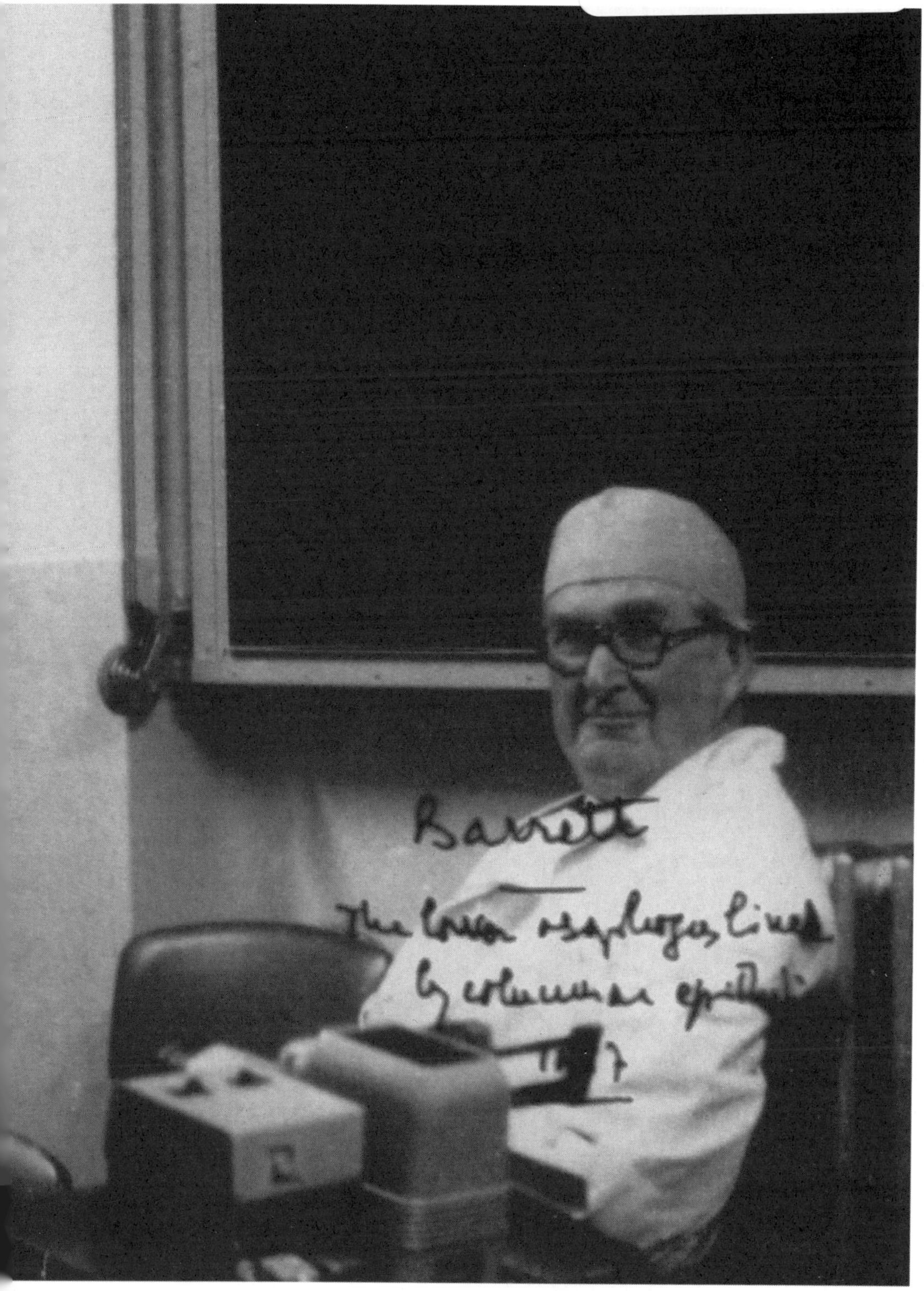

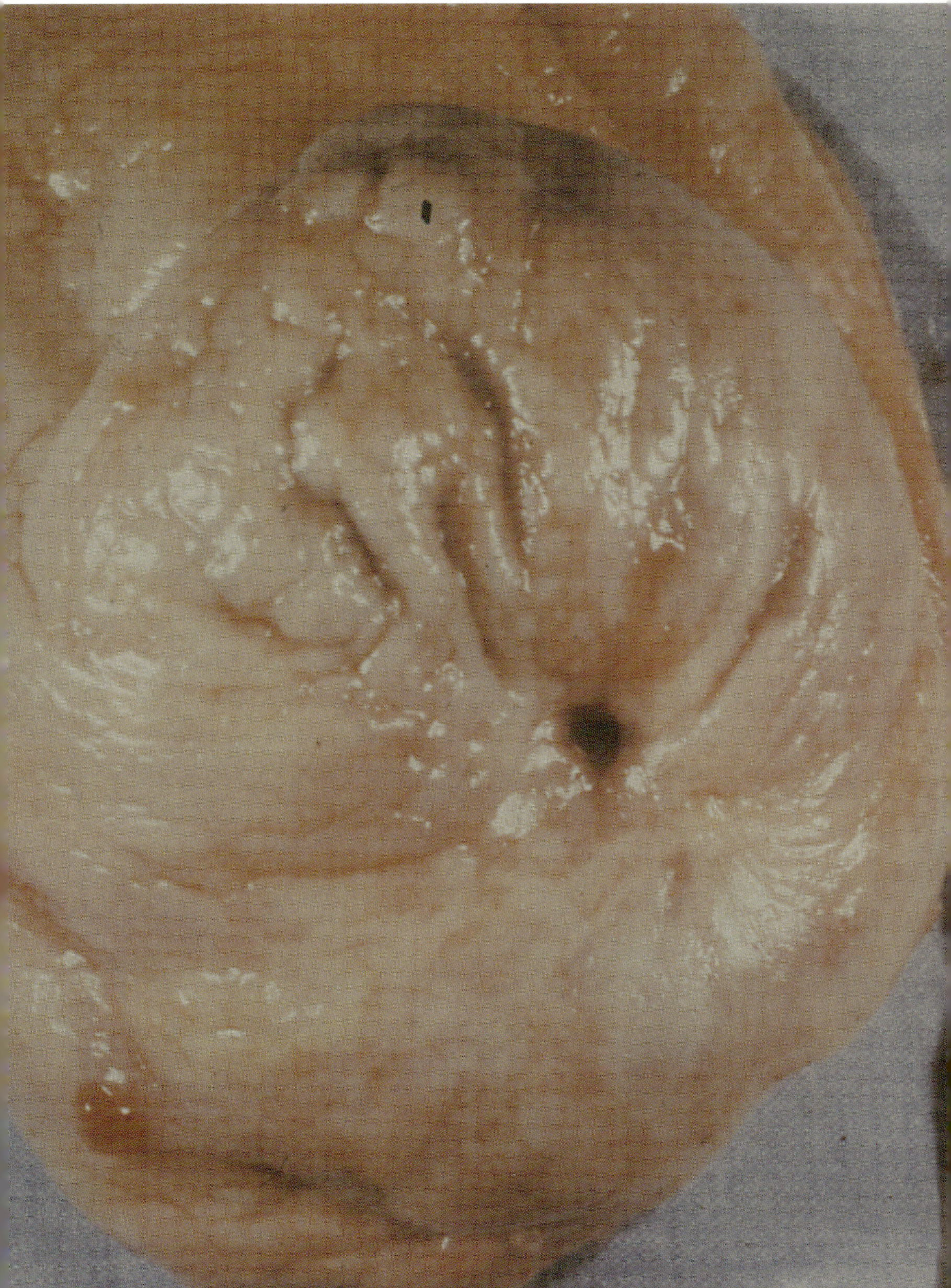

ISBN 2-7420-0384-3

Éditions John Libbey Eurotext
127, avenue de la République, 92120 Montrouge, France
Tél : 01 46 73 06 60
E-mail : contact@john-libbey-eurotext.fr
Site internet : http://www.john-libbey-eurotext.fr

John Libbey Eurotext Limited
42-46 High Street
Esther, Surrey, KT 10 9QY
United Kingdom

CIC Edizioni Internazionali
Corso Trieste 42
00198 Roma, Italia
Tel : (39) 06 841 26 73

© 2003, John Libbey Eurotext, Paris

Il est interdit de reproduire intégralement ou partiellement le présent ouvrage sans autorisation de l'éditeur ou du Centre Français d'Exploitation du Droit de Copie, 20, rue des Grands-Augustins, 75006 Paris.

O.E.S.O.

Organisation mondiale d'Études Spécialisées sur les maladies de l'Œsophage
World Organization for Specialized Studies on Diseases of the Esophagus

Barrett's esophagus
Columnar lined esophagus

250 questions - 250 answers

VOLUME II

Robert Giuli

Jörg Rüdiger Siewert
Daniel Couturier
Carmelo Scarpignato
Editors

John Libbey EUROTEXT

PREVIOUS BOOKS of O.E.S.O.

- 1985 : *Cancer of the esophagus*. 135 questions.
  Paris : Maloine, 430 p.
  R. Giuli Ed.

- 1988 : *Benign lesions of the esophagus and cancer*. Answers to 210 questions.
  Paris : Springer Verlag, 850 p.
  R. Giuli, R.W. McCallum Eds.

- 1991 : *Primary motor disorders of the esophagus*. 450 questions - 450 answers.
  Paris : John Libbey Eurotext, 1 220 p.
  R. Giuli, R.W. McCallum, D.B. Skinner Eds.

- 1994 : *The esophageal mucosa*. 300 questions - 300 answers;
  Paris : Elsevier, 1 200 p.
  R. Giuli, G.N.J. Tytgat, T.R. DeMeester, J.-P. Galmiche Eds.

- 1998 : *The esophagogastric junction*. 420 questions - 420 answers.
  Paris : John Libbey Eurotext, 1 600 p.
  R. Giuli, J.-P. Galmiche, G.G. Jamieson, C. Scarpignato Eds

Colour plates

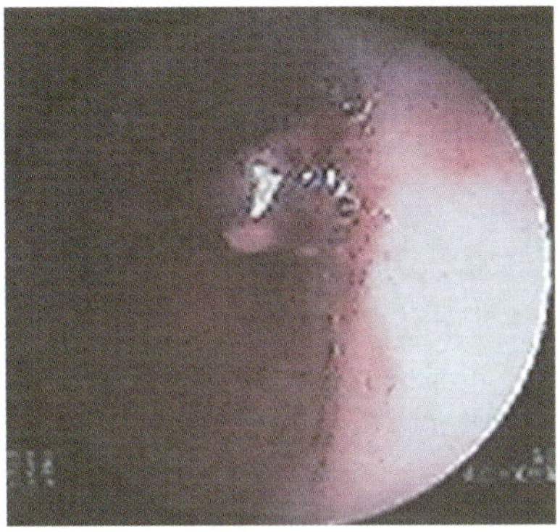

Figure 1. Patient 2 (*Table I*) with bleeding marginal ulcer which was injected. 48 hours later a perforation of distal esophagus occurred. **(See page 525.)**

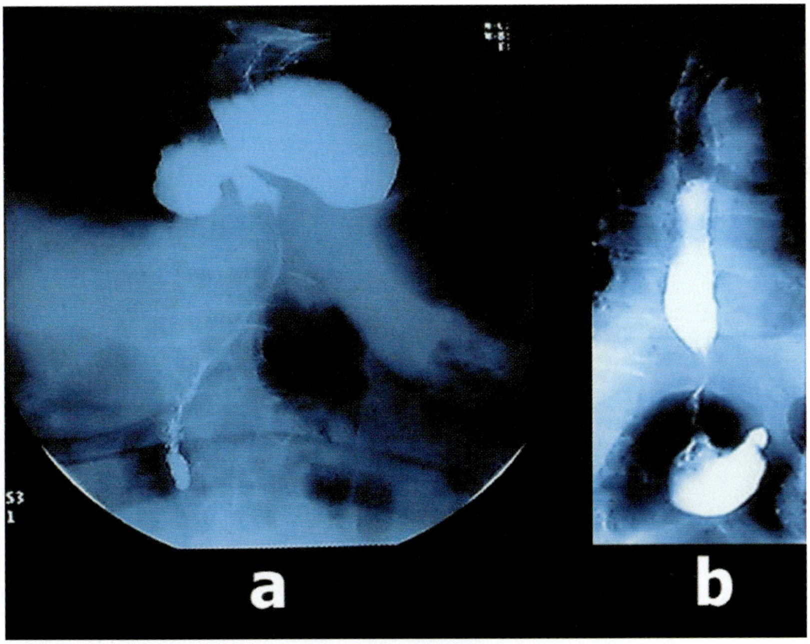

Figure 2. A. Patient 5. X-ray detected up side down stomach. **B.** Postoperative situs. **(See page 525.)**

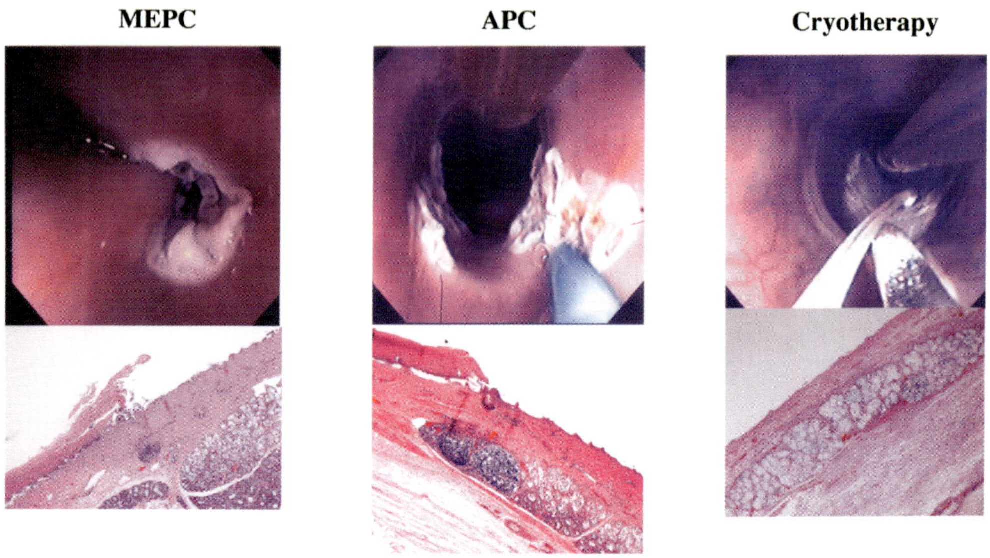

Figure 1. Endoscopy immediately and histology one hour post ablation. In all three there is complete epithelial ablation with an intact lamina propria. **(See page 628.)**

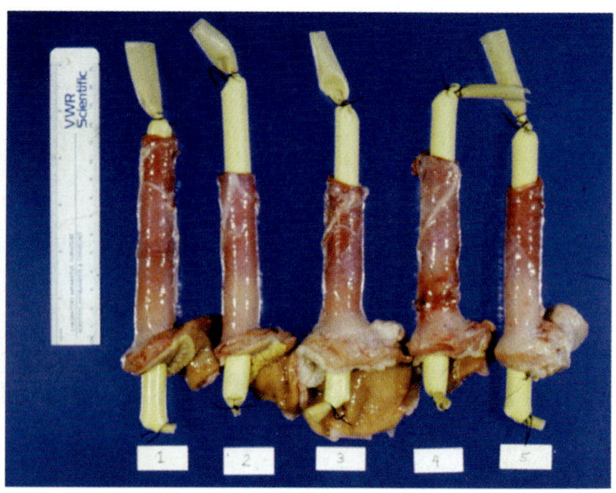

Figure 1. **(See page 631.)**

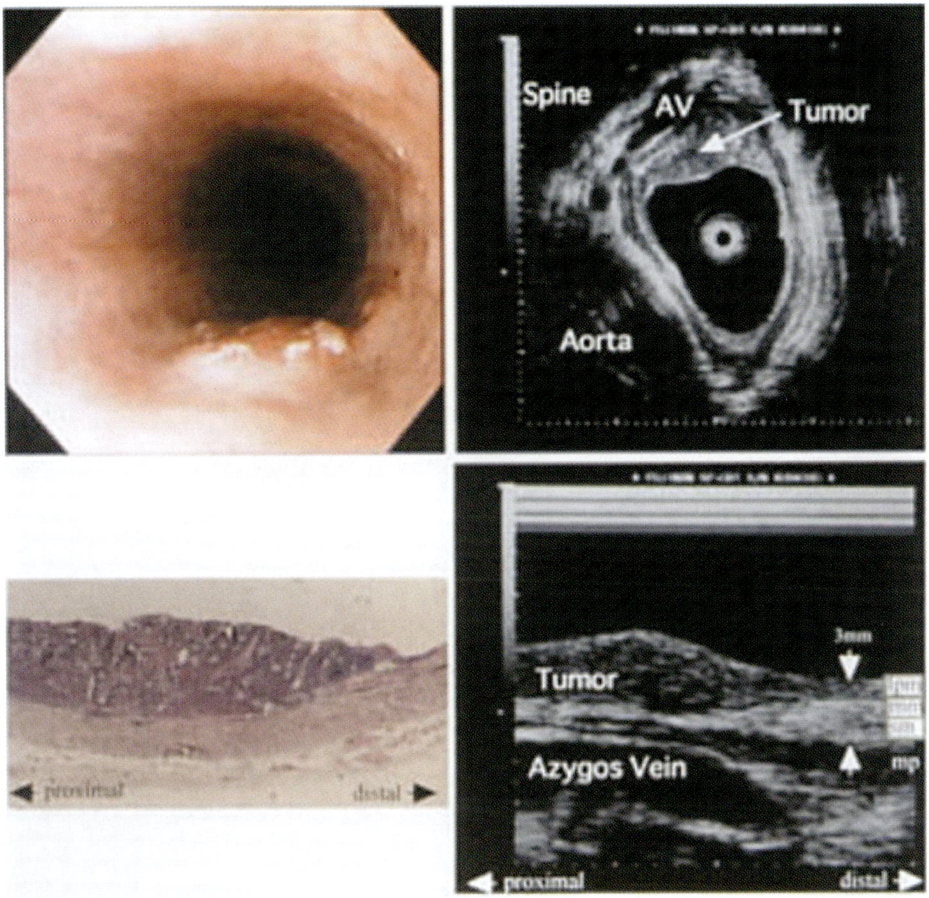

Figure 5. B. Ultrasonograms obtained by the soft balloon method. (See page 767.)

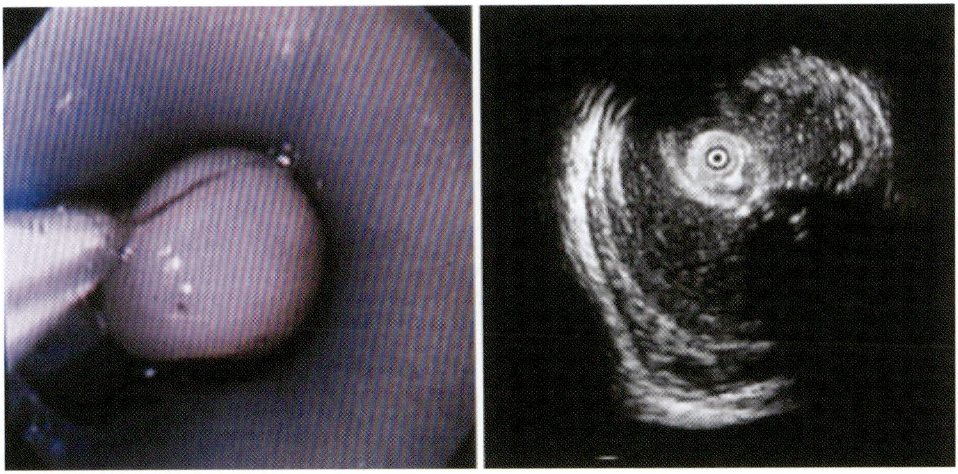

Figure 6. Endosonography during endoscopic resection (cited from [21] with permission) (See page 768.)

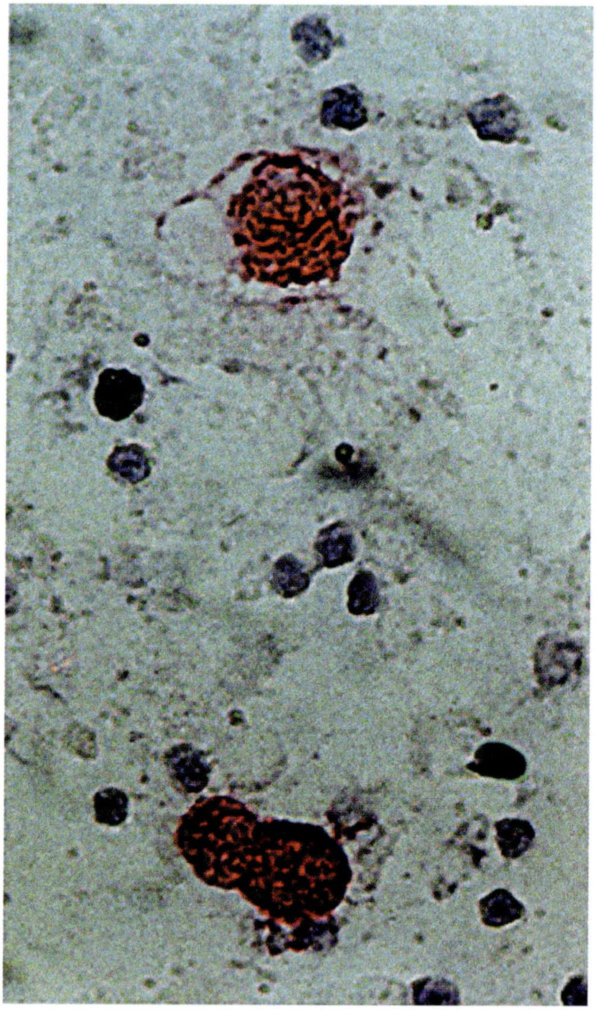

Figure 1. This is an example of tumor cells in a bone marrow aspirate from a patient with esophageal adenocarcinoma. Alkaline phosphatase anti-alkaline phosphatase staining for cytokeratin 18 demonstrates hyperchromatic tumor cells staining positive (red). **(See page 790.)**

Contents

VOLUME II

Treatments

Medical treatments

Surgical treatments

Screening and surveillance

Regression

Adenocarcinomas

Treatments

Medical treatments

Acid suppression in Barrett's esophagus: why and how?

C. Scarpignato, I. Pelosini, E. Molina (Parma)

Gastric juice that refluxes into the esophagus can injure esophageal squamous epithelium. When the injury heals through a metaplastic process in which an abnormal columnar epithelium replaces the injured squamous one, the resulting condition is called Barrett's esophagus [1]. This abnormal columnar epithelium is an incomplete form of intestinal metaplasia (IM), containing several columnar cell types with gastric, small intestinal, or colonic features. Although this so-called specialized IM may be more resistant to gastro-esophageal reflux (GER) than the native squamous mucosa, the metaplastic cells are predisposed to malignancy. Indeed, gastroesophageal reflux disease (GERD) and Barrett's esophagus are the most important risk factors for esophageal adenocarcinoma, a tumor whose frequency has increased dramatically during the last two decades in Western countries [2]. Recent studies suggest that the incidence of adenocarcinoma with Barrett's esophagus is 0.5% per annum, a rate that is low in absolute terms, but is more than 30-fold higher than that of the general population [3]. Studies of survival in patients with Barrett's esophagus have been done predominantly in older men, for whom the risk of death from common lethal disorders (*e.g.* myocardial infarction, stroke) far exceeds their 0.5% annual risk of esophageal adenocarcinoma [4]. A long-term study of young patients with Barrett's esophagus might show that the condition shortens life, but such study has not yet been published.

The pathogenesis of Barrett's metaplasia is not yet precisely understood; in particular, the key factors favouring its development are not known. Barrett's metaplasia is an acquired condition resulting from long-standing GERD. Barrett's esophagus is clearly associated with severe GER. Compared with patients with erosive and nonerosive GERD without Barrett's esophagus, patients with columnar-lined esophagus typically have greater esophageal acid exposure based on 24-hour pH monitoring [5-8]. However, there is some overlap and some studies found no difference in intraesophageal acid exposure time between Barrett's patients and patients with high-grade esophagitis [9]. Part of the increase in acid exposure in Barrett's patients may be related to the almost uniform presence of a hiatal hernia, which is typically longer and associated with larger defects in the hiatus than controls or patients with esophagitis alone [10]. In addition, patients with Barrett's esophagus have a lower basal esophageal sphincter pressure (LESP) compared with GERD patients without columnar metaplasia [6].

It has long been known that acid GER is accompanied by the reflux of duodenal contents, and there is increasing evidence from animal and human studies that duodeno-gastroesophageal reflux (DGER), consisting mainly of bile and pancreatic juice, might play a significant role in the development of Barrett's metaplasia and Barrett's carcinoma [11-13]. Clarification of the role of DGER reflux in the context of GERD was hampered for a long time by inadequate methods to detect it. Aspiration studies were not representative because of short testing periods; scintigraphy was semiquantitative at best, expensive, and combined with radiation exposure. In addition, pH monitoring alone does not represent DGER. The clinical introduction of ambulatory 24-hour bilirubin monitoring in 1993 allowed a quantitative measure of DGER for the first time [14]. Several studies using this new device have provided important insight into the role of DGER in causing esophageal mucosal injury in humans. These studies showed a significant but graded increase in both acid and DGER from normal controls to esophagitis and patients with columnar metaplasia, with the highest values in patients with Barrett's esophagus. Furthermore, it appears that DGER occurs most commonly in association with acid reflux. A pivotal study of Vaezi and Richter [15] in patients with and without complications of Barrett's esophagus [34] found increased reflux of bile and acid into the lower esophagus of both groups compared to healthy controls. More importantly, reflux of acid paralleled DGER, and both were significantly higher in patients with complicated Barrett's esophagus than in the uncomplicated group (*Figure 1*). Other investigators (*for review see* [12]) have subsequently confirmed the results of these studies.

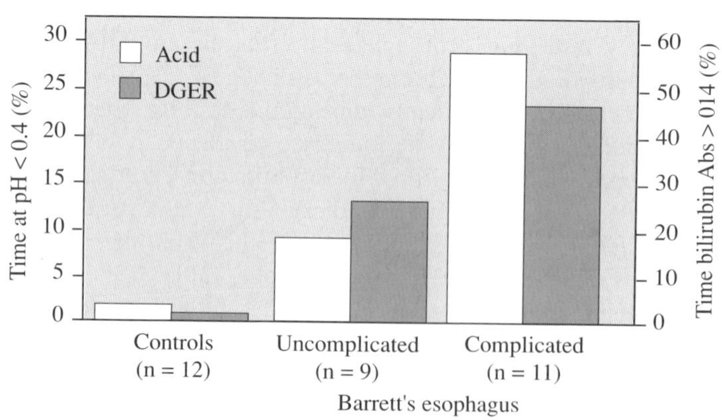

Figure 1. Acid and bile reflux in controls and in patients with uncomplicated and complicated Barrett's esophagus. Increase in both components of the esophageal refluxate was significantly ($p < 0.005$) higher in those patients with complication (from [34]).

Barrett's disease and the underlying GERD are intensively treated with the aim of reducing mortality from cancer arising from columnar metaplasia. Several management strategies have been proposed:

- antireflux therapy [16] or antireflux surgery [17] to reduce or even abolish GER and DGER;
- endoscopic ablation of Barrett's epithelium [18, 19];
- the use of non-steroidal anti-inflammatory drugs (NSAIDs) to inhibit cyclooxygenase (COX) isoenzymes and their effect on cellular proliferation [20, 21];
- regular endoscopic (and hystologic) surveillance [22, 23].

Although each strategy has a plausible rationale and some indirect evidence to support it, none has proved to reduce deaths from cancer in Barrett's esophagus. Furthermore, each entails expense, inconvenience, and variable risk [24]. Among the preventive strategies for cancer, only regular endoscopic surveillance has been recommended for routine clinical use by several medical societies, including the American College of Gastroenterology [25].

The aim of this paper is to review antireflux therapy in Barrett's esophagus and to present the latest developments in the field of antisecretory medications.

Treatment of gastroesophageal reflux disease in Barrett's esophagus

The primary goals of antireflux therapy, irrespective of the presence of Barrett's esophagus, are elimination of the symptoms and signs of reflux esophagitis, and prevention of GERD complications, such as peptic esophageal stricture and adenocarcinoma. Antireflux lifestyle modifications have traditionally been recommended for patients with GERD, including elevation of the head of the bed, avoidance of recumbency for several hours after meals, reduction in fat intake, and cessation of smoking, but little published data support the efficacy of these modifications [25]. And indeed the Genval Workshop Report [26] on reflux disease recently suggested that there is currently a significant overestimation of the likelihood that patients will derive adequate relief through alterations in lifestyle factors.

Modern medical therapy for GERD focuses on the suppression of gastric acid secretion through histamine H_2-receptor antagonists (H_2RAs) or proton pump inhibitors (PPIs) therapy [28], whereas surgical therapy is directed at correcting the underlying diathesis by creating a barrier to GER through fundoplication [29]. Medical and surgical therapies have been shown to be effective for healing the symptoms and signs of reflux esophagitis, and for limiting the peptic complications of GERD, although antireflux surgery is not devoid of morbidity [30] and, although very rarely, of mortality [29]. There is little doubt that antireflux surgery is an excellent management option for the properly selected patient in the hands of the skilled and experienced esophageal surgeon [29]. On the other hand, there is also little doubt that, as practiced, there has been substantial morbidity associated with the suboptimal utilization of antireflux surgery [30]. The risk of postoperative symptoms (especially dysphagia) creates considerable anxiety for surgeons, gastroenterologists, and patients alike [30]. As Watson and Jamieson [29] emphasize, experience does matter, especially in the arena of antireflux surgery. Whether or not you are likely to subject a patient to a Nissen fundoplication in the hands of an experienced surgeon, there is compelling evidence for not recommending that a patient be the "occasional case" of the nonspecialized surgeon. Results of surgical management are indeed operator-dependent.

On the contrary, no particular expertise is required for prescribing a pill (*i.e.* a proton pump inhibitor) whose undesirable effects, if any, are trivial and reversible [31].

Although for both medical [32] and surgical [17, 33] therapy some regression of the Barrett metaplasia has been reported, neither approach has been proved to decrease the risk of esophageal adenocarcinoma, even if the incidence of developing dysplasia or cancer following fundoplication appears to be less than with antisecretory treatment [34].

Acid suppression in Barrett's esophagus: H_2RAs or proton pump inhibitors?

H_2RAs have a relatively short duration of action and, depending on the individual agent and whether the patient is in a fed or fasting state, suppress acid for approximately 4-8 hours [35] Consequently, multiple daily doses of these agents are likely to be required. Furthermore, H_2RAs produce incomplete inhibition of post-prandial gastric acid secretion. Overall, these agents inhibit acid secretion by up to 70% over a 24-hour period [35, 36].

A further shortcoming is that tolerance to standard H_2RAs generally develops within 2 weeks of repeated administration, resulting in a decline in acid suppression [37]. This can be explained by a gastrin-induced increase in entero-chromaffin-like cell-derived histamine concentrations at the H_2-receptor on the parietal cell [38] and up-regulation of both gastrin and H_2-receptors (*Figure 2*). In contrast, PPIs control both basal and food-stimulated acid secretion and produce more complete and longer lasting acid suppression than H_2-blockers [39]. Such acid inhibition virtually abolishes the damaging peptic activity of gastric juice. In addition, tolerance to PPIs has not been observed, an advantage presumably attributable to the fact that they act at the final site of acid production, thereby blocking the effects of any compensatory mechanisms promoting acid secretion [38, 39].

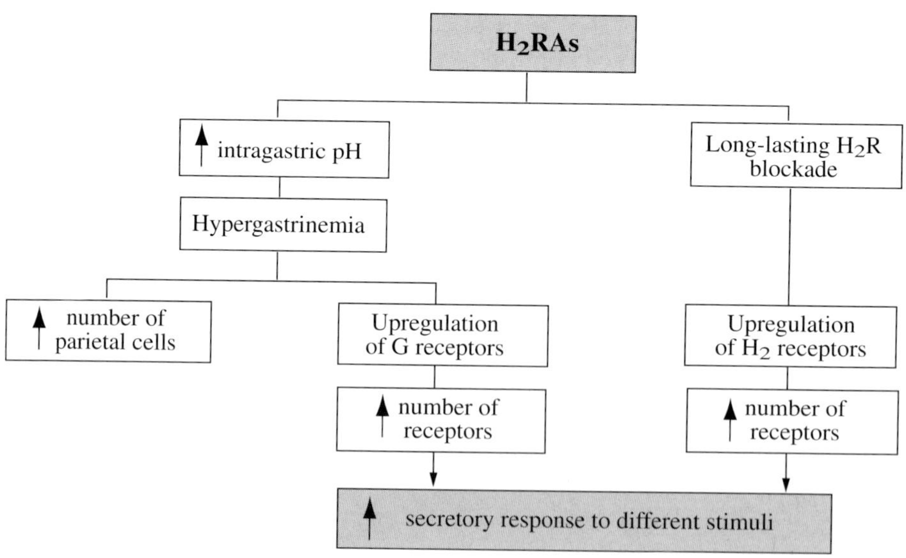

Figure 2. Mechanisms underlying the development of tolerance after short-term treatment with H_2RAs.

The appreciation that even twice daily PPIs are unable to control intragastric acidity during the night and that in both healthy subjects and GERD patients a "nocturnal acid breakthrough" (NAB, defined as a fall in gastric pH below 4 for more than 1 hour at night), does occur [40] has suggested the use of a bedtime dose of H_2RAs to improve acid control [41]. However, long-term use of these agents led to development of tolerance so that their effect on NAB lessened with prolonged therapy [42]. In addition, it must be emphasized that no study in patients with GERD has yet demonstrated that addition of H_2RAs to twice daily PPI therapy provides any further benefit above that derived from PPIs alone [43].

When used at the usual recommended dose, all available H_2 receptor antagonists (cimetidine, ranitidine, famotidine, nizatidine and roxatidine) are equally effective and have been found generally very safe [36, 44]. However, their efficacy is limited in more severe forms of GERD (such as the Barrett's esophagus) [44], where the superior efficacy and more rapid symptomatic relief provided by PPIs is well established [45].

Proton pump inhibitors for Barrett's esophagus: how effective are they?

Conventional-dose antisecretory therapy reduces, but fails to abolish, gastric acid secretion in most patients with Barrett's esophagus. Furthermore, the effect of this therapy of GERD symptoms in these patients does not accurately reflect the degree of acid suppression. Esophageal pH-monitoring studies frequently reveal pathologic acid reflux in patients with Barrett's esophagus rendered asymptomatic by PPIs administered in conventional dosages [46]. Approximately 80% of patients with Barrett's esophagus treated with a PPI twice daily experience NAB which is often associated with episodes of acid reflux [47]. Some individuals can achieve almost complete achlorydria by high-dose PPI therapy or by adding an H_2RA at bedtime to a regimen of a PPI administered twice daily [41], although such a benefit is not long-lasting [42]. Tailoring acid control individually with the help of pH-monitoring is feasible and effective not only in controlling symptoms but may also result on decreased length and development of squamous islands in patients with Barrett's epithelium [48].

Although the best way of decreasing DGER is an antireflux operation that corrects the defective barrier, aggressive acid suppression therapy with omeprazole 20 mg orally twice daily increases gastric pH, decreases gastric volume, and diminishes DGER to a degree similar to that of antireflux surgery [49, 50], without affecting duodenogastric reflux (DGR) [51]. It is worthwhile mentioning that, in experimentally-induced enterogastric reflux, animals treated with omeprazole had a significantly higher incidence of gastric cancer and esophageal hyperplasia [52]. Due to the potential harmful effect of duodenal contents in an anacid melieu [53], patients with Barrett's esophagus on long-term PPIs should be accurately monitored with the inclusion of gastric biopsies in their endoscopic surveillance program.

Concomitant symptomatic GERD is common in patients with Barrett's esophagus and manifests as heartburn, regurgitation, dysphagia, or chest pain. In patients with reflux esophagitis the degree of mucosal healing is directly related to the proportion of time during the 24-hour period for which the intragastric pH is maintained above 4 [54, 55]. As a consequence, numerous studies have documented the marked efficacy of PPIs in controlling symptoms of GERD and healing esophagitis and a large meta-analysis [56] clearly showed a distinct advantage – either in terms of healing or symptom relief – of PPIs over H_2-RAs (*Table I*), a finding confirmed in a recent Cochrane Review [57].

Table I. Mucosal healing and symptom relief in reflux esophagitis: results of a meta-analysis (from [56]).

7,635 patients	PPIs	H_2RAs
Overall healing (%)	83.6 ± 11.4	51.9 ± 17.1
Symptom-free proportion (%)	77.4 ± 10.4	47.6 ± 15.5
Healing rate (%/week)	11.7	5.9
Relief rate (%/week)	11.5	6.4

In patients with Barrett's esophagus, ulcers are located either within the metaplastic columnar mucosa, typically in the lower part of the esophagus, or higher up in the distal portion of the squamous esophagus near the squamometaplastic junction [58]. Regardless of their location, these ulcers cause reflux symptoms in 70% of cases, may contribute to anemia and gastrointestinal bleeding in 50% [58] and may actually result in a life-threatening esophagobronchial fistula [59]. PPIs heal these ulcers in 80-90% of cases, but recurrences are common [58].

Besides healing of esophagitis and ulcers, PPIs proved to be superior to H_2RAs also in the prevention of recurrence [60] and of peptic stricture formation [61, 62], which may occur in up to 70% of the patients with Barrett's ulcer at the squamo-metaplastic junction.

Can acid suppression by proton pump inhibitors be followed by regression of Barrett's metaplastic surface?

Regression of the metaplastic surface is considered an important end point in the management of patients with Barrett's esophagus. The risk of malignant transformation in Barrett's esophagus should be related, at least in part, to the extent of its mucosal involvement [63, 64]. The greater the length of tubular esophagus occupied by IM, the higher the number of predisposed cells undergoing molecular or genetic changes leading to dysplasia and adenocarcinoma. By contrast, a reduction in the surface or complete regression of IM would reduce or eliminate the risk of malignancy. To this end PPIs have been used either alone or in combination with an ablative endoscopic techniques.

Over the past decade, several studies using various PPI regimens as single therapy for variable time periods have yielded inconsistent results. Published clinical trials provide evidence of increases in squamous islands in the Barrett segment, but do not provide convincing data in support of complete regression of columnar metaplasia. In a review of prospective studies of the treatment of Barrett's esophagus with PPIs (with or without surgery), only 3 of 123 patients had apparent complete reversal of Barrett metaplasia [65]. It should be emphasized, however, that the extent of regression is difficult to assess because IM may underlie the islands of squamous epithelial regrowth. Sampling by endoscopic biopsy is useful in ruling out progression of columnar metaplasia to dysplasia or adenocarcinoma; on the contrary, complete regression of the lesion cannot be definitively proven by this technique.

While acid suppression with antireflux surgery or PPIs has proven insufficient to completely reverse Barrett metaplasia, ablation of the lesion followed by acid suppression may be a promising option. As long as acid reflux is controlled with high dose PPIs, it is possible to ablate the metaplastic and dysplastic columnar epithelium of Barrett's esophagus using thermal or photochemical energy and permit regeneration of squamous mucosa following tissue injury [66].

In summary, PPIs represent the cornerstone of the therapy of patients with Barrett's esophagus since they control symptoms, heal esophagitis and ulcers, and prevent recurrence and strictures. Although some regression of the metaplastic epithelium can occur during long-term (more than 2 years) treatment with PPIs, to this aim they are best viewed as adjuvant therapy after endoscopic ablation of the columnar epithelium. Nevertheless, the impact of PPI therapy on the natural history and evolution of Barrett's esophagus towards dysplasia and adenocarcinoma is unclear and further long-term studies evaluating both intraesophageal acid and bile reflux will be necessary [45].

Are currently available proton pump inhibitors all the same?

Although there are differences among PPIs concerning their pharmacokinetics, pharmacodynamics, influence by food and antacids as well as potential for drug interactions [67, 68], it is not always evident whether these often subtle differences are clinically relevant. Several comprehensive analyses of the available clinical trials concluded that – when used at equivalent doses in the treatment of various acid-related disorders – all the available agents are similarly effective [67, 69, 70]. These conclusions concerning "clinical" efficacy of PPIs are backed by similar results obtained in comparative "pharmacological" analysis [71]. Guidance from the National Institute for Clinical Excellence (NICE) does not differentiate between PPIs except on the grounds of price and accepted indications [72]. The physician's choice of one PPI over another must therefore rest with her/his interpretation of the clinical importance of the generally small differences among PPIs, their approval for treatment of specific clinical indications within the physician's practice jurisdiction, and the strength of the evidence based on the quantity and quality of the supporting clinical trials [69].

Shortcomings and limitations of current proton pump inhibitors

Although effective and safe, currently available PPIs are still far from the ideal antisecretory compound. An ideal drug should allow full acid control around the clock and dose-dependent and predictable pharmacokinetic and pharmacodynamic properties. These properties and the consequent clinical effects should also be reproducible in a wide range of patient populations [73]. Finally, an ideal agent will display high oral bioavailability, a rapid onset of action and few, if any, clinically relevant interactions with food or concomitantly administered drugs [74].

The so-called first-generation PPIs (omeprazole, pantoprazole and lansoprazole) have notable limitations. These drugs exhibit substantial interpatient variability in pharmacokinetics and may have significant interactions with other drugs. The time of dosing and ingestion of meals may also influence the pharmacokinetics of these agents as well as their ability to suppress gastric acid secretion. First-generation PPIs also have a relatively slow onset of pharmacological action and may require several doses to achieve maximum acid suppression and symptom relief, possibly limiting their usefulness in on-demand GERD therapy. First-generation PPIs may also fail to provide 24-hour suppression of gastric acid, and nocturnal acid breakthrough can occur even with twice-daily dosing [74].

Taking all the above considerations, it is clear that there is room for improvement and new generation PPIs could be able to overcome the limitations of first-generation compounds [75]. To obtain an ideal PPI capable of achieving full inhibition of acid control with the first dose different avenues can be pursued. One way is to develop a compound whose favorable metabolism would allow an enhanced delivery of the active form to the proton pump with consequent better inhibition of acid secretion. Exploiting the stereospecific catabolism of enantiomers follows that way.

The extension of plasma half-life is a critical factor in improving the onset of action of PPIs and thus compounds with half-life longer than that of current PPIs may be expected to display first-day efficacy. Such avenue can be pursued through the synthesis of new chemical entities with a molecular structure different from the current (*i.e.* substituted benzimidazole) one or designing a pro-drug which will release the PPI in the bloodstream [76]. Tenatoprazole (*Figure 3*), consisting of one imidazopyridine ring connected to a

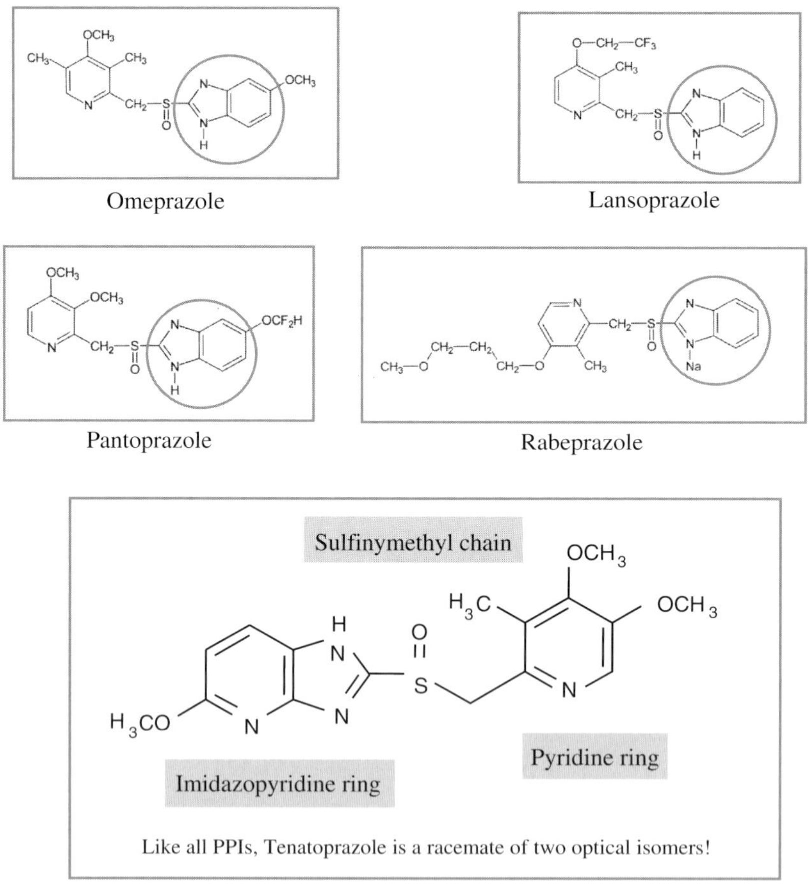

Figure 3. Chemical structure of the currently available PPIs (all benzymidazol derivatives) and of tenatoprazole (TU-199).

pyridine ring by a sulfinylmethyl chain, represents an example of a new chemical entity with extended half-life (about 8 hours compared to 1.0-1.5 hours) whereas compound D [76] is an investigational pro-PPI for very stable intravenous formulation that displays a longer duration of action in comparison with omeprazole. Some pro-drugs synthesized recently hydrolyze under physiological conditions (pH = 7.4) to provide PPIs with a half-life largely exceeding the 2 hours and are capable of providing sustained plasma concentration of the release PPI for a time longer than the currently used compounds [77].

Some interesting new PPI formulations have recently been patented [77]. An enteric coated extended release dosage form of a PPI provided an extended plasma concentration profile of the drug for a period of up to 12 hours. This pharmacokinetic profile is obtained with a formulation comprising a core material of a hydrophilic or hydrophobic matrix containing the PPI protected by enteric coating. An additional patent describes a multilayered tablet capable of releasing the PPI in discrete pulses separated in time (2 pulses of drug release at least 0.5 hour apart). The dosage form, which has one fraction with instant release of the drug and at least another fraction with a pulsed delayed release, is intended for once daily administration. The bioavailability and pharmacokinetic profile of these formulations have not yet been studied in humans and it is presently unknown whether they will assure a better and longer-lasting control of intragastric pH compared with the currently available PPI formulations.

The development of acid pump antagonists is another active area of research in controlling intragastric pH. Acid pump antagonists such as the imidazopyridines have thus far shown fast first day onset as well as improved control of daytime and nighttime intragastric pH with twice-daily dosing when compared to a once-daily PPI [76]. Although these drugs also target H^+, K^+-ATPase, they act *via* a distinct mechanism: they bind the extracytoplasmatic surface and act as reversible K^+-competitive antagonists [77]. They also display altered pharmacological properties and, unlike PPIs, do not require accumulation in the parietal cell space and acid activation. One drawback is the need for twice daily dosing since they inhibit the pump only for the duration of their presence in the blood: however, since these compounds are acid-stable, their plasma half-life may be readily prolonged with extended-release formulations [77]. One of such reversible antagonists, pumaprazole (compound also marked BY841), was found to be capable of elevating intragastric pH up to neutrality even upon a first administration while still displaying a limited, dose-dependent duration of action. Its onset and duration of action were similar to those of ranitidine, but its antisecretory efficacy proved to be significantly better [78]. Pumaprazole (100 mg b.i.d.) has already been studied in healthy volunteers where it raised the intragastric pH over a 24-hour period to a similar degree as omeprazole (20 mg o.d.), an effect more marked in *Helicobacter*-positive subjects [79].

In search of a better proton pump inhibitor

Rationalization within the pharmaceutical industry to combat escalating costs has included the close examination of research portfolios. Gastroenterology has been one of the casualties of this exercise and few companies currently retain a specific gastrointestinal research programme [80]. Astra-Zeneca (UK), who discovered the first PPI more than 20 years ago, synthesized and started the development of esomeprazole (the magnesium

salt of the S-isomer of omperazole) in 1990, making it available for clinical practice worldwide at the beginning of the third Millennium [81].
Taking into account that omeprazole comprises a racemic mixture of its two optical isomers, S-omeprazole and R-omeprazole (*Figure 4*), and that S-omeprazole is optically stable in humans with negligible inversion to the other isomer [82], the R & D team decided to follow the first of the avenues outlined above in order to obtain a PPI with improved acid control. By following the methodology (the so-called Sharpless expoxidation) discovered by K. Barry Sharpless, one of the three scientists who received the 2001 Nobel Prize in Chemistry [83], they set-up the stereoselective synthesis of esomeprazole [84] and were able to produce the isomer on large scale.

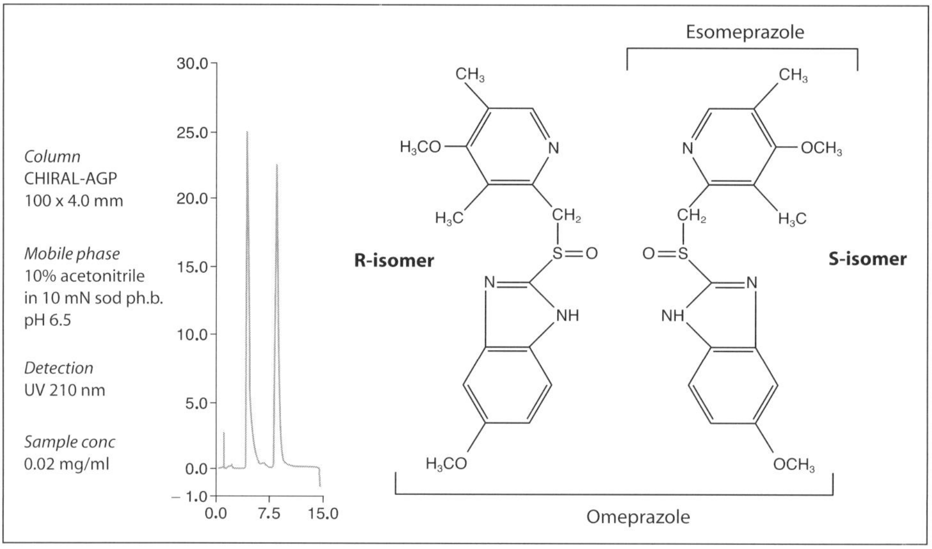

Figure 4. Omeprazole enantiomers and their separation by *chiral* HPLC.
Stereochemical separation of omeprazole isomers (http://www.registech.com:chiral:applications:omeprazole.htm)

In accordance with results of clinical trials in acid-related diseases [67, 69], where often different but somewhat equipotent doses of the different PPIs have been used, data from experimental pharmacological studies clearly show that – on a milligram basis – the available compound display the same potency and efficacy [71]. Since both R- and S-isomer of omeprazole are able to inhibit acid secretion in isolated gastric glands to the same degree [85], there should be no pharmacodynamic benefit in using one stereoisomer instead of the racemate. Both enantiomers (which are *chiral* sulfoxides) will give rise – within the secretory canaliculus – to the same reactive species, sulfenamide, which is *achiral* (*Figure 5*). There is therefore no pharmacodynamic reason why the racemate or any of its enantiomers should differentially interact with the proton pump [85].

Although the use of a PPI enantiomer does not confer any direct advantage *in vitro*, the pharmacokinetic (and pharmacodynamic) consequences of stereoselective drug metabolism might anyway affect drug activity *in vivo* [86, 87]. The metabolism of substituted

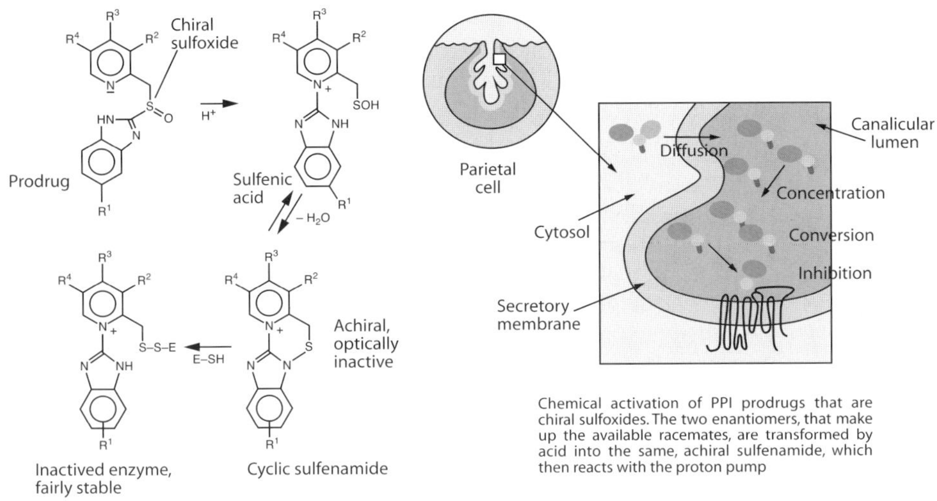

Figure 5. Chemical activation of PPIs within the parietal cell.

benzimidazoles, with exception of rabeprazole, is to a large extent dependent on hepatic cytochrome P-450 (CYP) isoforms, CYP3A4 and CYP2C19 [67, 68, 88]. These heme-containing enzymes are abundantly expressed in hepatocytes, where they exist in the smooth endoplasmic reticulum in association with a number of accessory proteins. There, the cytochromes P450 catalyze the multistep oxidation reactions that inactivate xenobiotics by the introduction or exposure of a functional group on their substrate. The dependence of most PPIs on metabolism by CYP2C19 makes them susceptible to alterations in bioavailability due to genetic polymorphisms affecting the activity of this enzyme [88, 89]. In particular, omeprazole is transformed in to three pharmacologically inactive metabolites, *i.e.* omeprazole sulphone and 5-hydroxy- plus 5-O-desmethyl-omeprazole, respectively. Studies performed in healthy volunteers [90] human liver microsomes and cDNA-expressed enzymes [91] have shown a significant stereoselectivity in the metabolism of omeprazole enantiomers. The R-isomer is almost exclusively metabolized (98%) *via* CYP2C19, 94% transforming to the 5-hydroxy metabolite, and 4% to the 5-O-desmethyl metabolite. Only 2% of the metabolism is *via* the CYP3A4 isoform. The S-isomer (esomeprazole) is metabolized primarily (73%) *via* the CYP2C19 isoform (46% going to the 5-O-desmethyl metabolite; 27% going to the 5-hydroxy metabolite), and by 27% *via* the CYP3A4 isoform to the sulphone metabolite (*Figure 6*). The intrinsic clearance (CL) of S-omeprazole is approximately one third of that of R-omeprazole, because of the considerably lower CL for formation of the 5-hydroxy metabolite (15 *versus* 43 µL • min/mg protein) *via* CYP2C19 [92]. This implies that the total metabolic clearance for S-omeprazole is lower than that for R-omeprazole, resulting in higher plasma levels of the S-isomer *in vivo*. These data suggest that, *in vivo*, S-omeprazole should undergo a lower first-pass effect thus leading to higher plasma levels and consequent better availability. Since the area under time-concentration curve correlates with secretory inhibition [93] the S-isomer should be capable of achieving a better acid control compared with the racemic mixture (*i.e.* omeprazole). The available *in vivo* pharmacokinetic, pharmacodynamic and clinical data all show that this is the case [94-98].

In a comparative study performed in healthy volunteers [99], esomeprazole (20 mg orally) proved to be significantly ($p < 0.05$) more effective in inhibiting pentagastrin-stimulated acid output than the same dose of omeprazole (45% *versus* 34%, respectively). More importantly, the intersubject variability (*Figure 7*) was found to be with esomeprazole remarkably less when compared with that of the racemate (11% *versus* 28%, respectively).

Being both ulcer and esophagitis healing strongly correlated with the time spent by intragastric pH above a threshold [100, 101], pharmacodynamic studies with esomeprazole have mainly focused on the drug effect on intragastric pH. A number of crossover studies, summarized by Scott *et al.* [97] and Johnson [98], have shown esomeprazole (20 or 40 mg daily) to be superior to omeprazole, lansoprazole and pantoprazole in maintaining intragastric pH > 4 when given orally for 5 days. Furthermore, while esomeprazole (20 mg daily) was as effective as rabeprazole 10 or 20 mg daily, the 40 mg dose was superior to rabeprazole 20 mg daily [97, 98].

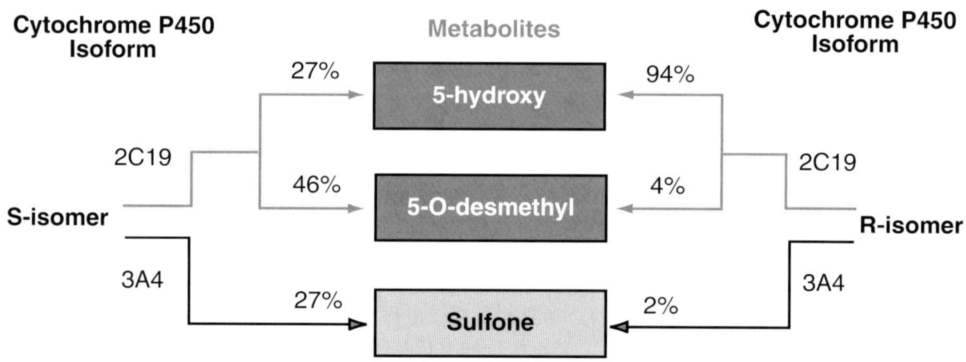

Figure 6. Stereospecific metabolism of omeprazole enantiomers by the hepatic cytochrome P450 (from [91]).

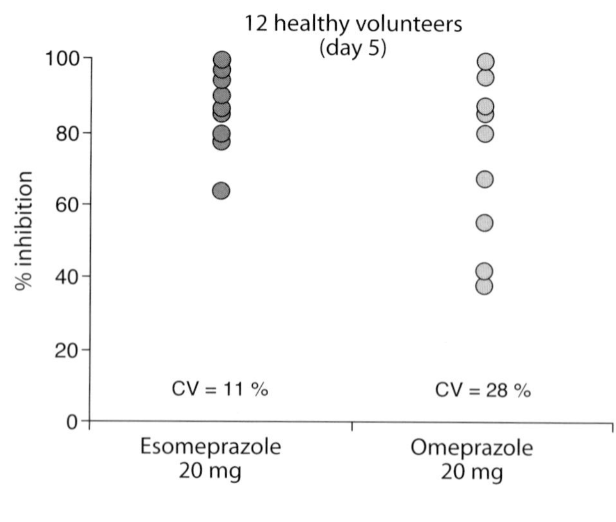

Figure 7. Inhibition of pentagastrin-stimulated acid secretion by esomeprazole or omeprazole: inter-subject variability (from [110]).

The more effective and predictable acid control achieved with esomeprazole compared with other PPIs may reflect peculiar pharmacokinetic properties of the drug, which shows an advantageous metabolism leading to a decreased first-pass effect and a lower systemic clearance compared with omeprazole. This, in turn, results in higher plasma levels with an enhanced delivery of the drug to the site of action (*i.e.* the parietal cell) and consequent blockade of a higher number of proton pumps in the secretory canaliculus [94].

Do these favorable pharmacokinetic properties translate in a better therapeutic efficacy in GERD? Two meta-analyses have indeed shown not only that esomeprazole achieves the highest healing rates of reflux esophagitis in the short-term [102] but also that esomeprazole 20 mg is the only step-down dose PPI able to show a significantly higher proportion of patients in remission of reflux compared with lansoprazole 15 mg [103]. The recently released consensus guidelines [104], developed under the auspices of the American Gastroenterological Association (AGA), clearly state that – while omeprazole, lansoprazole, pantoprazole and rabeprazole produce comparable rates of healing and remission in patients with erosive esophagitis – esomeprazole (40 mg) is slightly more effective than other PPIs in relieving heartburn and healing of erosive esophagitis.

Tenatoprazole has been designed in an attempt to obtain a PPI with a prolonged elimination half-life and a higher and sustained concentration in the gastric mucosa. Originally synthesized by Mitsubishi Pharma (Japan), the compound is now under active development by Negma-Gild Laboratories (France) [105]. Preclinical pharmacological studies have shown that the *in vivo* antisecretory potency of tenatoprazole, evaluated in different animal models (Shay rat preparation, acute fistula rats and Heidenhain pouch dogs) is 2-4 times higher than that observed with omeprazole [106, 107]. This higher potency is likely to be connected with a better bioavailability ranging from 77% to 88%. Conversely from omeprazole which delays gastric emptying [108], tenatoprazole is unable to affect emptying rate in rats [107]. In addition, experiments performed in gastric fistula dogs revealed an elevation of intragastric pH lasting longer (by 20%) than that observed with omeprazole or lansoprazole [109].

Pharmacokinetic studies, performed in Japanese subjects, showed a 7-fold longer half-life (7.6 hours and 13.7 hours after single and repeated administration of 20 mg, respectively), compared to the other PPIs. The area under the concentration – time curves, that reflect tissue exposure, were about 20-fold higher after single oral administration of 20 mg and 40 mg (24.50 and 67.76 mg • hr/ml, respectively) [110]. These pharmacokinetic properties translated in to a long-lasting antisecretory action. Indeed, inihibition of basal and tetragastrin-stimulated acid output in healthy volunteers was still significant 2 days after tenatoprazole administration (*Figure 8*). Intragastric pH-recordings, performed after repeated administration of 10 mg of the drug, did show that the time spent above pH 3 and pH 4 reached 96.7% and 88.0%, respectively, The most interesting finding was the prolonged effect of tenatoprazole during nighttime, since the % of pH holding time above 3 and 4 was almost identical during this period compared to daytime (94.7 % *versus* 98.3% and 86.3% *versus* 89.3%, respectively) [110].

Pharmacokinetics of tenatoprazole was recently investigated in *Helicobacter pylori*-negative healthy Caucasian subjects in a randomized, double-blind, dose-ranging study (10-80 mg, both single and repeated administration). A linear correlation between tenatoprazole dose and AUC was found, thus showing a linear pharmacokinetic pattern.The long half-life of tenatoprazole was confirmed for every dose, reaching 8.7 ± 2.6 hours for repeated administration of 40 mg [111]. Pharmacodynamic studies in healthy volunteers

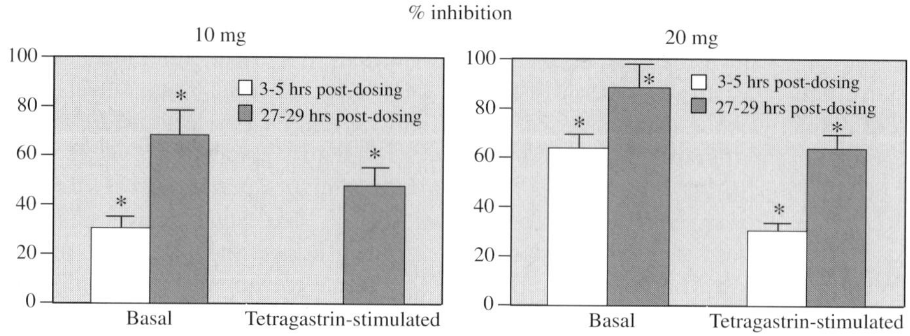

Figure 8. Effect of a single oral administration of tenatoprazole on acid secretion in healthy volunteers (from [110]).

showed an increase of intragastric pH with tenatoprazole 40 mg daily for seven days significantly higher ($p < 0.01$) than that observed with the same regimen of esomeprazole (*Figure 9*), the median pH being 4.7 ± 1.1 and 3.6 ± 1.4 respectively [112]. In addition, the time spent above pH 4 during nighttime after tenatoprazole administration was significantly longer than that observed with esomeprazole (*Table II*).
The available Japanese and European studies point out both pharmacokinetic and pharmacodynamic advantages of tenatoprazole over the existing PPIs. Whether these properties will translate in a better therapeutic efficacy remains to be seen.

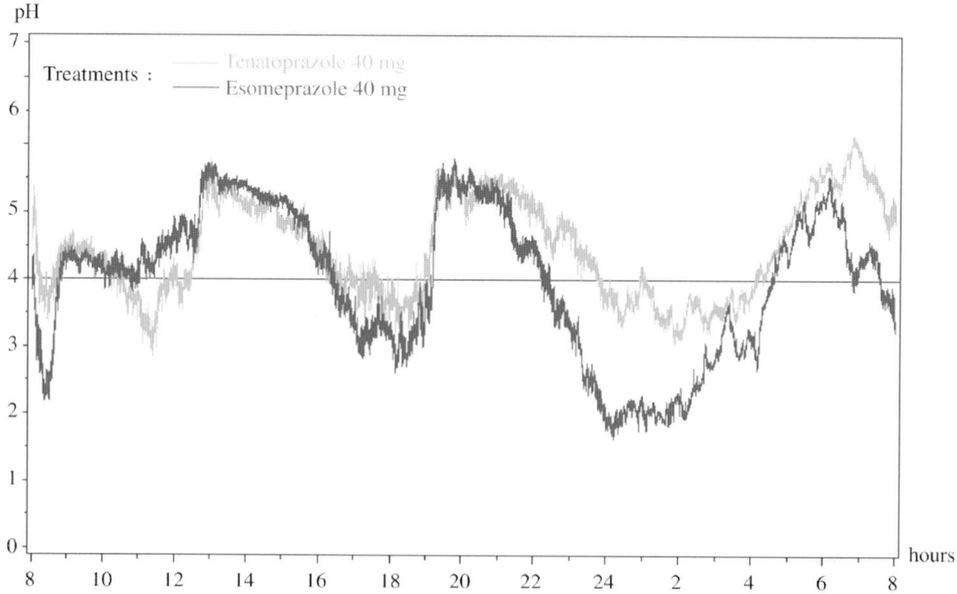

Figure 9. 24-hour median pH profiles in healthy volunteers receiving esomeprazole or tenatoprazole (from [112]).

Table II. Intragastric pH in healthy volunteers receiving esomeprazole or tenatoprazole: % time spent above pH 4 (from [112]).

	Esomeprazole 40 mg	Tenatoprazole 40 mg	Significance
Total (24 hours)	56.2 ± 16.5	63.3 ± 17.8	NS
Daytime	65.6 ± 17.7	62.2 ± 18.5	NS
Nightime	46.8 ± 19.7	64.3 ± 21.7	$p < 0.01$

Conclusions

It is now well established that profound acid suppression represents the mainstay of the medical management of patients with Barrett's esophagus and there is no doubt that PPIs are the preferred drugs to achieve this important goal. Not only do they control symptoms, heal esophagitis and ulcers, and prevent recurrence and strictures but might also hinder carcinogenesis. Some indirect evidence is indeed consistent with the idea that GERD promotes malignancy in established Barrett's esophagus, and that acid suppression might prevent cancer. Biopsy specimens of specialized intestinal metaplasia maintained in organ culture exhibit hyperproliferation and increased expression of COX-2 (a mediator of proliferation) when exposed to acid for only 1 hour, but not when exposed to acid continuously for up to 24 hours [113, 114]. Brief esophageal acid exposure also activates the mitogen-activated protein kinase pathways that can increase proliferation and decrease apoptosis in Barrett's esophagus [115]. These observations suggest that episodic esophageal acid exposure from GERD might stimulate hyperproliferation, suppress apoptosis and, possibly, promote carcinogenesis in Barrett's esophagus.

While no significant change in the proliferative activity of Barrett's esophagus (as assessed by *in vitro* labeling with 5-bromo-2-deoxyuridine) in 22 patients treated with omeprazole for 2 years [116], a recent study did show a significant reduction of proliferation markers after PPI therapy [117]. In this investigation, biopsy specimens were taken from 39 patients with Barrett's esophagus at baseline and after 6 months of therapy with PPIs given in doses sufficient only to eliminate GERD symptoms. The expression of PCNA (a proliferation marker) decreased and the expression of Villin (a differentiation marker) increased significantly in biopsy specimens from the 24 patients in whom PPIs normalized esophageal acid exposure, but not in the 15 with persistently abnormal acid reflux during PPI therapy [117]. It is evident that acid inhibition, if intensive and complete, may indeed function as chemopreventive therapy in Barrett's-related carcinogenesis. Reversal or elimination of columnar metaplasia may not be a necessary endpoint in the battle to prevent malignancy; chemoprevention with PPIs (with or without coxibs, selective inhibitors of COX-2) may be a more viable alternative [20]. To what extent acid exposure must be reduced to be beneficial is presently unknown, but it conceivable that the more profound acid suppression is, the more likely the reduction in cancer risk will be. In this connection effective and long-acting PPIs are welcome.

References

1. Spechler SJ, Goyal RK. The columnar lined esophagus, intestinal metaplasia, and Norman Barrett. Gastroenterology 1996;110:614-621.
2. Shaheen N, Ransohoff DF. Gastroesophageal reflux, Barrett esophagus, and esophageal cancer: scientific review. JAMA 2002;287:1972-1981.
3. Shaheen NJ, Crosby MA, Bozymski EM, Sandler RS. Is there publication bias in the reporting of cancer risk in Barrett's esophagus? Gastroenterology 2000;119:333-338.
4. Woloshin S, Schwartz LM, Welch HG. Risk charts: putting cancer in context. J Natl Cancer Inst 2002;94:799-804.
5. Neumann CS, Cooper BT. 24 hour ambulatory oesophageal pH monitoring in uncomplicated Barrett's oesophagus. Gut 1994;35:1352-1355.
6. Singh P, Taylor RH, Colin-Jones DG. Esophageal motor dysfunction and acid exposure in reflux esophagitis are more severe if Barrett's metaplasia is present. Am J Gastroenterol 1994;89:349-356.
7. Oberg S, DeMeester TR, Peters JH, Hagen JA, Nigro JJ, DeMeester SR, Theisen J, Campos GM, Crookes PF. The extent of Barrett's esophagus depends on the status of the lower esophageal sphincter and the degree of esophageal acid exposure. J Thorac Cardiovasc Surg 1999;117:572-580.
8. Vaezi MF, Richter JE. Role of acid and duodenogastroesophageal reflux in gastroesophageal reflux disease. Gastroenterology 1996;111:1192-1199.
9. Coenraad M, Masclee AA, Straathof JW, Ganesh S, Griffioen G, Lamers CB. Is Barrett's esophagus characterized by more pronounced acid reflux than severe esophagitis? Am J Gastroenterol 1998;93:1068-1072.
10. Cameron AJ. Barrett's esophagus: prevalence and size of hiatal hernia. Am J Gastroenterol 1999;94:2054-2059.
11. Vaezi MF, Richter JE. Double reflux: double trouble. Gut 1999;44:590-592.
12. Richter JE. Importance of bile reflux in Barrett's esophagus. Dig Dis Sci 2001;18:208-216.
13. Gutschow CA, Schroder W, Holscher AH. Barrett's esophagus: what is the poison - alkaline, biliary or acidic reflux? Dis Esophagus 2002;15:5-9.
14. Bechi P, Cianchi F. Technical aspects and clinical indications of 24-hour intragastric bile monitoring. Hepatogastroenterology 1999;46:54-59.
15. Vaezi MF, Richter JE. Synergism of acid and duodenogastroesophageal reflux in complicated Barrett's esophagus. Surgery 1995;117:699-704.
16. Fitzgerald RC, Lascar R, Triadafilopoulos G. Review article: Barrett's oesophagus, dysplasia and pharmacologic acid suppression. Aliment Pharmacol Ther 2001;15:269-276.
17. DeMeester TR. Surgical therapy for Barrett's esophagus: prevention, protection and excision. Dis Esophagus 2002;15:109-116.
18. Walker SJ, Selvasekar CR, Birbeck N. Mucosal ablation in Barrett's esophagus. Dis Esophagus 2002;15:22-29.
19. Urosevic P, Kiroff GK. Ablation of Barrett's epithelium: the promise and the problems. Dis Esophagus 2002;15:30-38.
20. Fennerty MB, Triadafilopoulos G. Barrett's-related esophageal adenocarcinoma: is chemoprevention a potential option? Am J Gastroenterol 2001;96:2302-2305.
21. Fennerty MB. Barrett's-related esophageal cancer: has the final hurdle been cleared, now paving the way for human chemoprevention trials? Gastroenterology 2002;122:1172-1175.
22. Sontag SJ. Preventing death of Barrett's cancer: does frequent surveillance endoscopy do it? Am J Med 2001;111(Suppl 8A):137S-141S.
23. Craanen ME, Blok P, Meijer GA, Meuwissen SG. Surveillance in Barrett's oesophagus: a critical reappraisal. Scand J Gastroenterol 2002;37(Suppl 236):4-8.
24. Spechler SJ. Managing Barrett's esophagus. Decisions have to be based on indecisive data. Br Med J 2003;326:892-894.
25. Sampliner RE, The Practice Parameters Committee of the American College of Gastroenterology. Practice guidelines on the diagnosis, surveillance, and therapy of Barrett's esophagus. Am J Gastroenterol 1998;313:1028-1032.
26. Meining A, Classen M. The role of diet and lifestyle measures in the pathogenesis and treatment of gastroesophageal reflux disease. Am J Gastroenterol 2000;95:2692-2697.
27. Dent J, Brun J, Fendrick AM, Fennerty MB, Janssens J, Kahrilas PJ, Lauritsen K, Reynolds JC, Shaw M, Talley NJ. An evidence-based appraisal of reflux disease management: Genval Workshop Report. Gut 1999;44(Suppl 2):1-16.
28. DeVault KR, Castell DO. Updated guidelines for the diagnosis and treatment of gastroesophageal reflux disease. The Practice Parameters Committee of the American College of Gastroenterology. Am J Gastroenterol 1999;94:1434-1442.
29. Watson DI, Jamieson GG. Antireflux surgery in the laparoscopic era. Br J Surg 1998;85:1173-1184.
30. Bruley des Varannes S, Gharib H. Reflux gastro-oesophagien: contreparties fonctionnelles de la chirurgie antireflux. Gastroenterol Clin Biol 2000;24:B17-B23.
31. Scarpignato C. New therapeutic modalities for benign esophageal disease: an overview. Digest Liver Dis 2001;33:260-265.
32. Sampliner RE. Reduction of acid exposure and regression of Barrett's esophagus. Dig Dis 2001;18:203-207.
33. Gurski RR, Peters JH, Hagen JA, DeMeester SR, Bremner CG, Chandrasoma PT, DeMeester TR. Barrett's esophagus can and does regress after antireflux surgery: a study of prevalence and predictive features. J Am Coll Surg 2003;196:706-712.

34. Klaus A, Hinder RA. Medical therapy versus antireflux surgery in Barrett's esophagus: what is the best therapeutic approach? Dig Dis 2000;18:224-231.
35. Colin-Jones DG. The role and limitations of H_2-receptor antagonists in the treatment of gastro-oesophageal reflux disease. Aliment Pharmacol Ther 1995;9(Suppl. 1):9-14.
36. Scarpignato C, Bruley des Varannnes S. Traitement médical du RGO par les antagonistes des récepteurs H_2 de l'histamine. Gastroenterol Clin Biol 1999;23:S78-S89.
37. Wilder-Smith CH, Merki HS. Tolerance during dosing with H_2-receptor antagonists. An overview. Scand J Gastroenterol 1992;27(Suppl 193):14-19.
38. Sandvik AK, Brenna E, Waldum HL. Review article: the pharmacological inhibition of gastric acid secretion: tolerance and rebound. Aliment Pharmacol Ther 1997;11:1013-1018.
39. Wolfe, MM, Sachs, G. Acid suppression: optimizing therapy for gastroduodenal ulcer healing, gastroesophageal reflux disease, and stress-related erosive syndrome. Gastroenterology 2000;118(2 Suppl 1):S9-S31.
40. Peghini PL, Katz PO, Bracy NA, Castell DO. Nocturnal recovery of gastric acid secretion with twice-daily dosing of proton pump inhibitors. Am J Gastroenterol 1998;9:763-767.
41. Xue S, Katz PO, Banerjee P, Tutuian R, Castell DO. Bedtime H_2 blockers improve nocturnal gastric acid control in GERD patients on proton pump inhibitors. Aliment Pharmacol Ther 2001;15:1351-1356.
42. Fackler WK, Ours TM, Vaezi MF, Richter JE. Long-term effect of H_2RA therapy on nocturnal gastric acid breakthrough. Gastroenterology 2002;122:625-632.
43. Cross LB, Justice LN. Combination drug therapy for gastroesophageal reflux disease. Ann Pharmacother 2002;36:912-916.
44. Tougas G, Armstrong D. Efficacy of H_2 receptor antagonists in the treatment of gastroesophageal reflux disease and its symptoms. Can J Gastroenterol 1997;11(Suppl B):51B-54B.
45. Triadafilopoulos G. Proton pump inhibitors for Barrett's oesophagus. Gut 2000;46:144-146.
46. Ouatu-Lascar R, Triadafilopoulos G. Complete elimination of reflux symptoms does not guarantee normalization of intraesophaeal acid reflux in patients with Barrett's esophagus. Am J Gastroenterol 1998;93:711-716.
47. Katz PO, Anderson C, Khoury R, Castell DO. Gastro-oesophageal reflux associated with nocturnal gastric acid breakthrough on proton pump inhibitors. Aliment Pharmacol Ther 1998;12:1231-1234.
48. Srinivasan R, Katz PO, Ramakrishnan A, Katzka DA, Vela MF, Castell DO. Maximal acid reflux control for Barrett's oesophagus: feasible and effective. Aliment Pharmacol Ther 2001;15:519-524.
49. Marshall RE, Anggiansah A, Manifold DK, Owen WA, Owen WJ. Effect of omeprazole 20 mg twice daily on duodenogastric and gastro-oesophageal bile reflux in Barrett's oesophagus. Gut 1998;43:603-606.
50. Menges M, Muller M, Zeitz M. Increased acid and bile reflux in Barrett's esophagus compared to reflux esophagitis, and effect of proton pump inhibitor therapy. Am J Gastroenterol. 2001;96:331-337.
51. Manifold DK, Marshall RE, Anggiansah A, Owen WJ. Effect of omeprazole on antral duodenogastric reflux in Barrett oesophagus. Scand J Gastroenterol 2000;35:796-801.
52. Wetscher GJ, Hinder RA, Smyrk T, Perdikis G, Adrian TE, Profanter C. Gastric acid blockade with omeprazole promotes gastric carcinogenesis induced by duodenogastric reflux. Dig Dis Sci 1999;44:1132-1135.
53. Theisen J, Nehra D, Citron D, Johansson J, Hagen JA, Crookes PF, DeMeester SR, Bremner CG, DeMeester TR, Peters JH. Suppression of gastric acid secretion in patients with gastroesophageal reflux disease results in gastric bacterial overgrowth and deconjugation of bile acids. J Gastrointest Surg 2000;4:50-54.
54. Bell NJ, Burget D, Howden CW, Wilkinson J, Hunt RH. Appropriate acid suppression for the management of gastro-oesophageal reflux disease. Digestion 1992;51(Suppl. 1):59-67.
55. Bell NJ, Hunt RH. Role of gastric acid suppression in the treatment of gastro-oesophageal reflux disease. Gut 1992;33:118-24.
56. Chiba N, De Gara CJ, Wilkinson JM, Hunt RH. Speed of healing and symptom relief in grade II to IV gastroesophageal reflux disease: a meta-analysis. Gastroenterology 1997;112:1798-1810.
57. van Pinxteren B, Numans ME, Bonis PA, Lau J. Short-term treatment with proton pump inhibitors, H_2-receptor antagonists and prokinetics for gastro-oesophageal reflux disease-like symptoms and endoscopy negative reflux disease (Cochrane Review). Cochrane Database Syst Rev 2001;CD002095.
58. Ollyo JB, Monnier PH, Fontolliet CH, Birchler R, Fasel J, Levi F, Gonvers JJ. L'ulcer de Savary: une nouvelle complication du reflux gastro-œsophagien. Schweiz Med Woschenschr 1988;118:823-827.
59. Nigro JJ, Bremner RM, Fuller CB, Theisen J, Ma Y, Starnes VA. Perforating Barrett's ulcer resulting in a life-threatening esophagobronchial fistula. Ann Thorac Surg 2002;73:302-304.
60. Vigneri S, Termini R, Leandro G, Badalamenti S, Pantalena M, Savarino V, Di Mario F, Battaglia G, Mela GS, Pilotto A, Plebani M, Davi G. A comparison of five maintenance therapies for reflux esophagitis. N Engl J Med 1995;333:1106-1110.
61. Smith PM, Kerr GD, Cockel R, Ross BA, Bate CM, Brown P, Dronfield MW, Green JR, Hislop WS, Theodossi A, et al. A comparison of omeprazole and ranitidine in the prevention of recurrence of benign esophageal stricture. Gastroenterology 1994;107:1312-1318.
62. Swarbrick ET, Gough AL, Foster CS, Christian J, Garrett AD, Langworthy CH. Prevention of recurrence of oesophageal stricture, a comparison of lansoprazole and high-dose ranitidine. Eur J Gastroenterol Hepatol 1996;8:431-438.

63. Menke-Pluymers MBE, Hop WC, Dees J, van Blankenstein M, Tilanus HW. Risk factors for the development of an adenocarcinoma in columnar-lined (Barrett's) esophagus. The Rotterdam Esophageal Tumor Study Group. Cancer 1993;72:1155-1158.
64. Cooper BT, Neumann CS, Cox MA, Iqbal TH. Continuous treatment with omeprazole 20 mg daily for up to 6 years in Barrett's oesophagus. Aliment Pharmacol Ther 1998;12:893-897.
65. Sampliner RE. Reduction of acid exposure and regression of Barrett's esophagus. Dig Dis 2000;18:203-207.
66. Overholt BF. Acid suppression and reepithelialization after ablation of Barrett's esophagus. Dig Dis 2000;18:232-239.
67. Stedman CAM, Barclay ML. Review article: comparison of the pharmacokinetics, acid suppression and efficacy of proton pump inhibitors. Aliment Pharmacol Ther 2000;14:963-978.
68. McColl KEL, Kennerley P. Proton pump inhibitors – differences emerge in the hepatic metabolism. Digest Liver Dis 2002;34:461-467.
69. Thomson ABR. Are the orally administered proton pump inhibitors equivalent? A comparison of lansoprazole, omeprazole, pantoprazole, and rabeprazole. Curr Gastroenterol Rep 2000;2:482-493.
70. Langman MJS. Which PPI? Gut 2001:49:309-310.
71. Kromer W, Horbach S, Lühmann R. Relative efficacies of gastric proton pump inhibitors: their clinical and pharmacological basis. Pharmacology 1999;59:57-77.
72. Guidance on the use of proton pump inhibitors in the treatment of dyspepsia. NICE, UK: Technology Appraisal Guidance No 7, 2000 (http://www.NICE.org.uk).
73. Huber R, Kohl B, Sachs G, Senn-Bilfinger J, Simon WA, Sturm E. Review article: the continuing development of proton pump inhibitors with particular reference to pantoprazole. Aliment Pharmacol Ther 1995;9:363-378.
74. Tytgat GN. Shortcomings of the first-generation proton pump inhibitors. Eur J Gastroenterol Hepatol 2001;13(Suppl 1):S29-S33.
75. Robinson M. New-generation proton pump inhibitors: overcoming the limitations of early-generation agents. Eur J Gastroenterol Hepatol 2001;13(Suppl 1):S43-47.
76. Sachs G. Improving on PPI-based therapy of GORD. Eur J Gastroenterol Hepatol. 2001;13(Suppl 1):S35-41.
77. Tonini M, De Giorgio R, De Ponti F. Novel therapeutic strategies in acid-related disorders. Expert Opin Ther Patents 2003;13:639-649.
78. Kromer W, Postius S, Riedel R. Animal pharmacology of reversible antagonism of the gastric acid pump, compared to standard antisecretory principle. Pharmacology 2000;60:179-187.
79. Martinek J, Blum AL, Stolte M, Hartmann M, Verdu EF, Luhmann R, Dorta G, Wiesel P. Effects of pumaprazole (BY841), a novel reversible proton pump antagonist, and of omeprazole, on intragastric acidity before and after cure of Helicobacter pylori infection. Aliment Pharmacol Ther 1999;13:27-34.
80. Parsons ME, Garner A. Review article: drug development in gastroenterology - the changing view of industry. Aliment Pharmacol Ther 1995;9:457-463.
81. Scarpignato C, Pelosini I, Lamarque D. Ésoméprazole : pharmacologie et développement d'un nouvel inhibiteur de pompe à protons. Hépatogastroenterology 2003;10:277-291.
82. Hassan-Alin M, Niazi M, Röhss K, Sthenoff H. Esomeprazole, the S-isomer of omeprazole, is optically stable in humans. Gastroenterology 2000;118(Suppl 2):A1244-1245.
83. The Nobel Foundation. Information for the Public. The 2001 Nobel Prize in Chemistry [http://www.nobel.se/chemistry/laureates/2001/public.htlm].
84. Cotton H, Elebring T, Larsson M, Li L, Sörensen H, von Unge S. Asymmetric synthesis of esomeprazole. Tetrahedron: Asymmetry 2000;11:3819-3825.
85. Kromer W. Relative efficacies of gastric proton-pump inhibitors on a milligram basis: desired and undesired SH reactions. Impact of chirality. Scand J Gastroenterol 2001;36(Suppl 234):3-9.
86. Eichelbaum M. Pharmacokinetic and pharmacodynamic consequences of stereoselective drug metabolism in man. Biochem Pharmacol 1988;37:93-96.
87. Tucker GT, Lennard MS. Enantiomer specific pharmacokinetics. Pharmacol Ther 1990;45:309-329.
88. Andersson T. Pharmacokinetics, metabolism and interactions of acid pump inhibitors-focus on omeprazole, lansoprazole and pantoprazole. Clin Pharmacokinet 1996;31:9-28.
89. Egan LJ, Murray JA. New perspectives in gastric acid suppression: genetic polymorphisms predict the efficacy of proton pump inhibitors. Dig Dis 2000;18:58-63.
90. Tybring G, Bottiger Y, Widen J, Bertilsson L. Enantioselective hydroxylation of omeprazole catalyzed by CYP2C19 in Swedish white subjects. Clin Pharmacol Ther 1997;62:129-137.
91. Äbelö A, Andersson TB, Bredberg U, Skanberg I, Weidolf L. Stereoselective metabolism by human liver CYP enzymes of a substituted benzimidazole. Drug Metab Dispos 2000;28:58-64.
92. Andersson T, Bredberg E, Sunzel M, Antonsson M, Weidolf L. Pharmacokinetics and effect on pentagastrin -stimulated peak acid output of omeprazole and its two optical isomers, S-omeprazole/esomeprazole and R-omeprazole. In: Abstract book from VII World Conference on Clinical Pharmacology and Therapeutics, Florence, Italy, July 15-20, 2002:241 (Abstract 935).
93. Junghard O, Hassan-Alin M, Hasselgren G. The effect of the area under the plasma concentration vs time curve and the maximum plasma concentration of esomeprazole on intragastric pH. Eur J Clin Pharmacol 2002;58:453-458.
94. Tonini M, Vigneri S, Savarino V, Scarpignato C. Clinical pharmacology and safety profile of esomeprazole, the first enantiomerically pure proton pump inhibitor. Digest Liver Dis 2001;33:600-606.

95. Vigneri S, Tonini M, Scarpignato C, Savarino V. Improving opportunities for effective management of gastro-esophageal reflux disease. Digest Liver Dis 2001;33:720-730.
96. Kale-Pradhan PB, Landry HK, Sypula WT Esomeprazole for acid peptic disorders. Ann Pharmacother 2002;36:655-663.
97. Scott LJ, Dunn CJ, Mallarkey G, Sharpe M. Esomeprazole. A review of its use in the management of acid-related disorders. Drugs 2002;62:1503-1538.
98. Johnson DA. Review of esomeprazole in the treatment of acid disorders. Expert Opin Pharmacother 2003;4:253-264.
99. Andersson T, Bredberg E, Sunzel M, Antonsson M, Weidolf L. Pharmacokinetics (PK) and effect on pentagastrin stimulated peak acid output (PAO) of omeprazole (O) and its 2 optical isomers, S-omeprazole/esomeprazole (E) and R-omeprazole (R-O). Gastroenterology 2000;118(Suppl. 2):A1210.
100. Burget DW, Chiverton SG, Hunt RH. Is there an optimal degree of acid suppression for healing of duodenal ulcers? A model of the relationship between ulcer healing and acid suppression. Gastroenterology 1990;99:345-51.
101. Bell NJ, Burget D, Howden CW, Wilkinson J, Hunt RH. Appropriate acid suppression for the management of gastro-oesophageal reflux disease. Digestion 1992;51(Suppl. 1):59-67.
102. Edwards SJ, Lind T, Lundell L. Systematic review of proton pump inhibitors for the acute treatment of reflux oesophagitis. Aliment Pharmacol Ther 2001;15:1729-1736.
103. Edwards SJ, Lind T, Lundell L. Systematic review of proton pump inhibitors for the maintenance of healed reflux oesophagitis. J Drug Ass 2002;5:165-178.
104. Peterson WL. Improving management of GERD. Evidence-based therapeutic strategies. Bethesda: AGA Press, 2002:1-28.
105. Anonimous. Tenatoprazole. Benatoprazole, TU 199. Drugs RD 2002;3:276-277.
106. Uchiyama K, Wakatsuki D, Kakinoki B, Takeuchi Y, Araki T, Morinaka Y. Effects of TU-199, a novel H^+, K^+-ATPase inhibitor, on gastric acid secretion and gastroduodenal ulcers in rats. Methods Find Exp Clin Pharmacol 1999;21:115-122.
107. Kakinoki B, Ono C, Yamazaki N, Chikamatsu N, Wakatsuki D, Uchiyama K, Morinaka Y. General pharmacological properties of the new proton pump inhibitor (+/-)-5-methoxy-2-[[(4-methoxy-3,5-dimethylpyrid-2-yl)methyl] sulfinyl]-1H-imidazo[4,5-b]pyridine. Methods Find Exp Clin Pharmacol 1999;21:179-187.
108. Waldum HL, Lehy T, Brenna E, Sandvik AK, Petersen H, Sognen BS, Bonfils S, Lewin MJ. Effect of the histamine-1 antagonist astemizole alone or with omeprazole on rat gastric mucosa. Scand J Gastroenterol 1991;26:23-35.
109. Uchiyama K, Wakatsuki D, Kakinoki B, Takeuchi Y, Araki T, Morinaka Y. The long-lasting effect of TU-199, a novel H^+, K^+-ATPase inhibitor, on gastric acid secretion in dogs. J Pharm Pharmacol 1999;51:457-464.
110. Negma-Lerads. Tenatoprazole (TU-199) Investigator's brochure. September 2001.
111. Domagala F, Ficheux H. Pharmacokinetics of tenatoprazole, a novel proton pump inhibitor, in healthy male caucasian volunteers. DDW 2003, Orlando, Abstract ID#102823.
112. Galmiche JP. Diurnal and nocturnal gastric acid control with tenatoprazole:a comparison with esomeprazole in healthy volunteers. In: Abstract Book of the Symposium "Night-time control of acid secretion: a challenge for a new PPI in acid-related diseases", held during the DDW, Orlando, May 2003.
113. Fitzgerald RC, Omary MB, Triadafilopoulos G. Dynamic effects of acid on Barrett's esophagus: an ex vivo proliferation and differentiation model. J Clin Invest 1996;98:2120-2128.
114. Shirvani VN, OLiatu-Lascar R, Kaur BS, et al. Cyclooxgenase 2 expression in Barrett's esophagus and adenocarcinoma: ex vivo induction by bile salts and acid exposure. Gastroenterology 2000;118:487-496.
115. Sotiza RF, Shewmake K, Terada LS, et al. Acid exposure activates the mitogen-activated protein kinase pathways in Barretts esophagus. Gastroenterology 2002;122:299-307.
116. Peters FT, Ganesh S, Kuipers EJ, et al. Effect of elimination of acid reflux ori epithelial cell proliferative activity of Barrett esophagus. Scand J Gastroenterol 2000;35:1238-1244.
117. Ouatu-Lascar R, Fltzgerald RC, Triadafilopoulos G. Differentiation and proliferation in Barrett's esophagus and the effects of acid suppression. Gastroenterology 1999;117:327-335.

What should be the minimal dosage and duration of treatment by proton pump inhibitors?

E.C. Klinkenberg-Knol (Amsterdam)

In the large majority of patients Barrett's esophagus is supposed to be the consequence of chronic acid gastroesophageal reflux. Over the past decade, acid suppression with proton pump inhibitors (PPI's) has become the mainstay of treatment of patients with Barrett's esophagus [1].

Reflux reducing treatment - that is, treatment with these acid inhibitory drugs, generally relieves symptoms adequately, and helps to prevent restenosis after instrumental dilation. Whether such treatment may also modify the risk of cancer development is however unknown. Although dysplasia is an important, if not the most important marker for cancer risk, the length of Barrett's epithelium also appears to be a risk factor for dysplasia or adenocarcinoma [2, 3]. Thus a decrease of cancer risk might be anticipated if treatment could induce a regression of Barrett's epithelium with restitution of squamous epithelium. This article will discuss the specific goals of PPI-therapy in Barrett's esophagus, including dosage and duration of treatment.

Concomitant symptomatic gastroesophageal reflux disease (GERD) is common in patients with Barrett's esophagus. PPI's, irrespective of dose or duration of treatment, provide the the greatest overall symptom relief [4]. As a group, however, patients with Barrett's esophagus have greater exposure to esophageal acid than other patients with GERD and control of symptoms may require higher than usual doses of PPIs [5]. Moreover, doses of PPI's that are sufficient to control symptoms do not normalize acid reflux in all patients [6]. On the other side, it has been noticed that eldery patients with Barrett's esophagus may be less symptomatic than the younger group [7].

Not only one tries to reach symptom relief, but also healing of coexistent esophagitis. Only after healing of esophagitis exact measurement and endoscopic judgement of Barrett's epithelium possible. Irrespective of dose or length of treatment, healing of esophagitis is best and faster achieved with PPIs [6].

Patients with Barrett's esophagus, as a group, are more likely to have recurrences because they have severe physiological abnormalities, such as low lower esophageal sphincter tone, impaired esophageal body peristalsis, and greater than average esophageal acid exposure [8]. Maintenance therapy with PPIs prevents relapses in more than 80% of patients with GERD, even with severe, resistant disease [9].

Long-term PPI therapy is also indicated for the healing and prevention of esophageal ulcers, located within the metaplastic columnar mucosa, or in the squamous esophagus near to the squamometaplastic junction. A frequently occurring complication of these squamous junction ulcers is peptic stricture formation. Also in this condition the use of PPIs has resulted in fewer dilatations and less dysphagia symptoms than high dose H_2 blockers [10].

Regression of the metaplastic surface is considered an important end point in the management of patients with Barrett's esophagus. The risk of malignant transformation in Barrett's esophagus should be related, at least in part, to the extent of its mucosal involvement [2, 3]. It is generally accepted that PPI therapy does not result in total regression of Barrett's esophagus, although pathological studies of patients with Barrett's esophagus, treated with PPIs, have shown that there is undoubted evidence of squamous re-epithelialization over and adjacent to Barrett's type mucosa. Recently, it has been shown that both macroscopic and microscopic squamous islands mainly derive from esophageal glands, normal structures within the esophagus [11]. Although these squamous islands may occur in untreated Barrett's esophagus, there is clear evidence that these islands are greatly increased in Barrett's esophagus treated with profound acid suppression. Over the past decade, several studies using various PPI regimens have yielded inconsistent results [12-16]. This is partly due to the impossibility to accurately measure the length and surface of the Barrett's epithelium. Moreover, the degree of control of intraesophageal pH and reflux of bile acids have been inadequately documented. Still, at least partial regression seems to occur early after therapy starts, usually in the first two years [16] with little or no evidence of further partial regression. With this incomplete replacement of Barrett's epithelium, endoscopic surveillance will still be necessary [17].

Recommendations for proton pump inhibitor therapy in Barrett's esophagus

The above mentioned end points of treatment in Barrett's esophagus, such as control of concomitant GERD and prevention of complications establish PPI's as the most important pharmacological agents in this condition.

Moreover, there are suggestions that sufficient treatment with PPI's will promote the regression of Barrett's epithelium and enhance the appearance of squamous islands, both possible factors for reducing the risk of adenocarcinoma.

Intensive antireflux therapy with PPI's, that is at least 20 mg omeprazole twice daily, must be initiated, as soon as Barrett's esophagus is diagnosed endoscopically. Ideally, the PPI dose should be titrated to obtain complete intraesophageal acid suppression [8]. Once the right dose of PPI's has been established, the duration of treatment will be infinite.

References

1. Castell DO, Katzka DA. Barrett's esophagus: continuing questions and controversy. Gastrointest Endosc 1999;49:S5-S8.
2. Iftikhar SY, James PD, Steele RJC, Hardcastle JD, Atkinson M. Length of Barrett's oesophagus:an important factor in the development of dysplasia and adenocarcinoma. Gut 1992;33:1155-1158.
3. Menke-Pluymers MBE, Hop WJC, Dees J, Blankenstein van M, Tilanus HW. Risk factors for the development of an adenocarcinoma in columnar-lined (Barrett) esophagus. Cancer 1993;72:1155-1158.
4. Chiba N, Degara CJ, Wilkinson JM , Hunt RH. Speed of healing and symptom relief in grade II to IV gastroesophageal reflux disease: a meta-analysis. Gastroenterology 1997;112:1798-1810.
5. Ouatu-Lascar R, Triadafilopoulos G. Complete elimination of reflux symptoms does not guarantee normalization of intra-esophageal acid reflux in patients with Barrett's esophagus. Am J Gastroenterol 1998;98:711-716.
6. Katzka DA, Castell DO. Successful elimination of reflux symptoms does not ensure adequate control of acid reflux in Barrett's esophagus. Am J Gastroenterol 1994;89:989-991.
7. Triadafilopoulos G, Sharma P. Features of symptomatic gastroesophageal reflux disease in elderly patients. Am J Gastroenterol 1997;92:2007-2011.
8. Stein HJ, Hoeft S, DeMeester TR. Functional foregut abnormalities in Barrett's esophagus. Thorac Cardiovasc Surg 1993;105:107-111.
9. Klinkenberg-Knol EC, Nelis F, Dent J, Snel P, Mitchell B, Prichard P, Lloyd D, Havu N, Frame M, Roman J, Walan A, and long-term study group. Long-term omeprazole treatment in resistant gastroesophageal reflux disease:efficacy, safety, and influence on gastric mucosa. Gastroenterology 2000;118:661-669.
10. Swarbrick ET, Gough AL, Foster CS, Christian J, Garrett AD, Longworthy CH. Prevention of recurrence of oesophageal stricture: a comparison of lanzoprazole and high-dose ranitidine. Eur J Gastroenterol Hepatol 1996;8:431-438.

11. Biddlestone LR, Barham CP, Wilkinson SP, Barr H, Shepherd NA. The histopathology of treated Barrett's oesophagus: squamous re-epithelialisation following acid suppression, laser and photodynamic therapy. Am J Surg Pathol 1998;22:239-245.
12. Cooper BT, Neumann CS, Cox MA, Iqbal TH. Contiuous treatment with omeprazole 20 mg daily for up to 6 years in Barrett's oesophagus. Aliment Pharmacol Ther 1998;12:893-897.
13. Malesci A, Savarino V, Zentelin P, Belicchi M, Mela GS, Lapertosa G, Bocchia P, Rhonchi G, Franseschi M. Partial regression of Barrett's esophagus by long-term therapy with high-dose omeprazole. Gastrointest Endosc 1996;44:700-705.
14. Wilkinson SP, Biddlestone L,Gore S, Shepherd NA. Regression of columnar-lined (Barrett's) oesophagus with omeprazole 40 mg daily: results of 5 years of continuous therapy. Aliment Pharmacol Ther 1999;13:1205-1209.
15. Sampliner RE. Effect of up to 3 years of high-dose lansoprazole on Barrett's esophagus. Am J Gastroenterol 1994;89:1844-1848.
16. Peters FTM, Ganesh S, Kuipers EJ, Sluiter WJ, Klinkenberg-Knol EC, Lamers CBHW, Kleibeuker JH. Endoscopic regression of Barrett's oesophagus during omeprazole therapy;a randomised double blind study. Gut 1999;45:489-494.
17. Sampliner RE, Steinbronn K, Gareval HS, Riddell RH. Squamous mucosa overlying columnar epithelium in Barrett's esophagus in the absence of antireflux surgery. Am J Gastroenterol 1988;83:510-512.

Should non-steroidal anti-inflammatory drugs be used for the reversal of Barrett's esophagus?

G. Morgan (Swansea)

There is good evidence that the consumption of non-steroidal anti-inflammatory drugs (NSAIDs) such as aspirin reduces the risk of colorectal cancer by about 50% [1]. This hypothesis is supported by over 20 epidemiological studies and experimental evidence. NSAIDs inhibit the cyclooxygenase (COX) enzyme and thus lead to a reduced synthesis of prostaglandin E_2 (PGE_2). COX inhibition is thought to be an important, if not exclusive, mechanism of colorectal cancer prevention since PGE_2 is produced in excessive amounts by colorectal cancers.

Compared with colorectal cancer, there is less evidence that aspirin and other NSAIDs reduce the risk of esophageal cancer. Similar to colorectal cancer, however, esophageal cancers also produce excessive amounts of PGE_2 [2]. Furthermore, three out of four experimental animal studies have demonstrated that NSAIDs reduce the incidence and multiplicity of esophageal cancers in rodents treated with esophagotropic carcinogens [3-6].

There is epidemiological evidence that aspirin reduces the risk of esophageal cancer. Funkhouser and Sharp [7] followed 14,407 United States residents for 12-16 years. Persons were classified as nonusers, occasional users or regular users of aspirin based upon their response to two questions at baseline examination. Occasional use was associated with a 90% decreased risk (relative risk, RR, 0.10 CI 0.01-0.76) although this was only based on 15 cases of esophageal cancer. No regular user of aspirin developed esophageal cancer. The authors called for further studies to determine whether aspirin protects against both esophageal adenocarcinoma and/or squamous cell carcinoma.

In a small hospital case-control study in Greece, Garidou *et al.* [8] found that the chronic intake of any analgesic was associated with 50% lower risk of esophageal adenocarcinoma and 40% lower risk of esophageal squamous cell carcinoma. This inverse association, however, was non-significant due to the small study size.

Farrow *et al.* [9] investigated the association between aspirin use and esophageal cancer using data from a population-based case-control study. There were 293 cases of esophageal adenocarcinoma, 221 cases of esophageal squamous cell carcinoma and 695 controls. Cases were aged 30-79 years and were diagnosed with cancer in three geographical areas with population based cancer-registries. Controls were selected by random digit dialling and through the rosters of the Health Care Financing System. They found that people who reported ever using at least one tablet of aspirin per week for six months or more had significantly lower risk of adenocarcinoma by 52% (RR 0.48 CI 0.32-0.70) and squamous cell carcinoma by 48% (RR 0.52 CI 0.31-0.87). Current use was even more strongly associated with lower risk of both adenocarcinoma (RR 0.37 CI 0.24-0.58) and squamous cell carcinoma (RR 0.49 CI 0.28-0.87). This study also showed that using at least one tablet of aspirin per week in the last 6 months reduced stomach cancer risk by 45%.

Most recently, Langman *et al.* [10] have conducted a large case-control study using the general practice research database in the United Kingdom. 12,174 cases of 9 types of cancer (including esophageal cancer) were identified and there were 34,934 controls. NSAIDs appeared to significantly lower the risk of stomach and esophageal cancer. With respect to the latter, the odds ratio was 0.64 (0.41 to 0.98) which is consistent with a 36% risk reduction.

NSAID chemoprevention of esophageal adenocarcinoma

The experimental and epidemiological data suggest that NSAIDs do reduce the risk of esophageal adenocarcinoma. On this basis, giving patients at high risk of esophageal adenocarcinoma NSAIDs is logical. Patients with Barrett's esophagus are therefore candidates for NSAIDs in order to lower their risk of developing esophageal adenocarcinoma.

NSAIDs are ulcerogenic to the gastrointestinal mucosa (particularly the stomach) and it is believed that this is related, at least in part, to PGE_2 inhibition. More recently, 2 forms of the COX enzyme have been identified. COX-1 is a constitutive enzyme responsible for diverse physiological functions including protection of the gastrointestinal tract, renal homeostasis, uterine function, etc. COX-2 is predominantly inducible and is responsible for the synthesis of inflammatory prostaglandins.

COX-2 is expressed in high amounts in Barrett's esophagus [11, 12]. COX-2 expression is thought to be an important predictor of colorectal cancer development and a similar deleterious role is likely in the esophagus. A number of selective COX-2 inhibitors, such as rofecoxib and celecoxib, are now marketed as potent anti-inflammatory drugs with fewer toxic effects on the gastrointestinal mucosa compared with older generation NSAIDs. These new selective agents are good candidates for cancer chemoprevention trials in Barrett's esophagus patients. The small potential of gastrointestinal toxicity can be further reduced by the addition of potent acid suppressant drugs such as proton pump inhibitors. Acid suppressants are widely used to alleviate symptoms in Barrett's esophagus patients and this practice further enhances the justification for undertaking COX-2 inhibitor cancer chemoprevention studies.

Sulindac may be alternative NSAID that could be studied for the chemoprevention of adenocarcinoma. Clinical studies have consistently shown that sulindac is effective in reducing the size and number of colorectal polyps in patients with familial adenomatous polyposis (FAP) [13]. FAP is associated with mutations to the tumor suppressor gene adenomatous polyposis coli (APC) and there may be some underlying genetic similarity between FAP and Barrett's esophagus which predisposes to cancer development [14]. Similar to COX-2 inhibitors, sulindac administration in Barrett's esophagus patients should be simultaneously given with an acid suppressant drug in order to reduce the risk of gastrointestinal toxicity.

There may be another benefit to giving Barrett's esophagus patients NSAIDs. There is evidence that patients with Barrett's esophagus are also at an increased risk of developing colorectal cancer [15]. NSAIDs would also be expected to reduce the increased risk of colorectal cancer.

Closing remarks

There is good evidence that NSAIDs reduce the risk of esophageal adenocarcinoma. Focussed cancer chemoprevention trials in Barrett's esophagus patients are therefore warranted. Potential NSAIDs for such chemoprevention trials include rofecoxib, celecoxib and sulindac and these agents should be given with an acid suppressant drug in order to minimise risk of gastrointestinal toxicity. It is not possible with current knowledge to predict whether NSAIDs would actually reverse Barrett's esophagus but clinical trials would be able to provide good evidence in answer to this specific question.

References

1. IARC Handbooks of Cancer Prevention. Volume 1. Non-steroidal anti-inflammatory drugs. Lyon: International Agency for Research on Cancer, 1997.
2. Botha JH, Robinson KM, Ramchurren N, Reddi K, Norman RJ. Human esophageal carcinoma cell lines: prostaglandin production, biological properties, and behaviour in nude mice. J Natl Cancer Inst 1986;76:1053-1056.
3. Rubio CA. Antitumoral activity of indomethacin on experimental esophageal tumors. J Natl Cancer Inst 1984;72:705-707.
4. Rubio CA. Further studies on the therapeutic effect of indomethacin on esophageal tumors. Cancer 1986;58:705-707.
5. Bespalov VG, Troyan DN, Petrov AS, Alexandrov VA. Inhibition of the esophagus tumour development by anti-inflammatory drugs indomethacin and dexamethasone. Pharmacol Toxicol 1989;52:67-70.
6. Siglin JC, Barch DH, Stoner GD. Effects of dietary phenthyl isothiiocyanate, ellagic acid, sulindac and calcium on the induction and progression of N-nitrosomethylbenzylamine-induced esophageal carcinogenesis in rats. Carcinogenesis 1995;16:1101-1106.
7. Funkhouser EM, Sharp GB. Aspirin and the reduced risk of esophageal cancer. Cancer 1995;76:1116-1119.
8. Garidiou A, Tzonou A, Lipworth L, Signarello LB, Kalapothaki V, Trichopolous D. Life-style factors and medical conditions in relation to oesophageal cancer by histologic type in a low-risk population. Int J Cancer 1996;68:295-299.
9. Farrow DC, Vaughan TL, Hansten PD, Stanford JL, Risch HA, Gammon MD, Chow WH, Dubrow R, Ahsan H, Mayne ST, Schoenberg JB, West AB, Rotterdam H, Fraumeni JF Jr, Blot WJ. Use of aspirin and other non-steroidal anti-inflammatory drugs and the risk of esophageal and gastric cancer. Cancer Epidemiol Bio Prev 1998;7(2):97-102.
10. Langman MJS, Cheng KK, Gilman R, Lancashire RJ. Effect of anti-inflammatory drugs on overall risk of common cancer: case-control study in general practice research database. Br Med J 2000;320:1642-1646.
11. Fu S, Ramanujam KS, Meltzer SJ, Wilson KT. Expression and localisation of inducible nitric oxide synthase and cyclooxygenase-2 in Barrett's esophagus. Gastroenterology 1997;114(2):A565.
12. Shirvani VN, Ouatu-Lascar R, Kaur BS, Omary B, Triadafilopoulos G. Cyclooxygenase 2 expression in Barrett's esophagus and adenocarcinoma: ex vivo induction by bile salts and acid exposure. Gastroenterology 2000;118:487-496.
13. Morgan G. Beneficial effects of NSAIDs in the gastrointestinal tract. Eur J Gastroenterol Hepatol 1999;11:393-400.

14. Fein M. APC gene alterations in Barrett's metaplasia are implicated at an early stage in the carcinogenesis of esophageal adenocarcinoma. Am J Gastroenterology 1997;97(2):359-360.
15. Morgan GP, Vainio H. The risk of oesophageal and colorectal cancers in Barrett's oesophagus: a pathophysiological hypothesis and potential of NSAID cancer chemoprevention. Eur J Cancer Prev 1998;7:195-199.

R.F. Souza (Dallas)

The incidence of esophageal adenocarcinoma has been increasing rapidly in the United States over the past two decades [1]. The major risk factors for adenocarcinoma of the esophagus are gastroesophageal reflux disease (GERD) and its sequella, Barrett's esophagus [1]. In Barrett's esophagus, squamous epithelium damaged by reflux esophagitis is replaced by a metaplastic, intestinal-type epithelium that is predisposed to malignancy [1, 2]. Cancers in Barrett's esophagus evolve through a sequence of genetic alterations in which the cells acquire the ability to proliferate without exogenous stimulation, to resist growth-inhibitory signals, and to avoid triggering the programmed cell death mechanism (apoptosis) that ordinarily destroys cells that acquire extensive genetic damage.

Clinical evidence suggests that nondysplastic Barrett's epithelium has both an increased proliferative rate and a reduced apoptotic rate. Cellular proliferation has been studied in biopsy specimens of Barrett's esophagus by measuring the incorporation of tritiated thymidine into cellular DNA, and by immunostaining for antigens associated with proliferation including Ki-67 and proliferating cell nuclear antigen (PCNA) [3]. Compared to gastric fundic and junctional-type epithelia, the specialized intestinal metaplasia (IM) of Barrett's esophagus has been found to exhibit increased proliferation by all of these methods [3]. Moreover, GERD has been established as a strong risk factor for esophageal adenocarcinoma, and recent studies suggest that GERD may increase cell proliferation in Barrett's esophagus [2]. Biopsy specimens of specialized IM maintained in organ culture demonstrate a significant increase in tritiated thymidine uptake when the explants are exposed briefly to acid, suggesting that the brief, episodic esophageal acid exposure typical of GERD may promote tumorigenesis by stimulating hyperproliferation in Barrett's esophagus [4]. Additionally, apoptosis has been studied in biopsy specimens of Barrett's esophagus by immunostaining for fragmented DNA using the TUNEL assay. Compared to biopsies of normal squamous esophagus, the specialized IM of Barrett's esophagus has been found to exhibit decreased apoptosis by this method [5, 6]. In addition, molecular evidence suggests that nondysplastic Barrett's epithelium has enhanced proliferation and decreased apoptosis. Multiple studies have shown that nondysplastic Barrett's esophagus overexpresses cyclin D1 and contains alterations in the p16 and p53 tumor suppressor genes [7-10]. These 3 genetic events act in concert to promote cell proliferation by promoting cell cycle progression and cell division. Nondysplastic Barrett's epithelium also demonstrates overexpression of cyclooxygenase-2 (COX-2) and inactivation of the adenomatous polyposis gene (APC) which act to decrease the rate of apoptosis [11, 12]. Taken together, this clinical and molecular evidence support the notion that nondysplastic Barrett's epithelium has both an enhanced rate of proliferation and a decreased rate of apoptosis.

Cyclooxygenases (COXs) are the key enzymes that mediate the production of prostaglandins from arachidonic acid. Two isoforms of COX have been identified, COX-1 and COX-2. COX-1 is expressed constitutively, whereas COX-2 can be induced by a number of agents including cytokines, growth factors, and tumor promoters [13, 14]. Data from both human and animal studies suggest an important role for COX-2 in gastrointestinal tumorigenesis [15, 16]. Studies *in vitro* have shown that overexpression of COX-2 reduces the rate of apoptosis [17]. Up-regulation of COX-2 has been observed in a number of human tumors including colorectal, pancreatic, and gastric adenocarcinomas [18-20] . Furthermore, overexpression of COX-2 has been detected in human esophageal squamous cell carcinomas and adenocarcinomas, and in the non-malignant, metaplastic epithelium of Barrett's esophagus, as discussed above [11, 21, 22].

A number of epidemiologic studies have concluded that the use of aspirin and other non-steroidal anti-inflammatory drugs (NSAIDs) may protect against the formation of gastrointestinal tumors [23-25]. However, it is not clear whether the antitumor effects of NSAIDs result from inhibition of COX-2, both COX-1 and COX-2, or from some COX-independent mechanism. What does appear clear, though, is that NSAIDs exert their antitumor by decreasing the rate of cell growth primarily by inducing apoptosis [26-29]. NSAIDs have been shown to reduce the formation of colorectal carcinomas in animal models, and to inhibit the formation of colonies by human colorectal carcinoma cell lines by enhancing the rate of apoptosis [30-32]. Moreover, by increasing the rate of apoptosis, treatment with NSAIDs has decreased both the number and size of colonic polyps in animal models and in patients with familial adenomatous polyposis [20, 33-35]. However, few data are available on NSAIDs exerting any effect on the rate of cellular proliferation by altering the cell cycle [36].

Based on the evidence above, NSAID use in patients with Barrett's esophagus is likely to increase the underlying rate of apoptosis, which is abnormally low, in nondysplastic Barrett's epithelium. However, the abnormally increased rate of cell cycle progression in nondysplastic Barrett's epithelium is unlikely to be altered by the use of NSAIDs. Therefore it is unlikely that NSAIDs will reverse Barrett's esophagus. On the other hand, NSAIDs may play role in decreasing the rate of progression of nondysplastic Barrett's mucosa to dysplastic mucosa and cancer. As Barrett's epithelium progresses to dysplasia and cancer, there is a progressive increase in COX-2 expression [22]. Moreover, the elevation of COX-2 during neoplastic progression in Barrett's esophagus most likely contributes to the development of these neoplastic lesions by maintaining a low rate of apoptosis [37, 38]. Recent studies suggest that this hypothesis is plausible. Treatment with both COX-2 selective and nonselective NSAIDs has been shown to decrease cell growth and induce apoptosis in Barrett's-associated adenocarcinoma cell lines [37, 38]. These studies provide an experimental basis for clinical studies designed to determine whether NSAIDs will be useful in altering the rate of neoplastic progression in patients with nondysplastic Barrett's esophagus.

Reference

1. Parker SL, Tong T, Bolden S, Wingo PA. Cancer statistics, 1997 (published erratum appears in CA Cancer J Clin 1997;47(2):68). CA Cancer J Clin 1997;47:5-27.
2. Lagergren J, Bergstrom R, Lindgren A, Nyren O. Symptomatic gastroesophageal reflux as a risk factor for esophageal adenocarcinoma. N Engl J Med 1999;340:825-831.
3. Gray MR, Hall PA, Nash J, Ansari B, Lane DP, Kingsnorth AN. Epithelial proliferation in Barrett's esophagus by proliferating cell nuclear antigen immunolocalization. Gastroenterology 1992;103:1769-1776.
4. Fitzgerald RC, Omary MB, Triadafilopoulos G. Dynamic effects of acid on Barrett's esophagus. An ex vivo proliferation and differentiation model. J Clin Invest 1996;98:2120-2128.
5. Katada N, Hinder RA, Smyrk TC, Hirabayashi N, Perdikis G, Lund RJ, et al. Apoptosis is inhibited early in the dysplasia-carcinoma sequence of Barrett esophagus. Arch Surg 1997;132:728-733.
6. Wetscher GJ, Schwelberger H, Unger A, Offner FA, Profanter C, Glaser K, et al. Reflux-induced apoptosis of the esophageal mucosa is inhibited in Barrett's epithelium. Am.J Surg 1998;176:569-573.
7. Arber N, Lightdale C, Rotterdam H, Han KH, Sgambato A, Yap E, et al. Increased expression of the cyclin D1 gene in Barrett's esophagus. Cancer Epidemiol Biomark Prev 1996;5:457-459.
8. Wong DJ, Barrett MT, Stoger R, Emond MJ, Reid BJ. p16INK4a promoter is hypermethylated at a high frequency in esophageal adenocarcinomas. Cancer Res 1997;57:2619-2622.
9. Barrett MT, Sanchez CA, Prevo LJ, Wong DJ, Galipeau PC, Paulson TG, et al. Evolution of neoplastic cell lineages in Barrett oesophagus. Nat Genet 1999;22:106-109.
10. Casson AG, Mukhopadhyay T, Cleary KR, Ro JY, Levin B, Roth JA. p53 gene mutations in Barrett's epithelium and esophageal cancer. Cancer Res 1991;51:4495-4499.
11. Wilson KT, Fu S, Ramanujam KS, Meltzer SJ. Increased expression of inducible nitric oxide synthase and cyclooxygenase-2 in Barrett's esophagus and associated adenocarcinomas. Cancer Res 1998;58:2929-2934.
12. Lord RV, Kawakami K, Brabender J, Danenberg D, Beer DG, Krasna MJ, Tamura G, Fleisher AS, Laird PW, Eads CA, Dannenberg PV. The presence of APC gene hypermethylation in the serum is a specific marker for esophageal adenocarcinoma. Proc AACR 2000;41:812.
13. Simmons DL, Levy DB, Yannoni Y, Erikson RL. Identification of a phorbol ester-repressible v-src-inducible gene. Proc Natl Acad Sci USA 1989;86:1178-1182.
14. Jones DA, Carlton DP, McIntyre TM, Zimmerman GA, Prescott SM. Molecular cloning of human prostaglandin endoperoxide synthase type II and demonstration of expression in response to cytokines. J Biol Chem 1993;268:9049-9054.
15. Subbaramaiah K, Telang N, Ramonetti JT, Araki R, DeVito B, Weksler BB, et al. Transcription of cyclooxygenase-2 is enhanced in transformed mammary epithelial cells. Cancer Res 1996;56:4424-4429.
16. Williams C, Luongo C, Radhika A, Zhang T, Lamps LW, Nanney LB, et al. Elevated cyclooxygenase-2 levels in Min mouse adenomas. Gastroenterology 1996;111:1134-1140.
17. Tsujii M, DuBois RN. Alterations in cellular adhesion and apoptosis in epithelial cells overexpressing prostaglandin endoperoxide synthase 2. Cell 1995;83:493-501.
18. Eberhart CE, Coffey RJ, Radhika A, Giardiello FM, Ferrenbach S, DuBois RN. Up-regulation of cyclooxygenase 2 gene expression in human colorectal adenomas and adenocarcinomas. Gastroenterology 1994;107:1183-1188.
19. Tucker ON, Dannenberg AJ, Yang EK, Zhang F, Teng L, Daly JM, et al. Cyclooxygenase-2 expression is up-regulated in human pancreatic cancer. Cancer Res 1999;59:987-990.
20. Steinbach G, Lynch PM, Phillips RK, Wallace MH, Hawk E, Gordon GB, et al. The effect of celecoxib, a cyclooxygenase-2 inhibitor, in familial adenomatous polyposis. N Engl J Med 2000;342:1946-1952.
21. Zimmermann KC, Sarbia M, Weber AA, Borchard F, Gabbert HE, Schror K. Cyclooxygenase-2 expression in human esophageal carcinoma. Cancer Res 1999;59:198-204.
22. Shirvani VN, Ouatu-Lascar R, Kaur BS, Omary MB, Triadafilopoulos G. Cyclooxygenase 2 expression in Barrett's esophagus and adenocarcinoma: ex vivo induction by bile salts and acid exposure. Gastroenterology 2000;118:487-496.
23. Thun MJ, Namboodiri MM, Calle EE, Flanders WD, Heath CWJ. Aspirin use and risk of fatal cancer. Cancer Res 1993;53:1322-1327.
24. Greenberg ER, Baron JA, Freeman DHJ, Mandel JS, Haile R. Reduced risk of large-bowel adenomas among aspirin users. The Polyp Prevention Study Group. J Natl Cancer Inst 1993;85:912-916.
25. Giardiello FM, Hamilton SR, Krush AJ, Piantadosi S, Hylind LM, Celano P, et al. Treatment of colonic and rectal adenomas with sulindac in familial adenomatous polyposis. N Engl J Med 1993;328:1313-1316.
26. Elder DJ, Halton DE, Crew TE, Paraskeva C. Apoptosis induction and cyclooxygenase-2 regulation in human colorectal adenoma and carcinoma cell lines by the cyclooxygenase-2-selective non-steroidal anti-inflammatory drug NS-398. Int J Cancer 2000;86:553-560.
27. Rahman MA, Dhar DK, Masunaga R, Yamanoi A, Kohno H, Nagasue N. Sulindac and exisulind exhibit a significant antiproliferative effect and induce apoptosis in human hepatocellular carcinoma cell lines. Cancer Res 2000;60:2085-2089.
28. Zhang G, Tu C, Zhang G, Zhou G, Zheng W. Indomethacin induces apoptosis and inhibits proliferation in chronic myeloid leukemia cells. Leuk Res 2000;24:385-392.
29. Li M, Lotan R, Levin B, Tahara E, Lippman SM, Xu XC. Aspirin induction of apoptosis in esophageal cancer: a potential for chemoprevention. Cancer Epidemiol Biomark Prev 2000;9:545-549.

30. Kawamori T, Rao CV, Seibert K, Reddy BS. Chemopreventive activity of celecoxib, a specific cyclooxygenase-2 inhibitor, against colon carcinogenesis. Cancer Res 1998;58:409-412.
31. Sheng H, Shao J, Morrow JD, Beauchamp RD, DuBois RN. Modulation of apoptosis and Bcl-2 expression by prostaglandin E2 in human colon cancer cells. Cancer Res 1998;58:362-366.
32. Molina MA, Sitja-Arnau M, Lemoine MG, Frazier ML, Sinicrope FA. Increased cyclooxygenase-2 expression in human pancreatic carcinomas and cell lines:growth inhibition by nonsteroidal anti-inflammatory drugs. Cancer Res 1999;59:4356-4362.
33. Stoner GD, Budd GT, Ganapathi R, DeYoung B, Kresty LA, Nitert M, et al. Sulindac sulfone induced regression of rectal polyps in patients with familial adenomatous polyposis. Adv Exp Med Biol 1999;470:45-53.
34. van Stolk R, Stoner G, Hayton WL, Chan K, DeYoung B, Kresty L, et al. Phase I trial of exisulind (sulindac sulfone, FGN-1) as a chemopreventive agent in patients with familial adenomatous polyposis. Clin Cancer Res 2000;6:78-89.
35. Oshima M, Dinchuk JE, Kargman SL, Oshima H, Hancock B, Kwong E, et al. Suppression of intestinal polyposis in Apc delta716 knockout mice by inhibition of cyclooxygenase 2 (COX-2). Cell 1996;87:809.
36. DuBois RN, Shao J, Tsujii M, Sheng H, Beauchamp RD. G1 delay in cells overexpressing prostaglandin endoperoxide synthase-2. Cancer Res 1996;56:733-737.
37. Aggarwal S, Taneja N, Lin L, Iannettoni MD, Orringer MB, Rehemtulla A, Beer DG. Indomethacin-induced apoptosis in esophageal adenocarcinoma cells involves upregulation of BAX and activation of caspase 9 independent of COX-2 expression. Proc Am Ass Cancer Res 2000;41:825.
38. Souza RF, Shewmake K, Beer DG, Cryer B, Spechler SJ. Selective inhibition of cyclooxygenase-2 suppresses growth and induces apoptosis in human esophageal adenocarcinoma cells. Cancer Res 2000;15:5767-5772.

What are the effects of therapy on length of Barrett's epithelium?

K.R. DeVault (Jacksonville)

The goals of gastroesophageal reflux disease treatment in patients with Barrett's esophagus include control of symptoms, healing and maintenance of healing of esophagitis and prevention of progression of the Barrett's esophagus toward cancer. The first two are fairly easy using either medical therapy with proton pump inhibitors (PPI) or with antireflux surgery. We have much less data on prevention of progression, but it would certainly appear that if a treatment resulted in regression of the length of Barrett's esophagus it might also decrease the risk for progression.

There have been several studies that address this issue. Sampliner reported on 27 patients followed for almost three years on lansoprazole 60 mg once a day [1]. There was no decrease in the length of Barrett's esophagus, but 62% of patients developed squamous islands. In a longer study, Sharma *et al.* followed 13 of these patients for a mean of 5.7 years on lansoprazole 30 mg twice daily [2]. There was no decrease in the length of Barrett's esophagus whether or not complete control of esophageal acid (as documented by pH testing on therapy) was obtained with the lansoprazole. A larger study of 47 patients treated with various doses of omeprazole also showed squamous islands, but no overall decrease in the length of Barrett's esophagus [3]. Conversely, Malesci *et al.* reported a 12-month study suggesting an overall decrease from 4.5 to 2.1 cm with 12 months of acid suppression [4]. These data demonstrate the most impressive decrease in length of Barrett's esophagus to date and have been difficult to replicate. Srinivasan *et al.* recently reported a series of 9 patients who had complete control of esophageal acid using a PPI twice daily along with a histamine blocker at night. This treatment resulted in a modest decrease in the mean length of Barrett's esophagus in these patients from 7.2 to 5.2 cm which reached statistical significance ($p < 0.001$) [5]. A randomized trial of raniditine 150 mg twice daily compared to omeprazole 40 mg twice daily showed a minimal decrease in length in the omeprazole, but not in the ranitidine group [6]. In fact, histamine blockers have not been able to produce either squamous islands or a decrease in the length of Barrett's esophagus in prospective studies. In an extensive review of the literature in regards to this subject, only 3 patients were identified with apparent complete reversal of Barrett's esophagus on medical (PPI) therapy [7].

There are many difficulties and challenges inherent in even attempting to study this question. A theme that arises from the positive studies is that more complete acid suppression is needed if we have any hope of affecting the length of Barrett's esophagus. How should this be assured? Some would suggest serial pH studies until a level of acid suppression is reached that results in a total lack of esophageal acid, while others would advocate giving everyone twice-daily PPI therapy along with a histamine blocker at bedtime. Both of these approaches are expensive and inconvenient, especially since they have not been proven to produce long-term benefit in Barrett's esophagus. On the other hand, symptom driven therapy will result in continued reflux of acid in many patients with Barrett's esophagus [8]. Squamous islands appeared to be more common than a decrease in length, but we have no data equating the appearance of either with a decrease in risk of Barrett's esophagus related cancer. In fact, Sharma *et al.* reported that intestinal metaplasia (IM) was present below most squamous islands [9]. IM has also been seen below the "new" squamous epithelium in cases where the length of Barrett's esophagus shortened.

In summary, partial regression and the appearance of squamous islands may occur with aggressive acid suppression in a proportion of patients with Barrett's esophagus, but total regression is rarely if ever seen. Additional prospective studies are needed to determine if there are other advantages of aggressive, perhaps complete control of acid which could include regression, but more importantly prevention of progression to malignancy.

References

1. Sampliner RE. Effect of up to 3 years of high-dose lansoprazole on Barrett's esophagus. Am J Gastroenterol 1994;89:1844-1848.
2. Sharma P, Sampliner RE, Camargo E. Normalization of esophageal pH with high-dose proton pump inhibitor therapy does not result in regression of Barrett's esophagus. Am J Gastroenterol 1997:92:582-585.
3. Cooper BT, Neumann CS, Cox MA, Iqbal TH. Continuous treatment with omeprazole 20 mg daily for up to 6 years in Barrett's oesophagus. Aliment Pharmacol Ther 1998;12:893-897.
4. Malesci A, Savarino V Zentilin P, et al. Partial regression of Barrett's esophagus by long-term therapy with high-dose omeprazole. Gastrointest Endosc 1996;44:700-705.
5. Srinivasan R, Katz PO, Ramakrishnan A, et al. Maximal acid reflux control for Barrett's oesophagus: feasible and effective. Aliment Pharmacol Ther 2001;15:519-524.
6. Peters F, Ganesh S, Kuipers E, et al. Endoscopic regression of Barrett's oesophagus during omeprazole treatment: a randomized double blind study. Gut 1999;45:489-494.
7. Sampliner RE. Reduction of acid exposure and regression of Barrett's esophagus. Dig Dis 2001;18:203-207.
8. Katzka DA, Castell DO. Successful elimination of reflux symptoms does not insure adequate control of acid reflux in patients with Barrett's esophagus. Am J Gastroenterol 1994;89:989-991.
9. Sharma P, Morales TG, Bhattacharyya A, et al. Squamous islands in Barrett's esophagus:What lies underneath? Am J Gastroenterol 1998;93:332-335.

How can length of Barrett's epithelium be mesured?

J.L. Barnett (Ann Arbor)

Why is it important to accurately measure the extent of Barrett's esophagus? It makes intuitive sense that the greater the surface area of intestinal metaplasia, the more cells available for possible malignant transformation. Several reports suggest that this is true; the longer the segment of Barrett's mucosa, the greater the risk of dysplasia and subsequent carcinoma [1-3]. Although any length of Barrett's mucosa puts the patient at risk for malignancy, perhaps careful classification of length, surface area and other shapes or patterns of metaplastic tissue may have prognostic value. This, in turn, could alter surveillance intervals or even determine who is an appropriate candidate for selected methods of ablation therapy. Certain aspects of the pathogenesis and natural history of Barrett's esophagus are still incompletely understood. Carefully mapping the subtleties of regression or progression with time will unable us to better understand the natural history of this metaplasia. Mapping is particularly important when we attempt to measure the response of Barrett's to medical or surgical acid reduction and to assess the effects of ablation therapy. Esophageal biopsies during surveillance are easy to deal with as long as dysplasia is absent, but when dysplasia is identified, a systematic surveillance mapping technique allows us to better focus repeat biopsies to areas of concern. Perhaps accurate mapping will allow focused endoscopic therapy for dyplasia or even carcinoma in the future.

Nuclear scintigraphy and radiographic techniques are usually too insensitive to detect Barrett's metaplasia let alone accurately measure it. Endoscopy allows direct visualization of the mucosa and confirmatory biopsy. Most endoscopists measure the extent of Barrett's by describing its length beginning distally at the gastroesophageal junction just above the top of the gastric folds to its proximal extent where the apparent columnar mucosa changes to squamous epithelium. Barrett's length is determined by reading the endoscope numerical marking at the incisors when the tip of the straightened instrument is located first at the distal and then at the proximal margin and then subtracting the difference. Although arguably sufficient for most clinical purposes, this measurement technique is somewhat crude and poorly reproducible. Was the bottom of the esophagus measured accurately (minimal inflation of the distal esophagus to avoid flattening of the gastric folds at the top of the hiatal hernia)? Is the endoscope straightened? Can the individual centimeter markings on the scope be accurately estimated when printed at only 5 cm increments? Does the endoscopist measure at the incisors or the bite-block? How flexed is the patient's neck? Even the concept of Barrett's length is misleading. One long tongue of metaplastic tissue may extend for a few centimeters but cover only 25% of the esophageal circumference. Multiple squamous islands may cover much of the Barrett's surface area but would not be reflected in a length measurement. Clearly more accurate mapping techniques should be considered for both clinical and research purposes.

One option is to employ a vital stain to enhance the endoscopist's ability to identify and measure Barrett's mucosa. The metaplastic mucosa is stained using toludine or methylene blue or alternatively, the adjacent squamous epithelium is stained with Lugol's iodine. This enhances tissue borders and indistinct patches of irregular mucosa. This technique of chromoendoscopy is discussed elsewhere.

A basic starting point to improve length measurement is to establish standards among endoscopists at least within each endoscopy unit. Attempt to use a standard neck flexion position, be diligent with placement of the scope tip at the distal and proximal margins of the Barrett's lining and use the same incisors or bite-block edge. In my experience, alterations in these measured landmarks produces variability of 1-3 cms or more among different endoscopists. A study of sequential endoscopic measurements of the lower esophageal sphincter and the proximal extent of Barrett's mucosa supports this impression. Approximately 10% of patients had a greater than 4 cm change in these landmarks at a 6-week repeat endoscopy! [4]. This is particularly relevant in group practices or academic centers where different endoscopists may perform the procedure at different times on the same patient. When standard criteria are used and followed, interobserver agreement for Barrett's length measurement was found to have a reliability coefficient of 0.92 (1.0 is perfect agreement) [5].

One simple way to compare the effects of therapy on the length of Barrett's epithelium from one exam to the next or to mark an area of concern for later reference is to create an artificial landmark. Sterilized India ink has been used for tattooing in various portions of the gastrointestinal tract including the esophagus. An ink stain is produced using a sclerotherapy needle. It has been used to mark the border of Barrett's mucosa prior to multipolar electrocoagulation ablation therapy [6]. Another group looked at long-term persistence of the India ink tattoo at the top of Barrett's epithelium and found good (easily visible with some minor fading) or excellent (maintains initial vibrant color) visibility of the tattoo in fifteen patients 36 months after placement. There were no tattoo-related complications [7]. India ink tattooing appears to be reliable, safe and permanent. However, although the ink tattoo is focal, it is precise like an ink line on paper might be. An irregular squamocolumnar junction, squamous islands or small focal abnormalities are not easily marked or circumscribed with the present tattooing technique.

Another simple solution to endoscope measurement limitations is to improve the endoscope itself by adding markings onto the shaft of the instrument. Eisen *et al.* modified a standard upper endoscope by adding circumferential lines at 1 cm intervals and longitudinal lines at 90 degree intervals [8]. This fine-tunes the endoscopist's length measurement and allows better rotational orientation so quadrants could be better isolated. Using this modified endoscope and toludine blue to stain the metaplastic epithelium, they performed biopsies at 1 cm intervals (labeled from the incisors) in each quadrant (labeled by endoscope rotation in 90 degree increments). Biopsy specimens were analyzed for epithelium type, presence and degree of dysplasia and a variety of biomarkers. This mapping endoscopy was repeated in 30-90 days and reproducibility was assessed. The epithelial type was reproducibly identified on the second exam with 94% agreement (566 of 602 biopsies). Dysplasia was found in 7 of 18 patients on the initial exam and reproduced in all on the second exam. All sites of dysplasia were within the same or the adjacent quadrant and centimeter level on both exams. Finally, 3 different biomarkers (ploidy status, p53, Ki-67) were re-identified on the second exam in the majority of patients (97%, 89%, 85%). Eight patients underwent a standard surveillance exam (4 quadrant biopsies every 2 cm with a standard endoscope). Five had dysplasia (3 low-grade, 2 high-grade) on the mapping exam, but only 2 were found to have dysplasia (both low-grade) on the standard exam. A careful mapping protocal such as this one seems reproducible, practical and possibly more sensitive than standard endoscopy. However, some of the benefit may have been derived from the use of shorter 1 cm (*versus* 2 cm) sampling intervals and motivated endoscopists involved in a study rather than refinements in the endoscope markings. Also, the added benefit of chromoendoscopy in this setting has yet to be teased out. As the authors point out, a randomized mapping trial using this technique is needed.

Kim *et al.* have taken a sophisticated, quantitative approach to mapping Barrett's esophagus [9]. They took endoscopic photographs of the esophagus and used a novel computer program to transform the photographs into two dimensional maps. The computer program corrects for the distortion of the endoscope lens, calculates the center of the circular photograph and ultimately recreates the three-dimensional cylindrical image and "unrolls" it into a flat image. The surface area of Barrett's metaplasia can then be calculated. The validated the program by creating color drawings rolling up into tubes to simulate Barrett's esophagus. The varied the color, shape, length, tube diameter, distance between photographs and endoscopist. The computer-generated surface area was then compared to the actual measured value. The calculated areas correlated with the actual areas quite well (r = 0.96) with an overall area of 5.2%. Accuracy was improved by decreasing the photographic interval from 4 cm to 2 cm, but was not significantly affected by color, shape, tube diameter or endoscopist. In patients, there was excellent correlation among computer technicians and among endoscopists. They then compared surface area calculations to length measurements in 17 patients with Barrett's esophagus [10]. Patients with a mean Barrett's length of 7 cm (3-13 cm) underwent sequential exams a mean of 14 months apart. The mean change in length correlation between the two exams was r = 0.90 compared to r = 0.99 for the area correlation (not significantly different), but the percent change in absolute length (27%) was significantly greater than the change in area (16%). In 53%, estimates of Barrett's progression or regression were discordant for the length and area measurements. Are surface area measurements alone superior to length measurements? Probably not because the numerical value is not enough. The number and size of squamous islands must be assessed as was done by this group. Progression at the squamocolumnar junction may be offset by the appearance of squamous islands leaving the overall surface area unchanged. This novel computerized photographic technique appears accurate and reproducible, but is expensive and not widely available.

In summary, careful measurements of metaplastic epithelium will allow us to better understand the pathogenesis, natural history and response to therapy of Barrett's esophagus. Refinements in the measurement of Barrett's esophagus include standardizing the basic technique of endoscopic length calculation, augmenting the markings on the endoscope shaft, making use of chromoendoscopy, tattooing, and computer image analysis using photography. Further experience and controlled trials are necessary to determine which of these techniques is most useful in a variety of clinical and research settings.

References

1. Iftikhar SY, James PD, Steele RJC, Hardcastle JD, Atkinson M. Length of Barrett's oesophagus: an important factor in the development of dysplasia and adenocarcinoma. Gut 1992;33:1155-1158.
2. Weston AP, Badr AS, Hassanein RS. Prospective multivariate analysis of clinical, endoscopic, and histological factors predictive of the development of Barrett's multifocal high-grade dysplasia or adenocarcinoma. Am J Gastroenterol 1999;94:3413-3418.

3. Rudolph RE, Vaughan TL, Storer BE, Haggitt, RC, Rabinovitch PS, Levine DS, Reid BJ. Effect of segment length on risk for neoplastic progression in patients with Barrett esophagus. Ann Intern Med 2000;132:612-620.
4. Kim SL, Waring JP, Spechler SJ, Sampliner RE, Doos WG, Krol WF, et al. Accuracy of esophageal measurements in Barrett's esophagus. Gastroenterology 1993;104:A117.
5. Sharma P, Morales TG, Sampliner RE. Short segment Barrett's esophagus - the need for standardization of the definition and of endoscopic criteria. Am J Gastroenterol 1998;93:1033-1036.
6. Sampliner RE, Fennerty B, Garewal HS. Reversal of Barrett's esophagus with acid suppression and multipolar electrocoagulation: preliminary results. Gastrointest Endosc 1996;44:523-525.
7. Shaffer RT, Francis JM, Carrougher JG, Root SS, Angueira CE, Szyjkowski R, Kadakia SC. India ink tattooing in the esophagus. Gastrointest Endosc 1998;47:257-260.
8. Eisen GM, Montgomery EA, Azumi N, Hartmann D, Bhargava P, Lippman M, Benjamin SB. Qualitative mapping of Barrett's metaplasia: a prerequisite for intervention trials. Gastrointest Endosc 1999;50:814-818.
9. Kim R, Baggott BB, Rose S, Shar AO, Mallory DL, Lasky SS, Kressloff M, Faccenda LY, Reynolds JC. Quantitative endoscopy: precise computerized measurement of metaplastic epithelial surface area in Barrett's esophagus. Gastroenterology 1995;108:360-366.
10. Kim R, Rose S, Shar AO, Weiner M, Reynolds JC. Extent of Barrett's esophagus metaplasia: a prospective study of the serial change in area of Barrett's measured by quantitative endoscopic imaging. Gastrointest Endosc 1997;45:456-462.

What are the effects of medical therapy on parietal cells? What are the consequences when medical treatment is stopped?

G. Tougas, R.H. Riddell, D.K. Driman (Hamilton)

Effects of acid suppression on gastrin secretion and gastric endocrine cells

The potent acid suppression resulting from the use of proton pump inhibitors (PPIs) has marked effects on gastric histology and physiology [1]. While most of the literature has been related to the effects of omeprazole therapy on gastric mucosal histology, there are reports confirming that the effects are likely observed with all PPIs and represent a class effect. Therefore for the purpose of the present discussion, all PPIs (omeprazole, lansoprazole, pantoprazole, rabeprazole, etc.) will be considered as being from the same class.

By inhibiting H^+, K^+-ATPase activity ("the proton pump") within parietal cells, PPIs dramatically reduce gastric acid secretion. This in turn will induce a predictable elevation in gastrin secretion and endocrine cells (particularly G cell) [2]. However the elevation is generally modest and will reach a plateau 2-4 folds above basal levels after several months of treatment. Only in patients with already elevated gastrin levels does therapy with a PPI result in more sustained gastrin increases [3]. It is important to differentiate between gastric endocrine cell hyperplasia and the occurrence of carcinoid tumors. While the former is common after long-term acid suppression, endocrine cell neoplasia and carcinoid tumors do not result from long-term PPIs, whatever the dose used.

Therefore, the prolonged use of a PPI, through the nearly complete inhibition of acid secretion from parietal cells, predictably induces a moderate gastric endocrine hyperplasia.

There is however no evidence linking the long-term use of a PPI to carcinoid neoplasia or endocrine tumors in the absence of an auto-immune pernicious anemia or a gastrinoma.

Effects of acid suppression on gastric mucosa and parietal cell mass

The prolonged use of a PPI profoundly increases the prevalence and distribution of chronic atrophic gastritis [4]. However, this effect of PPIs is only seen in patients with chronic *Helicobacter pylori* infection and associated atrophic gastritis. More recent studies, particularly from Kuipers *et al.*, have confirmed that in the absence of *Helicobacter pylori,* PPIs are not associated with an increased occurrence of atrophic gastritis than in control population.

On its own there is no evidence that acid suppression can increase the risk of gastric cancer, or that eradication of *Helicobacter pylori*, prior to the institution of long-term therapy with a PPI actually decreases the subsequent risk of developing gastric cancer.

More recent data have linked the chronic use of a PPI with an increased frequency of development of gastric polyps, particularly in the fundus [5]. Histologically, these polyps consist of poorly organized oxyntic mucosal cell clusters with scattered cysts found deep into the mucous neck cells. The increased risk of developing these relatively uncommon lesions appears to increase 10 fold in patients chronically receiving a proton pump (9/231 or 3.9%, *versus* 7/2072 or 0.3% in control subjects) [6]. There is anecdotal evidence to suggest that discontinuation of the PPI will lead to regression of the polyps although this has not been assessed prospectively. Thus far the neoplastic potential of these polyps has not been established but the evidence to date suggests that it is somewhat limited.

In patients without *Helicobacter pylori*, the prolonged use of PPIs actually produce parietal cell hypertrophy and hyperplasia, resulting in an effectively increased parietal cell mass [7]. In rats, omeprazole administration is associated with increased oxyntic mucosal thickness, a finding that has been attributed to sustained hypergastrinemia. A number of early reports have documented an increased parietal cell volume density and volume. Others have suggested that parietal cell hyperplasia also occurs. In a comprehensive study we have assessed the effects of long-term omeprazole therapy on gastric mucosal architecture and histology in *Helicobacter pylori* negative patients [7]. We compared the effects of omeprazole to the mucosal changes associated with ranitidine therapy as well. In this study, the use of a PPI was associated with marked and significant increases in parietal cell height, mass and number over control biopsies. Use of ranitidine increased parietal cell mass but had no discernible effect on the other parameters. For all parameters examined, the effect of omeprazole was greater than the effect of ranitidine. We were also able to establish a positive correlation between the duration of treatment (> 12 months *versus* < 12 months) and the magnitude of the changes in parietal cell height, mass and number.

It is likely that the parietal cell hyperplasia and hypertrophy we observe with omeprazole is due to a trophic effect resulting from the hypergastrinemia associated with the hypochlorhydria induced by a PPI. It also provides a physiological basis for the rebound hyperchlorhydria transiently associated with cessation of therapy with a PPI. There is evidence this effect is also observed with other PPIs as well, including lansoprazole.

The explanation for the apparent lack of effect of ranitidine is probably to be found in the much more modest acid secretory inhibition that can be achieved using a classical H_2 receptor antagonist at a standard dose. It is likely that the histological effects of acid secretory inhibition are dose dependent, although there are presently no data to support this assertion.

Only one study has so far examined the consequence of stopping PPI therapy on the gastric mucosal effects of these compounds. In a long-term study of the effects of lansoprazole on parietal cells, Stolte *et al.* have confirmed our previous observations of hypertrophy and hyperplasia [8]. As their follow-up was much longer, they were also able to observe that the longer the treatment with a PPI, the higher the prevalence of parietal cell hyperplasia. More importantly, they have found that parietal cell hypertrophy is entirely reversible and that parietal cell architecture returns to normal within three months of discontinuing lansoprazole. It is very likely that this is the case for all PPIs although this has yet to be specifically examined for other PPIs.

In summary, therapy with PPIs has a number of effects on gastric mucosa. These include well characterized effects such as gastric endocrine cellular hyperplasia, which is reversible and is not associated with an increased incidence of carcinoid tumors. In addition, it will alter the pattern of atrophic gastritis observed in *Helicobacter pylori* infected patients, with an increased severity of the inflammation in the body and a proximal extension of the atrophic mucosal changes initially confined to the antrum. Again, from the presently available literature, there is little evidence that this effect of PPIs and of acid suppression on gastric atrophy has any neoplastic potential on its own. The issues regarding the occurrence of gastric cancer in *Helicobacter pylori* patients however remain of significant concern.

In *Helicobacter pylori* negative patients, therapy with PPIs will induce significant parietal cell hyperplasia and hypertrophy. These effects are a consequence of the increased gastrin levels that result from the potent suppression of acid secretion induced by PPIs. They probably account for the rebound acid secretion seen in many patients upon discontinuation of therapy with PPIs. However, this mucosal effect is reversible and mucosal architecture returns to normal within three months of cessation of the PPI.

References

1. Fitzgibbons PL, Jamidar PA. The effects of long-term acid suppression on gastric mucosal histology. Am J Clin Pathol 1998;110:569-571.
2. Freston JW. Long-term acid control and proton pump inhibitors: interactions and safety issues in perspective.Am J Gastroenterol 1997;92:51S-57S.
3. Klinkenberg-Knol EC, Festen HPM, Jansen JBMJ, et al. Long-term treatment with omeprazole for refractory reflux esophagitis: efficacy and safety. Ann Intern Med 1994;121:161-167.
4. Kuipers EJ, Lundell L, Klinkenberg-Knol EC, et al. Atrophic gastritis and Helicobacter pylori infection in patients with reflux esophagitis treated with omeprazole or fundoplication. N Engl J Med 1996;334(16):1018-1022.
5. Graham JR. Omeprazole and gastric polyposis in humans. Gastroenterology 1993;104(5):1584.
6. Choudhry U, Boyce HW, Coppola D. Proton-pump inhibitor-associated gastric polyps. Am J Clin Pathol 1998;110:615-621.
7. Driman DK, Wright C, Tougas G, Riddell RH. Omeprazole produces parietal cell hypertrophy and hyperplasia in humans. Dig Dis Sci 1996;41(10):2039-2047.
8. Stolte M, Meining A, Seifert E, Alexandridis T. Treatment with lansoprazole also induces hypertrophy of the parietal cells of the stomach. Pathol Res Pract 2000;196(1):9-13.

Is development of gastric polyps during proton pump inhibitor therapy related to the length of treatment?

B.E. Schenk, A. Cats, E.J. Kuipers
(Zwolle, Amsterdam, Rotterdam)

Long-term treatment with proton pump inhibitors (PPI) is associated with increased serum gastrin levels. This increase is usually mild to moderate, but may be extreme, *i.e.* more than fourfold above the upper normal in some patients [1]. The increase of serum gastrin during PPI therapy is more pronounced in *H. pylori*-positive patients, in particular if atrophic gastritis of the corpus mucosa exists [1]. PPI therapy and the resulting serum gastrin increase are associated with histopathological changes of the gastric mucosa [2, 3]. First of all, gastrin has a trophic influence on the enterochromaffin-like (ECL) cells of the stomach [4]. ECL-cell hyperplasia is thus very common during treatment with PPI therapy [2, 5]. In some conditions with markedly increased serum gastrin levels, such as pernicious anemia and gastrinomas, ECL-cell hyperplasia may ultimately result in the development of gastric carcinoid formation. To our knowledge, this has however never been described during PPI therapy.

A second effect of PPI's on the gastric mucosa occurs in the presence of *H. pylori*. Colonisation with this bacterium is usually associated with an antral-predominant gastritis pattern, which pattern however changes into a corpus-predominant pan-gastritis during PPI therapy as a result of the acid-sensitivity of the bacterium. This pan-gastritis accelerates the progression to gland loss or atrophic gastritis. Such progression of corpus inflammation and atrophy, with a decrease of antral inflammation, was observed during profound acid suppressive therapy in *H. pylori*-positive patients exclusively [2, 6, 7]. A third effect of PPI's on the gastric mucosa is the development of prominent tonguelike intraluminal protrusions of the apical parietal cell cytoplasm and cystic dilation of the fundic glands (fundic gland hyperplasia) [8].

These effects of PPI therapy on the gastric mucosa, hypergastrinemia, parietal cell protrusion, ECL-cell hyperplasia, progression of *H. pylori* gastritis and the development of atrophy, may in theory all predispose to the formation of gastric polyps. In general populations, gastric polyps are rare, with an estimated prevalence of 1% to 3% in endoscopy and autopsy series. In some conditions, such as achlorhydria, atrophic gastritis, pernicious anaemia and gastric cancer, they occur more frequently. Fundic gland polyps were originally described in patients with familial polyposis [9-11]. In subjects without this condition, they appeared to be very rare with a prevalence of 0.084-1.9% [12-15], until Graham described the development of gastric polyps in patients during long-term treatment with omeprazole [16], which observation was soon confirmed by others [17, 18]. Endoscopically, the majority of these PPI-associated polyps are small (2-8 mm), sessile, multiple, with a partly translucent surface and usually located in the fundus or proximal in the gastric corpus. In most cases, these polyps appear to be fundic gland polyps, in some patients hyperplastic and inflammatory polyps occur [17, 18]. On histological examination, these polyps are composed of cystic, dilated fundic glands lined both with parietal and chief cells. Hyperplastic polyps, with a more irregular shaped and flat surfaced aspect upon endoscopy, display a dilated, elongated and branched foveolae with mucous cell lining on light and electron microscopy. A polymorph stromal inflammation, surrounding cystically dilated glands, was observed in the inflammatory polyps [19].

Data on the relation between dosage and duration of PPI treatment in relation to the occurrence of gastric polyps are scarce. In the series described by Graham, with annual endoscopical follow-up, twelve out of 33 patients developed gastric polyps after a mean treatment of 2.8 years [16, 20]. In 7 patients polyps developed within the first year of treatment, in 5 patients polyps were found after two to four years of treatment. Similar results were found by others. In a case study describing six patients developing polyps during treatment with 20 mg of omeprazole daily, polyps were noted after one year in 2 patients, after two years in 2 and after four and five years therapy in the remaining two patients [16]. Choudry *et al.* found a prevalence of gastric polyps of 7.3% (17/231 patients) after a mean treatment duration of 35 months (range: 3-98) with 20 mg omeprazole daily. Of the 15 polyps examined, 9 were fundic glands polyps, 4 hyperplastic polyps and 2 of the inflammatory type [17]. The interval of endoscopical follow-up in these patients was not specified in the study. Remarkably, several investigators observed disappearance of these polyps after discontinuation of omeprazole treatment, whereas they reoccurred after restarting this therapy. In a Dutch cohort followed for 4 years, gastric polyps were found in 27 of 163 of patients (17%) on long-term treatment with 40 mg omeprazole for gastro-esophageal reflux disease with annual endoscopical follow-up [19]. Two thirds of them were fundic gland polyps, the reminder were hyperplastic polyps. Comparison of those patients who developed polyps with those who did not showed no correlation between the formation of fundic gland polyps and the dose or duration of treatment, serum gastrin levels or *H. pylori* infection. Formation of hyperplastic polyps was associated with *H. pylori* infection. Polyp formation occurred gradually during follow-up, with most new cases diagnosed within one or two years after initiation of therapy. The number and size of these polyps may increase during ongoing therapy. Thus far, no PPI related gastric polyp became adenomatous, nor developed dysplastic or malignant changes. The clinical relevance of these polyps is as yet unclear, further prospective studies, addressing the mechanism of formation and its natural history are required.

In conclusion, gastric polyp formation during PPI therapy is not uncommon. The majority of these polyps consist of benign fundic glands polyps, which usually occur within the first two years of PPI treatment. At present, endoscopy surveillance of these polyps nor cessation of PPI treatment do not seems indicated.

References

1. Schenk BE, Kuipers EJ, Klinkenberg-Knol EC, Bloemena EG, Nelis GF, Festen HPM, Lamers CBHW, Meuwissen SGM. Hypergastrinemia and omeprazole therapy: influences of vagal nerve function, gastric emptying and Helicobacter pylori infection. Alim Pharm Ther 1998;12:605-612.
2. Klinkenberg-Knol EC, Festen HPM, Jansen JBMJ, et al. Long-term treatment with omeprazole for refractory reflux esophagitis: efficacy and safety. Ann Int Med 1994;121:161-167.
3. Lamberts R, Creutzfeldt W, Strüber HG, et al. Long-term omeprazole therapy in peptic ulcer disease; gastrin, endocrine cell growth, and gastritis. Gastroenterology 1993;104:1356-1370.
4. Tielemans Y, Hakanson R, Sundler F, et al. Gastrin stimulates the self-replication rate of enterochromaffinelike cells in the rat stomach. Gastroenterology 1989;96:723-729.
5. Eissele R, Brunner G, Simon B, et al. Gastric mucosa during treatment with lansoprazole: H. pylori is a risk factor for argyrophil hyperplasia. Gastroenterology 1997;112:707-717.

6. Kuipers EJ, Lundell L, Klinkenberg-Knol EC, et al. Atrophic gastritis and Helicobacter pylori in patients with reflux esophagitis treated with omeprazole or fundoplication. New Engl J Med 1996;334:1018-1022.
7. Berstad AE, Hatlebakk JG, Maartmann-Moe H, et al. Helicobacter pylori gastritis and epithelial cell proliferation in patients with reflux esophagitis after treatment with lansoprazole. Gut 1997;41:740-747.
8. Cats A, Schenk BE, Bloemena E, Roosedaal R, Lindeman J, Biemond I, Klinkenberg-Knol EC, Meuwissen SG, Kuipers EJ. Parietal cell protrusions and fundic gland cysts during omeprazole maintenance treatment. Hum Pathol 2000;31:684-690.
9. Nishiura M, Hirota T, Itabashi M, et al. A clinical and histopathological study of gastric polyps in familial polyposis coli. Am J Gastroenterol 1974;79;98-103.
10. Watanaba H, Enjoji M, Yao T, et al. Gastric lesions in familial adenomatosis coli: their incidence and histological analysis. Hum Pathol 1974;9:296-83.
11. Iada M, Yao T, Itoh H, et al. Natural history of fundic gland polyposis in patients with familial adenomatosis coli/ Gardner's syndrome. Gastroenterology 1984;86:1437-1442.
12. Lee RG, Burt RW. The histopathology of fundic gland polyps of the stomach. Am J Clin Pathol 1986;86:498-503.
13. Marcial MA, Villafana M, Hernandez-Denton J, Colon-Pagan JR. Fundic gland polyps: prevalence and clinicopathologic features. Am J Gastroenterol 1993;10:1711-1713.
14. Sipponen P, Laxen F, Seppala K. Cystic hamartomatous gastric polyps: a disorder of oxyntic glands. Histopathology 1983;7:729-737.
15. Kinoshita Y, Tojo M, Matsumoto T, et al. Incidence of fundic gland polyps in patients without familial adenomatous polyposis. Gastrointest Endosc 1993;39:161-163.
16. Graham JR. Gastric polyposis:onset during long-term therapy with omeprazole. Med J Aust 1992;157;287-288.
17. Stolte M, Bethke B, Seiffert E, et al. Observation of gastric glandular cysts in the corpus mucosa of the stomach under omeprazole treatment. Z Gastroenterol 1995;33:146-149.
18. El-Zimaity HM, Jackson FW, Graham DY. Fundic gland polyps developing during omeprazole therapy. Am J Gastroenterol 1997;92:1858-1860.
19. Choudry U, Boyce HW, Coppala D. Proton pump inhibitor-associated gastric polyps. Am J Clin Pathol 1998;110:615-621.
20. Graham JR. Gastric acne: omeprazole-induced fundic gland polyposis. Med J Aust 1998;168:93.
21. Schenk B.E. Studies on Helicobacter pylori and long-term profound acid suppression. Thesis 1999 Amsterdam, the Netherlands.

Can any correlation betweeen gastric polyps development and dysplasia be anticipated in Barrett's patients?

A.C. Svoboda, S. Tillisch-Svoboda, P.L. Morris (Santa Barbara)

The development of large (> 1 cm) non-neoplastic gastric polyps in patients undergoing surveillance endoscopy for Barrett's epithelium treated with continuous omeprazole for over one year, and polyp disappearance or size reduction by omeprazole discontinuation or dose reduction, prompted a review of all Barrett's patients followed by this investigator (Svoboda). The aim was to determine the incidence of gastric polyps in patients with Barrett's epithelium, the importance of length of esophageal columnar epithelium, and the influence of treatment on gastric polyp development. A retrospective review of Barrett's patient's records with attention to length of Barrett's segment, presence of dysplasia, treatment, gastric polyps, colon polyps and cancer, serum gastrin levels, and presence of *Helicobacter pylori* was carried out.

Case study

A 57-year-old white married moderately overweight male, with daily heartburn despite dietary restrictions and antacid usage, in December 1991 had ulcerative esophagitis (distal 3 cm) at endoscopy. Biopsies demonstrated intestinal metaplasia and Barrett's esophagus and H_2 receptor antagonists and prokinetic agents were initiated.

The patient returned for continued symptoms and Barrett's esophagus, and erosive esophagitis were confirmed. No gastric polyps were present. Therapy with omeprazole, 20 mg every morning was begun.

The patient did so well on omeprazole that he refused to stop the medication despite the fact that it was then only indicated for short-term therapy. Because of concerns about continued omeprazole usage follow-up endoscopy was advised in 6 months. At that time (May 1993) endoscopy showed 7-8 sessile fundal polyps 4-5 mm in diameter diagnosed on biopsy as hyperplastic polyps.

Omeprazole was discontinued and nizatidine 150 mg BID was begun. Because of both recurrent symptoms and the polyp history, endoscopy was repeated in 6 months (November 1993) with reintroduction of omeprazole when no gastric polyps were seen. In June 1994 endoscopy demonstrated both more (8-10) and larger (10-15 mm) gastric polyps with features of both fundal and hyperplastic polyps on multiple biopsies. Dose reduction of omeprazole to 20 mg every 2-3 days marginally controlled symptoms and endoscopy in December 1994 showed more (12-15) but smaller (6-9 mm) polyps.

During the follow-up period of this patient two additional patients on prolonged omeprazole therapy developed gastric polyps on follow-up. In each patient polyps disappeared or were smaller with omeprazole discontinuation or dose reduction. A review of patients under surveillance for Barrett's esophagus appeared warranted.

Method

A retrospective review of Barrett's patients' records with attention to length of Barrett's segment, presence of dysplasia, treatment, presence of gastric polyps, colon polyps and/or cancer, serum gastrin levels, and presence of *Helicobacter pylori*.

Barrett's esophagus was diagnosed by biopsy proven intestinal metaplasia (IM) with goblet cell hyperplasia at the gastroesophageal junction (GEJ) or in the tubular esophagus.

Findings

There were a total of 222 patients (137 males and 85 females). In 80 patients with long-segment Barrett's (over 3 cm of specialized columnar mucosa in the distal esophagus), the sex ratio was 59 males to 21 females, while in 142 patients with short segment Barrett's there were 78 males and 64 females. All moderate and severe dysplasia occurred in long segment Barrett's. In long segment Barrett's the mean age was 66 years with a range of 33-83 years. Average duration of known disease was 55 months with a range of 4-219 months. In short segment Barrett's the mean age was similar (68 years) with a range of 17-87 years. The average duration of known disease was 28 months with a range of 2-179 months.

As part of a concurrent study to determine the frequency of IM at the GEJ, 26 of 120 patients (21.6%) referred for endoscopy with no obvious Barrett's had IM on biopsy at the C-E junction.

Dysplasia in metaplastic tissue

Fifty-five Barrett's patients were reported to show dysplasia on at least one examination (26.8%). Low-grade dysplasia was predominant, occurring in 46 patients of whom 26 (31%) had long segment disease and 20 (16.5%) had short segment Barrett's. There was one (1) person with moderate (female) and eight (8) with severe dysplasia (1 female, 7 males). All moderate and severe dysplasia was found in long segment Barrett's. The longer the period of surveillance, the greater the likelihood of dysplasia developing. Dysplasia presence or severity, varied from one exam to the next, presumably because of sampling error although a protocol of four quadrant biopsies every one cm was employed in dysplasia follow-up.

Gastric polyps

Gastric polyp presence was recorded at each endoscopy with an estimate of number of polyps and size range. Gastric fundal polyps frequently occur between folds and adequate inflation of the stomach and careful retroflexion of the endoscope is necessary to avoid missing sessile lesions. The authors had a prior interest and previous publications relative to non-neoplastic gastric polyps providing a control group drawn from a very similar demographic population. This prior study was concerned with the frequency of parietal cell antibodies in endoscopic patients. Of 300 consecutive patients over the age of 40 having endoscopy, 14 or 4.7% were found to have non-neoplastic polyps generally against a background of partial atrophy or atrophic gastritis agreeing well with the 3-5% incidence in the endoscopic literature.

Gastric polyp occurrence in current study

At the time of diagnosis of Barrett's and prior to initiation of treatment, non-neoplastic (fundic gland or hyperplastic) polyps were present in 7 of 222 patients or 3.15%. While less frequent than controls this was not statistically significant. After proton pump inhibitor (PPI) therapy (omeprazole) the changes were dramatic. Polyps develop in 32 of 215 patients or 14.88% ($p = 0.0001$!). Of long segment Barrett's patients with polyps 14 (77%) were on PPIs. Of 62 patients without gastric polyps, 28 were on PPIs or 45%. This difference is significant ($p = 0.03$). Similarly in short segment Barrett's the number of those with polyps on PPIs (13/21 or 61.9%) was greater than those without polyps on PPIs (48/121 or 39.7%, $p = 0.10$) suggesting a trend. Polyps tended to be multiple, sessile and evenly distributed (on endoscopic biopsy) between fundic gland and hyperplastic polyps.

Other investigators have subsequently reported this association of proton pump use and gastric polyp development, especially in Barrett's patients. Presumably just as in pernicious anemia or atrophic gastritis with achlorhydria, high gastrin levels exert a trophic effect on gastric epithelium. However, in this study there were only two instances of serum gastrin elevation, one in short segment and the other in long segment Barrett's. Neither of these had gastric polyps or dysplasia. These polyps do not have a significant potential to become neoplastic and should not deserve endoscopic surveillance. However, additional examination of our data raised serious concerns. Not only did there appear to be an association between use of PPIs and subsequent non-neoplastic gastric polyp development, but those with long segment Barrett's who developed polyps were those most likely to develop dysplasia.

Of the 80 patients with long segment Barrett's, 18 developed polyps and dysplasia was present in 15 of these 18 (83.3%). Of those 62 without polyps, dysplasia was present in only 22 (25.5%). This is highly significant ($p = 0.001$!).

This risk in short segment Barrett's has not yet been demonstrated, in part because of short follow-up.

Conclusion

If gastric polyp development is associated with PPI usage and if polyps are a warning sign of dysplasia developing, can PPI usage be associated with dysplasia and progression to neoplasia? PPI usage is associated with gastric polyp development in both short and long segment Barrett's. Patients with Barrett's esophagus on prolonged use of omeprazole are more likely than controls to develop non-neoplastic gastric polyps ($p < .0001$). This is especially true with long segment (classical) Barrett's (p 0.0001 versus 0.131)

Patients with long segment Barrett's are more likely than short segment Barrett's to develop dysplasia. ($p < .0001$). All moderate and severe dysplasia occurred in long segment Barrett's.

A finding of gastric polyps is associated with a greater risk of esophageal dysplasia.

The development of gastric polyps during acid suppression therapy (especially with PPIs) in patients with long segment Barrett's is associated with a high and statistically significant risk of esophageal dysplasia. Careful surveillance is warranted and alternative therapy should be considered if polyps and dysplasia co-exist.

Bibliography

1. Svoboda AC. Is polypectomy indicated for gastric polyps? Am J Gastroenterol 1980.
2. Tillisch S, Svoboda A, Garrett R. Gastric polyps; use common sense, not surveillance. Am J Gastroenterol 1986;81:851.
3. Svoboda A, Tillisch-Svoboda S. Barrett's patients developing gastric polyps during acid suppression are at greater risk of esophageal dysplasia. Endoscopy 1996;28:S20.
4. El-Zimaity H, Jackson F, Graham D. Fundic gland polyps developing during omeprazole therapy. Am J Gastroenterol 1997;92:1858.
5. Choudhry V, Boyce HW, Coppola D. Proton pump inhibitor-associated gastric polyps. Am J Clin Path 1998;110:615.

Can intermittent therapy be envisaged in Barrett's esophagus?

S. Bank, P. Singh, A.C. Yao (New York)

The present study investigates the prevalence of carcinoma and high-grade dysplasia (HGD) in patients with Barrett's metaplasia and the incidence of progression to carcinoma, HGD or low-grade dysplasia (LGD) in patients with previously diagnosed Barrett's without therapy and with maintenance proton pump inhibitor (PPI) given either daily, or alternate days or intermittently. Although treating endoscopic esophagitis or reflux symptoms in patients with proven Barrett's is clearly recommended and desirable there is considerable controversy with regard to maintaining patients on acid suppressive therapy in asymptomatic patients without esophagitis. It now seems clear that acid suppressive therapy alone without ablation of the metaplastic mucosa or mucosectomy will not result in total replacement of Barrett's by squamous epithelium. There is however some evidence that maintaining patients on constant acid suppression may delay or prevent the occurrence of metaplasia in the Barrett's segment.

Material and methods

This study consists of two parts.

Part 1

A personal series of 120 patients with marked esophagitis unresponsive to H_2 receptor antagonists who were followed for 5-11 years on maintenance omeprazole after initial healing of the esophagitis with 20-60 mg of omeprazole. Fifty two of these had Barrett's at the initial and subsequent endoscopies. The number of patients, years of follow-up and the number in each year after 5 years are shown in *Table I*. *Table II* shows the follow-up from year 1 to years 5-11. Endoscopy with gastric or protocol esophageal biopsies were performed every 1-2 years, serum gastrin was drawn every 1-2 years and serum chemistry every 1-2 years. *Table III* shows the grade of esophagitis at the initial endoscopy using the Los Angeles grading system. It can be seen that most of the patients were Grade C

Table I. Patients with esophagitis (120 patients followed for 5-11 years).

Years	Nb of patients
10-11	16
8-9	20
6-8	32
5	52

Table II. Follow-up after initial healing of esophagitis.

Endoscopy	1-2 years
esophageal biopsies (protocol)	
gastric fundus biopsy	
Helicobacter pylori status, ECL cells	
gastric polyps	
Serum gastrin	1-2 years
Serum chemistry	1-2 years

Table III. Esophagitis at initial endoscopy.

LA - grade D	20%
LA - grade C	52%
LA - grade B	28%
Barrett's metaplasia	52
Gastric fundal type	10
Esophagitis (no metaplasia)	58
	120

(or severe) esophagitis even after conventional H_2 antagonist therapy. It also shows the number with Barrett's metaplasia at the initial endoscopy and those with esophagitis with no metaplasia. It is stressed that the maintenance therapy was only given after the esophagitis had healed at least to Grade B but mostly to normal and requiring anything from 20-60 mg of omeprazole to healing. At that time the omeprazole dosage was maintained according to the patient's symptoms and also on the basis of the findings on the yearly or two yearly endoscopy. *Table IV* shows the general maintenance dose required by the patients over the 5-11 years of their continuance in the study. It can be seen that 36% of patients required at least daily or bi-daily and sometimes 3 times a day omeprazole therapy to contain symptoms and healing. Of these, those with Grade D required at least 20 mg daily in most of the patients. On the other hand, alternate day therapy or even third or every fifth day therapy could contain symptoms and healing in 61% of patients. Occasionally there was some adjustment in the dose, either to increase or decrease but this rarely occurred and was left up to the patient. If an adjustment was required, it usually did not last for more than a week. Initially, the rationale for alternate day or intermittent therapy was based on three factors:

- the black box warning that daily maintenance therapy was not advised for more than two months;
- the cost factor in the United States of omeprazole;
- many patients refused to stop their therapy because of the consistently better results symptomatically than they were getting on the H_2 receptor antagonist or lifestyle changes.

Table IV. Omeprazole maintenance dose (after initial healing of esophagitis).

Frequency	Dose	% of patients
Daily	20 mg	31%
Daily	40-60 mg	5%
Alternate day	20 mg	44%
Every 3rd day or more	20 mg	17%

(50% of patients with initial LA grade D required at least 20 mg daily)

Part 2

The second part of the study was a questionnaire sent out to various gastroenterologists on Long Island, New York requesting them to respond on the number of Barrett's patients they had seen in their practice, the prevalent cases of carcinoma, HGD or LGD at the time of the first endoscopy, the incidence of carcinoma, HGD or LGD on follow-up of these patients and the incidence of carcinoma, HGD and LGD if the patients were retained on maintenance PPI therapy or not. Twenty two responses were received, some from institutional collections and some from individual gastroenterologists in the area. All in all there were 22 responses encompassing 1,126 cases of Barrett's esophagus. Sixteen of the 22 responders claimed that they were using daily or alternate day omeprazole therapy even in asymptomatic patients and 6 were treating only as symptoms arose.

Results

Part 1 - Personal series

Progression of the Barrett's to carcinoma or HGD or LGD on endoscopy after 5-11 years is shown in the *Table V*. It can be seen that there were no patients who progressed to carcinoma or to HGD in this rather small series and one patient developed questionable LGD which was sent out for confirmation and there was some controversy whether it was dysplasia at all or reactive dysplasia. The number of patients who developed Barrett's reversion to squamous islands was 6% but none reverted to total replacement of the Barrett's epithelium. For completeness, *Table VI* shows the incidence of changes after 5-11 years from esophagitis to Barrett's, carcinoma, HGD or LGD while on therapy. Again it can be seen that the progression from esophagitis to Barrett's in this series in 58 patients was again not found. The progression of esophagitis with or without Barrett's to carcinoma again 0% and the progression of esophagitis or Barrett's to HGD again 0% and even to LGD 0.8%.

Table V. Results after 5-11 years findings and progression.

Barrett's to carcinoma	0% (of 52)
Barrett's to high-grade dysplasia	0% (of 52)
Barrett's to low-grade dysplasia	1.8% (1 of 52)
Barrett's to squamous islands	6%

Table VI. Incidence of change after 5-11 years.

Progression from esophagitis to Barrett's (58 patients)	0%
Progression of esophagitis or Barrett's to carcinoma (120 patients)	0%
Progression of esophagitis or Barrett's to high-grade dysplasia (120 patients)	0%
Progression of esophagitis or Barrett's to low-grade dysplasia (120 patients)	0.8%

Table VII shows the prevalence of dysplasia and carcinoma in Barrett's, *i.e.* the finding of metaplasia or carcinoma at the initial endoscopy for heartburn, reflux, or other esophageal symptoms. It can be seen that carcinoma was detected at the initial endoscopy in two, HGD in 2, LGD in 2 and a controversial grade of medium grade dysplasia in a further 2 patients. Although the Gastrointestinal Division in our department were rather worried by this designation of

Table VII. Prevalence of dysplasia and carcinoma in Barrett's.

Carcinoma (resected)	2
High grade dysplasia (ablated)	2
"Medium" grade dysplasia	2
Low grade dysplasia	2
	8

"moderate" or "medium grade dysplasia" as an entity when the slides were sent out to two experts in the field the same report of medium or moderate grade dysplasia was returned. One can only assume that this designation falls somewhere between LGD and HGD.

Part 2

The results of questionnaires sent out to gastroenterologists in the Long Island area on the prevalence and incidence of carcinoma, HGD and LGD in their patients as can be seen from the *Table VIII*. Despite the largely increased number of cases compared to the personal series reported in Part 1, it is of interest that the results look very much the same from this much larger group. Of particular interest is the fact that at the initial endoscopy, carcinoma was found in some 4.5% of patients and HGD in about 4.9% with LGD in about 2.5%. So this is the prevalence of these findings in the 1,126 Barrett's patients. On the other hand, in those patients who were followed up either symptomatically, endoscopically or known to have developed lesions especially carcinoma, it can be seen that the incidence decreased dramatically. For carcinoma about 0.35%, HGD 0.4% and LGD just over 1%. Further, if the patients were maintained on daily or alternate day or more intermittent omeprazole therapy the incidence of carcinoma drops to .09%, the HGD to .35% and LGD to 1.24%.

Table VIII. Barrett's results of questionnaire. Long Island acid related studies (LIARS) group (22 responses, 1,126 cases).

	Carcinoma	High-grade dysplasia	Low-grade dysplasia
Initial endoscopy	4.53	4.97	2.49
Follow-up, no therapy	0.35	0.44	1.06
On omeprazole	0.09	0.35	1.24

16 of 22 responses, daily or alternate day proton pump inhibitor

Discussion

There is considerable controversy in the world literature with regard to (1) an observable change from esophagitis to Barrett's epithelium while under observation (2) to the prevalence and incidence of change of Barrett's epithelium to HGD or LGD or carcinoma and (3) whether maintenance therapy with PPIs will reduce or delay the development of dysplasia or carcinoma in patients with Barrett's if acid suppressive therapy is continued indefinetly. The results of the present study, both from a personal experience of daily or intermittent omeprazole therapy for Barrett's over 5-11 years failed to show any change to HGD or carcinoma, however, during the same period there was a prevalence of carcinoma or HGD diagnosed at the first endoscopy in the region of 5%. These initial results suggest that every patient with esophageal symptoms of any duration requires an initial endoscopy to diagnose or exclude carcinoma or HGD. On the other hand, if patients are maintained on therapy with a daily of intermittent use of PPI, endoscopic observation with biopsies could be delayed for 5 (or perhaps even 10 years) in the absence of increasing or symptoms or a change in the symptom pattern.

To substantiate this personal series, a questionnaire was sent out to members of the gastroenterological society regarding Barrett's metaplasia, there were 22 returns with 1,126 cases of Barrett's recorded and again it was evident that the prevalence of diagnosing carcinoma or HGD in Barrett's at the initial endoscopy was in the order of 5% for both carcinoma and 5% for HGD, whereas on follow-up of Barrett's the incident cases of carcinoma and HGD were considerably less and even reduced still further if the patients were maintained on omeprazole therapy. Clearly, if HGD or any dysplasia is diagnosed at the initial endoscopy, the whole pattern of therapy and/or surveillance must be drastically changed albeit the considerable diversity of opinion how to best handle these patients. What is clear however, is that the finding of HGD might already indicate submucosal carcinoma and that the patient has a 30-40% chance of developing carcinoma over the next 2-4 years. Thus, 1,126 cases of Barrett's conform to our own experience of a 5-11 year follow-up of 52 patients with Barrett's esophagus of a low incidence of death from HGD or carcinoma over the time span of these studies. However, even despite this low incidence of carcinoma or HGD one should still be vigilant with Barrett's esophagus if any change in symptoms occur or if a surveillance program is decided upon and there is a cellular change in the mucosal biopsies towards the dysplastic side.

The combined studies also suggest that maintenance omeprazole, even if given on alternate days or spread even longer to contain symptoms reveals a low incidence rate of carcinoma of HGD transformation. Clearly larger and longer studies need to be undertaken to see whether this holds true in the future.

Lastly, the fairly high prevalence of finding carcinoma and HGD in both the present series on the first endoscopy, begs the question whether we have not reached the point of screening for carcinoma, HGD, LGD or Barrett's epithelium in the population at large, for example, at the time that the patient has his first screening colonoscopy at the age of 50 which has recently been broadly publicized. It is estimated that there are some 130,000 new cases of cancer of the colon in the United States every year and only 10,000 cases of carcinoma of the esophagus. The question then arises whether it is cost effective to survey for carcinoma of the esophagus at least once during a patients lifetime after the age of 50. As upper endoscopy at this age is extremely safe when compared to colonoscopy and it would also be worth a study comparing the cost of screening upper endoscopy with that of colonoscopy and of the treatment of HGD or carcinoma when it occurs.

These results suggest that maintenance omeprazole albeit even given intermittently on alternate days or even longer may substantially reduce the conversion of Barrett's to high-grade dysplasia or carcinoma. Clearly larger scale studies are warranted. The difference between the prevalence and incidence cases begs the question of screening endoscopy after age 50.

References

1. Provenzale D, Schmit C, Wong JB. Barrett's esophagus: a new look at surveillance based on emerging estimates of cancer risk. Am J Gastroenterol 1999;94:2043-2053.
2. Drewitz DJ, Sampliner RE, Garewal HS. The incidence of adenocarcinoma in Barrett's esophagus: a prospective study of 170 patients followed 4.8 years. Am J Gastroenterol 1997;92:212-215.
3. Katz D, Rothstein R, Schned A, Dunn J, Seaver K, Antonioli D. The development of dysplasia and adenocarcinoma during endoscopic surveillance of Barrett's esophagus. Am J Gastroenterol 1998;93:536-541.
4. Streitz JMJ, Ellis FH, Tilden RL, Erickson RV. Endoscopic surveillance of Barrett's esophagus: a cost-effectiveness comparison with mammographic surveillance for breast cancer. Am J Gastrol 1998;93:911-915.

5. Shaheen NJ, Crosby MA, Bozymski EM, Sandler RS. Is there publication bias in the reporting of cancer risk in Barrett's esophagus? Gastroenterology 2000;119:333-338.
6. Weston AP, Sharma P, Topalovski M, et al. Long-term follow-up of Barrett's high-grade dysplasia. Am J Gastroenterol 2000;95:1888-1893.

What is the value of beta-carotene therapy in the treatment of Barrett's esophagus?

L.F. Johnson (Birmingham)

Beta-carotene is one of several antioxidant vitamins, found in dark-green leafy vegetables, and carrots, as well as yellow or red fruits and vegetables. As a precursor of vitamins A, which plays a role in the control of epithelial growth and differentiation, β-carotene has the potential to possibly neutralize the harmful effects of DNA-damaging free radicals. In fact, animal studies show that β-carotene protects rats and mice against experimental tumors that develop in squamous epithelia at sites such as skin and the buccal mucosa [1]. These data suggest that β-carotene might prevent esophageal cancer in humans by affecting precursor lesions such as Barrett's esophagus.

Epidemiologic data in humans show that patients with either squamous cell, or adenocarcinoma of the esophagus have low levels of β-carotene compared to age matched controls. In fact, the family members of these cancer patients also show the same low levels suggesting that a protracted diet deficient in β-carotene might have influenced some family members to have developed esophageal cancer [2]. Other epidemiologic data show that patients given β-carotene might be conferred protection from neoplasms at certain sites. For instance patients under high oxidation stress due to cigarette smoking appear to be somewhat protected by β-carotene at sites known to be affected by cigarette smoking [3].

If β-carotene confers protection against esophageal neoplasms one might expect to see alterations in cellular immunity in humans. In fact, humans given β-carotene for just three months, show an increase in the percentage of peripheral blood lymphocytes expressing natural killer cell markers as well as modest increases in percentage expressing transferrin and interleukin receptors [4]. Thus, β-carotene has been shown to alter cellular immunity in humans.

Even though epidemiologic and other data suggest that β-carotene, low in patient with esophageal cancer, alters cellular immunity, and might confer protection against the development of esophageal cancer, there is no data to support its effects on precursor lesions such as Barrett's esophagus. Fortunately, there is a study underway to address the impact of β-carotene in Barrett's esophagus [4].

References

1. Lieshout EM, Peters WH, Jansen JB. Effect of oltipraz, α-tocopherol, β-carotene and phenethylisothiocyanate on rat oesophageal, gastric, colonic, and hepatic glutatione, glutatione S-transferase and peroxidase. Carcinogenesis 1996;17:1439-1445.
2. Smith AH, Waller KD. Serum beta-carotene in persons with cancer and their immediate families. Am J Epidemiol 1991;133:661-671.
3. Terry P, Lagergren J, Weimin Y, Nyrén O, Wolk A. Antioxidants and cancers of the esophagus and gastric cardia. Int J Cancer 2000;87:750-754.
4. Prabhala RH, Garewal HS, Hicks MJ, Sampliner RE, Watson RR. The effects of 13-cis-retinoic acid and beta-carotene on cellular immunity in humans. Cancer 1991;67:1556-1560.

Can promotility agents maintain remission in Barrett's esophagus?

J.E. Richter (Cleveland)

Barrett's esophagus is characterized by very low lower esophageal sphincter pressure, decreased esophageal amplitude, dysmotility, and resulting increased gastroesophageal reflux. Therefore, the use of a promotility drug to correct these abnormalities is appealing. However, there is no evidence that promotility drugs can do this in Barrett's esophagus. In fact, this would be unlikely since the motility changes are usually the result of irreversible muscle damage.

The treatment of Barrett's esophagus today is best done with proton pump inhibitors (PPIs). These drugs predictably control reflux symptoms, heal esophagitis and esophageal ulcers, and prevent the relapse of symptoms and esophagitis. No data is available on the role of PPIs with prokinetic drugs in Barrett's esophagus. The only study suggesting a possible additive effect is the Italian investigation of Vigneri *et al.* [1] in 175 patients with reflux esophagitis, remission followed one of five drug regimen over one-year. Omeprazole maintained patients with esophagitis in remission 80% over the one-year period, while the addition of cisapride 10 mg QID increased remission rate slightly to 89%.

This question is irrelevant today, because cisapride, the most powerful prokinetic agent, has been removed from the market in the United States and Canada because of severe cardiac side-effects and deaths related to arrhythmias. Furthermore, the additional 9% relief gained by the addition of cisapride is not cost effective.

Reference

1. Vigneri S, Termini R, Leandro G, et al. A comparison of five maintenance therapies for reflux esophagitis. N Engl J Med 1995;33:1106-1110.

Can dysplastic mucosa develop under treatment?

E.C. Klinkenberg-Knol (Amsterdam)

Barrett's esophagus is a premalignant condition which develops as a sequelum of gastroesophageal reflux. In Barrett's esophagus the squamous epithelium is replaced by metaplastic columnar epithelium, to be divided histologically in gastric-cardia type, gastric-junctional type, and specialized intestinal type [1]. This stretch of metaplasia may extend from the cardia upwards over only a few centimeters as well as over the majority of the epithelial lining. In the metaplastic epithelium dysplasia can develop. Several grades can be distinguished, starting with no dysplasia, via indefinite for dysplasia, low-grade and high-grade dysplasia (HGD), to ultimately adenocarcinoma. The most reliable marker for (imminent or concurrent) malignancy is HGD. Adenocarcinoma develops in high-grade dysplastic specialized intestinal type metaplasia [2].

Proton pump inhibitors therapy in Barrett's esophagus [3]

There is increasing interest in the treatment strategies that reduce reflux, especially of acid, into the esophagus in an attempt to reduce the neoplastic potential of Barrett's esophagus. Proton pump inhibitors (PPIs) may result in minimal, partial or, even, in complete regression of Barrett's esophagus, but whether they reduce the neoplastic potential of the disease is still unknown.

Before considering the use of strong acid suppressive therapy for Barrett's esophagus it is important to understand the pathophysiology of acid suppression in this condition [4]. Intuitively, one would think that reduction in acid concentrations in the esophagus, by whatever means, shall reduce the inflammation, epithelial proliferation, mutagenic potential, and neoplastic risk in Barrett's esophagus. However, it has been argued that duodeno-gastroesophageal reflux (DGER), notably of bile acids and pancreatic trypsin, may be as important as acid and pepsin in the development of neoplastic change in Barrett's esophagus [5]. Probably acid and bile acids are synergistic in toxicity to the esophageal mucosa and their induction of Barrett's esophagus. Conjugated bile acids provoke esophageal damage at low pH levels, whereby unconjugated bile acids may be more toxic at neutral pH, the environment produced by powerful acid suppressing agents like the PPIs. So, under treatment with PPIs, the toxic effect of the unconjugated bile acids may perpetuate and these unconjugated bile acids may be a factor in the progression of the neoplastic sequence of Barrett's esophagus. Therefore, one could argue that antireflux surgery is the only really efficient therapy for Barrett's esophagus. However, acid suppression therapy with omeprazole 20 mg orally twice daily may diminish bile acid reflux by decreasing gastric volume to a similar degree as antireflux surgery.

At this moment the general believe is that acid reduction in the esophagus may lead to stabilisation of the Barrett's mucosa, not withstanding the possible effects of continued DGER. However, any pathological or molecular evidence of such an effect is lacking.

Changes of squamous re-epithelialization over and adjacent to Barrett's epithelium have been demonstrated after long-term treatment with PPIs [6]. The question whether this re-epithelialization is beneficial has not been answered. This squamous mucosa may conceal underlying Barrett's mucosa. This buried mucosa is possibly a neoplastic risk It may even result in the hiding of malignancy, with a crucial delay of diagnosis [7].

So, in conclusion, treatment with PPIs may result in partial or even complete regression of Barrett's esophagus. However, the question if PPIs reduce the neoplastic potential of the disease is far more important and is still unanswered.

References

1. Paul A, Trier JS, Dalton MD, Camp RC, Loeb P, Goyal RK. N Engl J Med 1976;295:476-480.
2. Miros M, Kerlin P, Walker N. Only patients with dysplasia progress to adenocarcinoma in Barrett's oesophagus. Gut 1991;32:1441-1446.
3. Triadafilopoulos G. Proton pump inhibitors for Barrett's oesophagus. Gut 2000;46:144-146.
4. Shepherd NA. Barrett's oesophagus and proton pump inhibitors: a pathological perspective. Gut 2000;46:147-149.
5. Vaezi MF, Richter JE. Bile reflux in columnar lined esophagus. Gastroenterol Clin North Am 1997;26:565-582.
6. Wilkinson SP, Biddlestone L, Gore S, Shepherd NA. Regression of columnar-lined (Barrett's) oesophagus with omeprazole 40 mg daily: results of 5 years of continuous therapy. Aliment Pharmacol Ther 1999;13:1205-1209.
7. Biddlestone LR, Barham CP, Wilkinson SP, et al. The histopathology of treated Barrett's oesophagus: squamous re-epithelialisation following acid suppression, laser and photodynamic therapy. Am J Surg Pathol 1998;22:239-245.

How should maintenance treatment be conducted?

B.T. Cooper (Birmingham)

Initial therapy for Barrett's esophagus

Initial treatment must be briefly considered. The metaplastic epithelium in Barrett's esophagus results from prolonged gastroesophageal reflux (GER) [1, 2] and probably does not cause symptoms [1]. Patients present with the symptoms of GER with or without associated reflux esophagitis or with the symptoms of complications of Barrett's esophagus *e.g.* benign ulcer, stricture, adenocarcinoma or bleeding [3]. Barrett's esophagus may be found in patients without esophageal symptoms during upper gastrointestinal endoscopy for other indications [3]. Barrett's esophagus patients with GER symptoms with or without reflux esophagitis are treated the same as other patients with GER with or without esophagitis [4-6]. Thus the treatment of choice is a proton pump inhibitor (PPI) for 8 weeks [7]. Because Barrett's esophagus patients may have elevated gastric acid secretion [8], they often require high doses of PPI *e.g.* omeprazole 40 mg daily or more. The aim is to completely relieve symptoms and heal any associated reflux esophagitis or benign ulceration in the Barrett's mucosa. As in reflux patients without Barrett's esophagus, this will be achieved in greater than 90% [7]. If the patient is well, re-endoscopy at the end of 8 weeks is not necessary except in patients with esophageal ulceration when healing should be checked. Patients with a Barrett's associated benign esophageal stricture may require dilatation at initial endoscopy or at the end of initial course of PPI therapy if dysphagia remains a problem. Like any patient who has resistant GER, Barrett's esophagus patients whose symptoms fail to respond over 8 weeks should be treated with more prolonged therapy, high dose PPIs, additional or alternative drugs or antireflux surgery as appropriate. In my unit antireflux surgery for continued reflux symptoms despite medical therapy has only been necessary in 0.3% of Barrett's esophagus patients.

Maintenance therapy for Barrett's esophagus

Aims

The aims of maintenance treatment in Barrett's esophagus are to control symptoms and if possible to induce the Barrett's epithelium to regress, to prevent dysplasia and to prevent complications. Further aims are to treat complications aggressively as they occur and to minimise the risks of drug therapy and monitor patients for their occurrence.

Maintenance treatment

Symptom control

Compared to GER patients without Barrett's esophagus, Barrett's esophagus patients tend to have severe impairment of lower esophageal sphincter (LES) tone [9] and therefore more acid reflux. Moreover, Barrett's esophagus patients are unlikely to get significant improvement in LES tone after acid suppressive treatment so symptomatic relapse is usual on cessation of effective antireflux medication. Therefore most patients are faced with the need to consider maintenance antireflux treatment to maintain symptom control. The drug which achieved control of GER symptoms can be offered as maintenance treatment. This means PPI therapy in most cases. Often the dose required to maintain symptom relief is less than that required to induce symptom relief, so that the patient initially treated with omeprazole 40 mg daily can be maintained on omeprazole 20 mg daily. However in my experience, it is unusual for Barrett's esophagus patients to remain well on omeprazole 10 mg daily. Unfortunately, complete symptom control does not necessarily mean that total control of acid reflux has been achieved [10, 11] and this may have other consequences (see below). Moreover, complete abolition of acid reflux can be difficult to achieve even with high doses of PPI [12]. Patients with Barrett's esophagus will probably require lifelong acid suppression to control GER symptoms, the only alternative being antireflux surgery. The latter may have cost advantages over maintenance PPI therapy in ordinary GER patients [13] and this may also be true for GER patients with Barrett's esophagus. However more data is needed. Few patients with Barrett's esophagus who are well on PPI therapy are willing to consider surgery as an alternative.

H_2 receptor antagonists often control GER symptoms in Barrett's esophagus patients [14] although high doses (*e.g.* ranitidine 600 mg daily or more) may be needed. These drugs can be effective treatment for patients intolerant of PPIs. Unfortunately, despite absence of GER symptoms, 14.6% of GER patients without Barrett's esophagus on maintenance treatment with ranitidine 150 mg bd have erosive esophagitis at endoscopy compared to only 4.5% of symptom free patients on maintenance treatment with omeprazole 20 mg daily [15]. A similar situation is likely in Barrett's esophagus patients so the Barrett's mucosa may still be exposed to significant acid with possible implications for complications such as dysplasia despite the absence of symptoms [10, 11].

Regression

This is an important aim of treatment of Barrett's esophagus patients and will be considered elsewhere in this volume (see p) in more detail. H_2 receptor antagonist therapy does not lead to regression [14] and the balance of evidence suggests that antireflux surgery does not either [16]. Lower dose PPI therapy (*e.g.* omeprazole 20 mg daily) does not reduce the length of the Barrett's esophagus segment over 6 years [16] whereas higher dose PPI therapy (*e.g.* omprazole 40 mg daily) causes a reduction in the length of the Barrett's esophagus segment in the first 2 years of therapy [17]. There is no further regression with time and complete abolition of Barrett's esophagus mucosa does not occur [17]. Even with lower dose PPI therapy, there is partial epithelialisation with islands of squamous epithelium in the Barrett's segment in 50% of cases [16]. Very high dose PPI therapy leading to more complete acid suppression might be expected to cause even further regression with greater squamous island formation but data is scarce so far and not encouraging [18]. However if this was shown to occur, it would be necessary to titrate PPI dose against 24 hour ambulatory esophageal pH results rather than against symptoms.

Ablation of the Barrett's mucosa by laser or photodynamic therapy followed by PPI therapy is an alternative approach [19, 20]. However this is not necessarily practical for all patients and may not ablate all metaplastic tissue [19]. It should be considered in patients with low-grade dysplasia.

Dysplasia

There is anecdotal evidence that Barrett's esophagus patients on maintenance PPI therapy are less likely to develop dysplasia [16]. However good controlled data is required.

Prevention of other complications

There is evidence from GERD patients without Barrett's esophagus that maintenance PPI therapy prevents relapse of esophageal ulcer and reduces restricturing in benign esophageal stricture after dilatation [21, 22]. Therefore it seems reasonable to conclude that maintenance PPI will prevent benign stricture and ulcer developing in Barrett's esophagus patients.

Many patients with Barrett's esophagus have *Helicobacter pylori* in their stomachs [23]. The bacteria does not influence esophageal acid reflux or GER symptoms [24]. The development of atrophic gastritis as a result of *H. pylori* may be accelerated in the presence of PPI induced acid suppression [25] although a recent study has not found this [26]. Therefore *H. pylori* eradication may be advisable if maintenance PPI therapy is to be given. There is no definite evidence that *H. pylori* is involved in the development of Barrett's esophagus or dysplasia but this is controversial. At present, if a patient with Barrett's esophagus is not taking a PPI long-term, the presence of *H. pylori* is not an indication for eradication.

Who should have maintenance therapy?

All patients should be offered treatment and the benefits should be balanced against the risks of drug side effects and the unknown effects of very long-term PPI therapy. However long-term omeprazole treatment (up to 11 years) is safe and efficient in GERD [27].

Patients need to know that possible benefits with regard to regression and lower risk of dysplasia with PPI therapy are unproven. A few patients have minor or occasional reflux symptoms which are easily controlled with regular or intermittent antacid or H_2 receptor antagonist therapy. They may not wish to have maintenance PPI therapy. Their choice must be respected.

Follow-up and monitoring

Ideally, patients should be seen in a specialist clinic yearly for assessment of symptom control and to monitor drug therapy. They should be seen at other times if there are problems with symptom control, new symptoms or problems with therapy. Patients should be offered surveillance endoscopy looking for cancer/dysplasia every 1-2 years provided they are potential candidates for active intervention should cancer/dysplasia be found. Endoscopy is needed more frequently if dysplasia has been found and at other times when new symptoms develop or if old symptoms relapse. However surveillance endoscopy in Barrett's esophagus patients is controversial because it may not be cost effective. This is considered elsewhere in this book (*see p. 654*).

There are a few gastroenterologists who are not convinced that Barrett's esophagus patients need either specialist follow up or surveillance endoscopy and they would see patients only if problems develop.

References

1. Sjogren RW, Johnson LF. Barrett's esophagus. Ann Intern Med 1982;97:103-107.
2. Tytgat GNJ, Hameetman W, Onstenk RR, Scotberg R. The spectrum of columnar lined Barrett's oesophagus. Endoscopy 1989;21:177-185.
3. Cooper BT, Barbezat GO. Barrett's oesophagus: a clinical study of 52 cases. Q J Med 1987;62:97-108.
4. Havelund T, Laursen LS, Anderson BN, et al. Omeprazole and ranitidine treatment of reflux oesophagitis. Br Med J 1988;296:89-92.
5. Bardhan KD, Morris P, Thompson M, et al. Omeprazole in the treatment of erosive oesophagitis refractory to high dose ranitidine and cimetidine. Gut 1990;31:745-749.
6. Lundell L, Backman L, Elstrom P, et al. Omeprazole or high dose ranitidine in the treatment of patients with reflux oesophagitis not responding to standard doses of H2 receptor antagonists. Aliment Pharmacol Ther 1990;4:144-155.
7. Sontag SJ, Schnell TG, Chejfec G, et al. Lansoprazole heals erosive reflux oesophagitis in patients with Barrett's oesophagus. Aliment Pharmacol Ther 1997;11:147-156.
8. Mulholland MW, Reid BJ, Levine DA, Rubin CE. Elevated gastric acid secretion in patients with Barrett's esophagus. Dig Dis Sci 1989;34:1329-1335.
9. Stein HJ, Hoeft S, DeMeester TR. Functional foregut abnormalities in Barrett's esophagus. J Thorac Cardiovasc Surg 1993;105:107-111.
10. Katzka DA, Castell DO. Successful elimination of reflux symptoms does not ensure adequate control of acid reflux in patients with Barrett's esophagus. Am J Gastroenterol 1994;89:989-991.
11. Ouatu-Lascar R, Triadafilopoulos G. Complete elimination of reflux symptoms does not guarantee normalisation of intra-oesophageal acid reflux in patients with Barrett's esophagus. Am J Gastroenterol 1998;93:711-716.
12. Fass R, Sampliner RE, Malagon IB, et al. Failure of oesophageal acid control in candidates for Barrett's oesophagus reversal on a very high dose of proton pump inhibitor. Aliment Pharmacol Ther 2000;14:597-602.
13. Lundell L, Dalenback J, Hattlebakk J, et al. Omeprazole or antireflux surgery in the long term management gastro-esophageal reflux disease: results of a multicentre trial. Gastroenterology 1998;114:A207.
14. Cooper BT, Barbezat GO. Treatment of Barrett's oesophagus with H2 blockers. J Clin Gastroenterol 1987;9:139-141.
15. Carlsson R, Galmiche JP, Dent J, et al. Prognostic factors influencing relapse of oesophagitis during maintenance therapy with antisecretory drugs: a meta analysis of long term omeprazole trials. Aliment Pharmacol Ther 1997;11:473-482.
16. Cooper BT, Neumann CS, Cox M, Iqbal TH. Continuous treatment with omeprazole 20 mg daily for up to 6 years in Barrett's oesophagus. Aliment Pharmacol Ther 1998;12:893-897.
17. Wilkinson SP, et al. Regression of columnar lined (Barrett's) oesophagus with omeprazole 40 mg daily :results of 5 years continuous therapy. Aliment Pharmacol Ther 1999;13:1205-1209.

18. Sharma P, Sampliner RE, Camargo E. Normalisation of esophageal pH with very high dose PPI therapy does not result in regression of Barrett's esophagus. Amer J Gastroenterol 1997;92:582-585.
19. Berensen MM, Johnson TD, Markowitz NR, Buchi KN, Samowitz WS. Restoration of squamous mucosa after ablation of Barrett's epithelium. Gastroenterology 1993;104:1686-1691.
20. Overholt BF, Panjehpour M. Photodynamic therapy in Barrett's esophagus. Sem Surg Oncol 1995;11:372-376.
21. Marks RD, Richter JE, Rizzo J, et al. Omeprazole versus H2 receptor antagonists in treating patients with peptic stricture and esophagitis. Gastroenterology 1994;106:907-915.
22. Smith PM, Kerr GD, Cockel R, et al. A comparison of omeprazole and ranitidine in the prevention of recurrence of benign oesophageal stricture. Gastroenterology 1994;107:1312-1318.
23. Cooper BT. Helicobacter pylori in Barrett's oesophagus. In: Guili R, Galmiche JP, Jamieson GG, Scarpignato C, eds. The esophago-gastric junction. Paris: John Libby Eurotext, 1998:963-966.
24. Peters FTM, Kuipers EJ, Ganesh S, et al. The influence of Helicobacter pylori on oesophageal acid exposure in GERD during acid suppressive therapy. Aliment Pharmacol Therap 1999;13:921-926.
25. Kuipers EJ, Lundell L, Klinkenberg-Knol EC, et al. Atrophic gastritis and Helicobacter pylori infection in patients with reflux esophagitis treated with omeprazole or fundoplication. N Engl J Med 1996;334:1018-1022.
26. Lundell L, Miettinen P, Myrvold HE, et al. Lack of effect of acid suppression therapy on gastric atrophy. Gastroenterology 1999;117:319-326.
27. Klinkenberg-Knol EC, Nelis F, Dent J, et al. Long term omeprazole treatment in resistant gastro-esophageal reflux disease: efficacy, safety and influence on gastric mucosa. Gastroenterology 2000;118:661-669.

Following all these questions, shouldn't the interest of prokinetics be strongly emphasized in the medical treatment of Barrett's esophagus?

D.O. Castell (Philadelphia)

The short answer to this question is a simple no. There are no studies in the literature documenting the effectiveness of any prokinetic agent in the treatment of patients with the severe form of esophageal injury and dysmotility that is typical of patients with Barrett's esophagus.

The potential goals of using a prokinetic agent in the patient with gastroesophageal reflux disease are two fold. The first is to attempt to decrease the amount of actual reflux. Although this can be achieved to some degree with prokinetic agents, the mechanism of the effect is not very clear. The effectiveness of prokinetic drugs to increase lower esophageal sphincter (LES) pressure is questionable. More importantly, there is no information that these agents will decrease the phenomenon of transient LES relaxations. In the patient with Barrett's esophagus who has poor contractile elements in the distal esophagus and LES, a prokinetic response is even less likely because of the poor basal muscle tone.

The second goal of a prokinetic agent would be to improve esophageal clearance. Here the likelihood of a positive response is even less. There is no convincing evidence that the prokinetic agents are effective in improving esophageal clearance in normal volunteers and even less convincing data that these drugs will work in the patient with defective contractile activity such as ineffective esophageal motility or the hypotensive LES.

All of the above supports the initial short answer to this question that a serious interest in prokinetic therapy in the patient with Barrett's esophagus should not be considered.

Surgical treatments

How long should medical treatment be continued before antireflux surgery?

H. Koop (Berlin)

Since the introduction of proton pump inhibitors (PPIs), medical therapy of gastroesophageal reflux disease (GERD) has become effective in almost all cases [1]. Even in severe, complicated reflux disease (*e.g.* associated with strictures or deep ulcers) profound acid inhibition achieved by PPIs is able to lead to complete healing. Individual dose adjustment is an essential factor for the success of treatment. If compliance can be assumed, failure of acid suppression therapy in GERD patients should make physicians cautious: results after antireflux surgery are often poor (or at least unpredictable) in such "refractory" cases. A detailed work-up to identify the individual pathophysiological alteration(s) is indispensable in these patients and a prerequisite for adequate therapeutic decisions. Most convincing results of antireflux surgery are observed in responders or at least partial responders to appropriate PPI treatment; not surprisingly, unreliable treatment concepts (*e.g.* employing H_2-receptor antagonists, prokinetic agents or even only life style alterations) do not satisfy the patients and are often a reason to ask for surgery.

If then medical therapy with few exceptions is able to control reflux disease also in the long run, the question arises in whom antireflux surgery should be performed. From the gastroenterologist's point of view, there are specific indications for surgery: preferentially, patients with massive volume reflux particularly during the night, with subsequent aspiration despite effective acid inhibition, should undergo surgery without delay before irreversible pulmonary diseases develop. Esophagitis due to biliary reflux (after partial gastric resection or total gastrectomy) cannot be effectively treated in the majority of patients and require surgery (high biliary reflux in otherwise unoperated patients as an indication for antireflux surgery is, however, viewed controversial). A further – though relative – indication for surgery is unwillingness of patients to take acid inhibitory drugs for years; however, patients should be extensively informed about possible complications of surgical procedures which frequently occur in non-specialized units [2] which often cannot be managed conservatively. As mentioned above, resistance to PPIs should make surgeons cautious to operate on since in this group of patients a significant number suffers from an "irritable esophagus syndrome" or other functional entities instead of true reflux disease.

Studies are available on medical treatment of GERD patients for 5 to 10 years [3, 4] which show that symptomatic control as well as maintaining healing can thus be achieved over long periods of time. The results from these studies indicate that PPIs even taken for a decade or longer are safe and increasing numbers of adverse events have not to be expected; thus, discontinuation due to side effects is a rare event. Serum gastrin elevations are moderate [4] and comparable to those in patients after vagotomy [5]. Furthermore, slight hypergastrinaemia is lacking clinical significance from the present point of view. One goal PPIs cannot achieve is total regression of Barrett's esophagus (though scattered squamous epithelial islands occur over time), but antireflux surgery cannot either.

There is some concern about long-term acid inhibition in patients with *Helicobacter pylori*-induced gastritis: some authors postulate that atrophy in the fundic region of the stomach progressively increases and that this process may eventually bear the potential risk of gastric malignancy [6]. Comparative trials in which patients were randomly assigned to either antireflux surgery or omeprazole treatment suggest that development of atrophy may slightly if at all be enhanced up to 5 years of PPI therapy [7], but there is no indication so far that dysplasia or gastric malignancy in the stomach are more frequent after long-term PPI therapy.

Should patients with GERD treated with PPIs advised to be treated for a minimum or maximum of time before they are transferred to surgery? The natural course of reflux disease varies in the single patient: some have daily symptoms whereas in others GERD takes an intermittent course. Therefore, the duration of therapy in the individual patient prior to surgery depends on the individual symptom profile. Medical treatment should last at least as long as its effect can be certainly evaluated (assessment seems possible during a 6-month period with occasional attempts to stop therapy where appropriate). Rapid recurrence of symptoms after temporary discontinuation of PPIs is a strong indicator for the need of effective and continuous prolonged antireflux therapy – either medical or surgical. As far as the maximum length is concerned, no upper limit can be defined. In particular, elderly patients are more cost-efficiently treated by PPIs; thus, surgery should generally be questioned in those patients. If a decision for surgery in younger patients is primarily based on economic considerations, delaying surgery does not make sense but should be performed as soon as the indication is clear. Economical consideration should, however, take into account that prices for drug treatment is likely to decrease over time thus making medical therapy probably more cost-effective in the future even in younger populations of reflux patients.

In conclusion, it seems difficult to define periods of conservative treatment prior to antireflux surgery. Within a period of 6 months it appears possible to evaluate the effects of PPI treatment and adjust the dose required in the given patient. In non-responders to medical therapy, a careful search for the nature of individual disease mechanisms should be performed.

References

1. Koop H. Reflux disease and Barrett's esophagus. Endoscopy 2000;32:101-107.
2. Rantanen TK, Halme TV, Luostarinen ME, et al. The long-term results of open antireflux surgery in a community-based health care center. Am J Gastroenterol 1999;94:1777-1781.
3. Koop H, Arnold R. Long-term maintenance treatment of reflux esophagitis with omeprazole. Prospective study in patients with H_2-blocker resistant reflux esophagitis. Dig Dis Sci 1991;36:552-557.
4. Klinkenberg-Knol EC, Nelis F, Dent J, et al. Long-term omeprazole treatment in resistant gastroesophageal reflux disease: efficacy, safety, and influence on gastric mucosa. Gastroenterology 2000;118:661-669.
5. Koop H, Frank M, Kuly S, et al. Gastric argyrophil (enterochromaffin-like), gastrin and somatostatin cells after selective proximal vagotomy in man. Dig Dis Sci 1993;38:295-302.
6. Kuipers EJ, Lundell L, Klinkenberg-Knol EC, et al. Atrophic gastritis and Helicobacter pylori infection in patients with reflux esophagitis treated with omeprazole or fundoplication. N Engl J Med 1996;334:1018-1022.
7. Lundell L, Havu N, Miettinen P, et al. No effect of acid suppression therapy over 5 years on gastric glandular atrophy. Results of a randomised study. Gastroenterology 2000;118:A213.

Can specific indications for mid (Toupet) fundoplication be defined?

M.K. Schilling, M.W. Büchler (Berne)

Advances in our knowledge of the pathology of gastroesophageal reflux disease (GERD) and the refinements of operative techniques have shifted the treatment of GERD from proton pump inhibitors (PPIs) or H_2-blockers to the surgical restoration of the lower esophageal sphincter (LES). While PPIs have been very effective in treating reflux symptoms and esophageal inflammation, they are unable to prevent oropharyngeal and pulmonary complications like laryngitis, hoarseness or asthma associated with GERD. Furthermore, epidemiological and experimental data suggest that in patients under gastric acid blockade, reflux of alkaline contents contributes to the development and/or propagation of Barrett dysplasia to gastroesophageal adenocarcinoma. The only effective means to prevent reflux of alkaline or acidic gastric contents, is therefore the restoration of the distal esophageal sphincter mechanism by a competent fundoplication. The question to know if fundoplication is best performed as a semicircular (Toupet) or circular wrap (Nissen-Rosetti) has been studied in several retro- and prospective trials (*Table I*), but the question of the specific indications for a semicircular fundoplication has not been studied in a scientifically conclusive *i.e.* inductive way. The best answer therefore has to be deducted from the outcome of prospective trials comparing Toupet *versus* Nissen-Rosetti fundoplication, but will remain preliminary, until prospective randomized trials with appropriate samples give sufficient evidence to stratify specific GERD subpopulations to either one or the other procedure.

The compilation of data depicted in *Table I and II* compares the two surgical procedures and the outcomes including complications after various follow-up periods.

Table I. Trials comparing Toupet (T) *versus* Nissen (N) fundoplication.

		Approach	Follow-up (years)	N/T n	Relapse	Heart burn	Acid regurgi-tation	Dysphagia	Flatulence	Gas bloat	LES length cm	LES tone mmHg	Authors preference
Thor	1989	Open	5	12/19			2/3	4/2		2/0			T, gas bloat, slip
Segol	1989	Open	2	18/16		0/1	1/0	1/0			3.3/2.9	9/12	N
McKernan	1994	Lap	0.3-1.1	14/14				2/0					T, dysphagia
Ottignon	1994	Open	2.8	43/28		2/3	2/2	15/3					T, motility
Lundell	1996	Open	> 3	65/72	3/4		8/9	7/10				18/13	T, herniation, flatulence
Lund	1997	Lap	0.5	16/46				7/4					T, dysphagia
Wetscher	1997	Lap	1.3	17/32				1/1			2.6/2.2	21/15	T improves esophageal contractility
Rydberg	1997	Open	3	15/18		0/0	0/0	0/0				20/14	T
Karim	1997	Lap	1.3	48/35		15/15	5/7						T
Laws	1997	Lap	2.3	23/17									=
Coster	1997	Lap	2.5/1	125/101				8/0				15/15	T, dysphagia
Rydberg1	1998		4.5	13/11					9/6		4/3	17/9	
Rydberg	1999	Open	3	53/53		3/7	3/7	5/3	33/16				-
Weber	1999	Open	1-8	102/154	8/9			20/11					T, dysphagia, bloating
TOTAL				548/570	11/13	20/26	21/28	56/34	42/22	2/0		16.3/13.3	
frequency					167/226	177/150	254/251	480/553	66/64	12/19			

Table II. Frequency of adverse symptoms after Toupet (T) or Nissen (N) fundoplication.

	TOTAL n	Relapse	Heartburn	Acid regurgitation	Dysphagia	Flatulence	Gas bloat
	N/T	N/T	N/T	N/T	N/T	N/T	N/T
Relative frequency (n)	548/570	11/167 13/226	20/177 26/150	21/254 28/251	56/480 34/553	42/66 22/64	2/12 0/19
Relative frequency (%)		6.6/5.8	11.3/17.3	8.3/11.2	11.7/6.1	63.6/34.8	16.7/0
p					0.01	0.03	
Odd-ratio					1.78	1.85	

Methods

A medline search for prospective trials comparing Toupet and Nissen fundoplication was performed. Surgical outcome including physiological parameters like LES pressure, residual symptoms and procedure specific symptoms were compiled and compared with Fischers exact test. The compilation was performed in order to obtain a guideline for sample sizes to detect outcome differences between the two procedures with a power of 0.9 and a α of 0.05.

Results

Between 1985 and 1999, a total of 14 trials comparing Nissen (548 patients) *versus* Toupet fundoplication (570 patients) were identified. Follow-up ranged from 3 months to 5 years. The relative frequency of a symptomatic relapse of GERD was 6,6% for Nissen and 5,8% for Toupet fundoplication. Patients having undergone Toupet fundoplication had a higher trend towards postoperative heartburn and acid regurgitation. However, postoperative dysphagia and flatulence were significantly lower in patients treated by Toupet fundoplication with an odd ratio of 1,78 for dysphagia and 1,85 for flatulence. The postoperative LES tone was 23% higher after Nissen than after Toupet fundoplication.

Discussion

A defective LES is the anatomic basis for GERD. Surgical restoration is the only means to restore that sphincter. As can be expected, a 360° wrap would increase the LES more than an incomplete (270°) one, and the compilation of studies shows that difference was 3 mmHg (*Table I*). Consequently, 1 out of 6 patients after a partial wrap but only 1 out of 9 patients after a total wrap experienced heartburn, and 1 out of 9 and 1 out of 13 patients had acid regurgitation after a partial and complete wrap respectively. The drawback of the higher LES tone achieved by a total wrap is dysphagia, which was experienced by 1 out of 9 patients after Nissen fundoplication, and by 1 out of 16 patients after a partial fundoplication. Moreover, the inability to regurgitate swallowed air after fundoplication caused flatulence in 2 out of 3 patients after Nissen and in 1 out of 3 patients after Toupet fundoplication.

In spite of scientific drawbacks in correct interpretation, one might conclude from those findings that patients with decreased esophageal propulsive force, may have difficulties to overcome the higher LES tone resulting from Nissen fundoplication and may benefit from Toupet fundoplication. Only prospective randomized trials stratifying patients for esophageal contractility could conclusively answer that question. In order to detect a 6% difference in dysphagia, acid regurgitation or heartburn with a power of 0,09 at a significance level of 0,05, a minimal number of 120 patients would be required.

References

1. Thor KB, Silander T. A long-term randomized prospective trial of the Nissen procedure versus a modified Toupet technique. Ann Surg 1989;210(6):719-724.
2. Segol P, Hay JM, Pottier D. Surgical treatment of gastroesophageal reflux: which operation to choose: Nissen, Toupet or Lortat-Jacob? A multicenter randomized trial. Gastroenterol Clin Biol 1989;13(11):873-879.
3. McKernan JB. Laparoscopic repair of gastroesophageal reflux disease. Toupet partial fundoplication versus Nissen fundoplication. Surg Endosc 1994;8(8):851-856.
4. Ottignon Y, Pelissier EP, Mantion G, Clement C, Birgen C, Deschamps JP, Carayon P, Gillet M. Gastroesophageal reflux. Comparison of clinical, pH-metric and manometric results of Nissen's and of Toupet's procedures. Gastroenterol Clin Biol 1994;18(11):920-926.
5. Lundell L, Abrahamsson H, Ruth M, Rydberg L, Lonroth H, Olbe L. Long-term results of a prospective randomized comparison of total fundic wrap (Nissen-Rossetti) or semifundoplication (Toupet) for gastro-oesophageal reflux. Br J Surg 1996;83(6):830-835.
6. Lund RJ, Wetcher GJ, Raiser F, Glaser K, Perdikis G, Gadenstatter M, Katada N, Filipi CJ, Hinder RA. Laparoscopic Toupet fundoplication for gastroesophageal reflux disease with poor esophageal body motility. J Gastrointest Surg 1997;1(4):301-308.
7. Wetscher GJ, Glaser K, Hinder RA, Perdikis G, Klingler P, Bammer T, Wieschemeyer T, Schwab G, Klingler A, Pointner R. Respiratory symptoms in patients with gastroesophageal reflux disease following medical therapy and following antireflux surgery. Am J Surg 1997;174(6):639-642.
8. Rydberg L, Ruth M, Lundell L. Does oesophageal motor function improve with time after successful antireflux surgery? Results of a prospective, randomised clinical study. Gut 1997;41(1):82-86.
9. Karim SS, Panton ON, Finley RJ, Graham AJ, Dong S, Storseth C, Clifton J. Comparison of total versus partial laparoscopic fundoplication in the management of gastroesophageal reflux disease. Am J Surg 1997;173(5):375-378.
10. Laws HL, Clements RH, Swillie CM. A randomized, prospective comparison of the Nissen fundoplication versus the Toupet fundoplication for gastroesophageal reflux disease. Ann Surg 1997;225(6):647-653.
11. Coster DD, Bower WH, Wilson VT, Brebrick RT, Richardson GL. Laparoscopic partial fundoplication vs laparoscopic Nissen-Rossetti fundoplication. Short-term results of 231 cases. Surg Endosc 1997;11(6):625-631.
12. Rydberg L, Ruth M, Abrahamsson H, Lundell L. Tailoring antireflux surgery:A randomized clinical trial. World J Surg 1999;23(6):612-618.
13. Weber TR. Toupet fundoplication for gastroesophageal reflux in childhood. Arch Surg 1999;134(7):717-720.

Compared to the Nissen valve, what is the effect of partial posterior fundoplication on gastric emptying?

T. Perniceni (Paris)

Delayed gastric emptying has been reported in 40% of patients with gastroesophageal reflux (GER) [1, 2], a finding that has been ascribed to an abnormally slow return of the proximal gastric tone to its basal value during the postprandial period [3]. Distension of the proximal stomach induces transient relaxation of the lower esophageal sphincter and may promote the occurrence of GER episodes. However, some studies found no relationship between delayed gastric emptying and GER [4-6]. In addition, it has been suggested that delayed gastric emptying in GER may be ascribable to reduced motility of the antrum [7]. Furthermore, one of the most common, although usually transient, unwanted effects of total or partial posterior fundoplication is a feeling of postprandial gastric fullness, which occurs in 25% of patients.

Scintigraphy has been used to investigate the effects of fundoplication procedures on gastric emptying. In a study of patients with GER, nausea, and a documented delay in gastric emptying, total fundoplication was followed by a significant reduction in the number of patients with nausea [8], suggesting that fundoplication enhanced gastric emptying [9]. Other scintigraphic studies evaluated solid and liquid emptying rates; most of them showed that both were increased after total or partial posterior fundoplication [10-13]. Persistent GER after fundoplication has been ascribed to persistent delay in gastric emptying [14]. It is important to note that Hill's procedure, which does not involve fundoplication, has no effect on gastric emptying. Total or partial fundoplication with vagotomy has been reported to enhance the emptying of liquids but not solids [11, 12].

The wall of the proximal stomach, which is used for fundoplication, contains baroreceptors and tension receptors sensitive to stretching. Physiologically, the postprandial period is characterized by gastric relaxation with no increase in intragastric pressure or parietal tone. This allows storage of food solids, which are secondarily redistributed to the antrum. This process is regulated by both nervous and hormonal factors [15]. Studies of the effects of total fundoplication on the stomach showed that compliance remained unchanged, but that postprandial relaxation was reduced [16, 17]. Similar findings were noted after partial posterior fundoplication [18] but not after implantation of an Angelchik prosthesis.

These disorders in proximal stomach relaxation combined with faster gastric emptying may explain the dyspeptic symptoms observed after fundoplication. There is no evidence that the type or rate of occurrence of these symptoms differ between total and partial posterior fundoplication. Intraoperative injury to the vagus nerves may contribute to the occurrence of dyspeptic symptoms.

References

1. Mc Callum RW, Berkowitz DM, Lerner E. Gastric emptying in patients with gastroesophageal reflux. Gastroenterology 1981;80:285-291.

2. Maddern GJ, Chatterton BE, Collins PJ, Horowitz M, Shearman DJC, Jamieson GG. Solid and liquid gastric emptying in patients with gastro-oesophageal reflux. Br J Surg 1985;72:344-347.
3. Penagini R, Hebbard G, Horowitz M, Dent J, Bermingham H, Jones K, Holloway RH. Motor function of the proximal stomach and visceral perception in gastro-oesophageal reflux disease. Gut 1998;42:251-257.
4. Shay SS, Eggli D, MC Donald C, Johnson LF. Gastric emptying of solid food in patients patients with gastroesophageal reflux. Gastroenterology 1987;92:459-465.
5. Keshavarzian A, Bushnell DL, Sontag S, Yegelwel EJ, Smid K. Gastric emptying in patients with severe reflux esophagitis. Am J Gastroenterol 1991;86:738-742.
6. Schwizer W, Hinder R, DeMeester TR. Does delayed gastric emptying contribute to gastroesophageal reflux disease? Am J Surg 1989;157:74-81.
7. Micali B, Albanese V, Baldari S, Cogliandolo A, Gulino FM, Scarpignato C. Vidange gastrique au cours du reflux gastro-œsophagien. Gastroenterol Clin Biol 1986;10:656-661.
8. Hui T, Fass S, Giurgiu D, Iida A, Tagaki S, Phillips E. Gastroesophageal disease and nausea. Does fundoplication help or hurt? Arch Surg 2000;135:545-549.
9. Viljakka M, Saali K, Koskinen M, Karhumäki L, Kössi J, Luostarinen M, et al. Antireflux surgery enhances gastric emptying. Arch Surg 1999;134:18-21.
10. Hinder RA, Stein HJ, Bremmer CG, DeMeester TR. Relationship of a satisfactory outcome to normalization of delayed gastric emptying after Nissen fundoplication. Ann Surg 1989;210:458-465.
11. Jamieson GG, Maddern GJ, Myers J. Gastric emptying after fundoplication with and without proximal gastic vagotomy. Arch Surg 1991;126:1414-1417.
12. Lundell L, Myers J, Jamieson GG. Delayed gastric emptying and its relationship to symptom of "gas bloat" after antireflux surgery. Eur J Surg 1994;160:161-166.
13. Maddern GJ, Jamieson GG. Fundoplication enhances gastric emptying. Ann Surg 1985;201:296-299.
14. Maddern GJ, Jamieson GG, Chatterton BE, Collins PJ. Is there an association between failed antireflux procedures and delayed gastric emptying? Ann Surg 1985;202:162-1655.
15. Notivol R, Coffin B, Azpiroz F, Mearin F, Serra J, Malagelada J. Gastric tone determines the sensitivity of the stomach to distension. Gastroenterology 1995;108:330-336.
16. Wijnhoven B, Salet G, Roelofs J, Smout APJM, Akkermans L, Gooszen N. Function of the proximal stomach after Nissen fundoplication. Br J Surg 1998;85:267-271.
17. Vu M, Straathof W, Schaar P, Arndt J, Ringers J, Lamers C, et al. Motor and sensory function of the proximal stomach in reflux disease and after laparoscopic Nissen fundoplication. Am J Gastroenterol 199;94:1481-1489.
18. Vu M, Ringers J, Arndt J, Lamers C, Masclee A. Prospective study of the effect of laparoscopic hemifundoplication on motor and sensory function of the proximal stomach. Br J Surg 2000;87:338-343.

What are the indications for an intra-thoracic Nissen fundoplication? What are the drawbacks of this technique?

C. Gutschow, R. Romagnoli, J.-M. Collard (Brussels)

The short esophagus: definition

Esophageal shortening may be defined as a longitudinal shrinkage of the esophageal muscle coat, so that the gastroesophageal junction (GEJ) is located above the diaphragm and cannot be replaced in the abdominal cavity even after extended mobilization of the esophageal tube up to the aortic arch through left thoracotomy.

Short esophagus (brachyesophagus) is to be distinguished from Barrett's esophagus (endobrachyesophagus), the latter consists of a columnar metaplasia of the distal esophageal mucosa with subsequent elevation of the squamous-glandular mucosal junction (z-line) but without any shortening of the esophageal muscle coat (*Figure 1*).

Esophageal shortening is associated with a long-standing gastroesophageal reflux disease (GERD) [1, 2] and is likely to reflect reflux-induced transmural inflammation. According to some authors, such a transmural injury might be linked to reflux of combined acid and duodenal juice into the esophagus, a condition in which bile salts act as a barrier-braker that allows acid to produce deep mucosal damage [3]. However, this hypothesis, although appealing, has not been confirmed yet by combined 24-hour esophageal pH- and bile measurements.

An irreducible cardia has been found in about 6% of patients referred for antireflux surgery [1, 4]. So, in a series reported earlier by our team, there were 25 patients with esophageal shortening among 340 patients (6.8%) referred to our department for antireflux surgery between September 1989 and July 1996 [5].

The best assessment method of the surgical irreducibility of the GEJ into the abdomen is to perform an upper gastrointestinal series in both the upright and supine positions and to consider the exact location of the junction between upper gastric folds and the unwrinkled surface of the esophageal tube. In this way, three different radiologic patterns may be defined (*Figures 2 and 3*).

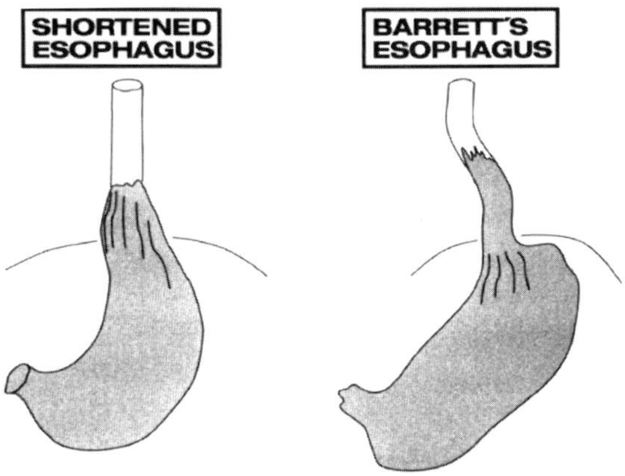

Figure 1. Distinction between short esophagus (brachy-esophagus, left) and Barrett's esophagus (endobrachyesophagus, right).

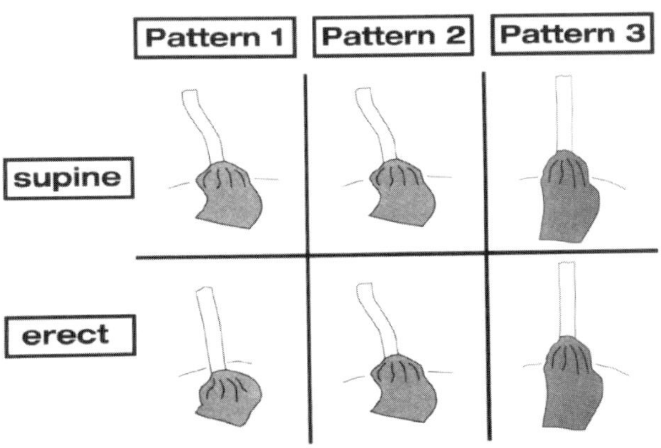

Figure 2. Diagram showing 3 different radiological patterns of sliding hiatal hernia.

Pattern 1

The junction between upper gastric folds and the unwrinkled esophageal surface is above the diaphragm in the supine position, but it spontaneously reduces below the diaphragm in the erect position (radiologically reducible cardia).

Pattern 2

The junction between upper gastric folds and the unwrinkled esophageal surface is above the diaphragm in both the erect and the supine positions, but the esophageal tube appears to be tortuous, so that it can be assumed that the cardia will be reducible into the abdomen after transhiatal surgical mobilization of the esophagus (radiologically irreducible but surgically reducible cardia).

Pattern 3

The junction between upper gastric folds and the unwrinkled esophageal surface is above the diaphragm in both the erect and the supine position, but the esophageal tube is straight, so that the cardia is unlikely to reduce into the abdomen following extended periesophageal dissection by thoracotomy (radiologically and surgically irreducible cardia).

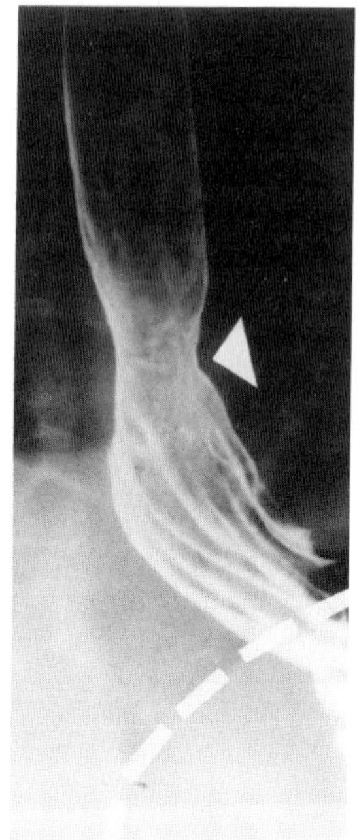

Figure 3. Radiograph taken in the erect position showing typical esophageal shortening (pattern 3) (arrow: intrathoracic GEJ; dashed line: diaphragm).

Surgical management

Various surgical procedures have been used to create an effective barrier against reflux of gastric contents into the lumen of a short esophagus. These include forward transposition of the hiatus [6], intrathoracic Nissen fundoplication [7], Collis-Belsey fundoplication [8], Collis-Nissen fundoplication [9], and transabdominal Maillet fundoplication [10] (*i.e.* a 360° fundic wrap placed around the subcardial area of the stomach). None of these procedures is ideal in such a way that the intrathoracic Nissen fundoplication leaves a gastric pouch in the chest, the Collis-Belsey or Collis-Nissen fundoplication creates a columnar-lined neo-esophagus above the subdiaphragmatic wrap, and the Maillet fundoplication combines both drawbacks. Another surgical modality consists of total duodenal diversion including distal gastrectomy and Roux-en-Y gastroenterostomy [11]. This procedure does not require any dissection of the fixed hiatal hernia (HH), but it exposes patients to postgastrectomy symptoms which may take over from those related to GERD. Of course, extreme shortening of the esophageal tube (*e.g.* location of the GEJ at the level of the carina) cannot be managed conservatively, but requires esophagectomy followed by gastric [12, 13] or colonic [2, 14] transposition.

Personal experience with intrathoracic Nissen fundoplication

Patients

Fifty-three patients with reflux-induced esophageal shortening were operated at the Louvain Medical School Hospital between 1986 and 2000. There were 17 women and 36 men ranging in age from 27 to 75 years (mean 51.1 years). Nine patients (18%) had a history of previous unsuccessful antireflux surgery, either transabdominal (n = 8) or transthoracic (n = 1). Reflux symptoms were present for a period ranging from 1 to 43 years (mean 16.3 years), which represented 31.2% of the patients' lifetime on average. The operation consisted of an intrathoracic Nissen fundoplication (n = 45), a subcardial 360°-fundoplication according to Maillet (n = 1), a duodenal diversion procedure combined with truncal vagotomy and antrectomy according to Holt and Large [15] (n = 4) and a subtotal esophageal resection (n = 3). The reason for esophageal resection in three patients was extreme shortening of the esophageal tube, one of these patients had had two previous antireflux procedures that eventually were ineffective against reflux. Patients who underwent a duodenal diversion procedure or a subcardial fundoplication according to Maillet had a reduced pulmonary function that precluded thoracotomy. One of these patients had a history of previous unsuccessful transabdominal fundoplication.

Surgical technique of intrathoracic Nissen fundoplication

The operation is done through a left thoracotomy in the seventh interspace, the eighth rib being cut posteriorly. Esophageal dissection is carried out from the hiatus up to the aortic arch. Care is taken to avoid injury to the vagi, especially in the presence of severe periesophagitis, which can make dissection extremely difficult. The fundus is dissected off the spleen through the hiatus by division of the short gastric vessels to bring a large amount of gastric tissue into the chest. The fundus is then wrapped counterclockwise around the lower esophagus, so that the suture line is located on the anterior aspect of the esophagus. A 50F Maloney bougie is introduced transorally by the anesthetist to prevent any narrowing of the esophageal lumen while constructing the wrap. Four to five interrupted nonabsorbable stitches are passed through the seromuscular layers of the left limb of the wrap, through the extramucosal layers of the esophagus and finally through the seromuscular layers of the right limb. They are tightened gently in order not to tear out the esophageal wall. A second covering row of interrupted stitches is placed over the first row, suturing the two limbs of the wrap. The 50F intraluminal bougie is removed and an 18F nasogastric catheter is introduced transnasally and secured. The wrap is anchored circumferentially to the crura before closure of the chest by placement of numerous non-absorbable stitches taking the extramucosal layers of the gastric wrap and the pleuromuscular layers of the crura.

As a consequence of acute complications related to the incarceration of the wrap into the hiatus during our initial experience with this procedure, some technical modifications have been introduced [7]:

- the hiatus, which is already enlarged because of the presence of a HH is widened further by either division of the left crus or diaphragmatic incision from the anterior margin of the crural sling;

- the stomach is handled carefully using the fingers, avoiding the use of forceps, especially the traumatizing Babcock clamps;
- a rather large amount of gastric tissue is used to create a very floppy wrap;
- particular care is taken to anchor the wrap to the crural sling; to do this, the surgeon pushes the left part of the diaphragm down with the left hand, mimicking diaphragmatic contractions like those that arise on cough, so that the anchorage sites can be precisely marked out on the wrap and no tension develops on the gastric wall in the postoperative course;
- the nasogastric catheter is removed only when the bowel movements resume to avoid acute distension of the newly constructed wrap in the early postoperative period;
- effervescent beverages and anti-inflammatory drugs are forbidden.

All 45 patients included in the current paper were operated on considering these technical modifications.

Postoperative complications

There was no postoperative death. A technical complication occurred during the immediate postoperative period in 2 patients, *i.e.* perforation (n = 1) or further herniation (n = 1) of the wrap into the chest. At follow-up, 4 patients needed reoperation because of either transhiatal herniation of the colon (n = 3), or further herniation of the fundoplication (n = 1) with subsequent compression of the heart and the lower lobe of the left lung (n = 1). The early postoperative perforation was managed by suturing of the gastric wrap with coverage of the suture line by omental fringes. The early herniation of the wrap into the chest was due to complete disruption of the suture line between the wrap and the hiatal sling, so that reanchorage was required. The late transhiatal herniations of the colon into the chest were managed by repositioning of the splenic flexure of the colon in the abdomen and reanchorage of the wrap to the hiatal sling. In the patient with further herniation of the fundoplication into the chest, the wrap was taken down with subsequent recurrence of reflux.

Three patients developed an ulcer within the fundoplication because of the intake of anti-inflammatory medications in spite of the fact that they were aware of the potential toxic effect of such medications on the gastric mucosa. In one of these patients, a gastropericardial fistula was suspected, although not clearly demonstrated [16]. All three were successfully treated by proton pump inhibitor therapy.

Clinical results

Forty-three of the 45 patients who underwent an intrathoracic fundoplication during the study period were suitable for a personal interview by the first author (Gutschow), so that they were asked for the presence of both residual reflux and surgery-induced symptoms (*Figure 4*). So, forty-two patients (97.7%) did not have any symptoms of reflux after a mean follow-up of 60.6 months (range: 1 to 161 months), and one patient complained of rare episodes of heartburn requiring intermittent intake of H_2-blockers. Surprisingly, the patient whose fundoplication had to be taken down did not have any reflux symptoms in spite of the presence of a massive radiological reflux at follow-up upper gastrointestinal series. Two patients (4.7%) had intermittent dysphagia for solids, and eight other patients

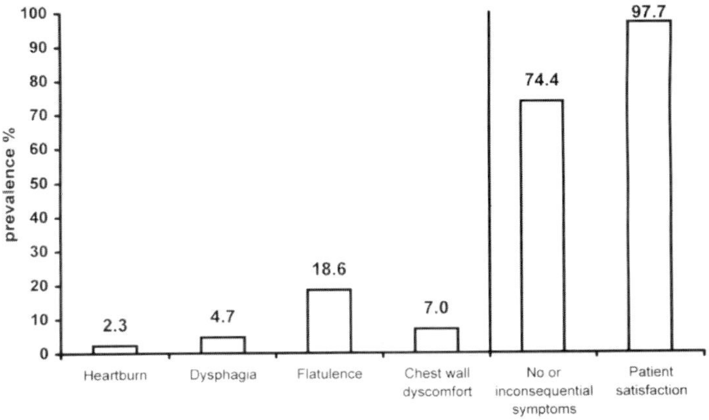

Figure 4. Clinical results in the 43 among the 45 patients with an intrathoracic Nissen fundoplication.

(18.6%) occasionally complained of a sensation of food passage which was considered inconsequential from their own standpoint. Socially disabling flatulence was present in 8 patients (18.6%), and 3 patients (7.0%) had residual chest wall discomfort at the level of the thoracic incision. Altogether, this made 32 patients (74.4%) with no or inconsequential symptoms, 10 patients (23.3%) without any reflux symptoms but with noticeable residual or surgery-induced symptoms, and one patient (2.3%) with both intermittent heartburn and chest pain. However, all patients interviewed – except the one whose fundoplication had to be taken down – would make the decision of an antireflux operation again.

Functional testing

Esophageal motility study

Esophageal motility was studied in 22 patients a few months after intrathoracic Nissen fundoplication. Lower esophageal sphincter (LES) pressure (mean ± sem) in these 22 patients increased from 5.5 mmHg ± 0.8 mmHg preoperatively to 17.2 mmHg ± 1.7 mmHg postoperatively ($p < 0.001$). Esophageal body motility study in 21 patients showed a normal pattern in 17 (81.0%), a dysmotility or dyscontractility pattern in 3 (14.3%), and it was not interpretable in 1 (4.7%) because of technical problems.

24-hour esophageal pH-monitoring

24-hour esophageal pH-monitoring was performed in 26 patients a few months after the operation. The percentage of total time intraesophageal pH < 4 dropped from 21.7% on the preoperative examination to 0.4% at early follow-up ($p < 0.001$). According to DeMeester's criteria [17], the prevalence of a pathologic intraesophageal 24-hour-pH study fell from 87.5% preoperatively to 0% at early follow-up.

Barium swallow study

Barium swallow study 3 to 4 weeks after the operation showed a normal intrathoracic wrap without any signs of radiological gastroesophageal reflux (GER). No patient had evidence of delayed emptying of the intrathoracic portion of the stomach.

Intrathoracic Nissen fundoplication controls pathologic GER into a short esophagus as does intra-abdominal Nissen fundoplication in patients with a normal-length esophagus. This is attested to by the fact that almost all patients have both no residual reflux symptoms and a normal exposure of the esophagus to acid at 24-hour pH monitoring at follow-up. These data indicate much better results than those achieved with antireflux procedures that create a neoesophageal tube such as the Collis-Nissen or the Collis-Belsey fundoplication [8, 9]. The main reason for the superiority of the intrathoracic Nissen fundoplication over the latter lengthening techniques is that the wrap is constructed around the lower esophagus above the intrathoracic GEJ rather than around the stomach.

Although used by many surgical teams 20 years ago [7, 18-20], there was a lot of controversy about the intrathoracic Nissen fundoplication because of the risk for the development of severe postoperative complications such as acute perforation of the wrap, its further herniation into the chest, or the development of gastric ulcers.

Actually, the absence of a phrenoesophageal membrane exposes the wrap to negative thoracic pressure, so that this "organized hiatus hernia" is further attracted up to the chest [21]. This situation is completely different from that of an unoperated hiatus hernia, which is located in its sac and remains submitted to positive abdominal pressure [22]. Sudden traction exerted by the diaphragm on the anchorage sites during coughing can tear out the gastric wall. Mimicking the diaphragmatic movements while anchoring the wrap appears to be the best way to plan the appropriate anchorage sites and prevent acute tension on the gastric wall.

Both mediastinal adhesions in relation to either a previous antireflux operation or reflux-induced periesophagitis can make intrathoracic dissection difficult, so as to predispose to damage to the gastric wall and vagal injury. The use of forceps while handling the fundus can also traumatize gastric tissue. Inadvertent truncal vagotomy may be responsible for delayed gastric emptying and impairment of the active relaxation of the stomach at meals, resulting in greater intragastric pressure with lower volumes [23]. On the other hand, a closed-loop phenomenon with subsequent increase in gastric pressure can arise in the case of intestinal obstruction. The role of devascularization of the fundus appears to be uncertain. Indeed, devascularization of the intrathoracic wrap is much less important than in a long gastric transplant as an esophageal substitute after subtotal esophagectomy. This gastric transplant is, in its way, a kind of hiatus hernia which is submitted to negative intrathoracic pressure, but perforation is very unusual because of the absence of a valve at the top. However, gastric distension and constriction of blood flow to the wrap resulting from too snug a closure of the hiatus obviously predispose to acute perforation of the wrap [24]. This situation is similar to Boerhaave's syndrome and requires an emergency thoracotomy. If the patient is reoperated on within the hours that follow the perforation, the defect can be sutured safely with maintenance of the wrap, but delayed rethoracotomy means take down of the fundoplication and replacement of as much gastric tissue as possible into the abdomen after closure of the perforation. Thoracic drainage alone, although proposed by some authors [25], seems to us to be hazardous.

Gastric ulcers that may develop in the intrathoracic fundoplication after intake of anti-inflammatory medications can be healed by acid-reducing therapy. In fact, gastric ulcers that were reported after both abdominal and thoracic fundoplications [19] are multifactorial in origin: vagal injury [26], gastrin release due to gastric distension [27] and bile reflux [28].

Conclusions

Surgical management of esophageal shortening is difficult because none of the techniques available is ideal. Performance of an intrathoracic Nissen fundoplication requires meticulous surgical technique to prevent the development of postoperative life-threatening complications such as acute perforation. Technical manoeuvres we have introduced more than 10 years ago should be taken into consideration by any surgeon who is unfamiliar with the procedure. These manoeuvres include further enlargement of the hiatus by either division of the left crus or performance of a 3-cm diaphragmatic incision radially from the anterior margin of the crural sling, manipulation of the gastric wall with the fingers rather than with traumatizing forceps, construction of a floppy wrap using a large amount of gastric tissue, careful anchorage of the wrap to the crural sling while mimicking diaphragmatic movements that arise on cough by pushing the left part of the diaphragm down, and removal of the nasogastric tube only after bowel movements resume.

In any case, misestimation of the surgical reducibility of the GEJ in a patient operated on for GERD leads to the placement of the fundoplication around the stomach instead of around the lower esophagus. This exposes to the risk for postoperative dysphagia, persistent heartburn and chest pain, because of subsequent herniation of the perigastric wrap into the chest, external compression of the herniated wrap secondary to partial disruption of the crura closure, or rather strangulation of the subcardial area of the stomach by the perigastric wrap [29-31].

References

1. Mattioli S, D'Ovidio F, Di Simone MP, Bassi F, Brusori S, Pilotti V, Felice V, Ferruzzi L, Guernelli N. Clinical and surgical relevance of the progressive phases of intrathoracic migration of the gastroesophageal junction in gastroesophageal reflux disease. J Thorac Cardiovasc Surg 1998;116:267-275.
2. Belsey RHR. Gastroesophageal reflux. Am J Surg 1980;139:775-781.
3. Gozetti G, Pilotti V, Spangaro M, Bassi F, Grigioni W, Carulli N, Loria P, Felice V, Lerro F, Mattioli S. Pathophysiology and natural history of acquired short esophagus. Surgery 1987;102:507-514.
4. Nissen R, Rossetti M. Die Behandlung von Hiatushernien und Refluxösophagitis mit Gastropexie und Fundoplicatio. Indikation, Technik und Ergebnisse. Stuttgart: Georg Thieme Verlag, 1959:138.
5. Collard JM, Romagnoli R, Otte JB. Are there specific complications related to intrathoracic Nissen fundoplication? What is the role of vagal injury, devascularization of the fundus and constriction of blood flow in acute complications following intrathoracic Nissen fundoplication? In: Giuli R, Galmiche JP, Jamieson GG, Scarpignato C, eds. The esophagogastric junction. Paris: John Libbey Eurotext, 1996:825-833.
6. Effler D, Ballinger C. Complications and surgical treatment of hiatus hernia and short esophagus. J Thorac Surg 1951;21:235-247.
7. Collard JM, De Koninck XJ, Otte JB, Fiasse RH, Kestens PJ. Intrathoracic Nissen fundoplication:long-term clinical an pH-monitoring evaluation. Ann Thorac Surg 1991;51:34-38.
8. Orringer MB, Sloan H. Collis-Belsey reconstruction of the esophagogastric junction:indications, physiology and technical considerations. J Thorac Cardiovasc Surg 1976;71:295-303.
9. Orringer MB, Orringer JS. The combined Collis-Nissen operation:early assessment of reflux control. Ann Thorac Surg 1982;33:534-539.
10. Maillet P, Baulieux J, Dumurgier C. A propos du traitement des brachy-œsophages acquis. Chirurgie 1976;102:519-524.
11. Herrington J, Mody B. Total duodenal diversion for treatment of reflux esophagitis uncontroled by repeated antireflux procedures. Ann Surg 1976;183:636-644.

12. Collard JM, Tinton N, Malaise J, Romagnoli R, Otte JB, Kestens PJ. Esophageal replacement: gastric tube or whole stomach? Ann Thorac Surg 1995;60:261-267.
13. Collard JM, Romagnoli R, Otte JB, Kestens PJ. The denervated stomach as an esophageal substitute is a contractile organ. Ann Surg 1998;227:33-39.
14. Otte JB, Lerut T, Collard JM, et al. Les plasties coliques de l'œsophage. Expérience chez 60 patients. Acta Chir Belg 1982;82:389-396.
15. Fékété F. Severe peptic esophagitis. Treatment by total duodenal diversion. Presse Med 1983;12:2239-2242.
16. d'Othée BJ, Gohy P, Sottiaux T, Collard JM. Pneumopéricarde et ulcère d'origine médicamenteuse au sein d'une valve antireflux intrathoracique. Gastroenterol Clin Biol 1998;22:251-253.
17. DeMeester TR. Prolonged oesophageal pH-monitoring. In: Read NW, ed. Gastrointestinal motility: which test? Petersfield, England: Wrighston Biomedical Publishing Ltd, 1989:41-51.
18. Mansour KA, Burton HG, Miller JI Jr, Hatcher CR Jr. Complications of intrathoracic Nissen fundoplication. Ann Thor Surg 1981;32:173-178.
19. Richardson J, Larson G, Polk H. Intrathoracic fundoplication for shortened esophagus. Treacherous solution to a challenging problem. Am J Surg 143:29-35.
20. Maher J, Hocking M, Woodward F. Supradiaphragmatic fundoplication. Long term follow-up and analysis of complications. Am J Surg 1984;147:181-186.
21. Balison J, McGregor A, Woodward E. Postoperative diaphragmatic herniation following transthoracic fundoplication. Arch Surg 1973;106:164-166.
22. DeMeester TR, Lafontaine E, Joelson BE, et al. Relationship of a hiatal hernia to the function of the body of the esophagus and the gastroesophageal ,junction. J Thorac Cardiovasc Surg 1981;82:547-558.
23. Davenport H. Physiology of the digestive tract. Chicago: Year Book Medical Publishers, 1982:52.
24. Meredith J, Kon N, Poole G, Pennell T. Physiologic effects of intrathoracic placement of Nissen fundoplication. Curr Surg 1985;42:32-34.
25. Burnett H, Read R, Morris W, Campbell G. Management of complications of fundoplication and Barrett's esophagus. Surgery 1977;82:521-530.
26. Bushkin F, Woodward E, O'Leary J. Occurrence of gastric ulcer after Nissen fundoplication. Am J Surg 1976;42:821-826.
27. Maher J, Cerda J. The role of gastric stasis in the genesis of gastric ulceration following fundoplication. World J Surg 1982;6:794-799.
28. Bremner CG. Gastric ulcer after the Nissen fundoplication: a complication of alkaline reflux. S Afr Med J 1977;51:791-793.
29. Collard JM, Verstraete L, Otte JB, et al. Clinical, radiological and functional results of remedial antireflux operations. Int Surg 1993;78:298-306.
30. Collard JM, Romagnoli R, Kestens PJ. Reoperations for unsatisfactory outcome after laparoscopic antireflux surgery. Dis Esophagus 1996;9:56-62.
31. Collard JM, Verstraete L, Romagnoli R. What are the consequences of herniation of the repair into the chest? Why are they different from the primary intrathoracic Nissen? In: Giuli R, Galmiche JP, Jamieson GG, Scarpignato C, eds. The esophagogastric junction. Paris: John Libbey Eurotext, 1996:796-798.

Is a floppy valve a good guarantee against postoperative dysphagia?

D.I. Watson (Adelaide)

Postfundoplication dysphagia

Whilst antireflux surgery, and in particular total fundoplication, is an effective treatment for gastroesophageal reflux disease, it is followed by troublesome dysphagia in some patients. This adverse outcome can spoil an otherwise good surgical result, and it will even require surgical revision in a small number of patients [1]. postfundoplication dysphagia can follow a range of problems, and in some patients the problem is due to more than one problem.

Many surgeons and gastroenterologists believe, perhaps at times simplistically, that this problem is due to the construction of an overly tight total fundoplication, and that the routine construction of a very loose total wrap (by fully mobilising the gastric fundus) or a partial fundoplication will prevent postoperative dysphagia. Unfortunately other problems can also contribute to dysphagia. For example, a narrow diaphragmatic hiatus due to the formation of dense perihiatal scar tissue [2], or even over tightening of the hiatus during hiatal repair, can be troublesome, and in our hospital narrowing of the hiatus due to perihiatal fibrosis has been the commonest problem requiring surgical revision.

Another potential cause of dysphagia can be the construction of a circumferential wrap in patients with absent esophageal body peristalsis (adynamic esophagus). Our preference in this situation is to perform a partial fundoplication procedure. A more serious problem is the formation of a total fundoplication in a patient with achalasia, who was misdiagnosed with reflux preoperatively. The use of esophageal manometry should prevent this problem. A further cause of early postoperative dysphagia can be "esophageal ileus". We have recently shown that esophageal motility is absent in most patients in the early period following laparoscopic fundoplication, but that normal motility returns at later follow-up [3]. This may explain some of the early dysphagia most patients experience following fundoplication.

Preventative strategies

A range of strategies for the prevention of postoperative dysphagia have been proposed. These include the construction of a short, loose total fundoplication with division of the short gastric vessels and full fundal mobilization – the so called "Floppy Nissen" procedure [4, 5]. This approach is discussed below. Other technical factors thought to be important include the use of a large (more than 50 Fr) bougie within the esophageal lumen for the calibration of an appropriately loose fundoplication [4]. Whilst there is evidence that this approach can be associated with less dysphagia, the passage of the bougie can occasionally cause perforation of the esophagus. The routine performance of some form of partial fundoplication also has its advocates [6, 7], and a variant of this approach is the concept of tailoring the type of fundoplication constructed to identifiable preoperative factors, such as esophageal motility [8].

Assessment of dysphagia

When considering the issue of dysphagia following fundoplication, it is important to consider exactly what the term dysphagia means, and to clearly define how the symptom of dysphagia is assessed. Widely differing rates of dysphagia are reported following a variety of antireflux procedures, and this variation is not due to surgical technique alone. Some surgeons consider difficulty swallowing of any degree to be significant and report their results accordingly, whereas others make subjective judgements about whether the symptom represents a significant clinical problem, and if it doesn't, they don't report it as dysphagia. Furthermore, there is a tendency for the operating surgeon to underestimate the true incidence of postoperative dysphagia in patients he has operated on. This is partly because most patients wish to please, or at least not upset their surgeon. Different outcomes are often elicited by an independent investigator, particularly if the investigator is not a medical practitioner. For these reasons, if reports of outcomes following surgery for reflux are to be meaningful, the assessment of dysphagia should be standardized and it should be assessed by someone who is independent from the operating surgeon. Furthermore, because surgeons have failed to reach a consensus view about how this symptom should be assessed and reported, any comparison of dysphagia rates for patients undergoing antireflux surgery in different institutions are essentially meaningless, and this is one of the greatest impediments to meaningful comparison of surgical outcomes from different institutions. Randomized comparisons of patients undergoing surgery in the same hospital, with independent follow-up by the same person should provide more reliable information about the true differences between different operative approaches.

Of relevance, in two of the randomized trials previously reported from the University of Adelaide Department of Surgery [9, 10], 6 different methods of assessing dysphagia were applied in all patients both before and after surgery. These comprised 3 yes/no answer questions, two 0 to 10 visual analogue scales, and a 0 to 45 dysphagia scoring system. Each of these methods elicited a different dysphagia rate, highlighting the fact that what question is asked will influence the outcome elicited. For example, whilst 31% of patients reported dysphagia for solid foods 6 months after surgery when asked a simple yes/no question, 38% of the same cohort of patients reported dysphagia when the 0 to 45 score was applied, a variation of 7% in the dysphagia rate elicited. Of interest, and often poorly recognized, 34% and 47% of the same group of patients respectively reported dysphagia before surgery when the same questions were asked, suggesting that dysphagia might actually be less common following total fundoplication than before surgery!

Floppy Nissen fundoplication

The construction of a floppy total (Nissen) fundoplication was first proposed by Donahue *et al.* [5] in 1977, and this concept was supported and popularised by subsequent reports from DeMeester *et al.* [4]. This entails full mobilization of the gastric fundus by dividing the short gastric vessels and posterior fundal attachments, thereby enabling a loose total fundoplication to be constructed which incorporates both the anterior and posterior fundal walls. The concept is appealing, as it achieves a very loose fundoplication, and prevents the erroneous construction of a tight or a twisted/rotated fundoplication. Unfortunately, arguments used to support this approach rely entirely on the results of uncontrolled case series or comparisons with historical controls. Furthermore, DeMeester *et al.* [4] often quoted study made two concurrent changes to the surgical technique applied (division of the short gastric vessels, and shortening of the fundoplication), and an attempt was then made to dissect out the contribution each change made to the differences seen between the different surgical groups, thereby making assessment of the impact of short gastric vessel division alone even more difficult. One could also argue that the progressive improvement in surgical outcome reported in his series could have been, at least in part, influenced by a learning curve phenomenon. In other words, as his experience grew, the clinical outcome improved, at least in part because of greater surgical experience. Such a learning curve phenomenon was associated with improved clinical outcomes following laparoscopic total fundoplication in our experience, without any change in surgical technique [11].

In the era of laparoscopic surgery the issue of division *versus* non division of the short gastric vessels has continued to be hotly debated, with a number of surgeons adding to the debate by comparing their laparoscopic experience with a total fundoplication performed initially without dividing the short gastric vessels, with their subsequent experience with dividing short gastric vessels [12]. In these studies, laparoscopic Nissen fundoplication was always commenced without dividing the short gastric vessels, and as laparoscopic experience grew, these surgeons began to divide the short gastric vessels. They then compared their experience with the two techniques, and found that dysphagia was more common in patients in whom the short gastric vessels had been left intact. From this it was concluded that the short gastric vessels should be divided so that a "floppy" total fundoplication could be constructed, and this would minimize the likelihood of postoperative dysphagia. However, such an analysis fails to take account of the effect of a learning curve bias, and this is likely to be significant in the early stages of a surgeon's experience with laparoscopic fundoplication [11].

The outcomes of two recently reported prospective randomized trials of division *versus* no division of the short gastric vessels during total fundoplication have both demonstrated no important outcome differences [9, 13]. These trials enrolled 50 and 102 patients undergoing either open or laparoscopic fundoplication respectively. In particular, the incidence and severity of postoperative dysphagia was not influenced be dividing the short gastric vessels. The open surgery study reported by Luostarinen *et al.* [13] did, however, report a higher incidence of postoperative para-esophageal hiatus herniation in patients who had their short gastric vessels divided, suggesting that division of the vessels could even worsen the outcome of total fundoplication! These randomized studies should provide more reliable evidence for the determination of the issue of dysphagia following total fundoplication. It is possible that the most important technical step necessary for the avoidance of postoperative dysphagia following a total fundoplication is to ensure a short loose wrap, irrespective of whether the short gastric vessels are divided or not.

Alternatives to total fundoplication

A range of alternatives to total fundoplication, in particular partial fundoplication techniques, have been proposed for the surgical correction of reflux, but with a reduced incidence of postoperative dysphagia. Unfortunately, until relatively recently, comparisons between these procedures and total fundoplication have been subject to the same problem of historical control bias described above. Four randomized studies have compared a posterior partial fundoplication technique with a total fundoplication, and whilst one of the smaller studies demonstrated a non-significant trend towards less dysphagia following posterior fundoplication [7], these studies have not demonstrated any overall reduction in the rate of dysphagia with follow-up to 5 years compared to the total fundoplication [14-16]. On the other hand, a recently reported randomised study of 107 patients followed for 6 months, has demonstrated less dysphagia following an anterior hemifundoplication, suggesting that this approach, or a variant of it, might offer a better strategy for the minimization of dysphagia following fundoplication [10]. Nevertheless, even in this study, 15% of patients still had some dysphagia for solid food 6 months after anterior fundoplication, even though it was usually not troublesome.

Conclusions

When answering the question of whether a floppy valve (a very loose total fundoplication) can provide a good guarantee against dysphagia following total fundoplication, it is important to realize that approximately 40% of patients undergoing antireflux surgery have dysphagia (of some degree) before surgery is performed, and that there is a small group of patents who will develop troublesome new dysphagia following antireflux surgery, even after a floppy total or a partial fundoplication. The evidence currently available from randomized trials suggests that division of the short gastric vessels does not reduce the risk of dysphagia, and furthermore, the construction of a posterior partial fundoplication is not likely to be a better strategy for dysphagia prevention. However, the alternative of an anterior partial fundoplication should be considered further, with the early results of one trial suggesting that this approach might provide a better strategy for improving the overall outcome of surgery for reflux. Whether it is appropriate to apply this approach more widely should await the outcome of further trials.

References

1. Watson DI, Jamieson GG, Game PA, Williams RS, Devitt PG. Laparoscopic reoperation following failed antireflux surgery. Br J Surg 1999;86:98-101.
2. Watson DI, Jamieson GG, Mitchell PC, Devitt PG, Britten-Jones R. Stenosis of the esophageal hiatus following laparoscopic fundoplication. Arch Surg 1995;130:1014-1016.
3. Jamieson GG, King DR, Myers JC, Watson DI. Early post-operative motility following laparoscopic fundoplication. Aust NZ J Surg 1999;69:A57.
4. DeMeester TR, Bonavina L, Albertucci M. Nissen fundoplication for gastroesophageal reflux disease. Evaluation of primary repair in 100 consecutive patients. Ann Surg 1986;204:9-20.
5. Donahue PE, Bombeck CT. The modified Nissen fundoplication - reflux prevention without gas bloat. Chir Gastroenterol 1977;11:15-27.
6. Watson A, Jenkinson LR, Ball CS, Norris TL. A more physiological alternative to total fundoplication for the surgical correction of resistant gastro-oesophageal reflux. Br J Surg 1991;78:1088-1094.
7. Thor KBA, Silander T. A long-term randomized prospective trial of the Nissen procedure versus a modified Toupet technique. Ann Surg 1989;210:719-724.
8. Kauer WKH, Peters JH, DeMeester TR, Heimbucher J, Ireland AP, Bremner CG. A tailored approach to antireflux surgery. J Thorac Cardiovasc Surg 1995;110:141-147.
9. Watson DI, Pike GK, Baigrie RJ, Mathew M, Devitt PG, Britten-Jones R, Jamieson GG. Prospective double blind randomised trial of laparoscopic Nissen fundoplication with division and without division of short gastric vessels. Ann Surg 1997;226:642-652.
10. Watson DI, Jamieson GG, Pike GK, Davies N, Richardson M, Devitt PG. A prospective randomised double blind trial between laparoscopic Nissen fundoplication and anterior partial fundoplication. Br J Surg 1999;86:123-130.
11. Watson DI, Baigrie RJ, Jamieson GG. A learning curve for laparoscopic fundoplication. Definable, avoidable, or a waste of time? Ann Surg 1996;224:198-203.
12. Hunter JG, Swanstrom L, Waring JP. Dysphagia after laparoscopic antireflux surgery. The impact of operative technique. Ann Surg 1996;224:51-57.
13. Luostarinen ME, Isolauri JO. Randomized trial to study the effect of fundic mobilization on long-term results of Nissen fundoplication. Br J Surg 1999;86:614-618.
14. Lundell L, Abrahamsson H, Ruth M, Rydberg L, Lonroth H, Olbe L. Long-term results of a prospective randomized comparison of total fundic wrap (Nissen-Rossetti) or semifundoplication (Toupet) for gastro-oesophageal reflux. Br J Surg 1996;83:830-835.
15. Walker SJ, Holt S, Sanderson CJ, Stoddard CJ. Comparison of Nissen total and Lind partial transabdominal fundoplication in the treatment of gastro-oesophageal reflux. Br J Surg 1992;79:410-414.
16. Laws HL, Clements RH, Swillies CM. A randomized, prospective comparison of the Nissen versus the Toupet fundoplication for gastroesophageal reflux disease. Ann Surg 1997;225:647-654.

What are the indications for a Collis gastroplasty in Barrett's patients?

L.L. Swanstrom (Portland)

Gastroesophageal reflux disease (GERD) can present as a mild, benign clinical condition or as an end-stage problem with irreversible destruction of the esophagus. Complications can include bleeding from esophagitis, peptic strictures, decreased motility, Barrett's esophagus and axial shortening. The relationship between all of these complicating factors, and their impact on clinical outcomes, has not been completely established. Both Barrett's and axial shortening of the esophagus have the same underlying patho-etiology and are probably interrelated clinically. Injury of the esophageal mucosa by endogenous or exogenous acid or alkaline substances is the initiating cause of both Barrett's and esophageal shortening. Such caustic exposure causes tissue damage starting with simple neutrophile infiltration of the mucosa and submucosa and progressing to transmutable inflammation and mucosal sloughing (ulceration). The degree of acute tissue damage depends on the responsible agent (strong bases such as lye lead to deeper and more profound tissue damage), and length of exposure time. The later point is clinically relevant for patients with esophageal motility disorders and GERD who are known to have more severe effects from their reflux due to delayed esophageal clearance [1]. Chronic repetitive injury, such as seen in GERD, lead to stimulation of local tissue fibroblasts and eventual deposition of non elastic fibrous scar tissue in the submucosa, circular muscle layer and even in the longitudinal muscle layer in advanced cases [2].

An additional contribution to esophageal shortening which is especially relevant for laparoscopic antireflux surgery is the association of Barrett's and transmural esophagitis. Extension of inflammatory changes into the peri-esophageal tissues results in hyperemia and fibrosis of the mediastinal fat. Clinically this can result in difficulty in freeing the mediastinal esophagus to obtain intra-abdominal length for the fundoplication [3].

Both Barrett's and axial shortening have been blamed for higher failure rates following antireflux surgery [4]. Risk factors for the presence of esophageal shortening include the length of GERD symptoms, large hiatal hernias (> 5 cm), and peptic strictures. Barrett's esophagus is also commonly listed as a short esophagus risk factor as well. These risk factors are not absolute and, in the majority of cases, the esophagus can be sufficiently mobilized by surgical dissection to achieve adequate length [3]. The incidence of refractory esophageal shortening requiring a gastroplasty was only 3.5-5% in two recent laparoscopic Nissen series [5, 6]. Because it is frequently asymptomatic, the population incidence of Barrett's esophagus is unknown. It is, however, a relatively common finding in patients with GERD, being found in 1% of patients on upper endoscopy, in 3-6% of patients with chronic GERD symptoms and in as many as 20% of patients when random biopsies are done [7]. Circumstantial evidence of an association between Barrett's and esophageal shortening can be found in our antireflux experience (*Table I*).

Table I. Relationship between Barrett's esophagus and esophageal shortening in the Legacy gastroesophageal reflux disease database.

Patients having elective antireflux surgery (4/94-11/99)	677	
Biopsy proven Barrett's	98 (14.5%)	
Patients requiring Collis gastroplasty	37 (5.5%)	
Expected incidence of Barrett's and Collis	5 of 37 (13.5%)	
Observed incidence	8 of 37 (22%)	p = .001

Surgical treatment

Treatment goals for Barrett's patients are geared to the preventing of dysplasia and possible progression to esophageal adenocarcinoma. The best treatment remains controversial but antireflux surgery offers some theoretical benefit over medical therapy; which has failed to impact the rapid increase in esophageal adenocarcinoma in spite of its wide spread usage [8]. The use of ablation therapy is potentially the ultimate solution but also requires the effective control of reflux to prevent recurrence. Once again the most effective option for reflux control remains a fundoplications [9].

The "gold standard" of treatment for esophageal shortening remains the Collis gastroplasty. This technique allows an antireflux procedure to be performed in the abdomen, around the "neo-esophagus", without tension. Except for severe end stage disease, where esophagectomy may be the best solution, techniques of laparoscopic Collis gastroplasty offer the best long-term results while preserving the minimally invasive approach favored by patients and referring physicians. There are two basic approaches described for endoscopic esophageal lengthening. We first described a combination thoracoscopic and laparoscopic approach in 1995 which requires the insertion of a single additional 12mm port in the right chest and which closely reproduces a standard open Collis [3]. Hunter's group popularized a totally laparoscopic approach that uses a circular stapler and a liner endoscopic stapler [5]. This technique replicates the vertical banded gastroplasty of Mason. Long-term results of these two laparoscopic procedures are good as summarized in *Table II*.

As was noted for open Collis gastroplasty, we have shown in follow-up studies that a significant number of postoperative patients test positive for esophageal acid exposure. This is undoubtedly related to endogenous acid secretion from the ectopic gastric mucosa of the neo-esophagus [6]. The impact of such acid exposure on preexisting Barrett's is unknown but is of obvious concern and calls for close postoperative follow-up.

Table II. Mean 13 month follow-up of laparoscopic Collis experience.

- 10/91-9/99 = 968 lap fundoplications
- **37 (3.8%)** Collis procedures - 14 PEH
  - 9 strictures
  - 14 redo
- **8 Barrett's**
- 31 (97%) symptom improvement
- No recurrent herniation
- 9/21 (43%) abnormal 24-hourr pH

Conclusion

There is a clinical association between the presence of Barrett's esophagus and esophageal shortening. The best treatment of the short esophagus in the face of GERD is the laparoscopic Collis gastroplasty and fundoplication. There are emerging indications that an effective antireflux procedure is the best treatment for Barrett's esophagus as well. The non physiologic nature of the Collis neoesophagus remains a concern but it is reassuring that exposure to acid alone does not seem to promote dysplastic progression in Barrett's [10].

References

1. Stein HJ, Hoeft S, DeMeester TR. Functional foregut abnormalities in Barrett's esophagus. J Thorac Cardiovasc Surg 1993;105:107-111.
2. Bremner RM, Crookes PF, Constantini M, DeMeester TR, Peters JH. The relationship of esophageal length to hiatal hernia in gastroesophageal reflux disease. Gastroenterology 1992;102:A45-46.
3. Swanstrom LL, Marcus DR, Galloway GQ. Laparoscopic Collis gastroplasty is the treatment of choice for the shortened esophagus. Am J Surg 1996;171:477-481.
4. DeMeester TR, Stein HJ. Surgical treatment of gastroesophageal reflux disease. In: Castell DO, ed. The esophagus. Boston: Little, Brown & Co., 1992:579-626.
5. Johnson AB, Oddsdottir M, Hunter JG. Laparoscopic Collis gastroplasty and Nissen fundoplication: a new technique for the management of esophageal foreshortening. Surg Endosc 1998;12:1055-1060.
6. Jobe BA, Horvath KD, Swanstrom LL. Postoperative function following laparoscopic Collis gastroplasty for shortened esophagus. Arch Surg 1998;133:867-873.
7. Walia S, Laycock WS, Hunter JG. Barrett's esophagus. Semin Laparosc Surg 1995;2:54-59.
8. Haag S, Nandurkar S, Talley NJ. Regression of Barrett's esophagus: the role of acid suppression, surgery, and ablative methods. Gastrointestinal Endosc 1999;50:229-240.
9. Farrell TM, Smith D, Metreveli RE, Johnson AB, Galloway KD, Hunter JG. Fundoplication provides effective and durable symptom relief in patients with Barrett's esophagus. Am J Surg 1999;178:18-21.
10. DeMeester TR. Barrett's esophagus. Surgery 1993;113:239-241.

What are the differences between the Watson and Lortat-Jacob antireflux procedures?

A. Watson (London)

Both the Lortat-Jacob and the Watson antireflux procedures share the common aims of reflux control without total fundoplication by placing particular emphasis on factors known to be relevant to the antireflux mechanism. However, there are some differences in technique and in the extent to which the procedures have been studied.

Techniques

Lortat-Jacob procedure

This procedure was described by Lortat-Jacob in 1948 to resemble the treatment of genital prolapse on the basis that many authors had compared the anatomy and function of the hiatal region to the pelvic corridor of the lavator ani. It comprised the following steps:
- freeing of the intra-abdominal esophagus, cardia, gastric fundus and their peritoneal attachments, with exposure of the right and left limbs of the crural sling;
- achievement of a long intra-abdominal segment of esophagus;
- approximation of the crural sling behind the esophagus;
- reattachment of the gastric fundus to the sub-diaphragmatic peritoneum;
- reconstruction of the angle of His;
- fixation of the right margin of the gastric fundus to the left margin of the esophagus.

Watson procedure

This was described by Watson in 1984 [1]. At this time, Nissen fundoplication was well established as the most commonly performed anti-reflux procedure with well-documented effective reflux control. However, many authors had expressed concern about the incidence of troublesome mechanical complications, including dysphagia, gas-bloat and inability to belch or vomit, occurring in up to 25% of patients [2-4]. Several partial fundoplication procedures had been described such as the Hill, Belsey, Toupet and Lind in the expectation that reducing the degree of fundoplication from 360° to 180-270° would reduce the incidence of troublesome mechanical complications. Although popular with their advocates, these procedures did not gain universal acceptance as the Hill and Belsey procedures were technically more demanding that the Nissen fundoplication (Belsey requiring a thoracotomy) and there was concern that the other partial fundoplication procedures offered less effective reflux control than total fundoplication.

The principals on which the Watson procedure was based had some similarities with those of the Lortat-Jacob procedure. It was believed that if the factors known to influence competence could be corrected and indeed accentuated, the degree of fundoplication could be reduced sufficiently to result in a very low incidence of troublesome mechanical complications, without compromising efficacy of reflux control achieved by total fundoplication.

The steps in performing the procedure are as follows:
- division of the phrenoesophageal ligament and mobilization of the cardia, intra-abdominal esophagus and exposure of the crural sling;
- achievement of a long (5-6 cm) segment of intra-abdominal esophagus by blunt trans-hiatal dissection;
- a crural repair performed behind the intra-abdominal esophagus;
- fixation of the long intra-abdominal esophagus to the crural sling;
- accentuation of the angle of His by suturing the supero-medial aspect of the gastric fundus to the superior arch of the crural sling;
- performance of a 120° anterolateral fundoplication.

Clinical studies and results

Lortat-Jacob procedure

Because of the time at which this procedure was described, most of the assessment was by clinical and/or radiological assessment, by which criteria the procedure was shown to be effective in over 90% of cases, although those studying the long-term results of the procedure have stated "the assessment of these (long-term results) has demonstrated some deterioration of the results of the Lortat-Jacob operation" [5]. This published report has referred to postoperative assessment by manometry and pH monitoring, although the report is relatively superficial. It refers to lower esophageal sphincter (LES) tone being normal (17 cm of water) and that "relaxation obviates only 50% of pre-existing sphincter tone". The intra-abdominal segment is reported as measuring 4.8 cm in length. pH monitoring measured over 3 hours was reported to confirm the absence of reflux although the report did not give any further details of the study protocol, nor the number of patients studied.

Watson procedure

This procedure has been studied extensively both by the initiator and several independent groups, after performance both by an open and laparoscopic approach.

A clinical and objective study was performed on 100 patients operated by an open approach, with pre- and postoperative symptomatic assessment by a non-surgical observer together with pre- and postoperative endoscopy, manometry and 24-hour ambulatory pH monitoring [6]. The results as shown in *Tables I and II*, show that the incidence of symptomatic improvement, symptomatic cure, healing of endoscopic esophagitis (where

Table I. "Physiological" antireflux procedure: clinical results.

Symptomatic improvement	Symptomatic cure	Healing of esophagitis	Restoration of normal pH profile
94 (65-96)	82 (32-80)	86 (63-91)	84 (83-85)

The values shown are percentages; values in parentheses are the range recorded in the literature for Nissen fundoplication

Table II. "Physiological" antireflux procedure: mechanical complications.

Gas bloat syndrome	Inability to belch or vomit	Transient dysphagia	Troublesome dysphagia
0 (11-54)	0 (5-50)	11 (19-86)	2 (4-24)

The values shown are percentages; values in parentheses are the range recorded in the literature for Nissen fundoplication present) and restoration of a physiological pH profile compared favourably with the best published results following Nissen fundoplication, but the incidence of troublesome mechanical complications was very low, with no gas bloat (onset of bloating not present preoperatively) and only a 2% incidence of troublesome dysphagia. Manometric studies, compared with those of 30 asymptomatic controls showed that postoperative resting lower esophageal sphincter pressure (LESP) and intra-abdominal length and LES relaxation were all comparable to values in control subjects. This is in contrast to published values following Nissen fundoplication in which postoperative resting LESP is significantly higher than that in controls [7] and there is impairment of LES relaxation [8] both producing an element of "supra-competence". It is believed that these differences explain the very low incidence of troublesome mechanical complications following the Watson procedure. These results have been confirmed by other workers, who have similarly found the procedure to be as effective as published results of Nissen fundoplication in reflux control but with a very low incidence of troublesome mechanical complications [9]. The durability of the procedure has been demonstrated by Campbell *et al.* [10], who performed pH monitoring five years after the Watson procedure. They showed that at 5 years, 81% of patients had a physiological intraesophageal pH profile, which is comparable to similar data published for Nissen fundoplication [11]. Several studies have alluded to the Watson procedure when performed laparoscopically. A study by Watson *et al.* showed symptomatic relief in 91% of patients and all patients who underwent post-operative pH monitoring were restored to a physiological pH profile [12]. Whereas several reports had shown an increased incidence of mechanical complications following Nissen fundoplication when performed laparoscopically, associated with greater impairment of LES relaxation [13], results in relation to the Watson procedure showed that the low incidence of troublesome mechanical complications seen at open operation was replicated when the procedure was performed laparoscopically, with levels of resting LESP and LES relaxation being comparable both to those obtained at open operation and indeed by inference, comparable to control values [13]. In a prospective randomized control trial between laparoscopic Nissen fundoplication and the Watson procedure performed laparoscopically, Watson *et al.* demonstrated equivalent reflux control, but a significant reduction in the incidence of mechanical complications and a faster rate of esophageal emptying following the Watson procedure [14].

Conclusion

Although the Lortat-Jacob procedure and the Watson procedure share some common technical aspects, including the achievement of a long intra-abdominal segment of esophagus, posterior crural repair and correction of the angle of His, there are some important technical differences but predominantly differences to the extent to which the procedures have been subject to objective evaluation, including durability and prospective randomized trials against Nissen fundoplication, by independent observers. Furthermore, the Watson procedure has been extensively performed laparoscopically and independent evaluation has shown the results to be equivalent to those obtained at open operation, and in a prospective randomized trial against laparoscopic Nissen fundoplication, has been found to be as effective in reflux control but with a significantly lower incidence of troublesome mechanical complications.

References

1. Watson A, Norris TL. A clinical and pathophysiological study of a simple, effective operation for the correction of gastro-oesophageal reflux. Br J Surg 1984;71:991.
2. Leonardi HK, Corzier RE, Ellis FH. Re-operation for complications of the Nissen fundoplication J Thorac Cardiovasc Surg 1981;81:50-56.
3. Mansour KA, Burton HG, Miller JI, Hatcher CR. Complications of intrathoracic Nissen funoplication. Ann Thorac Surg 1981;32:173-178.
4. Negre JB. Post fundoplication syndromes. Do they restrict the success of Nissen fundoplicaiton? Ann Surg 1983;198:698-700.
5. Goutallier P. The Lortat-Jacob procedure. In: Giuli R, McCallum RW, eds. Benign lesions of the esophagus and cancer. Berlin: Springer-Verlag, 1989.
6. Watson A, Jenkinson LR, Ball CS, Barlow AP, Norris TL. A more physiological alternative to total fundoplication for the surgical correction of resistant gastro-oesophageal reflux. Br J Surg 1991;71:1088-1094.
7. DeMeester TR, Johnson LF. Evaluation of the Nissen anti-reflux procedure by esophageal manometry and 24 hour pH monitoring. Am J Surg 1975;129:94-100.
8. Ireland AC, Holloway RH, Toouli J, Dent J. Mechanisms underlying the antireflux action of fundoplication. Gut 1993;34:303-308.
9. Park K, Zentler-Munro P, Smith C, Munro A. Evaluation of the Watson fundoplication. Br J Surg 1992;70:S96-79.
10. Campbell KL, Munro A. Efficacy and incidence of post-fundoplication symptoms at a median of five years following open Watson fundoplication. Br J Surg 1998;85:8.
11. DeMeester TR, Bonavina L, Albertucci M. Nissen fundoplication for gastro-esophageal reflux disease. Ann Surg 1986;204:9-20.
12. Watson A, Spychal RT, Brown MC, Peck N. Callander N. Laparoscopic "physiological" antireflux procedure: preliminary results of a prospective symptomatic and objective study. Br J Surg 1995;82:651-656.
13. Peters JH, Heimbucher J, Dauer WKH, Incarbone R, Bremner CG, DeMeester TR. Clinical and physiologic comparison of laparoscopic and open Nissen fundoplication. J Am Coll Surg 1995;180:385-393.
14. Watson DI, Jamieson GG, Pike GK, Davis N, Richardson M, Devitt PG. Prospective randomised doulbe blind trial between laparoscopic Nissen fundoplication and anterior particle fundoplication. Br J Surg 1999;86:123-130.

What is the current rate of gas-bloat syndrom following open and laparoscopic antireflux surgery?

M.I. Booth, T.C.B. Dehn (Reading)

Antireflux surgery has a well-established position in the treatment of gastroesophageal reflux disease. Postfundoplication symptoms are seen in a proportion of patients, and in some may undermine the success of the antireflux procedure. The term "gas bloat" describes symptoms caused by gaseous distension of the stomach due to an inability to vent gas from the stomach by belching. Upper abdominal discomfort and distension may be accompanied by sweating and dizziness. Symptoms are usually encountered after meals, and in particular after fizzy drinks. The term "gas bloat syndrome" is also used to encompass a range of related symptoms, including postprandial fullness, back, chest and shoulder tip pain, inability to belch to relieve bloating, inability to vomit, generalised abdominal bloating and increased passage of flatus. Most surgical series rely upon subjective assessment of symptoms with much variation in terminology, severity scoring and follow-up period. This inevitably contributes to the widely differing rates of gas bloat reported in the literature.

With each swallow, 10-20 mls of air is introduced into the stomach. In normal circumstances this air is vented by gastroesophageal, followed by esophagopharyngeal gas reflux, *i.e.* "belching". This process is stimulated by distension of the gastric fundus. In normal subjects the majority of gastroesophageal gas reflux episodes occur during spontaneous (*i.e.* non-swallow induced) transient lower esophageal sphincter (LES) relaxations, which occur more frequently in the upright position [1]. Gastroduodenal gas efflux seems to play a much smaller role in the emptying of gas from the stomach [2]. In patients with gastroesophageal reflux (GER) and a defective LES, gas reflux also occurs during periods of prolonged LES hypotension. GER patients may be prone to aerophagy as a result of swallowing in order to neutralize symptomatic acid reflux with saliva, a learned behaviour pattern that may persist following fundoplication and contribute to postoperative bloating.

A number of techniques have been employed to assess objectively the influence of fundoplication on subjects' ability to belch. Smith *et al.* [3] assessed belch volumes by distending patients' stomachs with carbon dioxide and collecting belched air in a closed container system. After antireflux surgery, patients had a lower volume of individual belches and a reduced overall amount of belched gas compared to volunteers. However, no association could be shown between the volume of gas belched and gas bloat type symptoms.

The yield pressure of the gastroesophageal junction (GEJ) has been used as an indicator of gastroesophageal competence before and after surgery. It is determined by measuring the intragastric pressure required to open the GEJ, thus allowing equalisation of gastric and esophageal pressures. Yield pressures are significantly lower in patients with esophagitis than in healthy controls, and fundoplication causes an increase in yield pressure [4] that is irrespective of a change in the basal LES pressure [5]. However, the relationship between yield pressure, fundoplication technique and postfundoplication symptoms has not been addressed.

Johnsson *et al.* [6] used the manometric appearance of equalization of gastric and esophageal pressures (the so-called "common cavity phenomenon") as a surrogate marker of gastroesophageal gas reflux in patients before and after open 360° fundoplication. Fundoplication reduced the number of common cavity episodes and the number of transient LES relaxations following gastric distension without affecting the basal LES pressure. Rydberg *et al.* [7] used similar methods to compare total (360° Nissen-Rossetti) fundoplication and posterior partial (270° or Toupet) fundoplication. Common cavity episodes occurred more frequently in patients who had a Toupet procedure than in those who had a total fundic wrap. In addition basal LES tone was significantly higher after a total wrap, as was the nadir LES pressure after water swallows. However no attempt was made to correlate these findings with the patients symptoms post fundoplication.

More recently, Tew *et al.* [8] found that half of their post-Nissen fundoplication patient group reported the ability to belch, but no patient had a common cavity associated with a belch urge. This was in contrast to a control group in whom 48% of belch urges produced a common cavity. This raises the possibility that when reporting the ability to belch postoperatively, patients are in fact describing the venting of air retained in the esophagus rather than true gastroesophagopharyngeal gas reflux. This may help explain the observed discrepancies between the ability to belch and the ability to relieve bloating by belching, the latter being of more importance clinically.

The role which gastric emptying plays in post fundoplication symptoms is unclear. A proportion of patients with GER have delayed gastric emptying preoperatively, and it has been suggested that failure to improve gastric emptying is a factor in the development of post fundoplication symptoms [9]. Delayed gastric-emptying of solids preoperatively may help predict those patients who develop long-term postoperative symptoms of bloating and early satiety [10].

Gas bloat following open antireflux surgery has been reported to occur in 0-41% of patients [11-13, 15, 16, 18-24] (*Table I*). Despite this, few randomized studies have involved a comparison of the relative incidence of gas bloat using different surgical techniques. The largest study to date randomized 137 patients to a 360° (Nissen-Rossetti) or a 270° (Toupet) fundoplication [11]. There were no intergroup differences in the incidence of bloating or post prandial fullness at any postoperative follow-up point between 3 and 60 months. Overall, the ability to belch was present in 80% of patients at 5 years postoperatively. Smaller studies of Nissen *versus* Lind [12], Nissen *versus* Nissen-Rossetti [13] and Nissen *versus* Hill *versus* Belsey markIV fundoplication [14] have also failed to show any significant differences. In a non-randomized study of Nissen fundoplication, DeMeester *et al.* [15] noted that patients with normal LES characteristics on manometry preoperatively were more likely to suffer from gas bloat and flatus, as were those with upright reflux alone. Uncontrolled studies of partial posterior or anterior fundoplication

Table I.

Author	Procedure(s)	N	F/U (months)	Gas bloat (%)	Inability to belch (%)	Inability to relieve bloat (%)
Watson [19]	LNF + sgv *versus* LNF	102	6	41 *versus* 35	53 *versus* 38	43 *versus* 35
Watson [18]	LAF *versus* LNF	107	6	19 *versus* 28	17 *versus* 36	17 *versus* 32
Watson [22]	LAF	26	3-10	0	0	n/a
Walker [12]	ONF *versus* OLF	52	3-33	35 *versus* 15	n/a	n/a
Luostarinen [13]	ONF + sgv *versus* ONF	50	6-53	8 *versus* 22	15 *versus* 26	n/a
Lundell [11]	ONF *versus* OTF	137	36-60	26	20	n/a
Watson [16]	OAF	100	17-66	0	0	n/a
Franzen [23]	OPPF	84	72-168	13	21	n/a
Luostarinen [20]	ONF	25	216-264	36	60	n/a
Grande [24]	ONF	157	36-240	7	n/a	n/a
DeMeester [15]	ONF	100	12-156	15	36	n/a

LNF: laparoscopic Nissen fundoplication; + sgv: with division of short gastric vessels;
LAF: laparoscopic anterior (partial) fundoplication; ONF: open Nissen fundoplication;
OLF: open Lind (posterior partial) fundoplication;
OTF: open Toupet (posterior partial) fundoplication; OPPF: open posterior partial fundoplication

[16, 17] have claimed a reduced rate of postfundoplication symptoms but these claims have yet to be confirmed in randomized controlled trials. Equally there have been few randomized trials comparing the incidence of postoperative symptoms following fundoplication performed open and laparoscopically, although in non-randomized studies the incidence of gas-bloat produced laparoscopically seems to mirror that produced by open surgery. Comparisons of different laparoscopic techniques with short-term follow-up suggest that patients are more likely to be able to belch and less likely to complain of increased flatus if they undergo anterior partial fundoplication as opposed to total fundoplication [18]. Division or preservation of the short gastric vessels in the formation of a laparoscopic 360° wrap does not appear to influence gas bloat symptoms [19] .

Information on longer term follow-up by necessity comes from studies of open fundoplication. These suggest that gas bloat can persist for many years following surgery. In their 20-year follow-up of 25 patients who underwent Nissen fundoplication, Luostarinen *et al.* [20] identified nine patients with bloating and fifteen who were unable to belch. However none of their patients cited these symptoms as a cause of unsatisfactory outcome. An earlier report from the same group showed that patients with impaired belching postoperatively had significantly greater increases in flatus, although these symptoms were described as severe by only 1 patient out of 109 [21].

Most patients with gas-bloat symptoms postfundoplication will describe their symptoms as minor in comparison to the GER symptoms for which they had their surgery, and can be managed with a combination of reassurance, and general advice (avoiding fizzy drinks, heavy meals, etc.). The perception that symptoms improve with time receives limited support from the literature, with it being equally likely that patients simply become more tolerant of their symptoms with time. Endoscopic balloon dilation of the GEJ is of proven benefit for post fundoplication dysphagia, but may also be helpful for gas-bloat. The occasional patient with intractable symptoms can be offered re-operation, with the option of converting a total to a partial fundoplication.

Other aspects of laparoscopic antireflux surgery (conversion rate, re-operation rate, postoperative dysphagia rates, etc.) have been shown to be dependent on surgical experience, both individual and institutional, and no doubt the same applies to gas-bloat symptoms. Regardless of this, severe post fundoplication bloating is rare, and minor degrees of bloating may be seen as an acceptable price to pay for a successful antireflux procedure.

References

1. Wyman JB, Dent J, Heddle R, Dodds WJ, Toouli J, Downton J. Control of belching by the lower oesophageal sphincter. Gut 1990;31:639-646.
2. McInally E, Kelly E, Inglefinger F. Mechanism of belching: effects of gastric distension with air. Gastroenterology 1964;46:254-259.
3. Smith D, King NA, Waldron B, Cullen PT, Millar B, Fenwick M, Campbell FC. Study of belching ability in antireflux surgery patients and normal volunteers. Br J Surg 1991;78:32-35.
4. McGouran RCM, Galloway JM, Wells FC, Hendrie ORS. Is yield pressure at the cardia increased by effective fundoplication? Gut 1989;30:1309-1312.
5. Ismail T, Bancewicz J, Barlow J. Yield pressure, anatomy of the cardia and gastro-oesophageal reflux. Br J Surg 1995;82;943-947.
6. Johnsson F, Holloway RH, Ireland AC, Jamieson GG, Dent J. Effect of fundoplication on transient lower oesophageal sphincter relaxation and gas reflux. Br J Surg 1997;84:686-689.
7. Rydberg L, Ruth M, Lundell L. Mechanism of action of antireflux procedures. Br J Surg 1999;86:405-410.
8. Tew S, Ackroyd R, Jamieson GG, Holloway RH. Belching and bloating:facts and fantasy after antireflux surgery. Br J Surg 2000;87:477-481.

9. Hinder RA, Stein HJ, Bremner CG, DeMeester TR. Relationship of a satisfactory outcome to normalization of delayed gastric emptying after Nissen fundoplication. Ann Surg 1989;210:458-465.
10. Lundell LR, Myers JC, Jamieson GG. Delayed gastric emptying and its relationship to symptoms of «gas bloat» after antireflux surgery. Eur J Surg 1994;160:161-166.
11. Lundell L, Abrahamsson H, Ruth M, Rydberg L, Lonroth H, Olbe L. Long-term results of a prospective randomized comparison of total fundic wrap (Nissen-Rossetti) or semifundoplication (Toupet) for gastro-oesophageal reflux. Br J Surg1996;83:830-835.
12. Walker SJ, Holt S, Sanderson CJ, Stoddard CJ. Comparison of Nissen total and Lind partial transabdominal fundoplication in the treatment of gastro-oesophageal reflux. Br J Surg 1992;79:410-414.
13. Luostarinen MES, Isolauri JO. Randomized trial to study the effect of fundic mobilization on long-term results of Nissen fundoplication. Br J Surg 1999;86:614-618.
14. DeMeester TR, Johnson LF, Kent AH. Evaluation of current operations for the prevention of gastroesophageal reflux. Ann Surg 1974;180:511-525.
15. DeMeester TR, Bonavina L, Albertucci M. Nissen fundoplication for gastroesophageal reflux disease. Evaluation of primary repair in 100 consecutive patients. Ann Surg 1986;204:9-20.
16. Watson A, Jenkinson LR, Ball CS, Barlow AP, Norris TL. A more physiological alternative to total fundoplication for the surgical correction of resistant gastro-oesophageal reflux. Br J Surg 1991;78:1088-1094.
17. Hill LD. An effective operation for hiatal hernia:an eight year appraisal. Ann Surg 1967;166:681-692.
18. Watson DI, Jamieson GG, Pike GK, Davies N, Richardson M, Devitt PG. Prospective randomized double-blind trial between laparoscopic Nissen fundoplication and anterior partial fundoplication. Br J Surg1999;86:123-130.
19. Watson DI, Pike GK, Baigrie RJ, Mathew G, Devitt PG, Britten-Jones R, Jamieson GG. Prospective double-blind randomized trial of laparoscopic Nissen fundoplication with division and without division of short gastric vessels. Ann Surg 1997;226:642-652.
20. Luostarinen M, Isolauri J, Laitinen J, Koskinene M, Markkula H, Lehtinen E, Uusitalo A. Fate of Nissen fundoplication after 20 years. A clinical, endoscopical, and functional analysis. Gut 1993;34;1015-1020.
21. Luostarinen M. Nissen fundoplication for reflux esophagitis. Long-term clinical and endoscopic results in 109 of 127 consecutive patients. Ann Surg 1993;217;329-337.
22. Watson A, Spychal RT, Brown MG, Peck N, Callander N. Laparoscopic "physiological" antireflux procedure: preliminary results of a prospective symptomatic and objective study. Br J Surg 1995;82:651-656.
23. Franzen T, Bostrom J, Tibbling Grahn L, Johansson KF. Prospective study of symptoms and gastro-oesophageal reflux 10 years after posterior partial fundoplication. Br J Surg 1999;86:956-960.
24. Grande L, Toledo-Pimental V, Manterola C, Lacima G, Ros E, Garcia-Valdecasas JC, Fuster J, Visa J, Pera C. Value of Nissen fundoplication in patients with gastro-oesophageal reflux judged by long-term symptom control. Br J Surg 1994;81:548-550.

Is gas-bloat syndrome likely to occur after medical therapy?

S.J. Spechler (Dallas)

The gas-bloat syndrome is a variably defined and poorly characterized constellation of symptoms that can occur after fundoplication surgery for the treatment of gastroesophageal reflux disease (GERD). Symptoms often ascribed to gas-bloat syndrome include increased abdominal girth, abdominal fullness, inability to belch, and inability to vomit. However, GERD often is associated with abnormalities in gastric emptying and with motility disturbances that can produce symptoms that mimic the gas-bloat syndrome. In the VA Cooperative Study on GERD conducted from 1986 through 1988, 247 patients with complicated reflux disease were randomized to receive either medical therapy in the form of antacids, histamine H_2-receptor blockers, metoclopramide, and sucralfate; or surgical therapy in the form of Nissen fundoplication [1]. During the first year, both groups were questioned regarding the frequency of gas-bloat symptoms. Results for the first year were on *Table I*.

There was a significant increase in the frequency of the symptoms of inability to belch and vomit, but no significant difference in the frequency of the symptoms of increased abdominal girth and abdominal fullness. In the recently published follow-up study of this group, results 10 to 13 years later were on *Table II* [2].

Long-term there was no significant difference in the frequency of any of these symptoms of gas-bloat syndrome between the medical and surgical groups. These results suggest that symptoms of gas-bloat are frequent in both medically- and surgically-treated patients with GERD. Unfortunately, the patients were not questioned regarding these symptoms prior to receiving therapy, so it is not possible to determine how many had these symptoms at baseline.

Table I.

	Medical group	Surgical group
Increased abdominal girth	47%	53%
Abdominal fullness	50%	56%
Inability to belch	10%	25%*
Inability to vomit	5%	19%*

*P < 0.05

Table II.

	Medical group	Surgical group
Increased abdominal girth	36%	34%
Abdominal fullness	41%	42%
Inability to belch	20%	29%
Inability to vomit	20%	32%

References

1. Spechler SJ. Comparison of medical and surgical therapy for complicated gastroesophageal reflux disease in veterans. Department of Veterans Affairs Gastroesophageal Reflux Disease Study Group. N Engl J Med 1992;326:786-792.
2. Spechler SJ, Lee E, Ahnen D, Goyal RK, Hirano I, Ramirez F, Raufman JP, Sampliner R, Schnell T, Sontag S, Vlahcevic ZR, Young R, Williford W. Long-term outcome of medical and surgical treatments for gastroesophageal reflux disease. Follow-up of a randomized controlled trial. JAMA 2001;285:2331-2338.

Should highly selective vagotomy be added to antireflux surgery?

H.J. Stein, W.K.H. Kauer, J.R. Siewert (Munich)

With wider use of laparoscopic antireflux surgery, failed antireflux procedures are likely to become more common. We analyzed the causes of failure, management strategies, and outcome in a consecutive series of 105 patients with failed antireflux procedures. The present series and the recently published experience by other authors show, that today recurrent reflux due to disruption of the initial antireflux repair is the most common cause of failure of antireflux surgery [1, 2]. In our experience, this is in most instances due to insufficient fundic mobilization, failure to fix the repair to the cardia, and the use of absorbable suture material. Our study furthermore indicates that denudation of the lesser cuvature, as is performed with proximal gastric vagotomy, results in a high risk for the socalled "telescope phenomenon" [3], consisting of slippage of a fundoplication onto the gastric corpus. In addition, disorders of gastric emptying and lower esophageal sphincter dysfunction may result from this combination of procedures. We therefore discourage the use of proximal gastric vagotomy in combination with antireflux surgery.

References

1. Martin CJ, Crookes PF. Reoperation for failed antireflux surgery. Aust N Z J Surg 1990;60:773-775.
2. Rieger NA, Jamieson GG, Britten-Jones R, et al. Reoperation after failed antireflux surgery. Br J Surg 1994;81:1159-1161.
3. Siewert JR, Lepsien G, Weiser HF, et al. Das Teleskop-Phänomen. Chirurg 1979;48:640-645.

Emergency surgery in Barrett's disease

J. Danis (Linz)

The central role of gastric acid in the pathogenesis of gastroesophageal reflux disease (GERD) is well established. The therapeutic advantage of proton pump inhibitors (PPIs) is evident across all grades of GERD. PPIs became first line therapy in the last ten years. They relieve acute clinical symptoms and result in complete and long lasting healing of the affected esophageal mucosa in 80-90% of patients within 8 weeks [1, 2]. Information about the fate of those patients who remained unhealed after acute failure of PPIs has not been reported, and there are also few information about those, who developed acute complications of Barrett's disease. In this series of patients, early surgery was required for ulcer bleeding, penetration and perforation or esophagus outlet syndrom, due to incarceration or acute ulcerous stenosis.

Patients and methods

Of the 844 GERD patients investigated in our endoscopy department, 757 (89,69%) healed after antisecretory therapy and prokinetics or became a "telephoner". Seven of them having significant bleeding from esophageal ulcers healed during conservative therapy. Thirteen of 844 patients (1,54%) examined in the Endoscopy Department of the General Public Hospital in Hainburg an der Donau, Austria, between 1st January 1991 and 31st August 2000 underwent early surgery (*Table I*).

Table I. Early surgery in Barrett's patients.

Patient	Diagnosis	Symptoms	Period	Operation	O/LS	Complications	Outcome
1. F 64 years	Hiatus hernia, perforated Cameron's ulcer, peritonitis	Retrosternal pain	3 hours	Ulcer excision, suture Nissen, drainage	Open		Excellent
2. M 56 years	Bleeding marginal ulcer after aetoxysclerol inj., esophagus perforation	Retrosternal pain	24 hours	Esophagectomy, gastrostomy 3M later retrosternal colon interposition	Open	Mediastinitis	Good
3. M 73 years	Acute ulcerous esophagus stenosis	Dysphagia, regurgitation	1 week	Modified balanced operation	LS	6-14 days postop. pneumonia	Excellent
4. M 72 years	Acute ulcerous haemorrhagic esophagitis	Haematemesis	48 hours			Irreversible haemorrhagic shock	Died
5. F 82 years	Up side down stomach	Dysphagia, regurgitation	1 week	Posterior crura repair, Toupet	LS		Excellent
6. M 48 years	Mesoaxial stomach volvulus	Intermitent dysphagia, regurgitation	2 months	Derotation, anterior fundopexy, pyloropexy	LS		Excellent
7. F 66 years	Incarcerated paraesophageal hernia ,ulcerous esophagitis	Gastric outlet syndrom	4 days	Posterior crura repair, Nissen	LS	4-9 days postop. pneumonia	Excellent
8. M 72 years	Up side down stomach	Dysphagia, regurgitation	2 days	Posterior crura repair, Toupet	LS		Excellent
9. F 81 years	Paraesophageal hernia, colon incarcerated	Ileus	4 days	Posterior crura repair, Nissen	Open		Excellent
10. F 63 years	Bleeding Barrett's ulcer	Haemorrhagic shock	6 days	Modified balanced operation	Open		Excellent
11. F 65 years	Penetrating marginal ulcer	Heartburn	14 days	Modified balanced operation	Open		Excellent
12. F 50 years	Up side down stomach	Dysphagia, regurgitation, anaemia	4 weeks	Posterior crura repair, Toupet	LS		Excellent
13. M 55 years	Bleeding Barrett's ulcer	Haemorrhagic shock	2 days	Modified balanced operation	LS		Excellent

The first type of the surgery performed (5 patients) was the modified "balanced" operation, with truncal or proximal selective vagotomy, hernia's sac removal, posterior diaphragmatic crura repair and a Nissen floppy wrap fundoplication, as described elsewhere [3]. Surgery was completed with extramucosal pyloroplasty. This operation was performed by laparotomy on three patients with ulcer bleeding (*Figure 1*) and laparoscopically in the next one who suffered from acute edematous stenosis of the esophagus.

The second type operation was done on patients with large paraesophageal hernia or upside down stomach. An anatomical reposition of the herniated/incarcerated part of the stomach (*Figures 2 and 3*), retroesophageal crura repair as well as a Nissen or partial Toupet fundoplication was performed laparoscopically in five of six patients. The trocar position was 5 cm supraombilical, under the xiphoid process, in the left and right hypochondrium and in the left mesogastrium (*Figure 4*). The lesser omentum was divided, diaphragmatic crura were prepared, the hernia sac margin was dissected with the Ultrasonic scissor (Auto suture) and the sac removed. The vagus nerve was identified and separated from the esophagus. The 3-9 retroesophageal, prevagal positioned stitches resulted in an esophagus-sized narrowing of the diaphragmatic hiatus. Surgery was completed with a total or partial fundoplication.

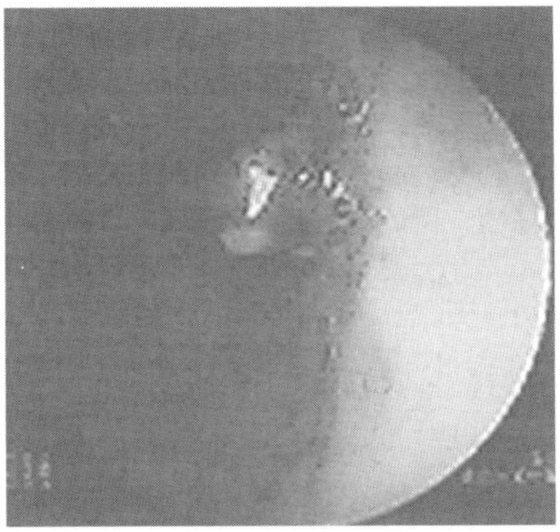

Figure 1. Patient 2 (*Table I*) with bleeding marginal ulcer which was injected. 48 hours later, a perforation of distal esophagus occurred. (See page V for colour figure.)

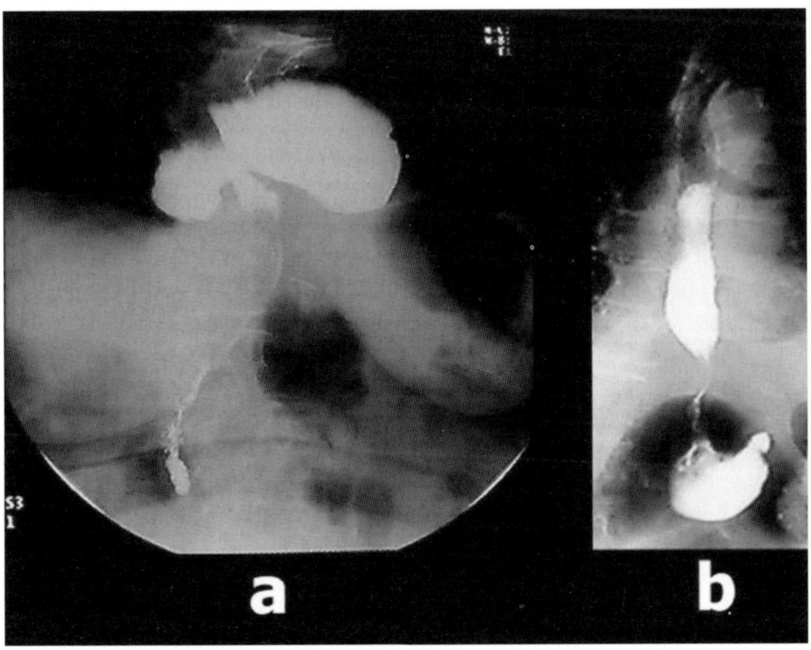

Figure 2.
A. Patient 5. X-ray detected up side down stomach.
B. Postoperative situs.
(See page V for colour figure.)

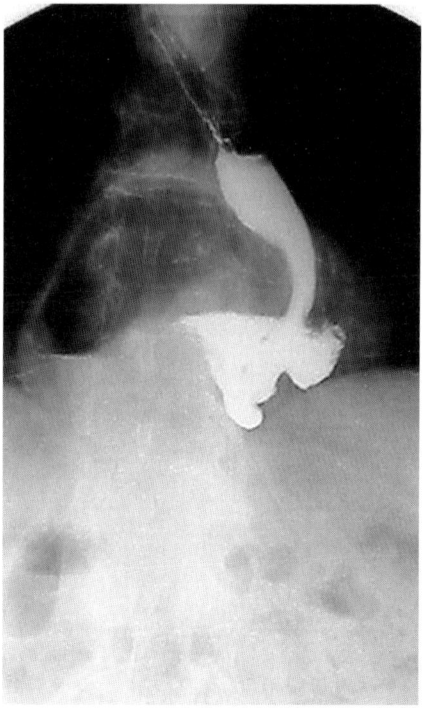

Figure 3. Patient 7 with incarcerated paraesophageal hernia.

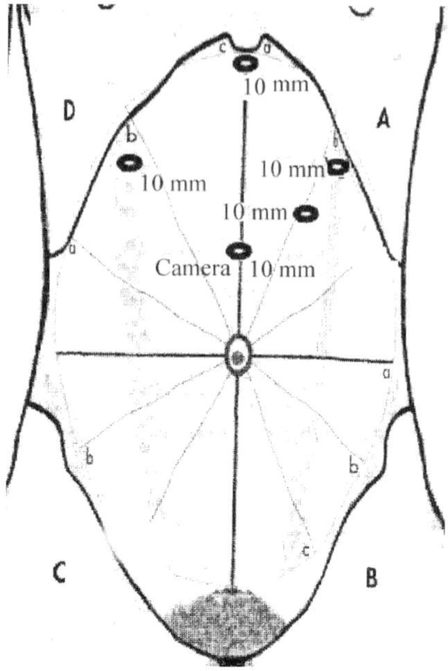

Figure 4. Position of the ports during laparoscopic fundoplication.

The 6th patient suffered from abundant vomiting and ulcerous esophagitis, as stated by gatroscopy. The symptoms ceased surprisingly after the gastroscopy. However, 24 hour later, the full symptomatology relapsed again, and an X-ray Barium examination of the stomach showed an organoaxial volvulus. Subsequent laparoscopy confirmed the X-ray findings but no hiatus hernia could be found. A laparoscopic derotation, with anterior fundopexy and laparoscopic pyloropexy on to pancreatic capsule were performed, using the same approach with five trocars as for the laparoscopic fundoplication. The stomach fundus was sutured firstly with diaphragm, starting on the anterior margin of the hiatus, continuing left anterolateral towards the abdominal wall as previously described [4]. The great curvature was sutured to the anterior abdominal wall with three stitches. Moreover, we fixed the pyloric channel on to the upper margin of the pancreas head capsule. The procedure was completed with plication of the lesser omentum.

In another patient, the bleeding marginal ulcer was treated by means of local injection of Aetoxysclerol® (Kreussel Pharma, Germany). However, a perforation of the ulcer occured within 54 hours, a diffuse mediastinitis developed, and an esophagectomy with cervical esophagostomy, gastrostomy, and mediastinal drainage was then performed. Four months later, esophageal reconstruction with retrosternal gastric tube and esophagogastric anastomosis was performed (Prof. Klepetko, AKH Wienna).

The remaining patient with bleeding Barrett's ulcer died immediately after initial gastroscopy, due to irreversible haemorrhagic shock. In this patient, a concomitant renal carcinoma was found at the autopsy. However, this finding had no link with the ulcerous esophagitis.

Discussion

Since starting laparoscopic treatment of GERD in June 1997, the indications for surgery increased dramatically: between June 7th 1997 and August 31st 2000, elective open surgery was performed in only two patients, and an elective laparoscopic fundoplication indicated in 72 patients. 1,42% required early surgery due to life-threatening complications despite therapy with PPIs and prokinetics. One patient died before surgery (0,12% out of 844).

In an emergency situation, the problem of decision-making as to the indication and choice of surgical procedure is predominant. Except gastric hyperacidity, our knowledge of the natural history of reflux esophagitis is still rather limited. Moreover, emergency patients are often underexamined. Indication for surgery is also supported by the so-called AFP criteria [5, 6] comprisisng the hiatus hernia (Anatomy-A), reflux (Function criterion-F), as well as the Pathology (P) of the distal esophagus. One group of the patients had a severe "non responding" form of GERD with continuous suffering. In the other group, a predominant anatomical impairment, with an incarcerated paraesophageal hernia or up side down stomach could be stated by means of routinely performed endoscopy and X-ray examination. Neither pH metry nor manometry were performed for these patients because of the priority to relieve the symptoms by means of antisecretory drugs and/or surgical control of the life-threatening complications. In emergency situation, we chose the "balanced" operation taking simultaneoustly into account various pathophysiological factors (cardia valve, acid secretion and reservoir emptying). The original procedure, described for the first time by Berman JK and Berman EJ in 1959 [7] was developed further and consists now in highly selective vagotomy with extramucosal pyloroplasty, posterior repair of the diaphragmatic crura with at least three stitches, and a Nissen floppy wrap or a Toupet fundoplication [3]. A next development of the "balanced" operation was the laparoscopic approach in one patient. The rationale for the "balanced" procedure was based on the fact that before the operation, except in the case of the great incarcerated hiatus hernia, we did not know which steps would be necessary to expect a good result. Partial performance of the technique only failed to control specific complications of the GERD [8].

Paraesophageal hernia, an uncommon type of stomach protrusion into the mediastinum, differs from the sliding one in the posterior anchoring of the cardia and its patency. Clinical manifestation may occur through intermittent gastric obstruction or true volvulus. Uncommon reports demonstrating the laparoscopic repair of a paraesophageal hernia are available: they are based mostly on case reports, and no surgical technique could be proposed as a method of choice: in order to narrow the hiatus, an anterior, anterolateral closure of the diaphragm was performed, or prosthetic material was used [9-12]. These techniques were previously used also in classical open surgery. However, the results were not satisfactory and recurrences occurred in 47% [13] The posterior crura repair was successively selected as the method of choice in axial hiatus hernia and this technique was also performed during laparoscopic surgery [14, 15]. An architecture impairment, namely a dehiscence of the diphragm may play a crucial role in the development of a paraesophageal hernia, as a consequence of the widening of the lower thorax aperture due to pulmonary obstruction disease, anatomical constitution, obesity, etc.

Some authors performing anterior crura repair did not construct any mechanical antireflux valve because the posterior cardia anchoring remained intact [10]. However, after anterior suture of the hiatus, the diaphragmatic arch can be retracted more distally and the His angle can be widened, and the intra-abdominal part of the esophagus reduced, both resulting in reflux recurrence [13].

The posterior crura repair paradoxically requires destroying the intact fixation of the esophagus, also resulting in reflux symptoms as found in 80% of 28 patients having undergone open surgery [16]. In comparison, only 18% morbidity was observed in 27 patients on whom an antireflux procedure was performed [17]. All our four patients operated by laparoscopy, with posterior crura repair and antireflux valve for giant paraesophageal hernia remain symptom-free 5-24 months after surgery.

Esophageal lesions resulting in mediastinitis are uncommon. Few reports demonstrate small series having sepsis, fistula or bleeding into the mediastinum [18, 19]. A therapeutic strategy comprises early esophagectomy or diversion/exclusion, intensive care and delayed reconstruction. One of our patients underwent reconstruction of the esophagus four months after the perforation.

In general, the prognosis of untreated complications of GERD is poor. However, a better awareness of the disease and suspicion of its presence are required to prevent delays or errors in diagnosis and allow for appropriate therapeutic decisions. Refined diagnostic including endoscopy, biopsy, pH- and manometry, as well as increasing indications of laparoscopic surgical procedures would enable to shift potential emergency patients to the elective group.

References

1. Vigneri S, Termini R, Leandro G, Badalamenti S, Pantalena M, Savarino V, Di Mario F, Battaglia G, Mela GS, Pilotto A, Plebani M, Davi G. A comparison of five maintenance therapies for reflux esophagitis. N Engl J Med 1995;333:1106-1110.
2. Pace F, Sangaletti O, Trapi E, Santalucia F, Bianchi Porro G. Short and long-term outcome of medically treated reflux esophagitis. Hepatogastroenterology 1995;42:131-134.
3. Danis J. The "Balanced" operation for life threatening complications of severe "non responding" form of gastroesophageal reflux disease. A case report. Hepatogastroenterology 1997;44:302-306.
4. Styger S, Demartines N, Zuber M, Harder F. Der chronischer Magenvolvulus. Chir Praxis 2000;57:231-234.
5. Siewert JR, Feussner H. The options for surgical therapy of reflux esophagitis. Gullet 1993;3:76-83.
6. Bancewicz J, Matthews HR, O'Hawan T, Adams JA. Comparison of surgically treated reflux patients in two surgical centres. In: Little AG, Fergusson MB, Skinner DB, eds. Disease of esophagus Vol II. Mount Kiscoe, New York: Future Publishing Company, 1991:177-180.
7. Bermak JK, Berman EJ. Balanced operation for esophagitis associated with hiatal hernia, hiatal hernia en masse and hiatal hernia with so called true congenitally short esophagus. Arch Surg 1959;78:889.
8. Braghetto I, Csendes A, Burdiles P, Korn O. Antireflux surgery, highly selective vagotomy and duodenal switch procedure: post-operative evaluation in patients with complicated and non complicated Barrett's esophagus. Dis Esophagus 2000;13:12-17.
9. Kuster GG, Gilroy S. Laparoscopic technique for repair of paraesophageal hiatal hernias. J Laparoendosc Surg 1993;3:331-338.
10. Kuvano H, Hashizume M, Ohta Sumiyoshi K, Sugimachi K, Haraguchi Y. Laparoscopic repair of paraesophageal hiatal hernia with gastric volvulus. Hepatogastroenterology 1998;45:303-306.
11. Paul MG, DeRosa RP, Petrucci PE, Palmer ML, Danovitch SH. Laparoscopic tension-free repair of large paraesophageal hernias. Surg Endosc 1993;11:303-307.
12. Watanabe G, Tanaka J, Odashima S, Kitamura M, Koyama K. Laparoscopic repair of paraesophageal hiatus hernia without fundoplication. Surg Today 1997;27:1093-1096.
13. Duda M, Dlouhy M, Gryga A, Rocek V, Kochner M, Herman J. Surgical treatment of patients with paraesophageal and mixed hiatal hernias. Rozhl Chir 1991;70;423-429.
14. Cuschieri A. Laparoscopic antireflux surgery and repair of hiatal hernias. J Laparoendosc Surg 1993;3:331-338.

15. Zacherl H, Danis J, Loncsar G, Grünwald M, Göschl P. Laparoskopische Chirurgie in einem Kreiskrankenhaus. Chir Praxis 2000;57.
16. Styger S, Ackermann C, Schuppiser JP, Tondelli P. Reflux disease following gastropexy for para-esophageal hiatal hernia. Schweiz Med Wochenschr 1995;125:1213-1215.
17. Perez Diaz MD, Turegano Fuentes F, Perez Morera A, Martinez Hijosa E, Calvo Serrano M, del Valle Hernandez E. Incarcerated giant hiatal hernia. Rev Esp Enferm Dig 1993;84:367-371.
18. Antoracci R, Perkins AB, Hillstrom M, Tung GA. General case of the day. Perforated Barrett ulcer of the distal esophagus. Radiographics 1996;16:197-199.
19. Guillem PG, Porte HL, Saudement A, Qandalle PA, Wurtz AJ. Perforation of Barrett's ulcer: a challenge in esophageal surgery. Ann Thorac Surg 2000;69:1707-1710.

What are the drawbacks of vagotomy and antrectomy associated to total duodenal diversion and Roux-en-Y reconstruction?

V. Schumpelick, B. Dreuw, K. Ophoff, N. Ponschek, M. Niewiera
(Aachen)

Today, more than 165 years after Beaumont discovered that the stomach could secrete hydrochloric acid, rarely contains bile in health but in situations of "violent passion" [1] duodenogastric reflux is still under discussion and the focus now lies on its role as a major cofactor for the development of Barrett's esophagus and carcinoma of the gastroesophageal junction [2-4]. Duodenal secretions mainly contain bile acids, pancreatic juice, lecithin, lysolecithin, bicarbonate and phospholipase A and B. The cytotoxic effect of bile acids [5] and lysolecithin [6] has been proven experimentally [3, 4, 7-10]. Whereas acid gastroesophageal reflux (GER) can be treated successfully with modern proton pump inhibitor therapy and a variety of open or laparoscopic antireflux procedures, treatment of duodeno-gastric reflux remains a therapeutic challenge [11, 12].

To prevent duodenal content from refluxing into the stomach (and consecutively refluxing into the esophagus), the duodenal juice has to be diverted from the stomach. There exists a variety of operations to achieve a duodenal diversion. Roux-en-Y gastrojejunostomy [13], suprapapillary Roux-en-Y duodenojejunostomy (so-called duodenal switch operation) [14] or interposition of a jejunal segment between stomach and duodenum [15]. To avoid stomal ulcerations, the classically performed Roux-en-Y gastrojejunostomy requires an additional antrectomy and vagotomy to reduce gastric acid secretion.

The surgeon has to keep in mind that a lot of possible side effects, disturbances of intestinal motility and pancreocibal asynchrony are accompanied with such procedures. Because of the ongoing discussion about the malignant potential of alkaline duodeno-gastroesophageal reflux, its presence in complicated gastroesophageal reflux disease [13, 16, 17] and attempts of treatment by Roux-en-Y diversion [13], we have reanalyzed a series of animal experiments and clinical studies carried out between 1981 and 1996. Initially, they were designed to analyze the risk of ulcer, extent of duodenogastric reflux, gastric acidity, gastric emptying, and motility of different types of gastrointestinal anastomosis, *e.g.* Roux-en-Y loop, jejunal interposition, Billroth I and II anastomosis [15, 18-29]. The results of these studies help for better understanding the effects of vagotomy, antrectomy and Roux-en-Y procedures on the upper gastrointestinal physiology.

Vagotomy

Vagotomy as a treatment for gastroduodenal ulcer was introduced by Dragstedt in 1943 [30]. Vagotomy coincides not only with a reduction of the cephalic phase of secretion but also with a significant reduction of the motor activity of the stomach, especially the antrum. This results in an initially increased evacuation of fluid meals and a delayed emptying of solid meals [31]. As a consequence of loss of antral acidification, serum gastrin is increased. In case of truncal vagotomy or injury of the Crow's Foot (antral branches of the vagus nerve), pyloric motility is disturbed with severe alteration of gastric emptying and stasis. Dissection of the hepatic branches may lead to gall stone formation and injury of the celiac branch to diarrhea.

Reduced gastric acidity after vagotomy impairs the natural resistance to bacterial overgrowth. This effect is enhanced by hypomotility, gastrointestinal stasis and failure of the interdigestive intestinal motility. Reduced gastric acidity with pH rise above 3 will reduce pepsin activity with impairement of the initial stage of protein digestion.

Gastric emptying after vagotomy

Electromyographic recordings in animal experiments implicate that after vagotomy the basal electrical rhythm (phase I of the migrating motoric complex) is disturbed [32, 33]. We studied the electrical and mechanical activity of the gastric wall after truncal vagotomy in 5 dogs. Activity was verified by means of implanted electrodes and pressure transducers. (for details see [34]).

Longlasting motility disturbances expressed as a disorganization of the basic electrical rhythm occurred in the gastric wall. According to the motility pattern periods of tachygastria and tachyarrhythmia were identified. Those periods interrupted the regular fasted motility and persisted in the postprandial period. Simultaneous registration of the mechanical activity of the gastric wall during disorders of the electrical rhythm revealed a complete absence of contractility. This may be one pathophysiological correlate for the frequently described delayed gastric emptying after vagotomy.

Cardiorespiratory effects after vagotomy

In another study on 38 urethan anesthetized guinea-pigs low frequency (1-30 Hz) electrical afferent stimulation of the abdominal vagus was performed before and after bilateral cervical vagotomy. Several cardiovascular and respiratory parameters were measured (for details see [35])

The electrical afferent stimulation of the abdominal vagus elicited cardiovascular and respiratory reflexes, which were eliminated by bilateral cervical vagotomy: two thirds of the animals showed a bradycardia with arrhythmia. Another third had no heart rate alteration. Biphasic blood pressure alteration with an initial decrease and a following increase was the most common blood pressure response. Longlasting stimulation resulted in a blood pressure increase of 25 to 30 mmHg in 75% of the animals. An acceleration of the respiratory rate was noted. A vago-vagal and/or vagosympathetic reflex is considered from this study. The clinical implication of these results for cardiorespiratory alterations following vagotomy are uncertain: it could be demonstrated, however, that there are retrograde effects of the abdominal vagus that will be unquestionably influenced by abdominal vagotomy.

Intragastric pH and ulcer risk after vagotomy and Roux-en-Y

We have performed a study on rats to investigate the influence of vagotomy and the length of the jejunal loop of a Roux-en-Y biliary diversion on gastric pH and stomal ulcer risk. One hundred and seventy male Wistar rats were operated on under general ether aneasthesia and divided in groups. After 1/3 resection of the stomach a Roux-en-Y loop of 3, 6, 9 and 15 cm was created with additional vagotomy in the 15 cm group. For controls a Billroth I and Billroth II anastomosis was performed and one group was gastrotomized only.

Ten months later the animals underwent endoscopy, gastric pH from samples by gastric tube and stimulated gastric secretion with injection of 2 mg/kg histamine s.c. The ulcer free animals got a 7 day stimulation by histamine before the examinations were repeated. All ulcers were finally confirmed by autopsy and histologic verification (for details see [18, 36]).

A high incidence of stomal ulceration was found in rats, which was directly related to the length of the interposed jejunal segment (*Figure 1*). The reflux free stomachs with long Roux-en-Y limb developed stomal ulcerations in 72.7% within 10 months, after additional histamine stimulation in 91%. The interval of ulcer manifestation could be shortened to 10 days by continuous histamine stimulation, while the differences between the groups remained unchanged. An additional vagotomy caused a significant reduction of the ulcer risk from 93% to 17% for the 15 cm long Roux-en-Y loop. The gastric pH was influenced by the length of the jejunal segment. An additional vagotomy caused a significant elevation

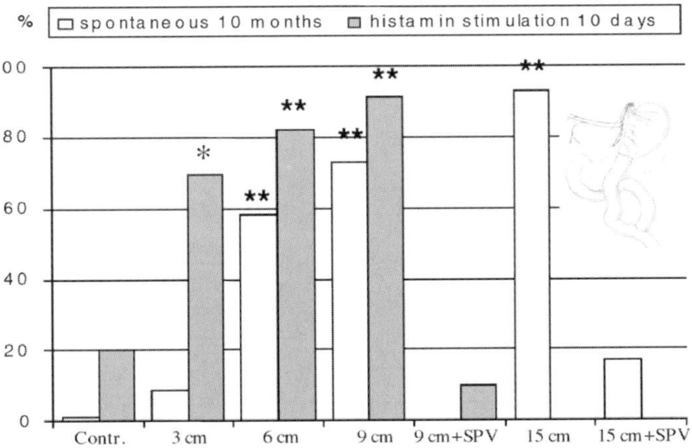

Figure 1. Ulcer incidence following Roux-en-Y gastrojejunostomy spontaneously 10 months after surgery and 10 days after histamine stimulation.
Note the significantly reduced but still existing ulcer incidence following additional vagotomy in the long, refluxfree loops of 9 and 15 cm length (values expressed as mean ± SEM, * $p < 0{,}05$, ** $p < 0{,}01$, compared to controls, Shi square test).

of the pH from 1,8 to 4,2 for the 15 cm long Roux-en-Y (*Figure 2*). Analysis of gastric secretion showed that secretion volume (*Figure 3*) and acid secretion (*Figure 4*) are not significantly influenced by the length of the Roux-en-Y limb. Only vagotomy significantly reduces acid secretion but not secretion volume. The complete results are summarized in *Table I*.

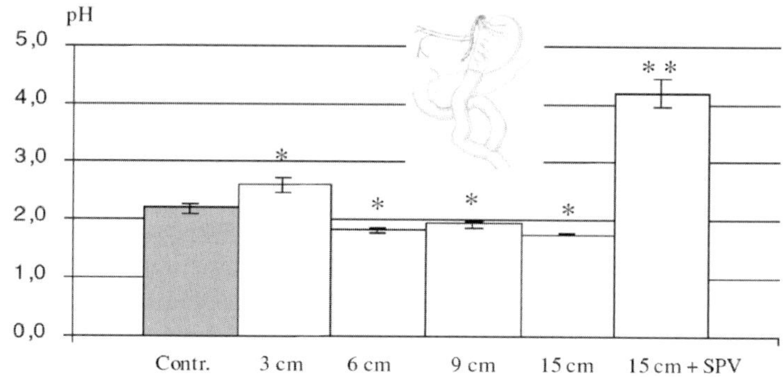

Figure 2. pH-values under fasting conditions following Roux-en-Y gastrojejunostomy of different lengths and additional vagotomy (values expressed as mean ± SEM, * p < 0,05, ** p < 0,005, compared to controls, Shi square test).

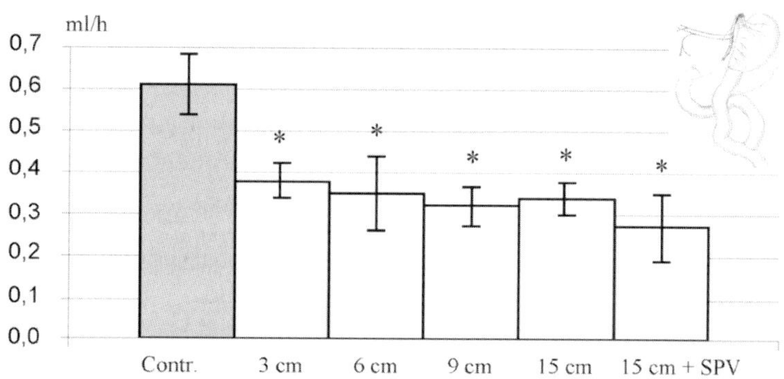

Figure 3. Analysis of gastric secretion following 1/3 resection and Roux-en-Y gastrojejunostomy of different lengths and additional vagotomy (* p < 0,01, compared to controls, Shi square test). Note that additionally vagotomy does not have a significant influence on the secretion volume.

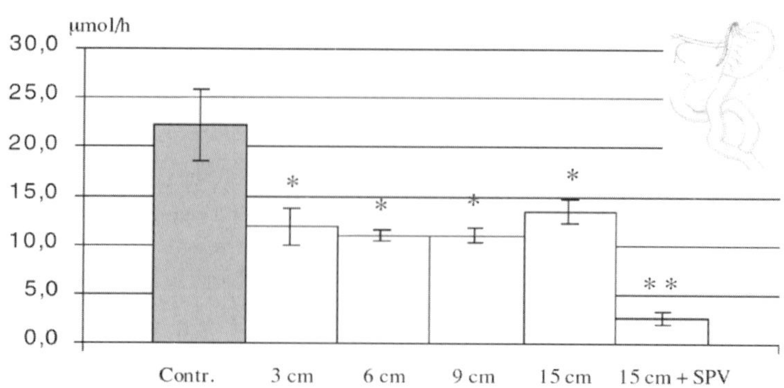

Figure 4. Analysis of gastric secretion following 1/3 resection and Roux-en-Y gastrojejunostomy of different lengths and additional vagotomy (* p < 0,01 compared to controls, ** p < 0,001 compared to all other groups). Note that additionally vagotomy significantly reduces the acid output.

Table I. Results of intraluminal pH, spontaneous and histamin stimulated ulcer incidence and analysis of gastric secretion following gastric resection of various extent and Roux-en-Y gastrojejunostomy (RYR) with and without additional vagotomy (SPV), Billroth I and II anastomosis and controls in rats.

Group	Intragastric pH Spontaneous		Ulcer incidence		Secretion analysis pH		Volume		Acid	
	pH	SEM	Spontaneous %	Histamine stim. %	pH	SEM	ml/h	SEM	umol/h	SEM
Controls	2,2	0,1	0	20	1,9	0,3	0,6	0,1	22,2	3,5
3 cm RYR	2,6	0,1	9	70	1,6	0,1	0,4	0,0	11,9	1,9
6 cm RYR	1,8	0,1	58	82	1,6	0,2	0,4	0,1	11,0	0,6
9 cm RYR	1,9	0,1	73	91	1,6	0,1	0,3	0,1	11,0	0,8
9 cm RYR + SPV				10						
15 cm RYR	1,8	0,0	93		1,8	0,1	0,3	0,0	13,4	1,3
15 cm RYR + SPV	4,2	0,2	17		3,0	0,1	0,3	0,1	2,7	0,8
Billroth I	3,3	0,3	0		2,3	0,3	0,4	0,1	12,9	2,3
Billroth II	3,0	0,2	0	58	1,8	0,1	0,4	0,0	11,4	1,8
Controls	2,2	0,1	0		1,9	0,3	0,6	0,1	22,2	3,5
1/3 resection + Roux Y	1,9	0,1	73		1,6	0,1	0,3	0,1	11,0	0,8
1/2 resection + Roux Y	1,9	0,1	64		1,9	0,1	0,3	0,0	7,8	1,2
2/3 resection + Roux Y	2,1	0,1	54		1,9	0,1	0,2	0,0	5,9	0,7
2/3 res. + Roux Y + SPV	4,5	0,3	20		3,3	0,2	0,2	0,0	2,6	0,6

We conclude from this study, that there is a protective role of the postresectional intestinogastric reflux on the gastrojejunal anastomosis concerning stomal ulceration. The gastric pH and the ulcer incidence are influenced by the length of the jejunal segment, the longer the segment, the more acid is the pH and the higher is the ulcer risk. A reflux preventive procedure utilizing a long Roux-en-Y duodenal diversion is therefore heavily ulcerprone and needs an additional vagotomy to lower the risk of stomal ulceration.

Antrectomy

In another study on 67 rats with the same design than the study mentioned above the influence of antrectomy and extent of gastric resection on intragastric pH and ulcer incidence for Roux-en-Y diversion was studied. The Roux-en-Y limb was chosen 9 cm long to achieve a reflux free condition. Five groups were created with 1/3, 1/2 , 2/3, 2/3 resection with additional vagotomy and one control group with gastrotomy only. The ulcer risk was significantly increased in all resection groups, but not in the group with additional vagotomy. The pH was low and not different from controls in the resection groups. Only after additional vagotomy the pH rose above pH 3. Gastric analysis showed that acid secretion per hour was significantly reduced in all resection groups, without differences between each other. Additional vagotomy resulted in a significanlty further reduction of acid secretion. Secretion volume was reduced by 1/3 and 1/2 gastric resection, and significanly more reduced by 2/3 resection without any additional effect of vagotomy. In summary this study showed that in case of reflux free condition with long Roux-en-Y, antrectomy has no effect on intragastric pH although it reduces acid secretion and secretion volume. Even more extended resection has little effect on secretion parameters and no effect on ulcer risk. Only additional vagotomy significantly increases gastric pH and reduces the risk for stomal ulceration.

Antrectomy will also result in a fall of the serum gastrin concentration, which removes the trophic effect of gastrin on the gastric mucosa [37].

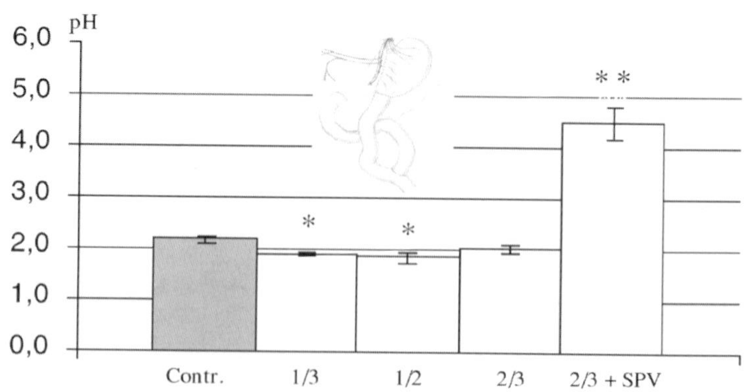

Figure 5. pH-values under fasting conditions following Roux-en-Y gastrojejunostomy of 9 cm length and different extent of gastric resection (values expressed as mean ± SEM, * $p < 0,05$, ** $p < 0,01$, compared to controls, Shi square test). Note that additional vagotomy has more effect on gastric pH than extent of resection.

Roux-en-Y loop

History

During the last 100 years, since Cesar Roux (1857-1934) began utilizing his "Loop-en-Y" procedure for gastric outlet obstruction, this technique fell into disfavour at the beginning of the 20th century due to a high incidence of postoperative stomal ulceration. Later, with additional vagotomy, it was revived in the 1950's and 1960's and was adapted for multiple applications. The greatest factor in its revival has been the treatment of postgastrectomy syndromes, including alkaline reflux gastritis, gastric atony, dumping and other syndromes as well as for the occasional treatment of complicated reflux esophagitis. Additionally, the Roux-en-Y anastomosis has been used to drain diverse organs as the biliary tract, pancreas and esophagus.

In the 1970's it became obvious that the Roux-en-Y procedure has more specific drawbacks. The main complication of loop-en-Y is the so-called Roux syndrome, secondary to gastric or efferent jejunal stasis, or both. Clinically, this symptom complex consists of epigastric fullness, nausea, intermittent or postprandial vomiting, or postprandial abdominal pain. These symptoms occur in up to 50% of all patients [38]. These complications limit the widespread use of Roux-en-Y gastrectomy for treatment of alkaline GER.

Duodenogastric reflux after Roux-en-Y

To investigate the amount of postresectional intestinogastricreflux following different types of gastrointestinal anastomosis, the duodenogastric reflux of bile acids and lysolecithin was studied in 48 pigs after Roux-Y-gastroenterostomy and compared to different types of gastroduodenostomy and jejunal interposition (for details see [39]).

The intragastric concentrations of bile acids and lysolecithin were found to be elevated after gastroduodenostomy compared to controls. An effective reflux prevention was possible by Roux-en-Y duodenal diversion of 50 cm length or by interposition of 25 cm of isoperistaltic jejunum. Bile acid and lysolecithin concentrations were lowest after Roux-en-Y diversion.

The results of this study underline that Roux-en-Y diversion has a low incidence of duodenogastric reflux. Thus this is an effective procedure to eliminate primary or secondary duodenogastric reflux.

Gastric emptying after Roux-en-Y

Gastric emptying is frequently delayed after Roux-en-Y gastrojejunostomy. It was shown that motility disturbances in the Roux-en-Y limb act as a functional outlet obstruction [40].

Intraluminal pressure recordings in patients with Roux-stasis syndrom showed that the motility is altered in the fasting as well as in the postprandial state [40]. These motility alterations are accompanied by disturbances of the transit [41]. Normal gastric emptying [42, 43] as well as delayed gastric emptying [38, 44] is described after Roux-en-Y. We studied the gastric emptying of Roux-en-Y gastrojejunostomy in an animal experiment using 12 female beagle dogs and a medium-viscosity nutrient meal (Meritene®). Four normal dogs were used as controls, 4 underwent a Billroth I gastrectomy and 4 a Roux-en-Y gastrectomy under general anaesthesia without additional vagotomy. Six weeks later, 8 strain gauge force transducers were implanted, 1 on the gastric remnant, 4 to the Roux limb and the duodenum, respectively, and 3 on the jejunum, beginning 30 cm distal to the ligament of Treitz. Gastric emptying was measured radiographically while motility was recorded simultaneously on a polygraph (for details see [21]).

Gastric emptying after Roux-Y gastrectomy was almost linear and not different from that in intact control dogs. In contrast to Roux-en-Y gastrectomy, emptying after Billroth I gastrectomy was initially accelerated and followed by a slow emptying phase. During the initial period, the segmenting activity of the Roux-en-Y limb significantly differed from the propulsive contractile pattern of the duodenum after Billroth I reconstruction. Force and frequency of gastrointestinal contractions were equivalent after both reconstruction procedures.

The results of this study showed that after gastric resection and Roux-en-Y anastomosis, the jejunal motility pattern is profoundly altered after the Roux-en-Y procedure and is responsible for the gastric emptying rate, which is slower than after Billroth I resection and comparable to normal gastric emptying. Our results further indicate that after subtotal gastrectomy, the intestinal contractile patterns are important determinants of gastric emptying.

Conclusion

The conventional Roux-en-Y duodenal diversion utilizing a long limb (50-60 cm) is an effective procedure to eliminate duodenogastric reflux. It caries an increased risk of stomal ulceration which makes an additional vagotomy and antrectomy necessary. Vagotomy and antrectomy cause a parasympathetic denervation of the intestinum, impaired gastric emptying, diminished gastric acid secretion, decreased size of the gastric reservoir, loss of the pylorus with changes in gastric emptying, interruption of neurohumoral relationships and feedback mechanisms of the stomach, duodenum, pancreas and the hepatobiliary system as well as a reduced trophic effect of gastrin on gastric mucosa. In combination with Roux-en-Y biliary diversion, the side effects of the Roux limb are added with negative effects on gastric emptying, loss of stimulation of the duodenal mucosa by chyme and, consecutively, a negative influence on the release of gastrointestinal hormones and digestive gland secretion (secretin, CCK-pancreozymin, GIP, motilin), alterations on motility patterns of the entire intestinal tract and a dissociation between the motility patterns of the bypassed duodenum and the rest of the gastrointestinal tract. Clinically this may result in epigastric fullness, nausea, intermittent or postprandial vomiting, or postprandial abdominal pain in a reasonable number of patients.

The suprapapillary Roux-en-Y duodenojejunostomy (duodenal switch) without vagotomy and antrectomy seems to entail less drawbacks [14], and therefore might be a better alternative than classical Roux-en-Y duodenal diversion. Because the preservation of a 3-7 cm segment of duodenum with its capability to secrete bicarbonates and neutralize gastric acid, the incidence of stomal ulcer is theoretically low and could be proven to be true in experimental [14] and clinical [45] work. This allows to make the loop long enough (50-60 cm) to prevent from alkaline reflux without fear for stomal ulceration. However, other side effects including pancreocibal asynchrony, duodenal hypomotility and bacterial overgrowth with possible alterations in digestion and assimilation may be the same as for conventional Roux-en-Y duodenal diversion. Therefore it should be restricted to the rare cases of otherwise untreatable patients as long as late results underline the initially optimistic results of duodenal switch [14, 45-48].

References

1. Beaumont W. Experiments and observations on the gastric juice and the physiology of digestion.Plattsburgh: Allen FP, 1933.
2. Attwood SE, Smyrk TC, DeMeester TR, Mirvish SS, Stein HJ, Hinder RA. Duodenoesophageal reflux and the development of esophageal adenocarcinoma in rats. Surgery 1992;111(5):503-510.
3. Fein M, Peters JH, Chandrasoma P, Ireland AP, Oberg S, Ritter MP, Bremner CG, Hagen JA, DeMeester TR. Duodenoesophageal reflux induces esophageal adenocarcinoma without exogenous carcinogen. J Gastrointest Surg 1998;2(3):260-268.
4. Pera M, Trastek VF, Carpenter HA, Fernandez PL, Cardesa A, Mohr U, Pairolero PC. Influence of pancreatic and biliary reflux on the development of esophageal carcinoma. Ann Thorac Surg 1993;55(6):1386-1392.
5. Grant R, Grossmann MI, Wang KJ, Ivy AC. The cytolytic action of some gastro-intestinal secretions and enzymes on the epithelial cells of the gastric and duodenal mucosa. J Comp Cell Physiol 1951;37:137.
6. Orchard R, Reynolds K, Fox B, Andrews R, Parkins RA, Johnson AG. Effect of lysolecithin on gastric mucosal structure and potential difference. Gut 1977;18(6):457-461.
7. Clark GW, Smyrk TC, Mirvish SS, Anselmino M, Yamashita Y, Hinder RA, DeMeester TR, Birt DF. Effect of gastroduodenal juice and dietary fat on the development of Barrett's esophagus and esophageal neoplasia: an experimental rat model. Ann Surg Oncol 1994;1(3):252-261.
8. Fein M, Ireland AP, Ritter MP, Peters JH, Hagen JA, Bremner CG, DeMeester TR. Duodenogastric reflux potentiates the injurious effects of gastroesophageal reflux. J Gastrointest Surg 1997;1(1):27-33.
9. Ireland AP, Peters JH, Smyrk TC, DeMeester TR, Clark GW, Mirvish SS, Adrian TE. Gastric juice protects against the development of esophageal adenocarcinoma in the rat. Ann Surg 1996;224(3):358-370.
10. Pera M, Cardesa A, Bombi JA, Ernst H, Pera C, Mohr U. Influence of esophagojejunostomy on the induction of adenocarcinoma of the distal esophagus in Sprague-Dawley rats by subcutaneous injection of 2,6-dimethylnitrosomorpholine. Cancer Res 1989;49(23):6803-6808.
11. Niemela S. Duodenogastric reflux in patients with upper abdominal complaints or gastric ulcer with particular reference to reflux-associated gastritis. Scand J Gastroenterol Suppl 1985;115:1-56.
12. Scudamore HH, Eckstam EE, Fencil WJ, Jaramillo CA. Bile reflux gastritis. Diagnosis, medical and surgical therapy. Am J Gastroenterol 1973;60(1):9-22.
13. Ellis-FH J, Gibb SP. Vagotomy, antrectomy, and Roux-en-Y diversion for complex reoperative gastroesophageal reflux disease. Ann Surg 1994;220(4):536-542.
14. DeMeester TR, Fuchs KH, Ball CS, Albertucci M, Smyrk TC, Marcus JN. Experimental and clinical results with proximal end-to-end duodenojejunostomy for pathologic duodenogastric reflux. Ann Surg 1987;206(4):414-426.
15. Schumpelick V, Stachow R, Schreiber HW. Late results of jejunal interposition. Scand J Gastroenterol 1984;92 227-231.
16. Stein HJ, Barlow AP, DeMeester TR, Hinder RA. Complications of gastroesophageal reflux disease. Role of the lower esophageal sphincter, esophageal acid and acid/alkaline exposure, and duodenogastric reflux. Ann Surg 1992;216(1):35-43.
17. Stein HJ, Kauer WK, Feussner H, Siewert JR. Bile reflux in benign and malignant Barrett's esophagus:e ffect of medical acid suppression and Nissen fundoplication. J Gastrointest Surg 1998;2(4):333-341.
18. Arlt G, Schumpelick V, Riechert B, Kloppel G. The ulcer risk in reflux preventive gastric operations. An experimental study. Scand J Gastroenterol Suppl 1984;92 125-128.
19. Begemann F, Schumpelick V. Problems in duodenogastric reflux assessment, using bile acid and lysolecithin measurement. Scand J Gastroenterol Suppl 1981;67 51-53.
20. Bolder U, Bares R, Arlt G, Hojabri K, Schumpelick V. Bile acid retention after Roux-en-Y biliary reconstruction demonstrated by tauro-23-(75Se)selena-25-homocholic acid. An experimental animal study. Scand J Gastroenterol 1990;25(7):681-688.
21. Buhner S, Ehrlein HJ, Thoma G, Schumpelick V. Canine motility and gastric emptying after subtotal gastrectomy. Am J Surg 1988;156(3 Pt 1):194-200.
22. Buhner S, Ehrlein HJ, Thoma G, Schumpelick V. Effects of nutrients on gastrointestinal motility and gastric emptying after Billroth-I gastrectomy in dogs. Dig Dis Sci 1988;33(7):784-794.
23. Ehrlein HJ, Thoma G, Keinke O, Tsiamitas C, Schumpelick V. Effects of nutrients on gastrointestinal motility and gastric emptying after distal gastrectomy with Roux-Y gastrojejunostomy in dogs. Dig Dis Sci 1987;32(5):538-546.

24. Ehrlein HJ, Buhner S, Thoma G, Schemann M, Keinke O, Tsiamitas C, Schumpelick V. Gastric emptying after Roux-Y and Billroth-I gastrectomy depends on viscosity of meal and contractile patterns of small intestine in dogs. Dig Dis Sci 1987;32(5):529-537.
25. Ehrlein HJ, Wulschke S, Thoma G, Schumpelick V. Gastrointestinal motility and gastric emptying after Billroth II gastrectomy in dogs. Dig Dis Sci 1989;34(8):1199-1210.
26. Schippers E, Willis S, Ruckdeschel G, Schumpelick V. Small intestinal myoelectrical activity and bacterial flora after Roux-en-Y reconstruction. Br J Surg 1996;83(9):1271-1275.
27. Schumpelick V, Begemann F. Amount of reflux in an operated stomach (author's transl). Dtsch Med Wochenschr 1981;106(16):497-500.
28. Schumpelick V, Schwoy M, Begemann F, Schreiber HW. Clinical results of jejunal transposition. Scand J Gastroenterol Suppl 1981;67:241-245.
29. Schumpelick V, Stemme D, Hofmann G, Begemann F. Intragastric bile acid and lysolecithin in gastroduodenal ulcer and gastric cancer. Scand J Gastroenterol Suppl 1984;92:172-177.
30. Dragstedt LR, Owens FM. Supradiaphragmatic section of the vagus nerves in the treatment of duodenal ulcer. Proc Soc Exp Biol Med 1943;53:152-156.
31. Wilbur BG, Kelly KA. Effect of proximal gastric, complete gastric, and truncal vagotomy on canine gastric electric activity, motility, and emptying. Ann Surg 1973;178(3):295-303.
32. Aeberhard P, Bedi BS. Effects of proximal gastric vagotomy (PGV) followed by total vagotomy (TV) on postprandial and fasting myoelectrical activity of the canine stomach and duodenum. Gut 1977;18(7):515-523.
33. Stoddard CJ, Waterfall WE, Brown BH, Duthie HL. The effects of varying the extent of the vagotomy on the myoelectrical and motor activity of the stomach. Gut 1973;14(8):657-664.
34. Schippers E, Vantrappen G, Braun J, Schumpelick V. Electromyographic and manometric studies of stomach motility after vagotomy. Z Gastroenterol 1991;29(11):581-584.
35. Paschen U, Schumpelick V. Effect of afferent abdominal vagus nerve stimulation on the blood circulation and respiration in the guinea pig. Z Gastroenterol 1977;15(4):254-263.
36. Schumpelick V, Arlt G, Riechert B, Klapdor R. Ulcer risk of reflux-preventing reconstruction following stomach resection – an animal experiment study. Z Gastroenterol 1984;22(11):630-643.
37. Rieu PN, Jansen JB, Joosten HJ, Biemond I, Yap SH, Lamers CB. Prospective comparison of gastric secretory function after gastrectomy with either Billroth II or Roux-en-Y anastomosis. Surgery 1989;105(3):331-336.
38. Hinder RA, Esser J, DeMeester TR. Management of gastric emptying disorders following the Roux-en-Y procedure. Surgery 1988;104(4):765-772.
39. Schumpelick V, Grossner D, Begemann F, Lauchart W. Prevention of reflux after gastro resection in the pig. Scand J Gastroenterol Suppl 1981;67 251-255.
40. Mathias JR, Fernandez A, Sninsky CA, Clench MH, Davis RH. Nausea, vomiting, and abdominal pain after Roux-en-Y anastomosis: motility of the jejunal limb. Gastroenterology 1985;88:101-107.
41. Perino LE, Adcock KA, Goff JS. Gastrointestinal symptoms, motility, and transit after the Roux-en-Y operation. Am J Gastroenterol 1988;83(4):380-385.
42. Donovan IA, Drumm J, Harding LK, Alexander-Williams J. Effect of Roux-en-Y reconstruction on the gastric emptying of a solid meal. Br J Surg 1987;74(6):491-492.
43. Pellegrini CA, Patti MG, Lewin M, Way LW. Alkaline reflux gastritis and the effect of biliary diversion on gastric emptying of solid food. Am J Surg 1985;150(1):166-171.
44. Hocking MP, Vogel SB, Falasca CA, Woodward ER. Delayed gastric emptying of liquids and solids following Roux-en-Y biliary diversion. Ann Surg 1981;(4):494-501.
45. Welch NT, Yasui A, Kim CB, Barlow AP, Hinder RA, DeMeester TR, Polishuk PV, Clark GW, Adrian TE. Effect of duodenal switch procedure on gastric acid production, intragastric pH, gastric emptying, and gastrointestinal hormones. Am J Surg 1992;163(1):37-44.
46. Csendes A, Braghetto I, Burdiles P, Diaz JC, Maluenda F, Korn O. A new physiologic approach for the surgical treatment of patients with Barrett's esophagus: technical considerations and results in 65 patients. Ann Surg 1997;226(2):123-133.
47. Hinder RA. Duodenal switch: a new form of pancreaticobiliary diversion. Surg Clin North Am 1992;72(2):487-499.
48. Klingler PJ, Perdikis G, Wilson P, Hinder RA. Indications, technical modalities and results of the duodenal switch operation for pathologic duodenogastric reflux. HepatoGastroenterology 1999;46(25):97-102.

What is the incidence of jejunal ulceration developed after Roux-en-Y gastrojejunostomy?

K.H. Fuchs, S.M. Freys, M. Fein, H. Tigges (Würzburg)

The most common application of partial gastric resection has been the treatment of gastric problems, such as peptic ulcer disease [1-5]. The application of partial gastric resection and Roux-en-Y reconstruction has been reserved in many centers only for severe cases, sometimes even after failed antireflux procedures. Follow-up data of a substantial series of patients of partial gastric resection and Roux-en-Y reconstruction after gastroesophageal reflux disease (GERD) is very limited. In the literature of gastric surgery after gastroduodenal ulcer disease, information about the Roux-en-Y reconstruction is only available in a few series. The most popular surgical therapy for gastroduodenal ulcers was a Billroth-II reconstruction or a Billroth-I reconstruction next to vagotomy. Ulcer recurrence after surgery for primary gastric ulcer is rather unusual and has been reported in less than 4% of the published cases [5]. In patients after surgery for duodenal ulcer recurrence is only marginally higher after resected cases. From several publications the recurrence rate of ulcers after subtotal gastrectomy without vagotomy lies in the area of 4-5% [4-6].

The reasons for ulcer recurrence after gastric resection and Roux-en-Y reconstruction are an insufficient distal antrum, in rare cases a retained Zollinger-Ellison syndrome or another reason for hypergastrinemia. Aggravating factors that also contribute to the development of recurrent ulcers at the anastomotic site can be excessive tobacco or alcohol use, ulcerogenic drugs such as non-steroidal anti-inflammatory drugs, or an emptying problem of the gastric remnant due to jejunal loop problems. Excessive enterogastric reflux of duodenal contents, especially bile and pancreatic juice, causes ulcerations in the gastric remnant or directly at the anastomotic area, but reflux usually does not occur following Roux-en-Y reconstructions. In extremely rare cases it has been observed in Roux-en-Y reconstructions with a very short efferent loop to the jejuno-jejunostomy.

The most important reason for a jejunal ulceration in a Roux-en-Y reconstruction after partial gastrectomy is an inadequate gastric resection. A substantial part of the stomach *i.e.* 2/3 of the gastric volume must be resected to reduce the acid producing capacity of the stomach sufficiently enough to give the jejunal mucosa the possibility to compensate for the remaining acid inflow at the anastomosis. In Europe, at least 60-80% of the gastric volume was resected when a Roux-en-Y reconstruction was considered [4, 7]. In the United States, partial gastrectomy with a Roux-en-Y reconstruction usually consisted of a maximum of 50% resection of the gastric volume usually combined with some form of a vagotomy [8]. The latter, however, often caused motility problems which became known as the Roux-en-Y syndrome. When considering a Roux-en-Y reconstruction, resection of two thirds of the stomach is needed without a combined vagotomy to achieve a sufficient acid reduction. If only half of the stomach is resected, the ulcer recurrence can amount up to 36% [4].

Twenty years ago only a few centers focussed their research interest on the Roux-en-Y reconstruction. Therefore, information on long-term results with this reconstruction method are lacking. Currently, the indication for a Roux-en-Y reconstruction and partial resection in patients with advanced GERD or with complex gastroduodenal ulcer disease and recurrence are extremely rare [9, 10]. Roux-en-Y reconstruction eliminates bile and pancreatic reflux components reaching the stomach. However, due to the complexity of the underlying functional disorder, successes in symptom reduction are variable. In some patients upper gastrointestinal symptoms can persist. It is very important to individually identify the causes of these problems because remaining symptoms and recurrent ulcerations such as jejunal ulcerations depend on the extent of resection, the grade of motility problems involved, and also the probability of remaining reflux problems.

The Roux-en-Y syndrome has been proposed as a motility disorder based on the jejunal limb causing abdominal pain, gastric stasis and vomiting. The ectopic pace-setter potential has been described after Roux-en-Y gastrectomies [8]. However, this syndrome does not appear in patients in whom partial gastrectomy is performed without vagotomy [3]. This has been proven in a prospective trial in that patients after Roux-en-Y reconstruction had no higher prevalence of symptoms or any bad outcome in gastric emptying compared to the control patients who were randomized with standard Billroth-II gastrectomy [11].

In our own study, 24 hours gastric pH monitoring was used to assess the acid environment in the gastric lumen *i.e.* the gastric 24 hours pH profile in several reconstruction procedures. *Figure 1* shows the reason for jejunal ulceration in the Roux-en-Y reconstruction. In the majority of the cases of patients with jejunal ulceration, there was a persistent gastric acidity documented in 24 hours gastric pH monitoring despite the fact that the stomach was partially resected [12]. As a consequence, one could recommend a 24 hours gastric pH monitoring investigation prior to any gastric surgery to determine the acid capacity of the stomach. If there is a severe persisting gastric acidity, preferably 70-80% of the gastric volume should be resected. Another step could be the assessment of the acidity of the gastric remnant after a partial gastric resection and Roux-en-Y reconstruction. If there is still, during the postoperative time, a persisting gastric acidity, additional medical coverage reducing an intraluminal acidity by proton pump inhibitors or H_2 blockers is advisable. In our series the jejunal ulceration rate after partial gastric resection and Roux-en-Y reconstruction with nearly an 80% reduction of gastric volume was below 1.5%.

In summary, jejunal ulceration after partial gastric resection and Roux-en-Y reconstruction depends on several factors. The most important reason for developing jejunal ulceration is a remaining acid capacity in the stomach that cannot be compensated by the jejunal mucosa. In literature this problem occurs in about 4-5% after gastric resection of 2/3 of the gastric volume. If only half of the stomach is resected, this rate can be as high as 36% in cases without combined vagotomy. A combined vagotomy does cause motility problems

Figure 1. Gastric pH in patients following partial resection.
PGA: persistant gastric acidity; R: recurrent ulcer.
Following Roux-en-Y reconstruction persistant gastric acidity is frequently found in patients with recurrent ulcer, while patients with no ulcer recurrence do not have persistant gastric acidity.

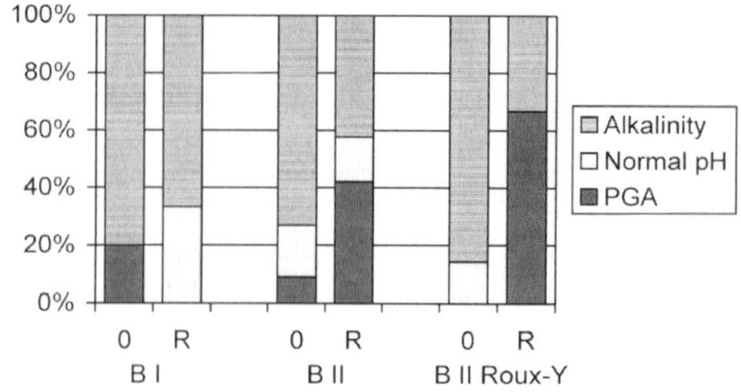

and, therefore, should be abandoned. The problem of jejunal ulceration after partial gastric resection and Roux-en-Y reconstruction can be limited to approximately 1% of the cases if a sufficient portion of the stomach is resected and the Roux-en-Y limb is long enough.

References

1. Goligher JC, Pulvertaft CM, deDombal FT, Conyers JH, Duthie HL, Feather DB, Latchmore AJC, Shoesmith JH, Smiddy FG, Willson-Pepper J. Five-to eight-year results of Leeds/York controlled trial of elective surgery for duodenal ulcer. Br Med J 1968;I:781.
2. Price WE, Grizzle JE, Postlethwait RW, Johnson WD, Grabicki P. Results of operation for duodenal ulcer. Surg Gynecol Obstet 1970;131:233.
3. Jordan PH, Condon RE. A prospective evaluation of vagotomy-pyloroplasty and vagotomy-antrectomy in the elective treatment of duodenal ulcer. Ann Surg 1970;172:547.
4. Herfarth Ch, Merkle N.Indikationen beim postoperativen Rezidivulcus nach Resektion. In: Blum AL, Siewert JR, eds. Ulcus-Therapie. Springer, 1982:672-680.
5. McAlhany, JC, Hanover TM, Taylor SM, Sticca RP, Ashmore JD. Long-term follwo-up of patients with Roux-en-Y gastrojejunostomy for gastric disease. Ann Surg 1994;219:451-457.
6. Berger T, Kock NG, Norberg PB. Truncal vagotomy with antrectomy or pyloroplasty for duodenal ulcer: a five-year follow-up study. Acta Chir Scand 1972;138:499.
7. Thiede A, Fuchs KH, Wirtz HJ, Hamelmann H. Roux-Y-Stapler-Rekonstruktion nach distaler Magenresektion. Langenbecks Arch Chir 1986;367:119-127.
8. Mathias JR, Fernandez A, Sninsky CA, Clench MH, Davis RH. Nausea, vomiting, and abdominal pain after Roux-en-Y anastomosis: motility of the jejunal limb. Gastroenterology 1985;88:101-107.
9. Washer GF, Gear MWL, Dowling BL, Gillison EW, Royston CMS, Spencer J. Randomized prospective trial of Roux-en-Y duodenal diversion versus fundoplication for severe reflux esophagitis. Br J Surg 1984;71:181.
10. Fekete F, Pateron D.What is the place of antrectomy with Roux-en-Y in the treatment of reflux disease? Experience with 83 total duodenal diversions. World J Surg 1992;16:349-353.
11. Rieu PNMA, Jansen JBMI, Joosten HJM, Lamers CBHW. Effect of gastrectomy with either Roux-en-Y or Billroth II anastomosis on small intestinal function. Scan J Gastroenterol 1990;25:185.
12. Fuchs KH, Selch A, Freys SM, DeMeester TR. Gastric acid secretion and gastric pH measurement in peptic ulcer disease. Prob Gen Surg 1992;9:138-151.

What are the mechanisms for abnormal bacterial proliferation in the upper gastrointestinal tract?

V. Schumpelick, B. Dreuw, K. Ophoff, N. Ponschek, D. Schubert (Aachen)

The normal stomach of a healthy volunteer is usually sterile without any bacterial growth in the fasting secretion [1]. The oral cavity however carries a characteristic microbial flora consisting of up to 30 different microbes. The most important of these are viridans streptococcus, staphylococcus, neisseria, apathogen coryne bacteriae and anaerobic microbes like *Leptotrichia buccalis*, *Bacteroides orali*s and actinomyces. In a hospital milieu, additional enteral bacteriae and yeasts can occur as a consequence of antibiotic therapy. Together with swallowed food these bacteriae and the microbes that are contained in the food reach the stomach, and under physiologic conditions, they leave the stomach within a few hours. Only the acid resisting mycobacteriae can be found in the stomach's fasting secretion. Bile, pancreatic juice and small bowel secretions are usually sterile or contain single saprophytic microbes. Only the terminal ileum may contain some sparse colonic microflora. This microbiologic situation may be altered by gastric surgery.

Up to 50% of patients following Roux-en-Y gastric resection suffer from a symptom complex called Roux-Y syndrom or Roux-stasis-syndrom [2]. At least part of the symptoms are thought to be generated by bacterial overgrowth in the upper gastrointestinal tract following these operations.

We have studied the bacterial overgrowth after different types of gastric resection in patients and experimentally in dogs after Roux-en-Y duodenal diversion.

The intragastric bacterial flora in 125 patients after different types of ulcer operations (Billroth I and II gastric resection, vagotomy with and without pyloroplasty and jejunal interposition) was correlated with pH value and histological state of gastric mucosa. Following vagotomy, most of the gastric juices were sterile. More than 60% of the resected stomachs were contaminated with fecal and oropharyngeal flora (*Table I*). There was a good correlation between bacterial overgrowth and pH value. Only 10-20% of the stomachs with pH values lower than 4.5 and more than 80% of the stomachs with pH values above 6 were bacterially contaminated (*Figure 1*). After vagotomy, oral type microbes predominated with almost no fecal type bacteriae, whereas after gastric resection fecal type and oral type microbes were almost equal distributed (*Table II*). Intragastric flora was found

Table I. Microbial flora in the stomach and upper part of the small bowel following gastric surgery.

Fecal type microbial flora	Bacteroides Petostreptococcus Bifidobacterium *E. coli* *Proteus vulgaris* *Klebsiella pneumoniae*	Enterobacter *Streptococcus fecalis* Clostridia *B. subtilis*
Oropharyngeal type microbial flora	Viridans-Streptococcus Staphylococcus Neisseria Corynebacteriae	Bacteroides Actinomyces *Leptotrichia buccalis*
Yeasts	*Candida albicans* *Candida parapsilosis* *Candida tropicalis*	*Torulopsis glabrata* *Candida krusei*

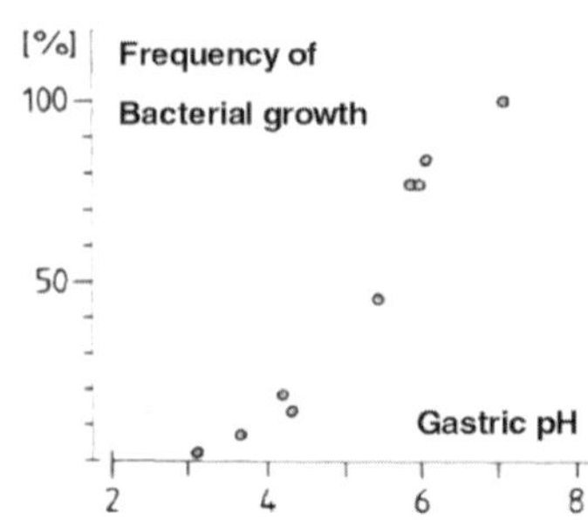

Figure 1. Intragastric pH and frequency of bacterial overgrowth in normals, after Billroth I and II gastric resection, vagotomy with and without pyloroplasty and jejunal interposition. Values are means of the groups studied. Note the clear correlation between gastric pH and bacterial growth.

Table II. Gastric pH and type of bacterial colonisation after different types of gastric surgery (Adapted from [3]).

	n	Colonisation		Stomach		mean pH	
		Fecal type	Oral type	Yeast	Steril	Basal	Stimulated
B-II-resection							
Retrocolic anastomosis	18	8	6	7	3	5,8	5,2
Antecolic anastomosis	18	7	1	3	9	5,4	5,0
Total	36	15	7	10	12	5,6	5,1
B-I-Resection							
Termino-terminal anast	25	13	8	15	0	6,0	4,3
Termino-lateral anast.	12	7	7	4	0	6,9	4,5
Supraduodenal termino-lateral anast.	3	2	1	3	0	7,5	5,2
Total	40	22	16	22	0	6,8	4,6
Vagotomy (VT)							
Selective proximal VT	11	0	2	0	9	4,2	1,9
S. total VT + pyloroplasty (Jaboulay)	15	0	1	3	11	3,7	1,9
S. total VT + pyloroplasty (Heineke-Mickulicz)	14	1	1	1	11	4,3	2,6
Total		1	4	4	31	4,1	2,1
Jejunum interposition							
Shorter than 15 cm	4	2	1	1	2	6,3	4,3
Longer than 15 cm	5	0	4	0	1	6,6	3,1
Total		2	5	1	3	6,5	3,7

in 90% of the stomachs with atrophic gastritis. Intragastric bacterial flora will support deconjugation of the bile acids and production of nitrosamine [3].

Experimentally, intestinal microflora was examined after partial gastrectomy and Roux-en-Y reconstruction in six dogs. Bacteriological analysis of 1 x 1 cm biopsy specimen from the stomach, duodenum and proximal jejunum were taken at the time of initial operation and 6 months later. In the first specimen, we did not find any bacteriae or only very low numbers. After six months however, high numbers of microorganisms were detected in the stomach, Roux limb, upper jejunum and duodenum with a predominance of fecal bacteria. The highest numbers were found near the gastrojejunal anastomosis (7,1 colony forming units) and the lowest in the gastric fundus (3.8 colony forming units). There were no significant differences of bacterial growth between the Roux limb, jejunum and duodenum. At all locations a typical fecal flora of about 50% aerobes and 50% anaerobes was present (*Table III*, [4]).

Table III. Evaluation of bacterial overgrowth 6 months after Roux-en-Y reconstruction and relative contribution of aerobic and anaerobic species.

	Anaerobic (%)	Aerobic (%)	Mean (SEM) bacterial flora (colony forming units)
Stomach			
Proximal	49	51	3.82 (2.24)
Distal	49	51	6.35 (1.05)*
Roux limb			
Proximal	51	49	7.08 (1.25)
Distal	47	53	6.79 (1.22)
Distal jejunum			
Proximal	54	46	6.23 (1.05)
Distal	49	51	5.84 (1.15)
Duodenum			
Proximal	58	42	5.53 (2.05)
Distal	50	50	6.31 (1.17)

* $p < 0.005$ (distal *versus* proximal stomach biopsy, Wilcoxon-Mann-Whitney *U* test)

Similar findings of bacterial overgrowth after Roux-en-Y reconstruction are reported in the literature [4-9].

This unphysiologic bacterial overgrowth may be facilitated by motility disturbances and pH alterations initiated by Roux-en-Y diversion. The motor motility complex usually functioning as a housekeeper with cleaning up the luminal content in the interdigestive phase, is altered and allows stasis and bacterial growth.

Reduced gastric acidity impairs the natural resistance to bacterial overgrowth. This effect is enhanced by hypomotility, gastrointestinal stasis and failure of the interdigestive intestinal motility.

The suprapapillary Roux-en-Y duodenojejunostomy (duodenal switch) without vagotomy and antrectomy leaves the stomach intact and has less complications than conventional Roux-en-Y diversion, experimentally [10] as well as clinically [11]. However, this procedure also bypasses the duodenum with possible duodenal hypomotility and pancreocibal asynchrony. Although not investigated yet after this type of operation, we expect the existence of some bacterial overgrowth in the blind duodenal limb and upper jejunum similar to the findings after conventional duodenal diversion. On the long run, at least some symptoms will develop from this situation. Therefore, duodenal diversion as a treatment for complicated gastroesophageal reflux and Barrett esophagus should be restricted to very selected patients, when other therapeutic options have failed.

References

1. Schassan HH. Bakteriologie des vagotomierten Magens. In: Schumpelick V, Begemann F, Werner B, eds. Refluxkrankheit des Magens, 1 ed. Stuttgart: Enke, 2000:130-133.
2. Hinder RA, Esser J, DeMeester TR. Management of gastric emptying disorders following the Roux-en-Y procedure. Surgery 1988;104(4):765-772.
3. Schumpelick V, Schassan HH. Bacteriology of the stomach after operation. Langenbecks Arch Chir 1980;350(4):271-279.
4. Schippers E, Willis S, Ruckdeschel G, Schumpelick V. Small intestinal myoelectrical activity and bacterial flora after Roux-en-Y reconstruction. Br J Surg 1996;83(9):1271-1275.
5. Bradley EL, III, Isaacs JT, Mazo JD, Hersh T, Chey WY. Pathophysiology and significance of malabsorption after Roux-en-Y reconstruction. Surgery 1977;81(6):684-691.
6. Dellipiani AW, Girdwood RH. The significance of abnormal bacterial proliferation in the gastrointestinal tract after gastric surgery. Scand J Gastroenterol 1967;2(3):161-168.
7. Greenlee HB, Gelbart SM, DeOrio AJ, Francescatti DS, Paez J, Reinhardt GF. The influence of gastric surgery on the intestinal flora. Am J Clin Nutr 1977;30(11):1826-1833.
8. Menge H, Simes G, Germer CT, Wagner J, Hahn H, Riecken EO. Qualitative and quantitative detection of bacterial flora in experimental blind loop syndrome of the rat. Zeitschrift Gastroenterol 1985;23(8):425-431.
9. Nielsen ML, Justesen T, Lenz K, Nielsen OV, Jensen SL. Bacterial flora of the small intestine and bile acid metabolism in patients with hepatico-jejunostomy Roux-en-Y. Scand J Gastroenterol 1977;12(8):977-982.
10. Welch NT, Yasui A, Kim CB, Barlow AP, Hinder RA, DeMeester TR, Polishuk PV, Clark GW, Adrian TE. Effect of duodenal switch procedure on gastric acid production, intragastric pH, gastric emptying, and gastrointestinal hormones. Am J Surg 1992;163(1):37-44.
11. DeMeester TR, Fuchs KH, Ball CS, Albertucci M, Smyrk TC, Marcus JN. Experimental and clinical results with proximal end-to-end duodenojejunostomy for pathologic duodenogastric reflux. Ann Surg 1987;206(4):414-426.

What are the consequences of duodenal hypomotility after total duodenal diversion and Roux-en-Y reconstruction?

V. Schumpelick, B. Dreuw, N. Ponschek, K. Ophoff, M. Niewiera (Aachen)

After gastric operations, about 20 to 30% of all patients complain of an abundance of postoperative gastrointestinal and vasomotor symptoms called "post-gastrectomy syndrome". In the beginning of this century, concepts as precipitated evacuation, dumping stomach, too narrow or too wide anastomosis predominate. In the thirties, the subdivision into early and late dumping syndrome follows. The description and treatment of the afferent loop syndrome in the middle of this century suggest the introduction of functional factors into the explanation of the post-gastrectomy syndrome. Then comes the recognition of the pathophysiological significance of the regurgitated duodenal content into the operated stomach, the postoperative alkaline reflux gastritis. Surgical correction of this symptom complex usually makes a duodenal diversion procedure necessary. Principally, diversion of duodenal content from the stomach can be achieved by standard Roux-en-Y gastrojejunostomy, Roux-en-Y Tanner-19 gastrojejunostomy, isoperistaltic jejunal interposition or suprapapillary duodenojejunostomy (duodenal switch procedure) [1]. Choosing a Roux-en-Y diversion will lead to a blind duodenal loop, excluded from the contact with gastric acid and the chemical and mechanical effects of the chymus. As a consequence, the alterations of upper gastrointestinal physiology generate clinical symptoms of nausea, vomiting, abdominal pain and epigastric fullness in up to 50% of patients following Roux-en-Y diversion [2]. To illuminate this situation, we will give a short brush up in gastric physiology and then present some previous studies focusing on duodenal motility.

Physiology of the stomach and duodenum

The main function of the stomach is to prepare ingested food for digestion, process foodstuff into fine particles and initiate the dispersion of fats, proteins and carbohydrates by breaking down cell walls. This requires specific motor and secretory activities.

Motor function

The motor function of the stomach results in storage, mixing and intermittent delivery of food into the small bowel. It is regulated by sympathetic and parasympathetic innervation. Activation of the parasympathetic vagus nerve results in contraction, activation of the sympathetic nerves results in relaxation and dilatation. The gastric motor pacemacer is localized high on the greater curve at the crossing of fundus and corpus. Food storage is enhanced by a process called receptive relaxation. Hereby, the upper portion of the stomach relaxes as the intake of food is anticipated. Solid food settles within the fundus along the greater curvature, whereas liquids pass rapidly along the lesser curve (The "*magenstrasse*"). The storage function is enhanced by the antrum which constantly returns material to the proximal stomach until it is reduced to a size of a few millimeters and ready for delivery into the duodenum. Evacuation is realized by a complicated regulation of proximal gastric contractions and duodenal relaxation, mediated by nervous and humoral parameters.

Secretion

About 800 cm^2 secreting surface of the gastric mucosa, of which 80% is localized in the fundus and corpus, produces 1,5 to 3 liters of secretion per day. Each mm^2 contains 100 pits (foveolus) with 3-7 glands, that is 40 x 109 glands. The amount of HCl production is directly correlated to the number of parietal cells. A total number of about thousand million parietal cells produce a basal acid output of 2-5 mmol per hour and a volume of 60-80 ml per hour. After maximal stimulation with pentagastrin, the maximal acid output is 20-25 mmol and 100-200 ml per hour.

The parietal cells produce intrinsic factor and hydrochloric acid with a concentration of 0,1 mol/liter and a pH of 1, the chief cells pepsinogen and cathepsin. Both are localized in the fundus and corpus. Mucous neck cells of the cardia and pylorus produce mucous and the Gastrin-producing cells (G-cells) of the antrum and cardia produce gastrin. Gastrin is a polypeptid that stimulates the parietal cells to secrete HCl and is released by mechanical dilatation of the antrum, vagal stimulation, intragastric amino acids, ethanol, proteins as well as bile acids. The surface cells contain abundant mucous granules within their apical surface and renew constantly a thin layer of mucous that protects the cells against the corrosive effect of the HCl. Additionally, they are thought to produce a sodium rich alkaline secretion. The Brünner glands of the duodenum secrete alkaline duodenal juice that neutralizes hydrochloric acid.

The gastric secretion is regulated by a complex feed back mechanism of stimulating and inhibitating mechanical, chemical, nerval and hormonal factors. Secretion is stimulated by antral distension, caffeine, ethanol, protein, roasting products, spices, bicarbonate or bile acids, vagal stimulation, gastrin, insuline, ACTH, STH, LTH, corticoids, androgens or parathyroid hormone. Secretion is inhibited by antral or duodenal acidification, stimulation of the sympathetic nerve, secretin, pancreozymin, glucagon, enterogastrin, bulbogastrin, GIP or VIP.

Gastric secretion consists of an interdigestive or fasting period and a digesting period. The latter consists of a cephalic, gastric and intestinal phase. Sensory contact with food stimulates the diencephalon and activates the vagus nerve. This leads to release of HCl and gastrin 5-7 minutes later and will last up to 3 hours (cephalic phase). Chemical, mechanical and thermic contact with ingested food in the stomach leads to gastrin release (gastric phase). Intestinal contact with chymus leads to additional gastrin release (intestinal phase, *Figure 4*).

To maintain the high endoluminal hydrogen ion concentration of pH 1 in comparison to the physiologic pH of 7,4 in the interstitial space, active and passive mechanisms are necessary; they are called the gastric mucosal barrier. Factors that are known to break down this barrier are acetylic acid, indometacin, ethanol as well as bile acids and lysolecithin and they may contribute to the development of corrosive gastritis and ulceration.

Vagal stimulation leads to gastrin release, acid secretion, receptive relaxation of the proximal stomach, rythmic antral contractions and coordinated relaxation of the pyloric sphincter.

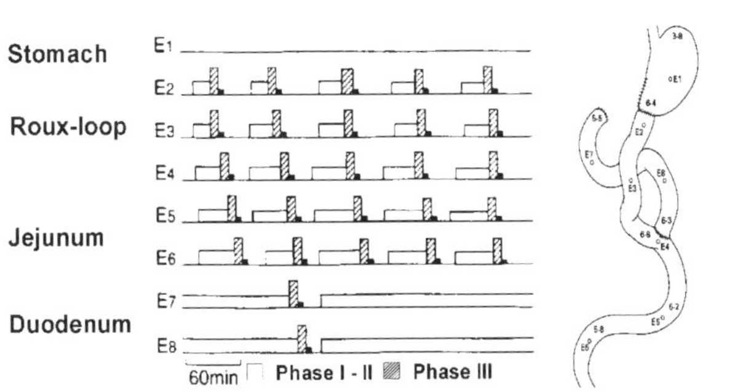

Figure 1. Scheme of the single phases of migrating motor complexes (MMC) in the interdigestive phase of intestinal motility after Roux-en-Y diversion. Phase III occurs regularly and is travelling along the Roux limb into the jejunum. Note the extremely reduced frequency of phase III in the duodenum. If phase III occurs in the duodenum it is not coordinated to the phase III of the Roux limb and jejunum.

The duodenum is the main site of secretin production and also produces other intestinal hormones like CCK-pancreozymin, motilin and gastric inhibitory peptid. Secretin release is initiated by duodenal acidification short after pyloric evacuation and is responsible for inhibition of gastric acid production and promoting pancreatic bicarbonate secretion. CCK-pancreozymin regulates pancreatic secretion of fluids rich in enzymatic contents, gall bladder contraction and excretion of bile to mix with the duodenal content. Simultaneously, gastric motility is inhibited to prevent from further gastroduodenal evacuation by CCK-pancreozymin and motilin.

Duodenal motility after Roux-en-Y

Disturbances of intestinal motility are known to develop in patients who have undergone Roux-en-Y gastric reconstruction. However, clinical and experimental findings to clarify the underlying pathophysiological correlate are not definite. Gastric emptying may be normal [3], accelerated [4] or delayed [2]. Manometric studies reveal that the intestinal motility after Roux-en-Y reconstruction is disturbed [5].

Previous studies revealed that bile salts are necessary to initiate normal intestinal motor motility complexes (MMC's). Diversion of bile from the gastrointestinal tract results in loss of MMC's. After reperfusion of bile salts into a peripheric vein or the portal vein MMC's are reestablished [6]. That means that diversion of bile does not influence the gastrointestinal motility pattern as long as the enterohepatic circle is maintained. For duodenal motility after Roux-en-Y, the transsection of the duodenum and creation of a blind loop is obviously more important. As reported by Code, transsection of the bowel generates a new pacesetter when the oral more frequent pacesetter potentials are missed [7]. In case of jejunal interposition the situation is different. It is known that in intestinal anastomosis VIP containing nerves grow in and lead to electromechanical docking [8].

Our own studies of electromyographic recording of motility after partial gastrectomy with Roux-en-Y reconstruction in dogs revealed no significant differences from controls in the Roux limb, but extensive changes in intestinal motility in the blind duodenal loop. The electromyographic pattern was characterized by an extreme loss of activity in the fasted and postprandial state. The basal electrical rhythm of the Roux limb was significantly decreased, while the frequency of phase III was increased ($p < 0.05$). The activity front of the migrating motility complex occurred only in 25% of the fasting studies and was not correlated in time

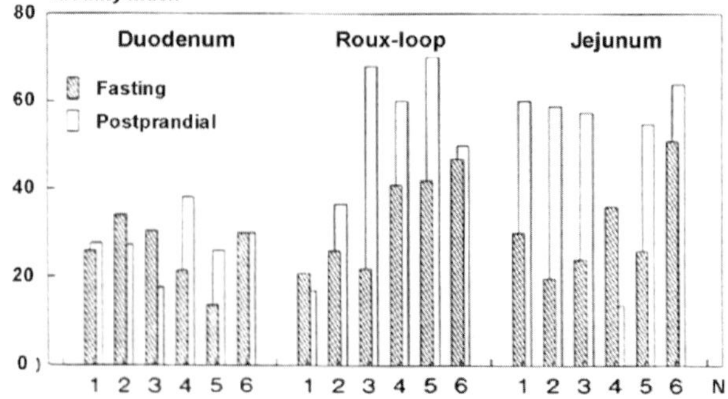

Figure 2. Calculated motility index after gastrojejunostomy and Roux-en-Y diversion in the duodenum, Roux limb and jejunum. Note the missing increase of the motility index in the duodenum compared to the Roux limb and jejunum in the postprandial period.

with motility patterns of connected small intestine (*Figure 1*). Food intake led to an increase in the mean (SEM) motility index in the Roux limb (from 46.1 (9.4) to 75.0 (21.5), $p < 0.05$), but not in the bypassed duodenum (from 27.0 (3.6) to 27.8 (4.1), p not significant, *Figure 2*) [9, 10]. This may be explained by exclusion of the duodenum from direct contact with food and gastric secretions, which are a decisive stimulus for postprandial motility in normal anatomic situation. The loss of the motility stimulus in the duodenum leads to duodenal hypomotility with delayed transport of bile and pancreas secretions. In our own patients, we could demonstrate, that the time before bile reaches the jejunum after stimulation is significantly delayed after Roux-en-Y diversion compared to jejunal interposition [11]. This finding is further supported by the report of decreased concentrations of trypsin and lipase in the jejunum of patients with Roux-en-Y duodenal diversion [12]. As a result, postprandial nausea, steatorrhoea or flatulence may be induced.

Another experimental study was conducted to evaluate the motility patterns after total gastrectomy while preserving or excluding the duodenal passage. Eight beagle dogs had total gastrectomy with jejunal interposition (n = 4) or Roux-en-Y reconstruction (n = 4). Motility patterns were detected with perfused manometry, sequential scintigraphic emptying studies, and a hydrogen breath test with lactulose. The preoperative studies of the same individuals served as controls. The emptying of the gastric substitutes was markedly accelerated compared with controls after 6 months (T50: 5.8-8.1 min). In the jejunal interposition group, intestinal transit was almost identical to preoperative controls whereas intestinal transit was significantly accelerated in the Roux-en-Y animals (controls: 101 ± 26 min, jejunum interposition: 104 ± 18.2 min, Roux-en-Y: 71.3 ± 13.4 min; $p < 0.01$, *Figure 3*). Pathologic motility patterns could be identified as the cause of this observations: Roux-en-Y dogs showed a marked increase of the intestinal motility index in the proximal jejunum ($p < 0.0001$) and a dissociation between the motility patterns of the duodenum and the gastric substitute (*Figure 4*). This part of the small bowel might generate two independent pacemarkers that both influence the lower intestinal parts after Roux-en-Y reconstruction [13].

Similar results could be verified in 68 disease free patients after jejunal gastric replacement (jejunal interposition: n = 40; Roux-en-Y reconstruction: n = 28). Patients with jejunal interposition showed a better weight gain (p = 0.001), a lower reflux rate (p = 0.01), a slower orocecal transit time (p = 0.05), a prompter bile flow after meal stimulation (p = 0.02), and lower peak glucose levels (p = 0.001). The emptying patterns of the different gastric substitutes were not different. A higher incidence of retrograde contractions in the

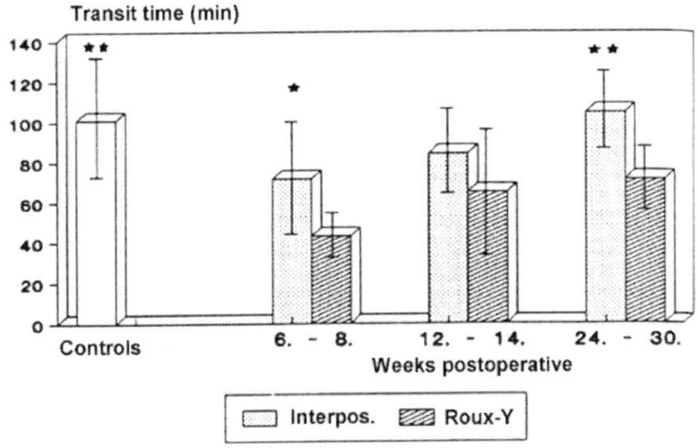

Figure 3. Orocecal transit time after total gastrectomy and jejunum interposition or Roux-en-Y diversion compared to controls. Values are expressed as medians ± SEM (*: p < 0,05, interposition compared to Roux-en-Y, **: p < 0,01, controls and interposition compared to Roux-en-Y).

Roux-en-Y group and a electromechanical dissociation between the duodenum and the gastric substitute were detected. The postoperative function of the jejunal gastric substitute does not mainly depend on it's emptying pattern or volume, but on the motility patterns of the entire intestinal tract which seem to be strongly influenced by the choice of duodenal diversion or not [13].

One major factor for the regulation of intestinal motility may be the amount and distribution of humoral receptors and cells that produce gastrointestinal hormones. To support this thesis, we studied the distribution of various enteroendocrine cells in the mucosa of the small bowel after total gastrectomy and Roux-en-Y diversion or jejunal interposition. All operated animals showed a marked decrease of VIP-positive cells in all locations. Bombesin/GRP-positive cells were reduced at all locations but increased in the duodenum of the Roux-en-Y group. Animals with Roux-en-Y diversion had a significant decrease of CCK-positive cells in the proximal duodenum and a decrease of motilin-positive cells in the distal duodenum. Motilin-positive cells in the lower jejunum and the terminal ileum were only found after Roux-en-Y diversion, but not in controls or after

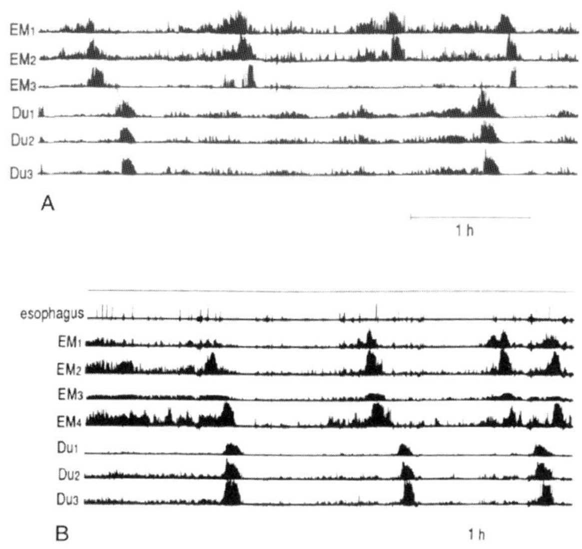

Figure 4. Eight channel perfused manometry of fasting motility after total gastrectomy and Roux-en-Y diversion (A) or jejunal interposition (B). EM: gastric replacement, Du: duodenum. Note the duodenal hypomotility and the dissociation of motility complexes between the gastric replacement and the duodenum after Roux-en-Y (A) compared to jejunal interposition (B) with intact migrating of the MMC.

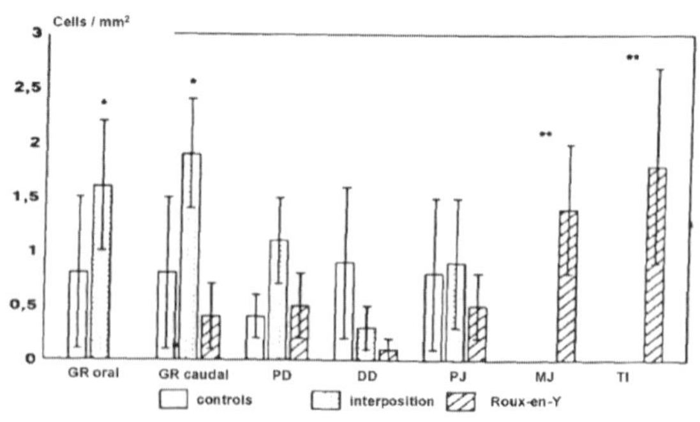

Figure 5. Frequency and distribution of motilin positive cells in controls and after total gastrectomy with jejunal interposition or Roux-en-Y diversion. (GR: gastric replacement; PD: proximal duodenum, DD: distal duodenum, PJ: proximal jejunum, MJ: middle jejunum, TI: terminal ileum, *: p < 0,05, controls and interposition compared to Roux-en-Y; **: p < 0,01, controls and interposition compared to Roux-en-Y).

jejunal interposition (*Figure 5*). These findings demonstrate that duodenal diversion does not only lead to duodenal hypomotility but will influence the motility of the whole gastrointestinal tract.

Conclusion

Total duodenal diversion will lead to duodenal hypomotility, because the contact of the duodenal mucosa with chymus and gastric secretions is lost. Duodenal hypomotility results in delayed transport of bile and pancreatic juice. Consequently the concentration of digestion ferments in the upper jejunum is decreased. This will result in digestion disorders with steatorrheoa, flatulence and abdominal pain as well as higher peak glucose levels. The interrupted oral pacemaker stimulus leads to the development of a second motility pacemaker localized in the duodenum which is not coordinated with the gastrojejunal motility. As a result, the orocecal transit time is accelerated and does allow only a shorter time for digestion. The negative effects caused by duodenal hypomotility are enhanced.

The reduced frequency of the MMC, usually functioning as a housekeeper with cleaning up the luminal content in the interdigestive phase, allows stasis which may lead to bacterial growth.

It is questionable up to today if the preservation of a few centimeters of proximal duodenum in case of duodenal switch operation is able to eliminate or significantly reduce these major side effects of Roux-en-Y diversion. The indication to such procedures therefore should be restricted to otherwise untreatable patients.

References

1. Klingler PJ, Perdikis G, Wilson P, Hinder RA. Indications, technical modalities and results of the duodenal switch operation for pathologic duodenogastric reflux. HepatoGastroenterology 1999;46(25):97-102.
2. Hinder RA, Esser J, DeMeester TR. Management of gastric emptying disorders following the Roux-en-Y procedure. Surgery 1988;104(4):765-772.
3. Britton JP, Johnston D, Ward DC, Axon AT, Barker MC. Gastric emptying and clinical outcome after Roux-en-Y diversion. Br J Surg 1987;74(10):900-904.
4. Pellegrini CA, Patti MG, Lewin M, Way LW. Alkaline reflux gastritis and the effect of biliary diversion on gastric emptying of solid food. Am J Surg 1985;150(1):166-171.
5. Perino LE, Adcock KA, Goff JS. Gastrointestinal symptoms, motility, and transit after the Roux-en-Y operation. Am J Gastroenterol 1988;83(4):380-385.
6. Kajiyama Y, Irie M, Enjoji A, Ozeki K, Ura K, Kanematsu T. Role of bile acids in duodenal migrating motor complexes in dogs. Dig Dis Sci 1998;43(10):2278-2283.
7. Code CF, Szurszewski JH. The effect of duodenal and mid small bowel transection on the frequency gradient of the pacesetter potential in the canine small intestine. J Physiol 1970;207(2):281-289.
8. Galligan JJ, Furness JB, Costa M. Migration of the myoelectric complex after interruption of the myenteric plexus: intestinal transection and regeneration of enteric nerves in the guinea pig. Gastroenterology 1989;97(5):1135-1146.
9. Schippers E, Willis S, Ruckdeschel G, Schumpelick V. Small intestinal myoelectrical activity and bacterial flora after Roux-en-Y reconstruction. Br J Surg 1996;83(9):1271-1275.
10. Schippers E, Schumpelick V. Motility disorders in the blind loop after Roux-en-y reconstruction. Electromyography studies in the animal experiment. Langenbecks Arch Chir 1994;379(2):99-104.
11. Bradley EL, III, Isaacs JT, Mazo JD, Hersh T, Chey WY. Pathophysiology and significance of malabsorption after Roux-en-Y reconstruction. Surgery 1977;81(6):684-691.
12. Fass J, Bares R, Hermsdorf V, Schumpelick V. Intestinal motility after jejunum interposition and Roux-Y reconstruction – an animal experiment study. Langenbecks Arch Chir 1993;378(4):239-248.
13. Fass J, Bares R, Staude M, Schumpelick V. Type of stomach replacement and intestinal motility after total gastrectomy. Leber Magen Darm 1993;23(5):194-203.

What information can be expected from intraoperative manometry in the surgical treatment of gastroesophageal reflux disease?

J. Chipponi, K. Slim, D. Pezet (Clermont-Ferrand)

It is now well established that the antireflux wrap (fundoplication) should be continent aiming to prevent postoperative reflux but also sufficiently floppy avoiding postoperative dysphagia. It seemed to us logical to assume that esophageal intraoperative manometry could be a reliable method to tailor the fundoplication and therefore to improve the functional results.

Patients and methods

The aim of this prospective study was to evaluate the esophageal intraoperative manometry (lower esophageal sphincter – LES) in the field of antireflux fundoplication.

Forty-eight patients were operated on for an intractable gastroesophageal reflux disease (GERD). All patients had preoperative and intraoperative manometry and 30 agreed to undergo a postoperative manometry with a mean postoperative follow-up of 20.7 months. Only these latter patients were included in the analysis.

Intraoperative measurements were done before any dissection of the hiatal crura and after partial and complete fundoplication.

The surgical procedures included 25 floppy-Nissen and 5 partial posterior fundoplications.

Results

Mean (sd) of intraoperative pressure and length of LES were 9.8 (5.3) mmHg and 2.9 (1.3) respectively. These values were not statistically different when compared with the preoperative values.

The simple dissection of the hiatus lead to a significant increase of LES pressure (LESP) which met 20.5 (8.2) mmHg.

LESP at the end of the procedure was 31.9 (11.5) mmHg after partial fundoplication and 38 (12) mmHg after complete (floppy) fundoplication. Postoperative values of LESP decreased with a mean rate of 50%, when compared with the values at the end of the procedures.

The analysis of the results for the 2 patients considered as failure cases because of an important dysphagia showed that the pressures measured at the end of the procedure were the highest, with increase of LESP 7.5 and 8.2 times higher than the preoperative values, whereas the mean increase for nondysphagic patients was 4.6 times.

The analysis of the results for patients considered as failure cases because of a recurrence of reflux (whether confirmed clinically or by a pH measurement) showed that the mean LESP at the end of the procedure was the lowest of the series (18.2 mmHg).

Postoperative mean LESP was also the lowest of the series (6 mmHg). This was significantly lower than the mean pressure for the other patients which was 11 mmHg.

Comments

The results of this prospective study allowed us to assert 2 hypotheses:
- first a fundoplication leading to a pressure increase lower than 6.6 times the values at the beginning of the procedure should not be followed by a dysphagia;
- taking into account the systematic decrease (50%) of LESP postoperatively, one can assume that the pressure should be over 23 mmHg at the end of the procedure, to prevent postoperative reflux recurrence.

Intraoperative manometry has been used initially by Hill [1]. It was considered as mandatory when performing the cardiopexy for reflux disease. The results of Hill were confirmed by Hermreck [2].

The increase of LESP after dissection of the hiatal crura and before any fundoplication has been reported by others like Jamieson [3]. The explanation of this phenomenon could be related to noncholinergic nonadrenergic inhibitor receptors of the esophagus which could be the damaged by the dissection.

The validity of intraoperative manometry as a method to assess fundoplication is controversial. Studies by DeMeester [4] and Jamieson [3], showed contradictory results related to other antireflux procedures. These authors considered that postoperative and uncertain decrease of LESP does alter the reliability of this method. According to Jamieson, intraoperative manometry cannot predict the postoperative functional results.

The lack of predictive value of intraoperative manometry regarding the likelihood of recurrent reflux seems logical since we all know that this failure could be related to mechanical problems such as the wrap breakdown or migration, or the performance of a too loose wrap.

On contrary, intraoperative manometry could be of value to predict (or better prevent) postoperative dysphagia. The performance of a too continent wrap is the main cause of postoperative dysphagia though some other factors (motor disorders of the esophagus, lack of transient relaxations) could also explain this complication.

Intraoperative manometry could be of interest during the performance of some fundoplications reputed to cause dysphagia such as the Nissen-Rossetti technique. It could also be used in multicentre clinical trials to objectively assess the respective techniques since we all know variations among surgeons in the technique of fundoplication. This approach allow the investigators to objectively assess LESP and LES length and to compare the results of each technique.

Conclusions

Due to the discordant results in the literature and the multiplicity of factors involved in the genesis of complications after surgical treatment of GERD, we cannot definitely recommend the intraoperative manometry to assess the fundoplications.

References

1. Hill LD Intraoperative manometry of lower esophageal sphincter pressure. J Thorac Cardiovasc Surg 1978;75:378-381.
2. Hemreck AS, Coates NR. Results of the Hill antireflux operation Am J Surg 1980;140:764-767.
3. Jamieson GG, Miers JC. The relationship between intraoperative manometry and clinical outcome in patients operated for gastroesophageal reflux. World J Surg 1992;16:337-340.
4. DeMeester TR. What is the role of intraoperative manometry. Ann Thorac Surg 1980;30:1-4.

What is the present rate for conversion after laparoscopic approach?

I. Cecconello, C. Eduardo Domene, S. Szachnowicz, J. Gama-Rodrigues (São Paulo)

The surgical treatment for Barrett's esophagus is not different from that used in non-complicated gastroesophageal reflux disease (GERD) [1]. However, there are many uncertainties remaining about its indications. Its main advantage are: the relief of symptoms, suppression of aggression of esophageal mucosa, and, eventually, preventing adenocarcinoma [2-4].

Deceiving long-term results of fundoplication have been reported in Barrett's esophagus. Some authors call attention to technical difficulties, as edema and shrinkage of the esophagus, leading to intraoperative complications and higher levels of conversion during a laparoscopic procedure [5-7].

In the Digestive Surgery unit of the University of São Paulo Medical School, 480 patients with GERD were operated on through video-laparoscopy from 1990 to march 2000. Age varied from 06 to 90 years (mean 44.3 years). The associated procedures were: cholecystectomy in 31 patients, proximal gastric vagotomy in ten and inguinal herniorraphy in five.

Ninety-three (93) patients had Barrett's esophagus, 17 with associated stenosis. In the preoperative evaluation, all the patients were submitted to barium upper gastrointestinal studies, endoscopy, esophagical manometry and 24 hour pH monitoring.

Nissen fundoplication was performed in 417 patients and Toupet procedure (270°) in 63. All Barrett's esophagus patients were submitted to a Nissen fundoplication [6]. The gastric fundus was mobilized in most of the cases by division of the short vessels, in order to perform an adequate fundoplication. Patients with stenosis were dilated preoperatively.

The morbidity was low and no death was observed. Considering all the cases, conversion to an open-procedure was necessary in two cases, due to a left pneumothorax, both without Barrett's esophagus.

Discussion

Laparoscopic surgery in Barrett's esophagus requires several specific features quoted by most of the authors. The literature on the subject is still lacking of prospective randomized studies, demanding similar indications and surgical approach in order to offer final patterned analysis for the treatment.

The conversion rates for Barrett's esophagus laparoscopic treatment is not different from those observed for non complicated GERD (*Table I*). In our experience also, there was no increase of the conversion rates, even in those patients with esophageal stenosis.

Table I. Laparoscopic fundoplication conversion rates. Patients with non-complicated gastro-esophageal reflux disease (GERD) and Barrett's esophagus with and without stenosis.

Authors	Non-complicated GERD	Conversion (%)	Barrett's esophagus	Conversion (%)	Barrett's esophagus + stenosis	Conversion (%)
Watson (1996*)	207	15 (7,2 %)	24	3 (12,5%)	7	0
Ritter (1997)	61	2 (3%)	17	0	–	–
Cadiere (1997)	211	3 (1,4%)	13	0	–	–
Farrell (1999)	496	0	74	0	–	–
Kiviluoto (1998)	179	0	21	0	8	0
Landreneau (1998)	126	2 (1,5%)	24	0	0	0
Ferguson (1998)	–	2 (3%)	0	0	–	–
Baulieux (1999)	–	–	9	0	–	–
Parini (1999)	41	0	1	0	0	0
Brandalise (2000)	739	4 (0,5%)	61	0	0	0
Our casuistic (2000)	387	2 (0,5%)	93	0	17	0
Total	2,447	30 (1,2%)	337	3 (0,9%)	32	0

* Statistically non-significant difference between conversions in Barrett's esophagus and non-complicated GERD.

There are only few studies that really separate the Barrett's esophagus cases. However, in other more important multicenter series, not sparing the cases, the presence of Barrett's esophagus is not quoted as a conversion factor [18-24].

The laparoscopic procedure gives easy access to the gastroesophageal junction, allows for safe dissection of the distal esophagus, and, when needed, upwards dissection of the esophagus through the diaphragmatic hiatus, to carry out a safe and tensionless valve confection even in cases which esophageal shrinkage.

On the other hand, some authors call attention to technical difficulties in patients with shortening of the esophagus or stenosis, thus rendering a Collis-Nissen procedure necessary in 10-20% of the cases [17].

When a patient with Barrett's esophagus is being operated, special care must be taken for the dissection. The parietal pleura is not rarely linked to the swollen area of the distal esophagus, making its release harder, and to be done with great care, to avoid perforation and pneumothorax formation. Dissection of the esophagus must also be performed very carefully. Esophageal perforation was not observed in our patients with Barrett's esophagus.

Conclusions

There are still controversies about the indications of the surgical treatment in Barrett's esophagus, the technical procedure to choose and the results. Laparoscopic fundoplication surely brings out a great benefit to the non-complicated GERD treatment, as well as for Barrett's esophagus patients:

- laparoscopic fundoplication for treatment of Barrett's esophagus does not present higher levels of conversion than non-complicated forms of GERD, even when associated with stenosis;
- laparoscopic treatment for Barrett's esophagus deserves some special attentions as:
  • careful dissection of the distal esophagus through the diaphragmatic hiatus, releasing an adequate length of abdominal esophagus to be involved in the fundoplication, even in the patients with short esophagus,
  • adequate release of the pleura that could be linked to the swollen periesophageal area,
  • care for esophageal dissection and isolation, mainly in the posterior face, in order to avoid esophageal perforation.

References

1. Waring JP. Barret's esophagus: current concepts in diagnosis and management. Medscape Gastroenterol 2000;2:3.
2. Navab F. Barrett's esophagus: clinical implications. Medscape Gastroenterol 2000;2:3.
3. Peters JH. The surgical management of Barrett's esophagus. Gastroenterol Clin North Am 1997;26(3):647-668.
4. De Meester SR, Campos GMR, DeMeester TR, Bremner CG, et al. The impact of antireflux procedure on intestinal mataplasia of the cardia. Ann Surg 1998;228(4);547-556.
5. Csendes A, Braghetto I, Burdiles P. Long-term results of classic antireflux surgery in 152 patients with Barrett's esophagus: clinical, radiologic, endoscopic, manometric, and acid reflux test analysis before and late after operation. Surgery 1998;123:645-657.
6. DeMeester TR, Attwood SE, Smyrk TH, Hinder RA. Surgical therapy in Barrett's esophagus. Ann Surg 1990;212:528-542.
7. Watson DI, Foreman D, Devitt PG, Jamieson GG. Preoperative endoscopic grading of esophagitis versus outcome after laparoscopic Nissen fundoplication. Am J Gastroenterol 1997;92:222-225.
8. Brandalise NA. Laparoscopic treatment for GERD. Data for publishing given by the author.
9. Farrell TM, Smith CD, Hunter JG, et al. Fundoplication provides effective and durable symptom relief in patients with Barrett's esophagus. Am J Surg 1999;178:18-21.
10. Cadiere GB, Himpens J, Rajan A, et al. Laparoscopic Nissen fundoplication: laparoscopic dissection technique and results. Hepatogastroenterology 1997;44:4-10.
11. Kiviluoto T, Siren J, et al. Laparoscopic Nissen fundoplication: a prospective analysis of 200 consecutive patients. Surg Laparosc Endosc 1998;8(6):429-434.
12. Landreneau RJ, Wiechmann RJ, Hazelrigg SR, et al. Success os laparoscopic fundoplication for gastroesophageal reflux disease. Ann Thorac Surg 1998;66:1886-1893.
13. Ritter DW, Vanderpool D, Westmoreland M. Laparoscopic Nissen fundoplication for gastroesophageal reflux disease. Am J Surg 1997;174:715-718.
14. Parini U, Fosson A, Murix EL, Liotta G. Laparoscopic treatment of gastroesophageal reflux. Chir Ital 1999;51(2):121-126.
15. Ferguson MK. Guidelines for laparoscopic antireflux procedure. Surg Endosc 1998;12(12):1451.
16. Baulieux J, Mabrut JY, Souquet JC, et al. Barret's esophagus and antireflux: a study of a series of 26 patients. Chirurgie 1999;124(4):398-405.
17. Morales TG, Sampliner RE. Barrett's esophagus: update on screening, surveillance and treatment. Arch Intern Med 1999;159:1411-1416.
18. Arnaud JP, Pessaux P, Ghavani B, et al. Fundoplicature laparoscopique pour reflux gastro-œsophaghien. Étude multicentrique de 1 470 cas. Chirurgie 1999;124:516-522.
19. Collet D, Cadiere GB. Conversions and complications of laparoscopic treatment of gastroesophageal reflux disease. Am J Surg 1995;169(6):622-626.
20. Dallemagne B, Weerts JM, Jeahes C, Markiewicz S. Results of laparoscopic Nissen fundoplication. Hepatogastroenterology 1998;45:338-345.

21. Zaninotto G, Molena D, Ancona E. A propective multicenter study on laparoscopic treatment of gastroesophageal reflux disease in Italy: type of surgery, conversions, complications, and early results. Surg Endosc 2000;14(3):282-288.
22. Frantzides CT, Richards C. A study of 362 consecutive laparoscopic Nissen fundoplications. Surgery 1998;124:651-655.
23. Johanet H, Bellouard A, Bokobza B. Laparoscopic cure of gastroesophageal reflux disease. Ann Chir 1999;53(5):382-386.
24. Hunter JG, Trust TL, et al. A physiologic approach to laparoscopic fundoplication for gastroesophageal reflux disease. Ann Surg 1996;223:673-687.

What are the indications for intraluminal suturing, Vicryl band ligation of the esophagus and submucosal teflon injection?

S.S. Kadirkamanathan, C.P. Swain (London)

Conventional antireflux surgical operations, which wrap the cardia around the esophagus such as a Nissen fundoplication, may be a poor choice of procedure to treat Barrett's esophagus. It is also difficult to perform effective surveillance of the cardioesophageal mucosal junction after surgery, since some tissue is buried in the wrap. There is no conclusive evidence of Barrett's regression following either medical or surgical therapy [1]. There have been case reports of adenocarcinoma of the esophagus following fundoplication, suggesting that antireflux surgery may not reverse the malignant potential of Barrett's esophagus [2]. Although laparoscopic antireflux surgery is very effective in curtailing reflux, the side effects can be quite troublesome. It is possible that combination of mucosal ablation and effective antireflux surgery might be an effective long-term treatment of Barrett's esophagus.

Endoscopic gastroplasty is a minimally invasive surgical procedure, which is performed at flexible endoscopy without laparotomy or laparoscopy [3]. This operation is similar to a Collis' gastroplasty, which was initially developed as a method for treating "short esophagus" which may be a synonym for or equivalent to a Barrett's esophagus [4].

Promising results have been reported in both European [5] and American series [6] using endoscopic sewing machine technology. Both the endoscopic sewing machine and the operative procedure for treatment of reflux have received Food and Drug administration (FDA) approval.

The results of endoscopic gastroplasty suggest that this operation can improve reflux symptoms and measured acid exposure of distal esophagus and increase lower esophageal sphincter (LES) length and pressure. These results were observed in 107 patients with gastroesophageal reflux disease. Patients with hiatus hernia larger than 2 cm were excluded and few patients with Barrett's esophagus were included. Four patients with Barrett's esophagus were treated in the above series had improved symptoms with decrease acid exposure. No attempt was made to ablate the Barrett's segment nor was regression observed following this treatment.

Good symptomatic results were obtained with endoscopic gastroplasty in 64 patients in a multicentre American study. Half the patients had stitches placed below the cardioesophageal junction in a linear configuration and the other half in a circumferential configuration. Patients with hiatus hernia > 2 cm and with Barrett's esophagus were excluded in this study.

Other endoscopic procedures for reflux have been considered. These include, band ligation, injection methods and thermal methods.

With Van Steigman, our group placed bands at the cardioesophageal junction and measured LES pressure and length and found no difference in studies in pigs. In comparison, endoscopic gastroplasty caused a significant increase in sphincter length and pressure in both pigs and dogs. Band ligation does not seem to be a promising method to treat reflux.

Placement of Vicryl scarf on the serosal aspect of the gastroesophageal junction has been shown to prevent experimental gastroesophageal reflux (GER) in animal models [7]. It is believed that it works by a mechanism similar to Angelchick prosthesis. No follow-up human studies have been reported.

Injection of collagen and teflon has been used by urologists for the treatment vesico-ureteric reflux for at least 15 years [8]. Injection of collagen was perhaps the earliest endoscopic method tried for the treatment of GER in animal models and in a few patients [9]. It was not pursued because of doubts about its long-term efficacy, the tendency of the collagen to disperse throughout the mediastinum, and because it was an expensive material.

Injection of sodium morrhuate at the cardioesophageal junction was used to treat reflux in experimental animal models [10]. It appears not to have been studied in man.

There has been renewed interest in injection for the treatment of reflux using new biocompatible inert polymers. Results of human studies are awaited.

There is a need for better less invasive endosurgical methods, which can prevent continuing acid related esophageal epithelial damage, which appears to be the stimulus for continuing intestinal metaplasia. It is possible that endoscopic gastroplasty or other flexible endoscopic procedures may offer a better option for surgical correction and monitoring of Barrett's esophagus. More work is required to establish whether this is the case.

References

1. Stein HJ, Feith M, Siewert JR. Malignant degeneration of Barrett's esophagus: clinical point of view. Rec Res Cancer Res 2000;155: 42-53.
2. Hakansson HO, Johnsson F, Johansson J, Kjellen G, Walther B. Development of adenocarcinoma in Barrett's oesophagus after successful antireflux surgery. Eur J Surg 1997;163:469-471.
3. Kadirkamanathan SS, Evans DF, Gong F, Yazaki E, Scott M, Swain CP. Antireflux operations at flexible endoscopy using endoluminal stitching techniques: an experimental study. Gastrointest Endosc 1996;44:133-143.
4. Collis JL. An operation for hiatus hernia with short esophagus. J Thoracic Surg 1957;34:768-778.
5. Swain CP, Park PO, Kjellin T, Gong F, Kadirkamanathan SS, Appleyard M. Endoscopic gastroplasty for gastro-esophageal reflux disease. Gastrointest Endosc 2000;51:AB144.
6. Filipi CJ, Edmundowicz SA, Gostout CJ Lehman GA, Raijman IL, et al. Transoral endoscopic suturing for gastro-esophageal reflux disease: a multicenter trial. Gastrointest Endosc 2000;51:AB143.
7. Feussner H, Horvath OP, Siewert JR. Vicryl scarf induced scarring around the esophagogastric junction as treatment of esophageal reflux disease. An experimental study in dog. Dig Dis Sci 1992;37:875-881.
8. Puri P, Guiney EJ. Endoscopic correction of vesicoureteric reflux secondary to neuropathic bladder. Br J Urol 1986;58:504-506.
9. O'Connor KW, Lehman GA. Endoscopic placement of collagen at the lower esophageal sphincter to inhibit gastroesophageal reflux: a pilot study of 10 medically intractable patients. Gastrointest Endosc 1988;34:106-112.
10. Donahue PE, Carvalho PJ, Davis PE, Shen YJ, Miidla I, Bombeck CT, Nyhus LM. Endoscopic sclerosis of the gastric cardia for prevention of experimental gastroesophageal reflux. Gastrointest Endosc 1990;36:253-256.

Are mechanical complications higher after laparoscopic Nissen than after the open approach?

W.K.H. Kauer, H.J. Stein, J.R. Siewert (Munich)

Gastroesophageal reflux disease (GERD) is a very common condition. The majority of patients who develop GERD are treated medically with proton pump inhibitors and prokinetic agents. However, 10% to 20% of these patients develop severe complications, such as Barrett's esophagus, and a significant number experience recurrence of their symptoms during long-term maintenance or after the treatment is terminated [1, 2]. Conventional surgical management of GERD with fundoplication as initially described by Nissen has been shown to be effective, durable, and superior to medical therapy [3-6]. Application of laparoscopy to surgical treatment of GERD has emerged in the last decade, and the number of patients who undergo antireflux surgery has significantly increased. Laparoscopic fundoplication has been shown to be safe and as effective as the open fundoplication, and has become the first surgical option [5, 6] since retrospective and prospective non-randomized studies have shown similar results for both techniques [7, 8].

However, in a multicentre randomized trial from the Netherlands [9] candidates for surgical treatment of GERD were randomly assigned to either laparoscopic or open 360° Nissen fundoplication. Primary endpoints were dysphagia, recurrent GERD, and intrathoracic hernia. Secondary endpoints were effectiveness and quality of life. They found that at the time of interim analysis, 11 patients in the laparoscopic group and one in the conventional group had reached a primary endpoint ($p = 0.01$). This difference was caused mainly by whether or not patients had dysphagia (seven patients in the laparoscopic group and none in the conventional group, $p = 0.016$). They came to the conclusion that although laparoscopic Nissen fundoplication was as effective as the open procedure in controlling reflux, the significantly higher risk of reaching a primary endpoint in the laparoscopic group led them stop the study.

At the present time more prospective randomized trials are needed to finally answer the above question.

References

1. Anvari M, Allen C, Born A. Laparoscopic Nissen fundoplication is a satisfactory alternative to long-term omeprazole therapy. Br J Surg 1995;82:938-942.
2. McKenzie D, Grayson T, Polk HC. The impact of omeprazole and laparoscopy upon hiatal hernia and reflux esophagitis. J Am Coll Surg 1996;183:413-418.
3. Spechler SJ. Comparison of medical and surgical therapy for complicated gastroesophageal reflux disease in veterans. N Engl J Med 1992;326:786-792.
4. DeMeester TR, Bonavina L, Albertucci M. Nissen fundoplication for gastroesophageal reflux disease. Ann Surg 1986;204:9-20.
5. Hinder RA, Filini CJ, Wetscher G, et al. Laparoscopic Nissen fundoplication is an effective treatment for gastroesophageal reflux disease. Ann Surg 1994;220:472-483.
6. Hunter JG, Trus TL, Branum GD, et al. A physiologic approach to laparoscopic fundoplication for gastroesophageal reflux disease. Ann Surg 1996;223:673-687.
7. Peters JH, Heimbucher J, Kauer WKH, et al. Clinical and physiological comparison of laparoscopic and open Nissen fundoplication. J Am Coll Surg 1995;180:385-393.

8. Eshraghi N, Farahmand M, Soot S, et al. Comparison of outcomes of open versus laparoscopic fundoplication performed in a single practice. Am J Surg 1998;175:371-374.
9. Bais JE, Bartelsmann JF, Bonjer HJ, et al. Laparoscopic or conventional Nissen fundoplication for gastroesophageal reflux disease: randomized clinical trial. The Netherlands Antireflux Surgery Study Group. Lancet 2000:355:170-174.

What is the rate of occurrence of vagal damage after antireflux surgery?

M. Luostarinen (Lahti)

Vagal nerve damage is possible during antireflux surgery. Some of the post-fundoplication symptoms are similar to the clinical symptoms or evoke vagal dysfunction (*Table I*) and, thus, vagal damage have implicitly been envisaged. Some single cases of vagal nerve damage with severe post-fundoplication symptoms have been described, but the true prevalence of this event is not yet known.

Table I. Symptoms and signs of vagal damage.

Diarrhea
Delayed gastric emptying of solid food
Enhanced gastric emptying of liquids
Dyspepsia
Gas bloat
Gastroparesis

How frequent are symptoms suggestive of vagal damage after antireflux surgery?

Diarrhea is very infrequent. In our long-term follow-up studies only one of the 134 patients complained from diarrhea 6 to 20 years after open antireflux surgery [1], and had undergone concomitant vagotomy during the operation. Increase of bloating has been reported by up to 22% of the patients in prospective studies and increase of flatus by 43% [2], these symptoms being occasionally disturbing in 10%. Bloating and flatus may be regarded as signs of vagal dysfunction, but it is more likely a question of normal postfundoplication physiology with changed belching ability [3, 4] with its consequences. Fundoplication have been shown to increase gastric emptying rate of both liquid and solids, which is not in agreement with functional disturbances caused by vagal damage [5-7]

Some evidence on true rate of vagal damage has recently been emerging: in two studies Wu *et al.* [6, 7] directly assessed vagal function in 24 patients (with Nissen fundoplication or Toupet's hemifundoplication) 6-12 months after antireflux surgery. Response of pancreatic polypeptide on insulin-induced hypoglycemia was used as a measure of vagal nerve integrity. Only one (4%) of these 24 patients had objective vagal damage.

In conclusion, larger studies are needed with more consecutive patients whith objective measurement of vagal function, before answering the question of the true rate of occurrence of vagal damage. Nevertheless, vagal dysfunction after antireflux surgery seems to be rare, but, in individual cases, it may be the reason for some of the postfundoplication symptoms.

References

1. Luostarinen M. Nissen fundoplication for gastro-oesophageal reflux disease: long-term results. Ann Chir Gynaecol 1995;84(2):115-120.
2. Luostarinen ME, Isolauri JO. Randomized trial to study the effect of fundic mobilization on long-term results of Nissen fundoplication. Br J Surg 1999;86(5):614-618.
3. Luostarinen M, Koskinen M, Reinikainen P, Karvonen J, Isolauri J. Two antireflux operations:floppy versus standard Nissen fundoplication. Ann Med 1995;27(2):199-205.
4. Johnsson F, Holloway RH, Ireland AC, Jamieson GG, Dent J. Effect of fundoplication on transient lower oesophageal sphincter relaxation and gas reflux. Br J Surg 1997;84(5):686-689.
5. Viljakka M, Saali K, Koskinen M, Karhumaki L, Kossi J, Luostarinen M, Teerenhovi O, Isolauri J. Antireflux surgery enhances gastric emptying. Arch Surg 1999;134(1):18-21.
6. Vu MK, Ringers J, Arndt JW, Lamers CB, Masclee AA. Prospective study of the effect of laparoscopic hemifundoplication on motor and sensory function of the proximal stomach. Br J Surg 2000;87(3):338-343.
7. Vu MK, Straathof JW, Schaar PJ, Arndt JW, Ringers J, Lamers CB, Masclee AA. Motor and sensory function of the proximal stomach in reflux disease and after laparoscopic Nissen fundoplication. Am J Gastroenterol 1999;94(6):1481-1489.

What are the late results of laparoscopic antireflux surgery?

G. Zaninotto, D. Molena, M. Costantini, G. Portale, M. Costantino, B. Gnoccato, E. Ancona (Padova)

Although, when surgery was compared to antacid and H_2-blocker therapies in the long-term treatment of gastroesophageal reflux disease (GERD) in 1975 by Behar [1] and in 1992 by Spechler [2], the overall findings suggested that antireflux surgery was consistently more effective than medical therapy, the introduction of proton pump inhibitor (PPI) – a powerful drug offering rapid symptom relief and curing esophagitis in the vast majority of patients – shifted the balance in favor of medical treatment [3]. In the last 10 years, antireflux surgery was consequently relegated to an ancillary role in the treatment of GERD: indications for it were relatively rare and limited to patients failing to respond to medical therapy or developing complications. A recent report from Lundell *et al.* showed, however, that surgery is even more effective than omeprazole in controlling GERD [4]. Surgery has also made substantial progress: thanks to a better understanding of the mechanism behind cardia competence, the surgical technique has been refined and become more effective with fewer side effects, allowing for a more efficient selection of patients suitable for antireflux surgery. The introduction of laparoscopic surgery has made surgery more acceptable to gastroenterologists and patients and the previous reluctance of physicians to refer patients for surgery has progressively decreased.

Long-term results of antireflux surgery

Laparoscopic antireflux surgery is feasible, with the same low mortality and morbidity and the same effectiveness (at least in the disease-specific short-term goal), as open surgery. Several authors [5, 6, 8] reported an > 90% improvement in symptoms and a 92-95% return to normal values in esophageal acid exposure measured by 24-hour pH monitoring. Follow-ups of up to 7 years are now available and they show a success rate higher than 90%. *Table I* shows the efficacy of laparoscopic fundoplication.

Table I. Efficacy of laparoscopic fundoplication for gastroesophageal reflux disease.

Author	Year	Patients	Operation	GERD recurrence (%)
Hinder [8]	1994	198	Nissen	7
Hunter [5]	1996	126	Nissen	3
Jones [9]	1996	85	Nissen	1.1
Dallemagne [10]	1998	127	Nissen	2.3
Peters [7]	1998	95	Nissen	4
Bell [11]	1999	138	Toupet	1
Padova	Unpubl.	199	Nissen	4

A prospective study was carried out in Italy on behalf of the Italian Society of Endoscopic Surgery and more than 600 patients were collected from 20 centers all over Italy in two years. The rate of intraoperative complications was 4.3% and only 1% were severe complications such as esophageal or gastric perforation. The early results on more than 300 patients are very promising: symptoms were controlled in 91% of patients and healing of severe esophagitis was achieved in 96% of patients. The patients' satisfaction after surgery collected on a visual-analog self-testing scale from 1 to 10 was between 8 and 10 in more than 80% of patients and less than 1% were dissatisfied with the outcome of the operation [6]. An important side-effect of laparoscopic antireflux surgery is dysphagia. It has been shown that transient dysphagia is common after surgery and is perhaps the sign of a well-made wrap; it generally resolves spontaneously in about 2 months. Persistent dysphagia has been reported in up to 10% patients and it seems to be related to the Nissen-Rossetti operation. Improved skills and certain technical modifications have resulted in a reduction of this most common side-effect of laparoscopic antireflux surgery. Complete mobilization of the gastric fundus by dividing the short gastric vessels enables a floppy, symmetrical wrap to encircle the distal esophagus [14]. Also, by mobilizing the gastric fundus, we avoid making the mistake of encircling the esophagus not with the upper part of the fundus, but with the gastric body. Gas-bloat syndrome and the inability to belch has an incidence ranging between 1% and 49% (*Table II*). It is necessary to assess preoperatively whether a

Table II. Incidence of gas-bloat after laparoscopic antireflux surgery.

Author	Year	Patients	Gas-bloat (%)
Hinder [8]	1994	198	7
Hunter [5]	1996	126	3
Horgan [15]	1997	232	30
Ritter [16]	1997	78	1
Anvari [17]	1998	260	49

patient already has any gastrointestinal motility disturbances. The floppy fundoplication should preserve the ability to belch and vagal nerve injury may be responsible when these symptoms persist postoperatively. One of the most important causes of failure in antireflux surgery, which is unlikely with open surgery, is wrap displacement into the chest (*Table III*). A more extensive dissection of the hiatus, fewer adhesions and earlier patient mobilization may play a part in the onset of this complication. Contributing factors may include inadequate closure of the diaphragmatic crura, a short esophagus and/or insufficient esophagus mobilization; in such cases, the use of a mesh to secure the hiatal closure and a Collis-Nissen operation to adequately lengthen the esophagus should be considered.

Table III. Incidence of anatomical displacement of laparoscopic fundoplication.

Author	Year	Patients	Fundoplication displacement (%)
Watson [18]	1995	253	17 (7%)
Anvari [17]	1998	260	49 (19%)
Soper [12]	1999	290	20 (7%)
Hunter [14]	1999	852	27 (3%)
Padova serie	Unpubi.	184	14 (8%)

In our experience of a consecutive series of 199 patients who underwent laparoscopic antireflux surgery, the overall success rate was 90%. The conversion rate was 5.5% and most of these were part of the first 50 cases. The most common reason for conversion was a large paraesophageal hernia or adhesions from previous operations. Intraoperative complications amounted to 3% and the most common were gastric wall perforations – occurring in 3 cases, repaired laparoscopically in 2/3 patients and requiring conversion to laparotomy in 1 (the postoperative course was uneventful in all 3 cases). The follow-up obtained in 184 patients with a median of 34 months (range 2-83) showed excellent/good results in 148 patients (80%). Failures are listed in *Table IV*. Additional endoscopic or surgical treatments were performed in 20/31 patients: 12 surgical repairs (9 laparoscopically and 3 with open surgery), 8 endoscopic dilations of the cardia and 3 endoscopic dilations of the pylorus), resulting in an improvement of symptoms in 17/20 patients (85%). Therefore, the overall success rate after primary or secondary treatment rose to 165 (90%). It is noteworthy that recurrent reflux symptoms were only recorded in 7 patients (4%); 2 of these had a Collis Nissen fundoplication repair because of esophageal stricture, 4 had a Nissen fundoplication and 1 a Toupet. The risk for GERD recurrence was higher in patients who had severe disease and shortening of the esophagus than in patients with a normal esophageal length (2/7 *versus* 4/181, $p < 0.001$).

Table IV. Causes of failure.

Postoperative dysphagia	9 patients (5%)
Fundoplication displacement	14 patients (8%)
Reflux recurrence	7 patients (4%)
Gas-bloat	4 patients (2%)
Patients dissatisfaction	2 patients (1%)

Conclusions

Laparoscopic antireflux surgery is a valuable treatment for patients with GERD; it should be performed by properly-trained surgeons with an appropriate background of esophageal physiology. Candidates for laparoscopic fundoplication should be assessed with particular attention to their overall gastrointestinal complaints – laparoscopic fundoplication is not always the answer. The surgical technique should be tailored to avoid postoperative side-effects and to increase the success rate.

References

1. Behar J, Sheahan DG, Biancani P, et al. Medical and surgical management of reflux esophagitis. A 38-month report on a prospective clinical trial. N Engl J Med 1975;293:263-268.
2. Spechler SJ. Comparison of medical and surgical therapy for complicated gastroesophageal reflux disease in veterans. The Department of Veterans Affairs Gastro-oesophageal Reflux Disease Study Group. N Engl J Med 1992;326:786-792.
3. Vigneri S, Termini R, Leandro G, et al. A comparison of maintenance therapies for reflux esophagitis. N Engl J Med 1995;333:1106-1110.
4. Lundell L, Miettinem P, Myrvold HE, et al Continued (5-year) follow-up of a randomized clinical study comparing antireflux surgery and omeprazole in gastroesophageal reflux disease. J Am Coll Surg 2001;192(2):172-181.
5. Hunter JG, Trus TL, Branum GD. A physiologic approach to laparoscopic fundoplication for gastroesophageal reflux disease. Ann Surg 1996;223:673-687.
6. Zaninotto G, Molena D, Ancona E. A prospective, multicenter study on laparoscopic treatment of gastroesophageal reflux in Italy: type of surgery, conversions, complications and early results. Surg Endosc 2000;14:282-288.
7. Peters JH, DeMeester TR, Crookes P, et al. The treatment of gastroesophageal reflux disease with laparoscopic Nissen fundoplication. Ann Surg 1998;228:40-50.
8. Hinder RA, Filipi CJ, Wetscher G, et al. Laparoscopic Nissen fundoplication is an effective treatment for gastroesophageal reflux disease. Ann Surg 1994;220:472-483.
9. Jones R, Canal DF, Inman MM, Rescorla FJ. Laparoscopic fundoplication: a three-year review. Am Surg 1996;62(8):632-636.
10. Dallemagne B, Weerts JM, Jeahes C, Markiewicz S. Results of laparoscopic Nissen fundoplication. Hepatogastroenterology 1998;45(23):1338-1343.
11. Bell RC, Hanna P, Mills MR, Bowrey D. Patterns of success and failure with laparoscopic Toupet fundoplication. Surg Endosc 1999;13(12):l 189-1194.
12. Soper NJ, Dunnegan D. Anatomic fundoplication failure after laparoscopic antireflux surgery. Ann Surg 1999;229(5):669-677.
13. Hunter JG, Smith CD, Branum GD, et al. Laparoscopic fundoplication failures: patterns of failure and response to fundoplication revision. Ann Surg 1999;230(4):595-606.
14. Hunter JG, Swanstrom L, Waring JP. Dysphagia after laparoscopic antireflux surgery. Ann Surg 1996;224:51-57.
15. Horgan S, Pellegrini CA. Surgical treatment of gastroesophageal reflux disease. Surg Clin North Am 1997;77(5):1063-1082.
16. Ritter DW, Vanderpool D, Westmoreland M. Laparoscopic Nissen fundoplication for gastroesophageal reflux disease. Am J Surg 1997;174(6):715-718.
17. Anvari M, Allen C. Laparoscopic Nissen fundoplication: two-year comprehensive follow-up of a technique of minimal paraesophageal dissection. Ann Surg 1998;227(1):25-32.
18. Watson A, Spychal RT, Brown MG, Peck N, Callander N. Laparoscopic "physiological" antireflux procedure: preliminary results of a prospective symptomatic and objective study. Br J Surg 1995;82(5):651-656.

Can antireflux surgery be considered as potentially reducing the risk of malignancy?

B. Gayet (Paris)

Gastroesophageal reflux (GER) is associated with an increased risk of cancer, particularly in patients with long-standing, frequent, and nocturnal reflux, as shown by a population-based case-control study in Sweden [1]. The risk increase is high for adenocarcinoma of the esophagus (odds ratio of up to 43.5) and smaller for adenocarcinoma of the cardia (odds ratio of up to 4.4). The incidences of esophageal adenocarcinoma and gastroesophageal reflux disease (GERD) have been increasing steadily for the last 20 years in industrialized countries. In France and in the United States, adenocarcinomas account for 50% of esophageal cancers in recent series as compared to only 10% and 20% two decades ago. The genesis of esophageal cancer involves several steps. GER causes intestinal metaplasia (IM), also called Barrett's esophagus, which can progress to low-grade then high-grade epithelial dysplasia. This sequence is believed to occur regardless of the length of Barrett's esophagus. It remains unclear whether GER can lead to carditis, defined as IM not visible by endoscopy, and to cancer of the cardia [2]. IM is found in 1% of patients undergoing endoscopy for any reason and in 3 to 10% of those undergoing endoscopy for reflux [2, 3]. The incidence of adenocarcinoma arising in Barrett's esophagus has recently been estimated at about 0.5% to 1% per year but the follow-up of the different prospective studies is quite short when compared with the life expectancy. Before discussing the potential ability of antireflux surgery to decrease the rate of malignant degeneration in patients with Barrett's esophagus, four comments are in order.

First, esophageal adenocarcinoma is widely believed to arise only within Barrett's esophagus, that is IM, and not within the other types of metaplasia.

Second, the definition of adenocarcinoma in Barrett's esophagus is not agreed on. Circumferential IM 3 cm or longer and a tumor within the metaplasia but away from the cardia clearly indicates malignancy in Barrett's esophagus. Uncertainty exists, however, when there is an adenocarcinoma arising within Barrett's esophagus but extending down to the cardia or an adenocarcinoma of the cardia with suprajacent Barrett's esophagus that shows no gross features of malignant degeneration or fails to meet classic criteria (*i.e.* that either is not circumferential or is circumferential but less than 2 cm long). Although these semiological distinctions are important when evaluating the literature, they should not deflect the clinician's attention away from the main issue: Barrett's esophagus is associated with an increase in the long-term risk of local degeneration with development of an adenocarcinoma in the involved segment or in the cardia.

Third, when evaluating the risk of malignant degeneration after antireflux surgery, care should be taken to exclude those patients in whom a malignancy present before the procedure is diagnosed only after the procedure. In patients with ulcerated lesions or extensive Barrett's esophagus, it can be difficult to rule out esophageal carcinoma with complete certainty. Adenocarcinoma diagnosed within six to 12 months after antireflux surgery should be classified as degeneration missed by the preoperative workup rather than as degeneration despite elimination of the acid and/or alkaline reflux. Furthermore, to improve the detection of malignancy, endoscopic vital staining should be performed before considering antireflux surgery in patients with Barrett's esophagus, and biopsies should be taken (a) from all atypical areas and (b) routinely at one- to two-centimeter intervals on opposite sides of the mucosa, moving the sampling sites 90° clockwise from one level to the next.

Fourth, the results of antireflux surgery deteriorate over time. Alleviation of reflux symptoms has been reported in 80% to 90% of patients ten years after antireflux surgery, whereas a normal pH recording has been found in fewer than 70% of patients in some studies, with the rate being lower in patients with Barrett's esophagus. This effect of time should be taken into account when evaluating the effect of eliminating acid and alkaline reflux on the risk of esophageal cancer.

The medical literature contains an abundance of case reports, retrospective studies, and even prospective studies showing that adenocarcinoma can occur after antireflux surgery [4-13]. Clearly, antireflux surgery fails to afford complete protection against esophageal adenocarcinoma. However, this does not mean that it affords no protection at all. Common characteristics in cases of adenocarcinoma in Barrett's esophagus after antireflux surgery are:

- absence of preoperative endoscopic vital staining performed using the above-described sampling technique;
- failure to evaluate the efficacy of the antireflux procedure by postoperative 24-hour pH recording, which is the only valid method;
- and failure to monitor efficacy over time by repeated pH recordings, annually for instance, which is difficult to achieve in asymptomatic patients.

To our knowledge, malignant degeneration in the absence of pH recording abnormalities has not been reported to date. Thus, there is an urgent need for studies evaluating the results of pH recordings at diagnosis of adenocarcinoma in Barrett's esophagus in patients with a history of antireflux surgery.

Table I. Occurrence of esophageal carcinoma in Barrett's esophagus according to the treatment and its result. Long-tem results from a randomized study [14].

Treatment	N° of adenocarcinomas per patient-years
Medical therapy	1/116
Antireflux surgery	1/319
Failed antireflux surgery	1/91
Successful antireflux surgery	0

Four studies found a reduction in the risk of malignant degeneration after effective antireflux surgery [14-17].

Ortiz *et al.* conducted a randomized study comparing antireflux surgery (Nissen procedure) and proton pump inhibitor (PPI) therapy in patients with Barrett's esophagus [14]. Median follow-ups were five years and four years in these two groups, respectively (range, 1-11 years in both groups). No cases of dysplasia or cancer occurred after successful antireflux surgery defined as absence of reflux by pH recording.

Katz *et al.* studied 102 patients with uncomplicated Barrett's esophagus. Follow-up was 563 patient-years. Adenocarcinoma developed in four patients (risk 1/141 patient-years) and high-grade dysplasia in four (overall risk, 1/70 patient-years), but none of these eight patients had had antireflux surgery.

Spechler *et al.* conducted a follow-up study of a prospective randomized trial comparing medical therapy (n = 165) and antireflux surgery (n = 82) in patients with severe GER (16). Only half these patients were available for the follow-up study. Esophageal adenocarcinoma developed in one patient in each group, yielding a risk of 1/437 patient-years in the nonsurgical group and 1/746 patient-years in the surgical group. However, only 108 patients had Barrett's esophagus, yielding a cancer risk of 1/259 patient-years, and outcome differences across treatments were not studied in the subgroup with Barrett's esophagus. Furthermore, the antireflux surgery failure rate was probably high, as 62% of patients continued to use antireflux medications after surgery, and only 10 of the 82 surgical patients underwent pH recordings postoperatively.

In a review, DeMeester *et al.* concluded that a functioning fundoplication seemed associated with protection against progression of Barrett's esophagus and that nonsurgical and failed antireflux surgery were associated with progression to dysplasia and adenocarcinoma [17]. In a previous article, the same group reported a study of 60 patients with IM of the esophagus (n = 45) or cardia (n = 15). Median follow-up was 25 months after antireflux surgery. Loss of IM occurred in 73% of the patients with involvement of the cardia only and in 4.4% of those with Barrett's esophagus. High-grade dysplasia or cancer did not occur in any of the patients.

In conclusion, whether antireflux surgery reduces the risk of esophageal adenocarcinoma in Barrett's esophagus remains unclear. A randomized study comparing no treatment, PPI therapy, and antireflux therapy might provide the information needed to settle this issue. Given the low rate of malignant degeneration, a large sample size would be needed to keep the risk of Type II error lower than 5%. However, there is firm evidence that antireflux surgery fails to protect completely against malignant degeneration, probably because about 10% of patients have persistent reflux initially and this rate increases over time. The answer to the question asked in the title of this article is probably "yes" provided the procedure ensures lasting (lifelong?) elimination of acid and alkaline reflux. When seeking to determine whether this warrants antireflux surgery in all patients with Barrett's esophagus, several factors should be considered. The potential benefit to the patient depends on the incidence of degeneration and on the magnitude of the risk reduction provided by antireflux surgery. Available data indicate that the incidence is about 0.5% and that the magnitude of the risk reduction is probably at least 5%. Thus, to prevent one case of esophageal adenocarcinoma, 400 patients would have to undergo antireflux surgery (1/(0.50-0.25%)). This number-needed-to-treat might be acceptable if surgery were inexpensive and caused no mortality or morbidity. The median mortality rate ranged from 0% to 0.4% in a metaanalysis of 21 136 surgically treated patients, a figure similar to the risk reduction provided by antireflux surgery [18]. Furthermore, among the adenocarcinomas that arise in patients receiving appropriate follow-up, some are amenable to curative surgery. Finally, the morbidity and long-term sequelae associated with surgery should be taken into consideration. For instance, in the above-mentioned study by Spechler *et al.* [16], the only significant difference after ten years was unexplained excess cardiac mortality in the surgically treated patients as compared to the nonsurgically treated patients. Although this finding requires confirmation, it should be borne in mind.

Finally, the data in the literature raise more questions than they provide answers. In patients with Barrett's esophagus, what is the best antireflux procedure? What is the magnitude of the risk reduction? What is the mean time to occurrence of a significant risk reduction? What is the incidence of degeneration in patients with Barrett's esophagus and in those with IM not visible endoscopically? After reflux surgery, should patients with Barrett's esophagus be monitored by endoscopy alone, according to current standard practice, or also by routine pH recordings? How often should follow-up endoscopy be performed? Endoscopic ablation of IM by plasma argon laser or dynamic phototherapy and, in patients with persistent reflux, lifelong PPI therapy have not been validated in patients with a history of antireflux therapy [19].

Studies providing strong evidence to support or disprove a risk-reduction effect of antireflux therapy are impatiently awaited, particularly as the incidence of esogastric adenocarcinoma is rising sharply in industrialized countries. Until such studies are published, it is reasonable to conclude from the available data that antireflux surgery can reduce the risk of malignant degeneration in the individual patient but that the evidence does not support routine antireflux surgery in all patients with Barrett's esophagus. During endoscopy to evaluate GER, routine collection of biopsies from the cardia is essential to help us improve our understanding of reflux-associated malignancies.

References

1. Lagergren J, Bergstrom R, Lindgren A, Nyren O. Symptomatic gastroesophageal reflux as a risk factor for esophageal adenocarcinoma. N Engl J Med 1999;340:825-831.
2. DeMeester SR, Campos GM, DeMeester TR, Bremner CG, Hagen JA, Peters JH, Crookes PF. The impact of an antireflux procedure on intestinal metaplasia of the cardia. Ann Surg 1998;228:547-556.
3. Pera M. Epidemiology of esophageal cancer, especially adenocarcinoma of the esophagus and esophagogastric junction. Rec Res Cancer Res 2000;155:1-14.
4. Holscher AH, Bader M, Siewert JR. Can antireflux surgery prevent malignant degeneration of Barrett esophagus? Dtsch Med Wochenschr 1985;110:551-555.
5. Agha FP. Progression of Barrett's mucosa to adenocarcinoma after antireflux surgery: radiologic-pathologic correlation. Dysphagia 1987;2:117-122.
6. Polepalle SC, McCallum RW. Barrett's esophagus. Current assessment and future perspectives. Gastroenterol Clin North Am 1990;19:733-744.

7. Williamson WA, Ellis FH Jr, Gibb SP, Shahian DM, Aretz HT. Effect of antireflux operation on Barrett's mucosa. Ann Thorac Surg 1990;49:537-541.
8. Streitz JM Jr, Ellis FH Jr, Gibb SP, Balogh K, Watkins E Jr. Adenocarcinoma in Barrett's esophagus. A clinicopathologic study of 65 cases. Ann Surg 1991;213:122-125.
9. Li H, Walsh TN, Hennessy TP. Carcinoma arising in Barrett's esophagus. Surg Gynecol Obstet 1992;175:167-172.
10. McDonald ML, Trastek VF, Allen MS, Deschamps C, Pairolero PC, Pairolero PC. Barrett's esophagus: does an antireflux procedure reduce the need for endoscopic surveillance? J Thorac Cardiovasc Surg 1996;111:1135-1138.
11. Hakansson HO, Johnsson F, Johansson J, Kjellen G, Walther B. Development of adenocarcinoma in Barrett's oesophagus after successful antireflux surgery. Eur J Surg 1997;163:469-471.
12. Yau P, Watson DI, Devitt PG, Game PA, Jamieson GG. Laparoscopic antireflux surgery in the treatment of gastroesophageal reflux in patients with Barrett esophagus. Arch Surg 2000;135:801-805.
13. Cameron AJ. Management of Barrett's esophagus. Mayo Clin Proc 1998;73:457-461.
14. Ortiz A, Martinez LF, Parilla P, Morales G, Molina J, Bermejo J, Liron R, Aguilar J. Conservative treatment versus antireflux surgery in Barrett's oesophagus: long-term results of a prospective study. Br J Surg 1996;83:274-278.
15. Katz D, Rothstein R, Schned A, Dunn J, Seaver K, Antonioli D. The development of dysphagia and adenocarcinoma during endoscopic surveillance of Barrett's esophagus. Am J Gastroenterol 1998;93:536-541.
16. Spechler SJ, Lee E, Ahnen D, Goyal RK, Hirano I, Ramirez F, et al. Long term outcome of medical and surgical therapies for gastroesophageal reflux disease. Follow-up of a randomized controlled trial. JAMA 2001;285:2331-2338.
17. DeMeester SR, DeMeester TR. The diagnosis and management of Barrett's esophagus. Adv Surg 1999;33:29-68.
18. Gayet B. Traitement chirurgical du reflux gastro-œsophagien : modalités et résultats de la chirurgie cœlioscopique. Gastroenterol Clin Biol 1999;23:S145-154.
19. Mc Carthy M, Wilkinson ML. Treatment of Barrett's esophagus by endoscopic laser ablation and antireflux surgery. Gastrointest Endosc 1999;49:129-130.

How to interpret postoperative progression of Barrett's esophagus in asymptomatic patients with documented 24-hour pH studies?

I.G. Martin (Auckland)

What happens to a segment of Barrett's esophagus following symptomatically successful antireflux surgery? What factors might be implicated in progression or regression of the Barrett's segment. What is the role of ongoing reflux as perhaps demonstrated by 24 hour pH studies? These factors need to be taken into account when considering the two forms of progression that may be encountered:

- has the Barrett's esophagus changed in length?
- has the Barrett's esophagus changed in character?

Other authors are specifically addressing the issue of whether antireflux surgery reduces the risk for the development of adenocarcinoma and therefore this point will not be addressed here although obviously it is linked to both of the above questions. Comments made in this paper will be confined to the area of disease progression.

What is the significance of a change in length of Barrett's esophagus after antireflux surgery?

Although we are considering disease progression it is useful to consider at this point the reported effects of antireflux surgery upon the extent of Barrett's esophagus in general. With good control of reflux it is hoped that the lower esophageal environment will return to normal and the stimulus which led to the development of the Barrett's esophagus will be removed. If this is the case then will the Barrett's esophagus "regress" to a normal squamous phenotype?

The first point to make is that almost all of the published observational studies have looked at long segment (> 3 cm) Barrett's esophagus and therefore any conclusions made for this group may not be true for patients with short segment disease. That having been said, these observational studies would suggest that even after successful antireflux surgery complete regression is rarely if ever seen and that the majority of patients continue with a clearly identified Barrett's segment. In a recent review summarising the English language literature DeMeester & DeMeester [1] identified 11 series following patients with Barrett's esophagus after antireflux surgery. From a total of 340 patients, 74% showed no change in the length of the Barrett's segment, 9% showed progression either in length (4%) or histology (5%) and 17% regression (12% partial). Only 4% of these patients had apparent complete regression. It has been our own experience that complete regression is very uncommon and that a static length of Barrett's mucosa is the most frequently seen outcome even after symptomatically and physiologically successful surgery. There is also no doubt that partial squamous re-epithelialization, most commonly with small islands occurs frequently. What is not known is the significance of this partial regression – what we and others have noted is that often if you biopsy these squamous islands you observe Barrett's type mucosal glands beneath the squamous surface. The significance or not of these buried glands is far from clear.

What of short segment Barrett's esophagus? The literature in this area is limited but interesting. One series has demonstrated that 73% of patients with intestinal metaplasia (IM) at the gastroesophageal junction (GEJ) but no visible Barrett's segment had loss of this IM following antireflux surgery, compared to just 4% of patients in whom a Barrett's segment was visible [2]. In this study no patient with IM at the GEJ only progressed to having a macroscopic Barrett's segment.

It would seem therefore that around 1 in 20 patients with Barrett's esophagus will progress in length after surgery. What are the implications of this finding? The simple answer is that we do not know. Around 10% of patients with documented reflux esophagitis and abnormal pH studies will develop Barrett's esophagus over a 3 year period when treated medically [4], but the majority of patients with preexisting Barrett's will show no change in the length of their segment. Others [5], have suggested that there is a relationship between the length of Barrett's esophagus and both lower esophageal sphincter status and the degree of esophageal acid exposure. Although this study was both substantial and provocative it did not present sequential data to truly answer the question as to whether significant ongoing or worsening reflux lengthens a Barrett's esophagus. There is very little data in postsurgical patients with which to answer this question, but what there is perhaps points towards an association with a lengthening Barrett's segment and recurrent or ongoing reflux. In one series [3], nine of 56 patients with Barrett's esophagus treated with antireflux surgery progressed in length; of these nine patients 4 were symptomatic and had documented evidence of recurrent reflux on 24-hour pH studies (5 were asymptomatic and were not tested).

What then are the implications of an increase in length of Barrett's esophagus in an otherwise asymptomatic patient? Using the available evidence it is likely that the patient has either recurrent or ongoing reflux which should be documented on a 24-hour pH study. What then? It is difficult to justify re-operation in the face of an asymptomatic patient but we do know that ongoing inflammation and acid exposure are powerful stimuli to proliferative change in Barrett's mucosa [6] and consideration must be given to commencing proton pump inhibitor (PPI) therapy even in the absence of symptoms.

Has the Barrett's segment changed in character?

What is meant by a change in character? I use this expression to indicate disease progression not reflected by a change in length but by the development of dysplasia (low or high-grade), carcinoma or perhaps even the expression of molecular markers known to be associated with the risk of development of carcinoma.

Up to 10% of patients who have previously undergone antireflux surgery with no evidence of dysplasia preoperatively will develop low-grade dysplasia (LGD) on follow-up. A smaller percentage will develop high-grade dysplasia (HGD) and around 3% adenocarcinoma [1]. Most of the carcinomas will develop within the first five years of antireflux surgery.

What are the implications of this form of progression? Certainly any patient who develops dysplasia should on first principles be placed on PPIs and rebiopsied. The subsequent strategy for the management of both low and high-grade dysplasia should be along the same lines as has been suggested for patients who have not previously undergone surgery. Currently we would recommend repeat endoscopic surveillance in 6 months for a patient with LGD and for confirmed HGD in a fit patient surgical resection and mucosal ablation in a less fit individual.

Are we in a position to use molecular markers as an indicator of disease progression? The answer in my opinion is currently no. The most explored marker p53 really mirrors histological changes of progression and no other marker has sufficient data behind it to make it a clinically useful tool. It does throw up the question that should a reliable marker of disease progression (current or future progression) be identified, how could it be utilised in a patient who has already undergone surgery.

In summary therefore the implications of histological progression in a post surgical patient are the same as in a patient who has not undergone surgery and the management strategy should be based upon the best available evidence from the general Barrett's literature.

References

1. DeMeester SR, DeMeester TR. Columnar mucosa and intestinal metaplasia of the esophagus: fifty years of controversy. Ann Surg 2000;231:303-321.
2. DeMeester SR, Campos GM, DeMeester TR, et al. The impact of an antireflux procedure on intestinal metaplasia of the cardia. Ann Surg 1998;228:547-556.

3. Sagar PM, Ackroyd R, Hosie KB, Patterspn JE, Stoddard CJ, Kingsnorth AN. Regression and progression of Barrett's oesophagus after antireflux surgery. Br J Surg 1995;82:806-810.
4. McDougall NI, Johnston BT, Collins JS, McFarland RJ, Love AH. Disease progression in gastro-oesophageal reflux disease as determined by repeat oesophageal pH monitoring and endoscopy 3 to 4.5 years after diagnosis. Eur J Gastroenterol Hepatol 1997;9:1161-1167.
5. Oberg S, DeMeester TR, Peters JH, Hagen JA, Nigro JJ, DeMeester SR, Theisen J, Campos GM, Crookes PF. The extent of Barrett's esophagus depends on the status of the lower esophageal sphincter and the degree of esophageal acid exposure. J Thorac Cardiovasc Surg 1999;117:572-580.
6. Fitzgerald RC, Omary MB, Triadafilopoulos G. Dynamic effects of acid on Barrett's esophagus: an ex vivo proliferation and differentiation model. J Clin Invest 1996;98:2120-2128.

What are the compared effects of medical *versus* surgical treatment on Barrett's strictures?

R.M. Bremner, C.G. Bremner (Los Angeles)

Barrett's strictures represent the end of the spectrum of reflux disease and the management of these problems is often complex and difficult. The aims of treatment of reflux esophageal strictures are to 1) provide complete and sustained relief of symptoms, 2) avoid stricture recurrence, 3) prevent gastroesophageal reflux disease (GERD) related complications. Successful antireflux treatment should accomplish all these goals without the need to take further medications.

Proton pump inhibitor (PPI) therapy has been shown to be more effective than histamine antagonists in the treatment of reflux esophagitis [1], and any comparison with surgical therapy should be made with PPI therapy.

Treatment with PPIs will decrease the esophageal exposure to acid and "bile", while surgery will repair the defective lower esophageal sphincter and reduce the hernia when present. Hiatal hernia is present in 85% of peptic strictures, and medical therapy will not treat this defect.

Symptomatic relief of symptoms with PPI does not imply complete control of gastroesophageal reflux.

Castell *et al.* have demonstrated this by repeated pH monitoring, and have shown better results if the dosage is adjusted accordingly [2]. Failure to adjust the dosage by this method may explain some of the unsatisfactory results of PPI therapy. In one series of 137 patients dilatation and PPI therapy gave freedom from dysphagia in only 50% of patients [3] at one year follow-up, and in another series there was still a need to re-dilate 30% of patients after 12 months therapy [4]. Six months therapy with PPI therapy is reported to cost $ 1,744; this may also be an important consideration in the patient's choice of therapy [5].

Results of antireflux surgery should be assessed at least two years after the operation because recurrences are more likely to occur after this period [6]. Csendes sounded this warning particularly to those assessing results of laparoscopic fundoplication.

In studies prior to PPI therapy, antireflux surgery gave consistently better results than therapy with histamine antagonist receptor treatment [7-9]. The current question is whether PPI therapy will be a match for surgery, and there are already some guiding results.

Ortiz *et al.* [8] used H_2-receptor antagonists until 1992 and then used omeprazole to treat 27 patients with Barrett's esophagus, and compared the results with patients treated by antireflux surgery (32 patients). Eight of 17 patients in the medical group and 2 of 13 in the surgical series still had a stricture after 5 years. Klinger *et al.* [10] reported on the results of laparoscopic surgery in 102 patients (7 Barrett's) who were refractory to medical therapy. The patients had been treated with H_2-receptor antagonists or PPI therapy. A total of 253 dilatations before surgery decreased to 29 after surgery in the mean observation period of 26 months prior to surgery and 25 months after surgery. Before surgery 13.5% also had frequent pneumonia, whereas no pneumonia was recorded after surgery. Lundell *et al.* compared the results of 310 patients enrolled in a multi-center trial comparing omeprazole with antireflux surgery. antireflux surgery was very effective in controlling GERD, and was better than omeprazole [11], although once increased doses of omeprazole were given the results were comparable.

There is also concern about recent reports of disappointing long-term results following antireflux surgery for Barrett's esophagus with stricture and shortening. Csendes reported on the late results of antireflux surgery in 35 Barrett's strictures; 61.5% (16 of 26 patients) still had a Visick 111 or 1V score [6]. However the antireflux procedure was not uniform in all cases (Hill or Nissen) which makes the comparison difficult. antireflux surgery in DeMeester's series of Barrett's strictures gave good results in 76% of 26 patients [12]. The longest follow-up of the Nissen fundoplication performed for Barrett's esophagus was reported from Finland [13]. After a median follow-up of 20 years in 46 patients, Luostarinen [13] concluded that the Nissen fundoplication gave reasonably good long-term results provided the Nissen was intact. Nineteen of 25 patients assessed stated that they would repeat the operation if given the choice again. Unsatisfactory results of antireflux surgery were recorded by Bonavina *et al.* especially in patients with a long, hard stricture, ineffective partial wrap, short esophagus or scleroderma [14].

It is quite possible therefore, that uncomplicated Barrett's esophagus treated by a full 360° fundoplication will give excellent results. The results of either fundoplication or medication for advanced disease (stricture, shortening) may not be as satisfactory: antireflux surgery for Barrett's esophagus should therefore be done before complications develop.

References

1. Silvis SE, Farahmand M, Johnson JA, et al. A randomized blinded comparison of omeprazole and ranitidine in the treatment of chronic esophageal stricture secondary to acid peptic esophagitis. Gastrointest Endosc 1996;43 (3):216-221.
2. Hatlebakk JG, Katz PD, Castell DO. Medical therapy management of the refractory patient. Gastroenterol Clin North Am 1999;28(4):847-860.
3. Smith PM, Kerr GD, Cockel R, et al. A Comparison of omeprazole and ranitidine in the prevention of recurrence of benign esophageal strictures. Gastroenterology 1994;107:1312-1318.
4. Richter JE. Peptic strictures of the esophagus. Gastroenterol Clin North Am 1999;28:(4) 875-891.
5. Marks RD, Richter JE, Rizzo J, et al. Omeprazole versus H2-receptor antagonist in treating patients with peptic stricture and esophagitis. Gastroenterology 1994;106:907-914.
6. Csendes A, Braghetto L, Burdiles P, et al. Long-term results of classic antireflux surgery in 152 patients with Barrett's esophagus: clinical, radiologic, endoscopic, manometric and acid reflux test analysis before and late after operation. Surgery 1998;123:645-657.

7. McEntee GP, Stuart RC, Nolan M, Hennessy TPJ. An evaluation of surgical and medical treatment of Barrett's oesophagus. Gullet 1991;1:169-172.
8. Ortiz A, de Haro LFM, Parilla P, et al. Conservative treatment versus antireflux surgery in Barrett's oesophagus: long-term results of a prospective study. Br J Surg 1996;83:274-278.
9. Attwood SE, Barlow AP, Norris TL, Watson A. Barrett's esophagus: effect of antireflux surgery on symptom control and development of complications. Br J Surg 1992;79:1050-1053.
10. Klinger PJ, Hinder RA, Cina RA, et al. Laparoscopic antireflux surgery for the treatment of esophageal strictures refractory to medical therapy. Am J Gastroenterol 1999;94 (3):632-636.
11. Lundell L, Dalenback J, Hatlebak J, et al. Omeprazole or antireflux surgery in the long term management of gastroesophageal reflux disease: results of a multicenter randomized clinical trial. Gastroenterology 1998;114:A207.
12. DeMeester TR, Attwood SEA, Smyrk TC, et al. Surgical therapy in Barrett's esophagus. Ann Surg 1990;212:528-542.
13. Luostrarinen M, Isolauri J, Laitinen J. Fate of Nissen fundoplication after 20 years. A clinical, endoscopical, and functional analysis. Gut 1993;34:1015-1020.
14. Bonavina L, Segalin A, Fumagalli U, Peracchia A. Surgical management of benign stricture from reflux esophagitis. Ann Chir Gynecol 1995;84 (2):175-178.

Can any of these treatments avoid complications of Barrett's disease?

E.C. Kinkenberg-Knol (Amsterdam)

The treatment of Barrett's esophagus is aimed at several different targets which include symptom relief, healing of esophagitis, and ultimately prevention of long-term complications such as peptic stenosis. These objectives are nowadays well achieved by medical acid suppression using either H_2-blocking agents or preferentially proton pump inhibitors (PPIs), and by antireflux surgery. In these aspects Barrett's esophagus is not essentially different from gastroesophageal reflux disease (GERD) in general. However, whether or not profound acid suppressive therapy or antireflux surgery also have a preventive effect on the long-term complications of Barrett's esophagus, in particular the development of dysplasia and adenocarcinoma is still under debate. The risk for esophageal adenocarcinoma in Barrett patients correlates with the severity of GERD, the length of the Barrett segment, and the local presence of dysplastic intestinal metaplasia (IM). This cancer risk might therefore be decreased by reduction of the length of the Barrett segment, preferentially leading to complete reversion of the metaplasia into normal squamous epithelium, or by decreasing the precancerous character with retention of metaplasia. As Barrett metaplasia results from chronic gastroesophageal reflux, Barrett regression can theoretically be obtained by antireflux treatment, either medical or surgical, or by mucosa ablation by *e.g.* electrocoagulation, argon plasma coagulation, laser therapy and photo dynamic therapy. We will compare the treatment modalities in the prevention of neoplastic complications.

Therapy for regression of metaplasia

Medical therapy [1]

Barrett's metaplasia results from chronic exposure of the distal esophagus to gastric acid and bile acids. Profound acid inhibition will prevent the reflux of gastric acid [2]. At the same time reduction of the gastric volume will lead to reduction of duodeno-gastro-esophageal reflux [3].

The question is: once IM of the esophagus occurs, can it be induced to revert to normal tissue or to regress with medical therapy? To date, 16 studies have been published that explore this issue [4]. Consistent regression has not been noted, although some shortening of the Barrett's segment has been described. Also the appearance of "squamous islands" has been reported. Complete regression is very rare and was only noted in 2 of 190 patients treated with PPIs and none with H_2-blockers. The question then is whether profound acid suppression can bring about changes for the better in the retained metaplastic epithelium. Several markers have been studied in this respect. Biomarkers of cancer risk, indicating epithelial cell proliferation or differentiation, do show impovement [5]. However, more molucular studies are required to assess whether the neoplastic potential is likely to be maintained in an environment of profound acid suppression.

Surgical therapy [6]

Does antireflux surgery promote healing or regression of the metastatic epithelium and does it halt the progression to dysplasia and cancer? There are conflicting reports about whether Barrett's mucosa regresses following antireflux surgery. A review of the English language literature since 1977 documents follow-up of 340 patients after antireflux surgery. Complete regression occurred in only 13 patients, whereas in 256 (75%) of the 340 patients the Barrett's epithelium remained unchanged. Thus regression of traditional Barrett's esophagus cannot be reliably predicted [7] or anticipated following antireflux surgery. The other question of importance is whether Barrett's esophagus progresses to high-grade dysplasia or cancer after surgical treatment of reflux disease. Review of the English language literature since 1975 revealed 11 series and a total of 346 patients with Barrett's esophagus followed after fundoplication. Patients were found to have esophageal carcinoma after antireflux surgery in only 7 of the 11 reports, 79% of the cancers developing within 5 years of fundoplication.The remaining cancers took 5-10 years after fundoplication, but in each case patients had signs of recurrent reflux. Thus a functioning fundoplication seems to provide protection from progression of Barrett's esophagus to adenocarcinoma in patients where this process has not started prior to the surgical procedure.

Ablation therapy

Theoretically the ideal treatment for a patient with Barrett's esophagus is one that will restore the normal squamous mucosa and eliminate the cancer risk associated with the intestinalisation of the cardiac-type mucosa. Currently neither medical nor surgical therapy reliably offers this. However, a number of experimental techniques for mucosal ablation show promise. It is evident from animal studies [8] and epidemiological human studies that IM develops under acidic conditions. The chance of success to achieve reversal of metaplastic epithelium into squamous epithelium by mucosal ablation, with a lasting effect, seems to depend on adequate acid suppression during and after the endoscopic treatment. However, the exact level of acid suppression necessary for reversal of Barrett's esophagus is not clear. Some series report reversal with persisting abnormal pH acid exposure [9], whereas others report the need to increase the dose of PPI to achieve reversal or recurrence of Barrett's esophagus with discontinuation of medication.

In summary, the evidence as it exists today would support the notion that the best treatment for a patient with established Barrett's esophagus is abolishment of acid reflux into the esophagus either by sufficient acid suppression or by a well-constructed antireflux procedure with periodically surveillance thereafter. If during surveillance low-grade dysplasia persists or develops, mucosal ablation should be considered.

References

1. Stollman N. The columnar-lined (Barrett's) esophagus. Can progression to cancer be prevented? Postgrad Med 2000;107:59-65.
2. Triadafilopoulos G. Proton pump inhibitors for Barrett's oesophagus. Gut 2000;46:144-146.
3. Shepherd NA. Barrett's oesophagus and proton pump inhibitors: a pathological perspective. Gut 200046:147-149.
4. Haag S, Nandurkar S, Talley NJ. Regression of Barrett's esophagus: the role of acid suppression, surgery, and ablative methods. Gastrointest Endosc 1999;50:229-240.
5. Peters FTM, Ganesh S, Kuipers EJ, et al. Epithelial cell proliferative activity of Barrett's esophagus: methodology and correlation with traditional cancer risk markers. Dig Dis Sci 1998;43:1501-1506.
6. DeMeester TR. Antireflux surgery in the management of Barrett's esophagus. J Gastrointest Surg 2000;4:124-128.
7. DeMeester SR, DeMeester TR. Columnar mucosa, intestinal metaplasia and adenocarcinoma of the esophagus and cardia: 50 years of controversy. Ann Surg 2000;231:303-321.
8. Bremner CG, Lynch VP, Ellis FH. Barrett's esophagus: congenital or acquired? An experimental study of esophageal mucosal regeneration in the dog. Surgery 1970;68: 209-216.
9. Kovacs B, Chen Y, Lewis TD, DeGuzman LJ, Thompson KS. Successful reversal of Barrett's esophagus with multipolar electrocoagulation despite inadequate acid suppression. Gastrointest Endosc 1999;9:547-553.

What is the current state of the trials comparing medical and surgical treatments in Barrett's esophagus? The Spanish experience

P. Parrilla, A. Ortiz, L.F. Martínez de Haro, V. Munitiz (Murcia)

Treatment for Barrett's esophagus is controversial. Conservative therapy with antisecretory drugs should be maintained for life [1]. Patients occasionally require large doses of antisecretory drugs to control the symptoms and cure the endoscopic lesions, which is expensive and may lead to the appearance of side-effects. Furthermore, this treatment does not modify the defective mechanical condition of the lower esophageal sphincter (LES) [2,

3] and the impaired motor activity of the esophagus, which means it does not prevent the alkaline reflux [4, 5] involved in the development of Barrett's esophagus and its complications. On the other hand, antireflux surgery which has proved effective in preventing reflux in 80-90% of patients with long-term follow-up [6-8], does not lead to disappearance of Barrett's esophagus either, as has been reported by most authors [9-13], with progression to adenocarcinoma in some cases [14, 15]. In this context, we compared the two types of treatment in a long-term prospective study [16], evaluating the progression or regression of the metaplastic segment, changes in the type of epithelium, percentage of patients in whom dysplasia appeared or developed from mild to severe, and the evolution of strictures and/or ulcers and other inflammatory phenomena. The study included 59 patients. Randomization was performed using a random number sequence before assessment. Two groups of patients were formed (medical treatment, n = 27; antireflux surgery, n = 32), which were homogeneous with regard to epidemiological, clinical, endoscopic, histological, manometric and pHmetric data (*Tables I and II*). Medical treatment for all patients (n = 27) consisted of hygiene, diet and postural measures associated with antisecretory drugs (H_2 antagonists initially and omeprazole from 1992 onwards for all) and periodical dilatations in patients with stenosis. Median follow-up was 4 years (range, 1-11). Surgical treatment in 30 patients consisted of a short Nissen fundoplication (1.5-2 cm) over a 48-50 french bougie and in the remaining two, when esophageal shortening prevented the achievement of a sufficient length of intra-abdominal esophagus, a Collis-Nissen procedure was performed. The abdominal approach was used in all patients. Dilatations were carried out before and after operation in patients with stenosis. Median follow-up was 5 years (range, 1-11). All patients underwent annual clinical,

Table I. Age, sex clinical, endoscopic and histological data of patients. Values in parentheses are percentages except where stated.

	Group I (n = 27) Conservative treatment	Group II (n = 32) Surgical treatment
Age (years) median (range)	40 (12-78)	32 (10-71)
Sex (M:F)	20:7	20:12
Duration of symptoms (years) median (range)	19 (2-50)	15 (1-50)
Symptoms		
Heartburn	24 (89)	29 (91)
Regurgitation	20 (74)	24 (75)
Dysphagia	14 (52)	16 (50)
Haemorrhage	6 (22)	10 (31)
Endoscopic data		
Esophagitis	13 (48)	22 (69)
Barrett´s ulcer	4 (15)	4 (12)
Stricture	17 (63)	13 (41)
Length of Barrett's segment (cm) median (range)	4 (3-12)	5 (3-14)
Types of epithelium		
Specialized	7 (26)	7 (22)
Junctional	4 (15)	4 (12)
Fundic	0	0
Two or more types	16 (59)	21 (66)
Dysplasia	0	0

Table II. Manometric and pH-metric data before treatment. Values are median (range).

	Group I (n = 27) Conservative treatment	Group II (n = 32) Surgical treatment
Manometric data		
Total length of LES (cm)	2 (1-4.5)	2 (1.5-4)
Abdominal length of LES (cm)	0 (0-1.7)	0.5 (0-2)
Resting pressure of LES (mmHg)	6.2 (0-16)	8.2 (0-19)
Amplitude of contractile waves (mmHg)	27 (0-101)	35 (9.5-147)
Percentage of simultaneous waves	6 (0-100)	0 (0-100)
Percentage of interrupted waves	0 (0-100)	0 (0-72)
pH-metric data		
Percentage of time with pH < 4	17 (1-76)	17.2 (3-83)

LES: lower esophageal sphincter

endoscopic and histological assessment. To check the efficiency of the antireflux procedure, operated patients underwent pHmetric and manometric controls 1 and 5 years after surgery.

In the authors's experience, conservative and surgical treatment proved equally effective in controlling symptoms (89% of satisfactory results after medical treatment *versus* 91% in patients following antireflux surgery). However, as in a previous report [17], the same was not true when evaluating associated endoscopic lesions, as the percentage of patients with esophagitis and persistent stenosis was significantly higher in the patients undergoing medical treatment than in those receiving antireflux surgery (*Table III*). In the same way, surgical treatment also proved more efficient in stabilizing the length of the metaplastic segment (*Table III*). Total regression of the metaplastic segment was not observed in any patient although, as can be seen in *Figures 1 and 2*, partial regression was noted in 8 of the patients undergoing antireflux surgery and in only 2 of the patients treated conservatively. Conversely, extension of the Barrett's esophagus was more frequent after

Table III. Endoscopic and histological findings before and after treatment.

	Medical		Surgery	
	Before treatment	After treatment	Before treatment	After treatment
Endoscopic data				
Esophagitis	13	7	22	1
Barrett's ulcer	4	0	4	0
Stricture	17	8	13	2
Length of Barrett's segment (cm) median (range)	4 (3-12)	5 (3-12)*	5 (3-14)	4.5 (3-13)
Histological data				
Mild dysplasia	0	5	0	0
Severe dysplasia	0	1	0	1**

* p < 0.01; ** for this patient the percentage of time with pH < 4 was 37 % 1 year after surgery

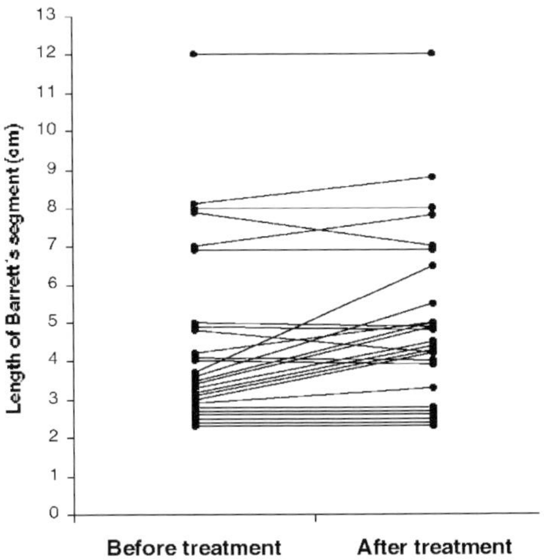

Figure 1. Length of Barrett's segment before and after medical treatment.

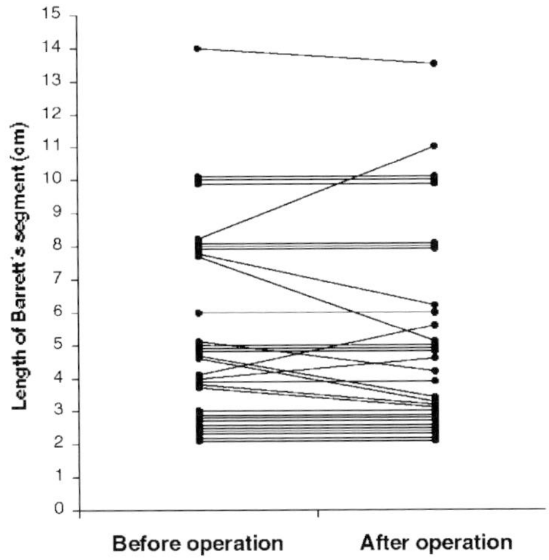

Figure 2. Length of Barrett´s segment before and after surgical treatment.

conservative treatment. Nevertheless, regression of the metaplasia is difficult to assess as it can occur circumferentially or leaving islands or metaplastic tongues among normal epithelium. The presence of regenerating squamous epithelium overlying residual columnar mucosa has also been reported [18], for which reason biopsies of insufficient depth may not detect residual columnar epithelium. Furthermore, after antireflux surgery the distance between the incisors and squamocolumnar junction may be modified by the surgical manoeuvres, which means the cardia must also be taken as a reference point. All these methodological problems explain why there are not conclusive data on the regression of Barrett's esophagus, although it has been reported occasionally, more frequently after antireflux surgery [18, 19].

The appearance of dysplastic changes in addition to Barrett's esophagus, and especially their disappearance after treatment, must be assessed with caution. The patchy nature of the lesion may lead to sampling error that can lead to false-negative biopsies, for which reason any study to assess dysplasia must include multiple biopsies along the whole of the metaplastic segment and in different sectors of the circumference. In this study, dysplastic changes appeared in 7 patients (12%) (2 severe dysplasias), 6 (10%) undergoing medical treatment and 1 (2%) following antireflux surgery. The latter received a Nissen procedure for Barrett's esophagus with inflammatory lesions. One year after surgery, clinical evaluation was fair and 24-hour pH monitoring showed 37% of time with pH < 4, for which reason the patient was treated with H_2 antagonists and given an annual endoscopic control. Six years later, high-grade dysplasia (HGD) was detected . In this patient as well as in the patient with HGD undergoing medical treatment an esophageal resection was performed and the presence of carcinoma *in situ* was confirmed in both cases. The rate of malignancy was one in 127 patient/years for the medical treatment group and one in 160 patient/years for the surgical treatment group, with no significant differences; however, it must be noted that the pHmetric monitoring performed in the patient from the surgical treatment group, one year after surgery, revealed failure of the antireflux procedure, with a percentage of time with pH < 4 of 37% (*Table III*). *Table IV* shows that antireflux surgery improved the

Table IV. Manometric and pH-metric data before and after surgery (n = 32).

	Preoperative	Postoperative
Manometric data		
Total length of LES (cm)	2 (1.5-4)	3.5 (2.5-5)*
Abdominal length of LES (cm)	0.5 (0.2)	3 (0-3.8)*
Resting pressure of LES (mmHg)	8.2 (0-19)	16.5 (5.5-29)*
Amplitude of contractile waves (mmHg)	35 (9.5-147)	42 (20-136)*
Percentage of simultaneus waves	0 (0-100)	0 (0-75)
Percentage of interrupted waves	0 (0-72)	0 (0-66)**
pH-metric data		
Percentage of time with pH < 4	17.2 (3-83)	1 (0-37)***

Values are median (range)
LES: lower esophageal sphincter; * $p < 0.01$; ** $p < 0.05$; *** $p < 0.001$

mechanical condition of the LES and the quality of esophageal peristalsis. The median percentage of time with pH < 4 in the postoperative controls was 1%, although it must be noted that 5 of 32 patients demonstrated pathological rates of reflux (median: 12%, range 5-37%). When combining the 5 patients in whom antireflux surgery failed with the medical treatment group (n = 32) and they were compared with the 27 patients with successful antireflux surgery, it could be seen that dysplastic changes appeared in 7 of the former (which means a rate of malignancy of 1/82 patient/years) and in none of the latter (zero rate), with statistically significant difference ($p < 0.05$).

In our opinion, although the clinical results are similar with both types of treatment, the endoscopic and histological modifications in this series, despite the small number of cases and methodological limitations, question the advantages of the systematic conservative approach in the initial management of patients with Barrett's esophagus.

These results are supported by a recent study [20] in which we quantified, using 24-hour esophageal monitoring and Bilitec™ 2000, the alterations that proton pump inhibitors treatment and Nissen fundoplication produce in the rates of acid reflux of duodenal contents to the esophagus in patients with Barrett's esophagus. This was a prospective study in which 10 patients underwent medical treatment consisting of omeprazole in doses of 40 mg/day for a minimum of 1 year (median: 13 months; range, 12-16 months) and 10 antireflux surgery (Nissen fundoplication), each type of treatment being indicated totally at random. The median follow-up was 12 months (range, 12-17 months). After treatment all the patients underwent clinical assessment, endoscopy with multiple biopsies, 24-hour pH monitoring and Bilitec™ 2000 study. The results obtained with 24-hour esophageal pH monitoring and Bilitec™ 2000 revealed that in the medical treatment group pathological acid reflux persisted in 2 patients and reflux of duodenal contents in 8 (*Figure 3*). Conversely, after surgery, both acid reflux and the reflux of duodenal contents disappeared in all but 1 case, in which a failure ocurred in the fundoplication (*Figure 4*). In view of these results it seems clear that medical therapy does not successfully control the reflux of biliopancreatic contents to the esophagus or even, in some cases, acid reflux even if the patient is asymptomatic.

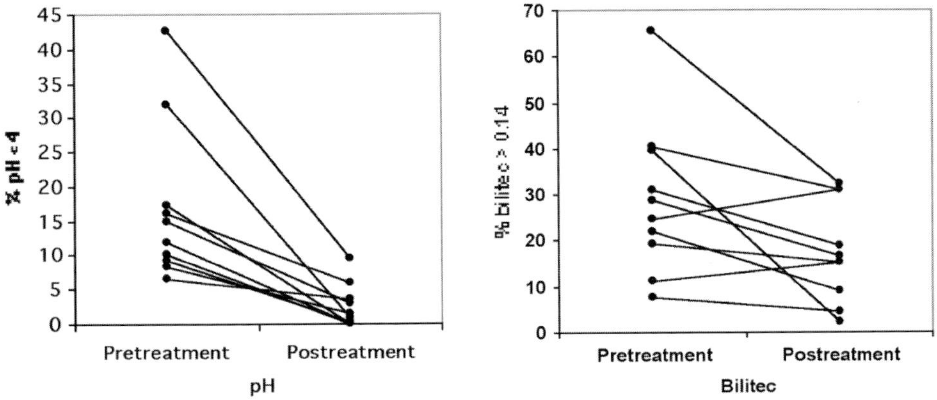

Figure 3. Percentages of pH and Bilitec™ of 10 patients treated with 40 mg/day omeprazole, before and after treatment. Discontinued line shows normal value, pH (4.5 %) and Bilitec™ (5.3 %).

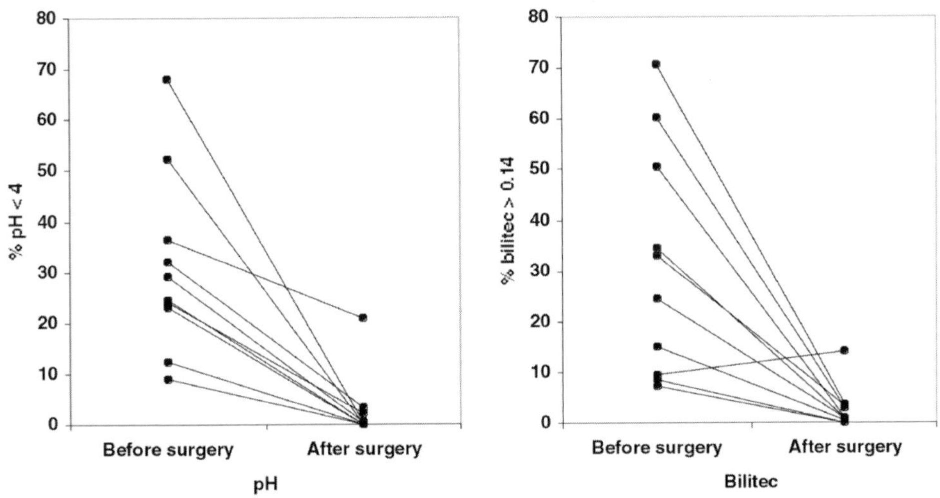

Figure 4. Percentages of pH and Bilitec™ of 10 patients operated with a Nissen fundoplication, before and after surgical treatment. Discontinued line shows normal value, pH (4.5%) and Bilitec™ (5.3%).

In conclusion, antireflux surgery should be considered the therapeutic method of choice especially because a lifetime or high doses of medication will be necessary and the results of medical therapy are inferior to antireflux surgery since the latter not only controls the reflux symptoms but also both the acid and biliopancreatic reflux. Conservative treatment would only be indicated in elderly patients or with organic disease that increase the risk of surgery. This should be corroborated by further studies with a larger number of patients and longer follow-up.

References

1. Hetzel DJ, Dent J, Reed WD, et al. Healing and relapse of severe peptic esophagitis after treatment with omeprazole. Gastroenterology 1988;95:903-912.
2. De Meester TR, Attwood SE, Smyrk ThC, Therkildsen DH, Hinder RA. Surgical therapy in Barrett's esophagus. Ann Surg 1990;212:528-542.
3. Fiorucci S, Santucci L, Farroni F, Pelli MA, Morelli A. Effect of Omeprazole on gastroesophageal reflux in Barrett's esophagus. Am J Gastroenterol 1989;84:1263-1267.
4. Attwood SE, DeMeester TR, Bremner CG, Barlow AP, Hinder RA. Alkaline gastroesophageal reflux: implications in the development of complications in Barrett's columnar-lined lower esophagus. Surgery 1989;106:764-770.
5. Gillen P, Keeling P, Byrne PS, Healy M, O'Moore RR, Hennessy TPJ. Implication of duodenogastric reflux in the pathogenesis of Barrett's oesophagus. Br J Surg 1988;75:540-543.
6. DeMeester TR, Bonavina L, Albertucci M. Nissen fundoplication for gastroesophageal reflux disease. Evaluation of primary repair in 100 consecutive patients. Ann Surg 1986;204:9-20.
7. Donahue PE, Samelson S, Nyhus LM, Bombeck CT. The floppy Nissen fundoplication. Effective long-term control of pathologic reflux. Arch Surg 1985;120:663-668.
8. Martínez de Haro LF, Ortiz A, Parrilla P, García JA, Aguayo JL, Morales G. Long-term results of Nissen fundoplication in reflux esophagitis without strictures. Clinical, endoscopic, and pHmetric evaluation. Dig Dis Sci 1992;37:523-530.
9. Mangla JC. Barrett's epithelium: regression or no regression? N Engl J Med 1980;303:529-530.
10. Naef AP, Savary M, Ozzello L. Columnar-lined lower esophagus: an acquired lesion with malignant predisposition. Report on 140 cases of Barrett's esophagus with 12 adenocarcinomas. J Thorac Cardiovasc Surg 1975;70:826-835.
11. Wellinger J, Ollyo JB, Savary M, Fontolliet C, Chapuis G. Surgical treatment of Barrett's esophagus: a propos of 110 cases. Helv Chir Acta 1989;55:695-698.
12. Bremner CG, Hamilton DG. Barrett's esophagus: controversial aspects. In: DeMeester TR, Skinner DB, eds. Esophageal disorders: pathophysiology and therapy. New York: Raven Press, 1985:233-239.
13. Williamson WA, Ellis FH Jr, Gibb SP, Shahian DM, Aretz HT. Effect of antireflux operation on Barrett's mucosa. Ann Thorac Surg 1990;49:537-542.
14. Hamilton SR, Hutcheon DF, Ravitch WJ, Cameron JL, Paulson M.Adenocarcinoma in Barrett's esophagus after elimination of gastroesophageal reflux. Gastroenterology 1984;86:356-360.
15. Bushkin FL, Neustein CL, Parker TH, Woodward ER. Nissen fundoplication for reflux peptic esophagitis. Ann Surg 1977;185:672-675.
16. Ortiz A, Martínez de Haro LF, Parrilla P, et al. Conservative treatment versus antireflux surgery in Barrett's oesophagus: long-term results of a prospective study. Br J Surg 1996;83:274-278.
17. Spechler SJ. Comparison of medical and surgical therapy for complicated gastroesophageal reflux disease in veterans. The Department of Veterans Affairs Gastroesophageal Reflux Disease Study Group. N Engl J Med 1992;326:786-792.
18. Skinner DB, Walther BC, Ridell RH, Schmidt H, Iascone C, De Meester TR. Barrett's esophagus. Comparison of benign and malignant cases. Ann Surg 1983;198:554-565.
19. Brand DL, Ylvisaker JT, Gelfand M, Pope CE 2nd. Regression of columar esophageal (Barrett's) epithelium after antireflux surgery. N Engl J Med 1980;302:844-848.
20. Parrilla P, Ortiz A, Martínez de Haro LF, Munitiz V, Molina J, Bermejo J. Proton pump inhibitors do not control duodeno-gastro-oesophageal reflux in patients with Barrett's oesophagus. Submitted for publication (2000).

The Italian experience

R. Ferraris, M. Morino and GOSPE
(Gruppo Operativo per lo Studio delle Precancerosi Esofagee)
(Turin)

Barrett's esophagus is a premalignant condition leading to adenocarcinoma of the esophagus. It is generally not subject to spontaneous or therapeutically induced regression [1]. Data on the incidence of esophageal adenocarcinoma indicate an alarming increase of this type of tumor [2]. Furthermore, the incidence data of adenocarcinoma in Barrett's esophagus in Italy, as recently reported by the GOSPE (Gruppo Operativo per lo Studio delle Precancerosi Esofagee), were similar to the other western countries [3]. A variable success of the Barrett's esophagus mucosal ablation with a complete restitution of the normally lined esophageal squamous epithelium has been recently obtained by coupling laser-endoscopic technique with gastric acid suppression following high dose of proton pump inhibitors (PPIs), or following antireflux surgery [4-6].

The laser technique requires multiple sessions and is associated with major complications as esophageal perforation or stenosis [7], and, in addition, is an expensive treatment. Other endoscopic techniques alternative to the laser technique have been recently used: *i.e.* the multipolar electrocoagulation [8] and the Argon plasma coagulation (APC) technique [9, 12]. In particular, the APC technique seems to be free of therapeutic hazard because of a limited action to the superficial part of the mucosa. It is cheaper, and at least equal to the laser therapy on superficial lesions; furthermore, it may require a lesser number of therapeutical sessions [10].

The aim of the present paper is to report the results of endoscopic ablation of Barrett's esophagus using APC and to compare medical (PPIs) *versus* surgical laparoscopic control of gastroesophageal reflux combined with APC of Barrett's esophagus.

Material and methods

From November 1996 to November 1999, 42 patients with histologically proven intestinal type Barrett's esophagus and symptomatic gastroesophageal reflux disease (GERD) were treated with endoscopic APC in a multicentric Italian trial (GOSPE - Barrett's esophagus ablation project).

All patients had a 24 hour pH-metry and esophageal manometry. The length of Barrett's esophagus varied from 2 to 11 cm endoscopically measured (mean length 4.1 cm). All the patients were previously included in a regular endoscopic and histological surveillance program as already reported [3, 13]. A grid form for topographic assessment of Barrett's esophagus similar to that described by Luman [5] was used: the exact limits of the metaplastic tissue was firstly defined for each patient, whereas the tissue ablation area and the biopsy sites were subsequently recorded. The study was approved by the local ethical committee. Written informed consent was obtained from all the patients selected for the study.

Suppression of GERD has been obtained before the endoscopic Barrett's esophagus ablation, either by medical (omeprazole 40 mg per day, 17 patients) or by surgical laparoscopic fundoplication according to clinical indication and preference of the patient. The surgical procedure was performed by the experienced surgical teams involved in the present study. The efficacy of surgical and medical treatments was checked by 24 hour pH-metry. Esophageal manometry was also performed 3 months after surgery. Endoscopic ablation of the Barrett's mucosa was performed by APC technique (Erbe; Tubingen - Germany) using 30-50W setting as suggested by Heler [14]. The APC beams were given starting from the squamocolumnar junction and proceeding to the gastroesophageal junction. The tongues of Barrett's esophagus were treated first, then half a column of the metaplastic esophageal circumference was coagulated. Particularly in extensive circumferential Barrett's esophagus, the "half circumferential" technique of ablation was

Table I. Results of endoscopic Barrett's esophagus ablation with argon plasma coagulation in a medical (PPI) or surgical gastroesophageal reflux controlled environment.

Patient	N°	Sex F	Sex M	Age (years)	Length of Barrett's esophagus pre-ablation (cm)	Number of sessions	Follow-up (months)	Histological follow-up: Squamous epithelium	Histological follow-up: Squamous epithelium + fundic Barrett mucosa	Histological follow-up: Specialized columnar epithelium
Surgical	25	12	13	51.5 (26-77)	4.1 (2-11)	2.9 (2-6)	9.7 (1-27)	22/25 88%	1/20 4%	2/20 8%
PPI	17	4	13	62.9 [43-79]	4.1 [2-8]	2.7 [1-6]	6.3 [1-12]	10/17 59%*	1/17 6%	6/17 35%*

* Statistically significant

used, acting as an inner control of the efficacy of the ablation in the course of successive sessions of treatment. As suggested by Sampliner [8], the above hemicircumferential technique of Barrett's esophagus ablation may also reduce the theoretical risk of complicating circumferential stenosis. Barrett's esophagus was coagulated until the colour of the mucosa appeared white. The ablated area was carefully mapped on the grid form previously described. The endoscopic APC sessions were performed at 30 day intervals until completed Barrett's esophagus ablation was achieved. Complete ablation was defined as the visual evidence of a complete coagulation of the residual metaplastic mucosa during the last session treatment, as also judged by the aid of the grid form. The duration of the treatment was approximately 15 to 20 minutes per session.

Histological follow up after ablation was performed for all the patients. Biopsies were taken one month following the completion of APC treatment and thereafter at 3-6 month intervals, depending on the compliance of the patients. Biopsy sampling was performed extensively by jumbo biopsy forceps at the sites of previously designed Barrett's esophagus using the grid form as a topographic reference. The biopsy sampling protocol included one biopsy every 2 cm at each of the four quadrants throughout the previous Barrett's segment. Biopsies were processed with the high iron diamine/alcian blue staining in the majority of the cases, allowing to the identification of type III intestinal metaplasia (IM) [15].

Results

Table I shows the mean results of endoscopic ablation of Barrett's esophagus by APC in the two groups of patients.

Histological follow-up after ablation was ranging from 1 to 27 months (mean follow-up 8.4 months). Histologically, squamous re-epithelialization was observed in 33 out of the 42 patients, 22/25 in the surgical group and 11/17 in the medical group of patients. Small islands of IM were observed under the neo-squamous epithelium in 7 patients. Recurrence of large visible metaplastic areas of Barrett's esophagus was seen in only one patient (of the medical group), three months after Barrett's esophagus ablation.

Thus, the global failure rate of the APC procedure was 19%: 8% in the surgical group and 35% in the group of patients treated with omeprazole. A regrowth of a mixed squamous and gastric type mucosa in the distal esophagus has been observed in 2 patients. There were no significant complications related to the APC treatment.

Discussion

Regression of specialized columnar epithelium in Barrett's esophagus following endoscopic laser therapy or multipolar coagulation has been reported with contrasting results [5, 6]. Less information is available with the recently developed APC technique [11, 12]. It has also been postulated that better results in Barrett's esophagus ablation could be expected in a reflux-free environment created by successful antireflux surgery rather than under medical treatment or no therapy at all [6, 12]. Data from our follow-up study show that endoscopic APC of Barrett's esophagus in a GERD controlled environment can restore a persistent squamous lining in the majority of patients, better in the surgical than in the medical group. Uncomplete eradication of specialized columnar epithelium should be considered as a failure of treatment, the malignant potential of residual patches being presumably unchanged. We think that these small islands of specialized columnar epithelium are deep remnants of the original Barrett's esophagus mucosa rather than a newly regrowth of intestinal epithelium. Whether these residual islands of specialized columnar epithelium could be at risk of cancer is to be established: only prospective, long-term follow-up studies with large number of patients could demonstrate an actual reduction in the mortality for adenocarcinoma following Barrett's esophagus ablation.

In conclusion, endoscopic APC treatment of Barrett's esophagus in a GERD controlled environment is safe and effective in the majority of the patients treated. Surgical therapy of GERD may produce a better histological pattern of re-epithelialization after ablation. Small islands of IM under the new squamous epithelium may persists in few patients, indicating that ablation of Barrett's esophagus must be the matter of controlled clinical trials.

References

1. Spechler SJ, Goyal RK.Barrett's esophagus. N Engl J Med 1986, 315:362-371.
2. Pera M, Cameron AJ, Trastek VF, et al. Increasing incidence of adenocarcinoma of the esophagus and esophagogastric junction. Gastroenterology 1993;104:510-513.
3. Ferrraris R, Bonelli L, e GOSPE. Incidence of Barrett's adenocarcinoma in an Italian population: an endoscopic surveillance programme. Eur J Gastroenterol Hepatol 1997, 9:881-885.
4. Berenson MM, Johnson TD, Markowitz NR, et al. Restoration of squamous mucosa after ablation of Barrett's esophageal epithelium. Gastroenterology 1993;104:1686-1691.
5. Luman W, Lessels AM, Palmer KR. Failure of Nd-YAG photocoagulation therapy as treatment for Barrett's esophagus - a pilot study. Eur J Gastroenterol Hepatol 1996;8:627-630

6. Salo JA, Salminen JT, Kiviluoto TA, et al. Treatment of Barrett's esophagus by endoscopic laser ablation and antireflux surgery. Ann Surg 1998;227:40-44.
7. Bremner RM, Mason RJ, Brenmer CG, et al. Ultrasonic epithelial ablation of the lower esophagus without stricture formation. A new technique for Barrett's ablation. Surg Endosc 1998;12:342-346.
8. Sampliner RE, Fennerty B, Garewal HS. Reversal of Barrett's esophagus with acid suppression and multipolar electrocoagulation:preliminary results. Gastrointest Endosc 1996;44:532-535.
9. Farin G, Grund KE. Technology of Argon-Plasma-Coagulation with particular regard to endoscopic application. End Surg 1994;2:71-77.
10. Sessler MJ, Becker HD, Flesch I. Therapeutic effect of argon plasma coagulation on small malignant gastrointestinal tumors. J Cancer Res Clin Oncol 1995;121:235-238.
11. Barham CP, Jones RL, Biddlestone LR, Hardwick RH, Shepherd NA, Barr H. Phototermal laser ablation of Barrett's oesophagus: endoscopica and histological evidence of squamous re-epithelialisation Gut 1997;41:281-284.
12. Van Laethem JL, Cremer M, O Peny M, Delhaye M, Deviere J. Eradication of Barrett mucosa with argon plasma coagulation and acid suppression: immediate and mid term results. Gut 1998;43:747-751.
13. GOSPE. Barrett's esophagus: epidemiological and clinic results of a multicentric survey. Int J Cancer 1991;48:364-368.
14. Heler SK, Heler LM, Josephs M, et al. Argon plasma coagulation:comparison to other candidate therapies for Barrett's ablation using the canine esophagus. Washington: AGA Abstract book, 1997.
15. Filipe MI, Lake BD. Histochemistry in pathology. London: Churchill Livingstone, 1983.

Ablation therapy

What is the profile of the best potential candidates for ablation therapy? The powerful influence of the hiatal hernia

S.J. Sontag (Hines)

Although the long-term results of ablation therapy of Barrett's adenocarcinoma are not yet known, several concerns have already surfaced as to the best potential candidates for ablative therapy. One factor is almost universally accepted: ablative therapy should be confined to those patients in whom the adenocarcinoma has been detected early and shown to be confined to the esophageal mucosa. Ablative therapy still should be considered as unproven therapy.

Hypothesis

Without hiatal hernia (HH), Barrett's esophagus cancers or gastroesophageal junction (GEJ) cancers are difficult to prevent and are difficult to diagnose. Once diagnosed, theyare difficult to ablate and to cure.

We base this hypothesis on a relatively small body of literature from the endoscopy clinic at Hines VA hospital, Hines Illinois, much of which indirectly suggests that the presence of HH has a determining effect on the diagnosis and outcome of esophageal cancer. We used the following definitions.

Definitions

- Hiatal hernia: gastric mucosal folds above the diaphragmatic hiatus for at least 2 cm during quiet respirations.

• Short segment Barrett's esophagus (SSBE):
- 1 cm or less of intestinal mucosa belonging to the tubular esophagus squamocolumnar junction approximately in proper area;
- irregular Z-line (squamocolumnar junction interrupted);
- tiny red tongues or spicules of intestinal metaplasia (IM).
• Long segment Barrett's esophagus:
- greater than 1 cm of intestinal mucosa belonging to the tubular esophagus;
- greater than 1cm of Barrett's esophagus;
- tongues, islands or circumferential IM.

Methods

For 17 years, patients with Barrett's esophagus were diagnosed in the ambulatory outpatient endoscopy clinic at Hines Veterans Affairs Hospital, Hines, IL. The clinic developed an organized patient recall system and employed a full-time computer data enterer. Endoscopies and biopsies, as well as all mapping and location measurements, were performed by one of two endoscopists using predefined criteria that were designed specifically for the screening and surveillance program. All data were recorded on preprinted data sheets. The configuration of the Barrett's esophagus and HH as well as details of all abnormalities were drawn and mapped by hand on to one of twenty-two different upper gut figures that adjusted for HH size and shape. All data were reviewed and verified before being entered into the computer database storage system. The program was continued for a subsequent 3 years in the combined inpatient/outpatient endoscopy clinic.

Results

Figure 1 shows the prevalence of HH according to the length of Barrett's esophagus in 1,099 patients with Barrett's esophagus. Without a HH, less than 5% of Barrett's esophagus patients had a segment of IM greater than 1 cm.
Our data also showed the following:
- 60% of all Barrett's esophagus have short segment (1 cm or less of IM);
- 89% of all Barrett's esophagus with low-grade dysplasia have short segment;
- 40% of all Barrett's esophagus with high-grade dysplasia (HGD) have short segment;
- 15% of all prevalent Barrett's esophagus cancers have short segment;
- 9% of all incident Barrett's esophagus cancers have short segment.

Thus, since the absence of HH is directly related to the presence of SSBE (1 cm or less), and SSBE has the potential to harbor HGD and adenocarcinoma, biopsy of the short segments, irregular squamocolumnar junctions, blips and tongues is critical to the early diagnosis of Barrett's cancer.

Often discussed, but rarely published, is the difficulty in obtaining biopsies from a normally snug GEJ, which is most often found when HH is absent. In fact, adequate biopsies of such short segments may require retroflexion of the endoscope - a maneuver that makes biopsy somewhat more difficult.

Finally, without HH, gastroesophageal reflux symptoms may not occur, and the motivating factor for early endoscopy may not be present. It is quite possible that the

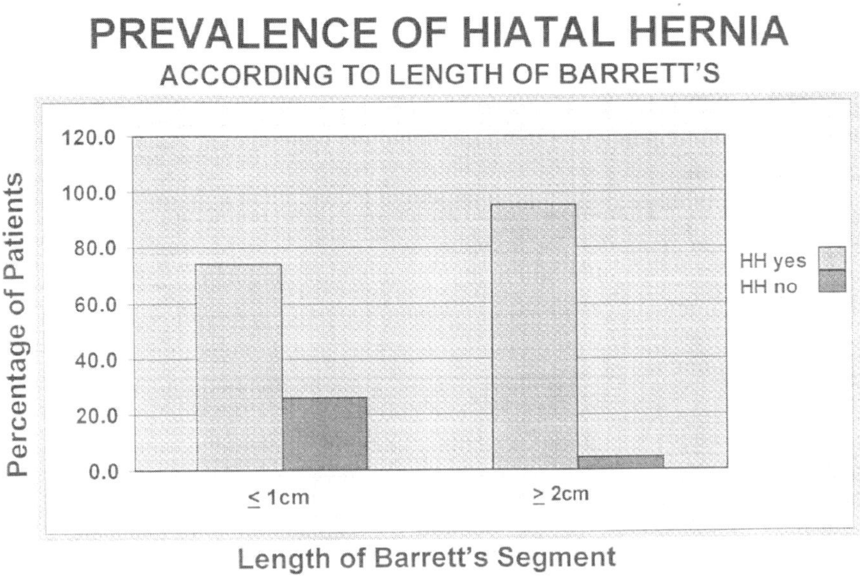

Figure 1. Shows the prevalence of hiatal hernia according to the length of Barrett's esophagus in 1,099 patients with Barrett's esophagus from the Hines VA 20-year data base. Without a hiatal hernia, less than 5% of Barrett's esophagus patients will have a segment of intestinal metaplasia greater than 1 cm.

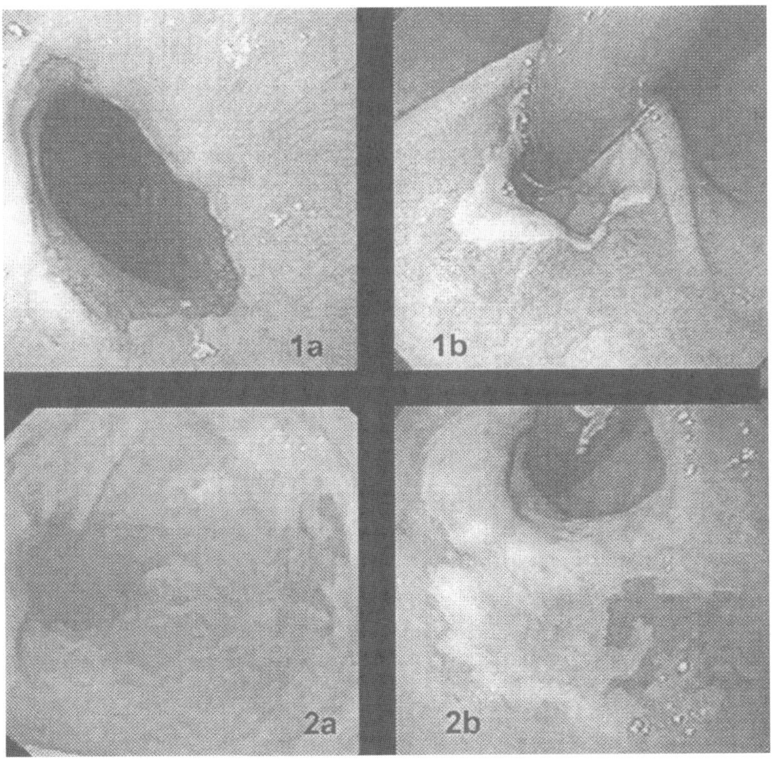

Figure 2. Shows the forward (a) and retroflexed (b) views of a patient without hiatal hernia (1a, 1b) and with hiatal hernia (2a,2b). Both patients had high-grade dysplasia. In the forward viewing photos (1a, 2a), the minimal abnormalities at the squamo-columnar junction could easily be missed, and tissue from 1a - without hiatal hernia - may be considerably more difficult to obtain than from 2a, where the hiatal hernia allows more flexibility and leeway.

absence of reflux symptoms without HH causes patients to present with adenocarcinoma in a later stage than those with reflux symptoms and HH. This concept is in need of study.

In conclusion:
- absence of HH almost guarantees absence of Barrett's esophagus longer than 1 cm;
- absence of HH permits only Barrett's esophagus that is short segment;
- absence of HH may mask the subtle, difficult to see, short segment ;
- HGD may appear at the squamocolumnar junction as a "blip";
- 10% of Barrett's esophagus harboring HGD or adenocarcinoma are in SSBE;
- ignoring the SSBE may result in missed diagnoses.

What is the rate of squamous epithelialization following KTP laser ablation? What is the necessary length of treatment?

H. Barr (Gloucester)

The potassium titanyl phosphate (KTP) laser emits light in the green at a wavelength of 532 nm. This laser line is produced from a neodymium yttrium aluminium garnet (Nd YAG) laser which has been frequency doubled by the insertion of the KTP crystal across the 1,064 nm infrared beam of the Nd YAG laser. The KTP laser has proved to be very useful for the ablation of superficial tissue with little risk of deeper damage. The ideal depth of damage to fulfil the criteria for successful re-epithelialization is yet to be established, since the nature of the injury and healing is still under investigation.

Considerations on the depth of damage

First, the depth of the metaplastic Barrett's epithelium has been measured at 0.5 mm (range 0.42-0.58) in fixed histological sections [1]. Using optical coherence tomography we have measured the epithelium at approximately 0.45 mm in freshly excised tissue. The tissue was preserved by freezing in liquid nitrogen and then thawed to room temperature for measurement [2]. Clearly, in order to destroy all the metaplastic tissue the depth of destruction must exceed this. Secondly, the nature of the injury produced must be considered, since columnar-lined metaplastic change is an injury response. It occurs following the chemical inflammation produced by gastroesophageal reflux disease. In a canine model of reflux disease it was thought that the deep esophageal gland could be the source of the metaplastic cells (*Figure 1* and *Figure 2*). Following reflux control the partial neo-squamous regeneration that occurred was thought to occur from the squamous lined gland duct [3]. However, recent studies in a rodent model, which has no deep esophageal glands, suggests that these glands and their ducts may not be crucial [4]. It appears likely

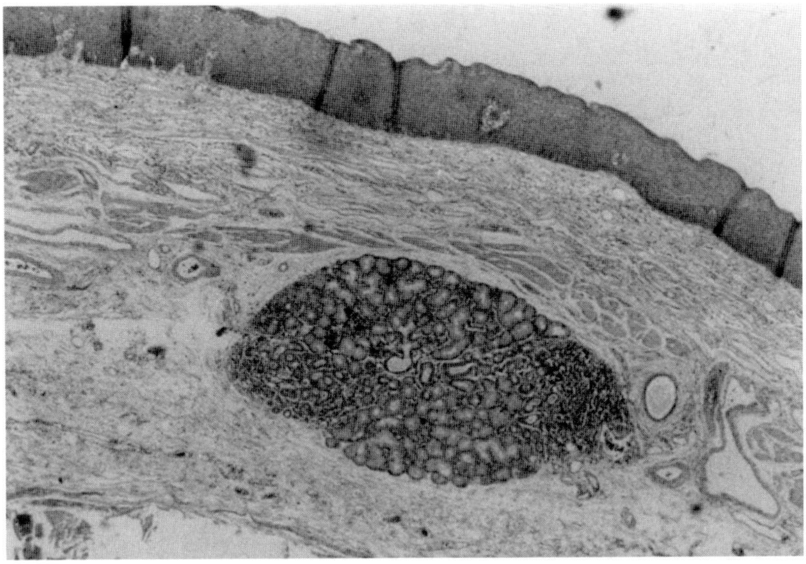

Figure 1. Squamous epithelium above a deep esophageal gland.

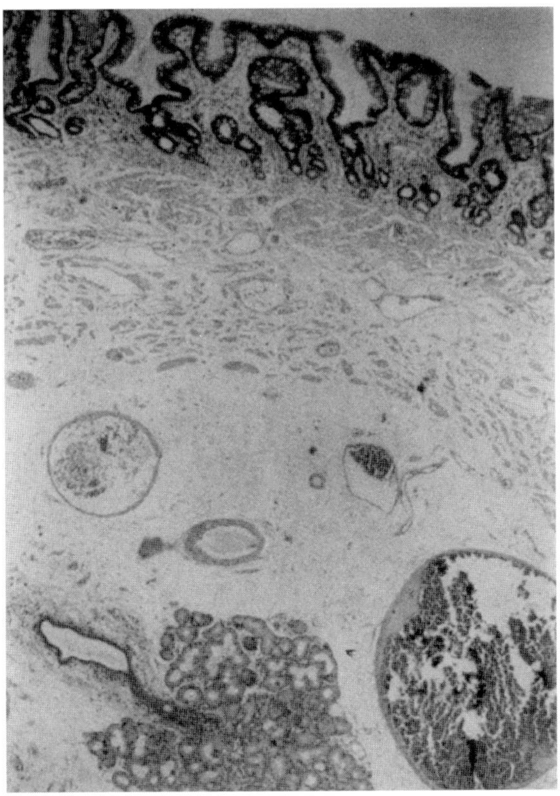

Figure 2. Specialized intestinal metaplastic epithelium (Barrett's) above a deep esophageal gland.

that there is a pluripotential stem located deep in the gland epithelium and in the basal layer of the squamous epithelium that can regenerate to columnar or squamous cells depending on the environmental circumstances.

KTP laser photothermal ablation of Barrett's esophagus

We have used a thermal imaging system to measure the depth of penetration and the thermal profile in tissue produced using the KTP and various other lasers (diode and Nd YAG) at various powers and energies. The purpose was to find parameters of between than 60-100°C (coagulative necrosis + vaporisation) on the luminal (mucosal) surface with less than 37°C (no risk of full thickness necrosis) on the external surface [5, 6].

Irradiation with the KTP laser, power 15-20 W for 1 second pulses produced surface temperatures of greater than 65°C with external temperature of 21°C. It was extremely difficult to generate high temperatures on the external surface of the esophagus using this laser. The diode laser (25 W for 5 seconds) could produce surface temperatures of 90°C but with an external temperature of 38°C. The Nd YAG laser tended to produce worrying temperatures through to the external surface at energy levels that were sufficient to produce thermal destruction on the mucosa. The KTP laser has proved to be very effective in treatment and eradication of metaplastic and dysplastic Barrett's epithelium, when combined with control of gastroesophageal reflux with proton pump inhibitor therapy [5, 7]. Neo-squamous epithelium was restored in 70% of patients with eradication of dysplasia and intestinal metaplasia. However, in 30% the neo-squamous epithelium covered metaplastic glands [5]. The rate of re-epithelialization is fairly rapid with healing occurring within 2-4 weeks although biopsy is essential since the visible endoscopic appearances can be very deceptive.

The nature of squamous re-epithelialization

As indicated the endoscopic appearance can be misleading since several areas identified by the endoscopist as neo-squamous following KTP ablation proved to be entirely columnar after histological examination [8]. In addition up to one third of patients will have buried glands under squamous surface. This remains a worrying scenario since cancer has been seen to occur after various mucosal ablation techniques and the oncogenic potential of the epithelium remains and cannot be ignored [2]. Since the aim is to prevent progression to cancer, partial ablation of the epithelium is an inadequate endpoint [9]. At present it must be recommended that all the Barrett's epithelium is ablated, and more importantly surveillance of the ablated segment must continue since malignant degeneration has been noted to occur.

Conclusion

There is rapid neo-squamous re-epithelialization after KTP laser ablation and reflux control. However residual metaplasia is common and repeat treatment often necessary. It is vitally important to maintain surveillance. Partial regression can not be considered an end point and the risk of malignant degeneration remains. It is recommended that all patients, even after apparent complete eradication, must have further endoscopic and full biopsy surveillance.

References

1. Ackroyd R, Brown NJ, Stephenson TJ, Stoddard CJ, Reed MW Ablation treatment for Barrett oesophagus:what depth of tissue destruction is needed. J Clin Pathol 1999;52:509-512.
2. Barr H. Barrett's esophagus: treatment with 5-aminolaevulinic acid photodynamic therapy. Gastrointest Endosc Clin North Am 2000;10:421-437.
3. Li H, Walsh TN, O'Dowd G, Gillen P, Byrne PJ, Hennessy TPJ. Mechanisms of columnar metaplasia and squamons regeneration in experimental barret's esophagus. Surgery 1994;115:176-181.
4. Van den Boogert J, Van Hillegersberg R, De Bruin RWF, Van Velthuysen MLF, Tilanus HW. A rat model for Barrett's oesophagus and prospects for photodynamic therapy. Eur J Gastroenterol Hepatol 1997;9:A53.
5. Barham CP, Jones RL, Biddlestone LR, Hardwick RH, Shepherd NA, Barr H. Photothermal laser ablation of Barrett's oesophagus: endoscopic and histological evidence of squamous re-epithelialisation. Gut 1997;41:281-384.
6. Dix T, Barr H. Photothermal ablation of metaplastic columnar-lined (Barrett's) oesophagus, experimental studies for safe endoscopic laser therapy. Prog Biomed Optics 1996;2922,:275-280.
7. Gossner L. May A, Stolte M, Seitz G, Hahn EG, Ell C. KTP laser destruction of dysplasia and early cancer in columnar-lined Barrett's esophagus. Gastrointest Endosc 1999;49:8-12.
8. Biddlestone LR, Barham CP, Wilkinson SP, Barr H, Shepherd NA. The histopathology of treated Barrett's esophagus. Am J Surg Pathol 1998;22:239-245.
9. Sampliner DB, Fass R. Partial regression of Barrett's esophagus-an inadequate endpoint. Am J Gastroenterol 1993;93:1794-1795.

What information can be drawn from available data regarding argon plasma coagulation for Barrett's esophagus?

J.L. Barnett (Ann Arbor)

Theoretically, the destruction of Barrett's mucosa would eliminate the subsequent development of esophageal adenocarcinoma. The goal of endoscopic ablative therapy is to completely destroy metaplastic tissue, and while preventing significant esophageal acid exposure, allow normal squamous mucosa to replace it. Short segment Barretts's esophagus would seem to be particularly amenable to endoscopic therapy because destruction of a smaller surface area would appear to have a lower tendency to produce complications such as chest pain, odynophagia and stricture and fewer endoscopic sessions should be required.

A variety of thermal, chemical and mechanical modalities may be employed including lasers, multipolar electrocoagulation, heater probe, photodynamic therapy, cryotherapy, ultrasonic therapy, and endoscopic mucosal resection. This short review discusses the available data regarding the electrocautery technique of argon plasma coagulation (APC) for Barrett's esophagus (not short segment specifically).

The APC consists of an electrosurgical generator combined with an argon gas delivery system both controlled by microprocessors. Argon, an inert noncombustible gas, is delivered through either a 2.3 mm (7Fr) or 3.2 mm (10Fr) endoscopic probe. Voltage ionizes the gas at the probe tip forming an electrically conductive plasma. When the distal tip of the probe is within 2-5 mm of the target, the current arcs to the tissue producing thermal injury. Because of the inability of dessicated devitalized tissue to conduct current, the depth of injury is usually < 3 mm depending on application time and wattage setting. The potential advantages of this non-contact application of energy for Barrett's compared to contact devices such as the multipolar electrocoagulation probe and the heater probe include no sticking effect or buildup of debris on the probe tip, the ability to "paint" a larger surface and good visual control of coagulation. The potential advantages over laser devices are lower cost, portability and a more limited depth of tissue injury. A disadvantage of the APC is mild gastric distention due to argon gas insufflation.

The first report using the APC for Barrett's esophagus was published by Dumoulin *et al.* in 1997 [1]. They partially treated 2 patients with long segment nondysplastic Barrett's using a 2 l/min gas flow rate at a power setting of 50 watts. Just over one half of the total length of tissue was treated beginning at the proximal margin and burning circumferentially 1 cm per session (monthly). The squamous mucosa successfully replaced the metaplastic tissue and the only complications were mild dysphagia and retrosternal discomfort. Since that report, there have been at least 5 other published series using the APC for ablation of Barrett's esophagus (*Table I*) [2-6]. A total of 112 patients were enrolled all requiring at least a 2 or 3 cm length of metaplastic tissue be present. Only a few patients had low or high-grade dysplasia. All were treated with potent, usually double-dose, proton pump inhibitor acid suppression therapy. The technique of APC varied though most seemed to use a power setting in the neighborhood of 50 watts with an argon gas flow rate of 1-2 l/min. One to ten sessions were required usually spaced 4-6 weeks apart with a median of about 3 per patient to ablate the Barrret's mucosa. Some were more conservative and averaged one session per cm of tissue treated. Some cauterized circumferentially and others treated 2-4 cm long, 1 cm wide strips, but purposefully left untreated mucosal bridges between the coagulated tissue strips hoping to avoid stricture formation. Minor complications of transient retrosternal discomfort and dysphagia or odynophagia were common, but more serious problems such as severe chest pain lasting days, severe esophagitis or stricture were seen in approximately 5% of patients. In one series of 30 patients, 2 esophageal perforations occurred including one death [3]. Both occurred early in their experience and were thought related to the probe being pushed through the esophageal wall. Residual metaplastic tissue either visible or underlying squamous mucosa was seen in at least one patient in every series and ranged from 7% to approximately 40% of the patients. Furthermore, the series with the longest follow-up identified relapsing islands of Barrett's metaplasia in 47% at 12 months [5].

An additional 200 or so patients reported in abstract form have been treated with the APC for Barrett's esophagus (*Table II*) [7-13]. Results are similar to the previously published reports. Transient chest pain and dysphagia are common but usually mild, although one group reported moderate-severe chest pain and odynophagia 3-10 days postprocedure in 54% including high fevers, stricture, effusion and pneumomediastinum. A small but definite minority develop recurrent Barrett's after a short follow-up of < 1 year. In two series totaling 40 patients, long-term inhibition of acid suppression was achieved surgically. After 7-12 months of follow-up, 8% developed recurrent metaplastic tissue [10,

Table I. List of published trials using the argon plasma coagulation for ablation of Barrett's esophagus.

	Nb of patients	Barrett's length (dysplasia)	F/u months	PPI Rx	Technique	Nb sessions	Complications	Residual Barrett's?
Dumoulin [1]	2	8, 10 cm	6	Omep 20 BID	50 W, Q 4 weeks	5 & 7	Mild chest pain/ dysphagia	Residual Barrett's esophagus in both
Byrne [3]	30	> 3 cm (4 LGD, 3 HGD)	9 (6-18) or surg	Omep 20 BID Q 4-6 weeks	Strips	1-7 (3.1)	Chest pain, odynoph. 2 perforations 1 death (3 dropouts)	Residual underlying Barrett's esophagus in 30%
Mork [4]	15	2-8 cm (2 LGD)	9 (7-13)	Omep 60 or Lanso 90 daily	60 W, 50% circum Q 4-6 weeks	1-8 (3.1)	Mild chest pain, 1 severe chest pain, (2 dropouts)	Residual underlying Barrett's esophagus in 1 (7%) Recurrence in 1
Van Laethem [5]	31	> 3 cm (5 LGD)	12	Omep 40 QD	Q 4-6 weeks	1-4 (2.4)	Mild dysphagia in most 2 strictures, 1 severe eoph (3 dropouts)	Residual underlying or persistent Barrett's esophagus in 12 (39%) Relapsing Barrett's esophagus in 47% at 1 year
Grade [6]	10	2-5 cm	3	Lanso 70 QD	60 W, 50% circum Q 4-6 weeks	1-3 (1.7)	Mild chest pain 44% Mild odynophagia 10% (1 dropout)	Residual underlying Barrett's esophagus in 2 (22%)
Martin [2]	26	> 2 cm				3-10		Residual underlying Barrett's esophagus in ? 9

Table II. List of abstracts using the argon plasma coagulation for ablation of Barrett's esophagus.

	Nb of patients	Barrett's length (dysplasia)	F/u months	PPI Rx	Technique	Nb sessions	Complications	Residual Barrett's?
Stucker [7]	21	8						
Porthun [8]	8	2-11 cm (1 LGD)	1	Lanso 30 QD	60 W	4-9	Upper abdominal pain	No Barrett's esophagus
Schulz [9]	73		12 (2-51)	Omep 40 TID	90 W	1-5 (2)	3 mild strictures (4%)	Residual Barrett's esophagus in 1 (2%)
Hashiba [10]	10	1-10 cm	7	Surgery	70 W	1-6 (2)	Mild CP, dysphagia	Residual Barrett's esophagus in 1 (10%)
Rahmani [11]	18	1-18 cm	2	Omep/Lanso 40-60 QD	45 W	1-3 (1.7)	CP-mild 12/18 Severe 3/18 Mild bleed 1/18	Residual Barrett's esophagus in 4 (25%)
Pereira-Lima [12]	24	0.5-7 cm (9 LGD, 1 HGD)	2	Omep 60	65-70 W	1-4 (2)	Mod-sev CP 13/24 Effus., strict. 3/24 Pn-mediastinum 1/24	No Barrett's esophagus
Tigges [13]	30		12	PPI + surgery later	Hosp 1 day Gen anesth.	1-7 (3)		Recurrent Barrett's esophagus in 2 (4%)

13]. The largest and apparently most successful series reported to date consisted of 73 patients followed for a median of 12 months (range 2-51 months) [9]. More aggressive APC power settings (90 watts) and acid suppression during healing (omeprazole 40 mg x 3 daily) were employed compared to most previous series. A median of only 2 sessions (range 1-5) were required to ablate the metaplastic tissue and in only 1 of 70 was squamous regeneration not achieved. Mild strictures developed in 4% requiring a single dilation. After a median of 1 year follow-up, no patient developed recurrent Barrett's although the examination interval was every 6 months.

Additional experience and shared techniques may help to limit serious complications while minimizing the number of sessions necessary to ablate Barrett's esophagus. Is a high power setting in conjunction with particularly potent acid suppression the answer? Should the coagulation involve 50% of the lumen or be fully circumferential? Should it be limited to just a few centimeters length of tissue per session? Is the "strip technique" designed to avoid strictures by cauterizing strips of tissue but leaving intervening lanes of normal tissue (to be then treated at the subsequent session) the best method? None of these series using APC were limited to short segment Barrett's and, in fact, most specifically excluded these patients. Intuitively, one would think that the short Barrett's patient would be ideal for APC endoscopic therapy: technically easiest to completely treat with the fewest sessions and the lowest complication rates. The major questions that characterize all forms of endoscopic ablation therapy remain. Is the complication rate acceptable? Is ablation cost-effective or even medically effective? Postablation follow-up to date is painfully short. What is the incidence of redevelopment of metaplastic tissue at 5 years postablation? The issue of residual Barrett's under regenerated squamous tissue remains perhaps the major concern. The variable occurrence reported to date may have as much to do with the aggressiveness (number, depth and frequency) of follow-up biopsies as to with the technique of ablation itself. Already a case of low-grade dysplasia progressing to high-grade dysplasia after apparent squamous re-epithelialization achieved with APC therapy has been described [14]. An even more disturbing report is a case of intramucosal adenocarcinoma developing under squamous epithelium 18 months after APC destruction of previously nondysplastic Barrett's [15].

References

1. Dumoulin FL, Terjung B, Neubrand M, Scheurlen C, Fischer HP, Sauerbruch T. Treatment of Barrett's esophagus by endoscopic argon plasma coagulation. Endoscopy 1997;29:751-753.
2. Martin WR. Treatment of a Barrett esophagus with argon plasma coagulation with acid suppression - a prospective study. Z Gastroenterol 1999;37:779-784.
3. Byrne JP, Armstrong GR, Attwood SEA. Restoration of the normal squamous lining in Barrett's esophagus by argon beam plasma coagulation. Am J Gastroenterol 1998;93:1810-1815.
4. Mork H, Barth T, Kreipe HH, Kraus M, Al-taie F, Jakob F, Scheurlen M. Reconstitution of squamous epithelium in Barrett's oesophagus with endoscopic argon plasma coagulation:a prospective study. Scand J Gastroenterol 1998;33:1130-1134.
5. Van Laethem JL, Cremer M, Peny MO, Delhaye M, Deviere J. Eradication of Barrett's mucosa with argon plasma coagulation and acid suppression:immediate and mid-term results. Gut 1998;43:747-751.
6. Grade JF, Shah IA, Medlin SM, Ramirez FC. The efficacy and safety of argon plasma coagulation therapy in Barrett's esophagus. Gastrointest Endosc 1999;50:18-22.
7. Stuker D, Dopieralski A, Zindel C, Farin G, Grund KE. Argon plasma coagulation (APC) for ablation of Barrett's epithelium: first clinical results in 21 patients. Gastroenterology 1998;114:A296.
8. Porthun M, Brand B, Thonke F, Bohnacker S, Seitz U, Binmoeller KF, Schrenck TV, Matsui U, Soehendra N. Endoscopic therapy of Barrett's esophagus using argon plasma coagulation (APC). Gastroenterology 1998;114:A260.

9. Schulz H, Miehlke S, Antos D, Schentke KU, Vieth M, Stolte M, Bayerdoerffer E. Ablation of Barrett's epithelium by endoscopic argon plasma coagulation used in combination with high-dose omeprazole. Gastroenterology 1999;116:A306.
10. Hashiba K, Brasil HA, Moribe D, D'Assuncao MA, Armellini ST, Cappellances CA. Is argon plasma coagulation (APC) effective in Barrett's esophageal mucosa ablation therapy? Gastrointest Endosc 1999;49:AB52.
11. Rahmani EY, Rex DK, Sherman S, Imperiale T, Lehman GA. Barrett's esophagus ablation using argon plasma coagulation. Gastrointest Endosc 1999;49:AB54.
12. Pereira-Lima JC, Lopes CV, Toneloto EB, Rynkowski C, Blaya C, Busnello JV. Does high power setting argon plasma coagulation (APC) ablate Barrett's esophagus without letting metaplastic mucosa underneath the new squamous epithelium? Gastrointest Endosc 1999;49:AB53.
13. Tigges H, Fuchs KH, Maroske J, Fein M, Thiede A. Combination of endoscopic argon plasma coagulation (EAPC) and antireflux surgery for treatment of Barrett's esophagus. Gastrointest Endosc 2000;51(A)3716.
14. Maass S, Martin WR, Spiethoff A, Riemann JF. Barrett esophagus with severe dysplasia in argon beam therapy. Z Gastroenterol 1998;36:301-306.
15. Van Laethem JL, Peny MO, Salmon I, Cremer M, Deviere J. Intramucosal adenocarcinoma arising under squamous re-epithelialisation of Barrett's oesophagus. Gut 2000;46:574-577.

What are the indications of argon beam plasma coagulation for eradication of Barrett's esophagus?

M. Kahaleh, J.-L. Van Laethem, J. Devière (Brussels)

Barrett's esophagus is associated with gastroesophageal reflux disease (GERD) and 10 to 20% of patients with GERD may develop this condition [1, 2]. Patients with Barrett's esophagus have an increased risk of developing adenocarcinoma of the esophagus, although the exact importance of that risk is difficult to appreciate, it is estimated 30 to 125 times greater than in the general population [2-4]. Even if the overall incidence of malignant transformation is relatively low, adenocarcinoma arising in Barrett's esophagus often manifest at an incurable stage [5] and their incidence in Western Europe and the United States is increasing [6], hence a lot of emphasis has been put on its precursor. Endoscopic surveillance of patient with Barrett's esophagus has been instituted to identify patients at high risk for developing adenocarcinoma by detecting dysplasia, the presumed morphologic precursor lesion [7]. Due to the high cost or routine endoscopic follow-up with biopsies, attempt to reverse Barrett's esophagus has been proposed to eliminate the need of surveillance and the risk of adenocarcinoma. High dose omeprazole and antireflux surgery were disappointing in inducing significant reversal [8-11].

Argon plasma coagulation (APC) combined with acid suppression has been used in several studies for the eradication of Barrett's esophagus (*Table I*), the aim behind this technique is to induce injury to the metaplastic epithelium in an acid suppressed environment in order to induce partial regression of Barrett's esophagus segments and squamous reepithelialization arising from pluripotential precursor cells in the treated areas [12-15].

We previously reported a study analyzing the immediate and mid term result of this treatment in 31 patients [13], 5 of them having low-grade dysplasia (LGD). Patients underwent a mean of 2.4 APC sessions (range: 1-4) combined with omeprazole 40 mg/day.

Table I. Argon plasma coagulation for eradication of Barrett's esophagus.

Authors	Patients (number)	Squamous reepithelialization	Underlying intestinal metaplasia	Follow-up (months)
Byrne 1998 [12]	27	70%	30%	9
Van Laethem 1998 [13]	31	61%	39%	12
Mork 1998 [14]	15	87%	13%	8
Schulz 2000 [15]	70	98%	2%	12

After one year of follow-up we eradicated Barrett's esophagus in 19 patients (61%). Even in those patients, occasional persistence of not macroscopically detectable intestinal metaplasia was found, visualized at histology underlying the new squamous epithelium. This major problem associated with this treatment has been reported in all series with an incidence of 2 to 39% [12-15] after only one year. We also recently reported a case of superficial adenocarcinoma arising underneath the squamous epithelium 18 months after complete reepithelialization [16]. This stresses the need for maintenance of surveillance even after achievement of squamous reepithelialization and questions the justification of such treatment. In addition especially in cases of circumferential Barrett's esophagus, APC is associated with significant complications. Mild chest discomfort posttreatment has been described from 18% to 46%, in the study by Byrne *et al.* [12] of twenty-seven patients treated, esophageal perforation occurred in two of them, one of whom died post-operatively. In our serie [13], one patient experienced esophageal bleeding requiring transfusion. Mild strictures resolved after balloon or bougie dilatation has been reported from 4.5% to 6.4% [12-13]. For these reasons, APC for non dysplastic or LGD Barrett's esophagus should still be considered as experimental and performed in the setting of carefully monitored clinical studies. It is only with the availability of long-term studies that the question concerning potential cancer risk reduction will be effectively addressed.

In patients with Barrett's esophagus associated with severe dysplasia, APC has disclosed some effectiveness in patients not candidate for surgery [17] but it is clearly challenged by other techniques including mucosectomy [18, 19] and photodynamic therapy [20].

References

1. Falk GW, Richter JE. Reflux disease and Barrett's esophagus. Endoscopy 1996;28:13-21.
2. Phillips RW, Wong RKH. Barrett's esophagus: natural history, incidence, etiology and complications. Gastroenterol Clin North Am 1991;20:791-816.
3. Lagergren J, Bergström R, Lindgren A, Nyren O. Symptomatic gastroesophageal reflux as a risk factor for esophageal adenocarcinoma. N Engl J Med 1999;340:825-831.
4. Spechler SJ, Robbin AH, Rubin HB, et al. Adenocarcinoma and Barrett's esophagus: an overrated risk? Gastroenterology 1984;87:927-933.
5. Paraf F, Flejou JF, Pignon JP, et al. Surgical pathology of adenocarcinoma arising in Barrett's esophagus: analysis of 67 cases. Am J Surg Pathol 1995;19:183-191.
6. Paraf F, Devessa SS, Kneller RW, et al. Rising incidence of adenocarcinoma of the esophagus and gastric cardia. JAMA 1991;265:1287-1289.
7. Hamilton SR, Smith RR. The relationship between columnar epithelia dysplasia and invasive adenocarcinoma arising in Barrett's esophagus. Am J Clin Pathol 1987;87:301-312.
8. Chen LQ, Nastos D, Hu CY, et al. Results of the Collis-Nissen gastroplasty in patients with Barrett's esophagus. Ann Thorac Surg 1999;68:1014-1020.

9. Gore S, Healey CJ, Sutton R. Regression of columnar-lined (Barrett's) oesophagus with continuous omeprazole therapy. Aliment Pharmacol Ther 1993;7:623-628.
10. Deviere J, Buset M, Dumonceau JM, et al. Regression of Barrett's epithelium with omeprazole. N Eng J Med 1989;320:1497-1498.
11. Malesci A, Savarino V, Zentili P, et al. Partial regression of Barrett's oesophagus by long term therapy with high dose omeprazole. Gastrointest Endosc 1996;44:700-757.
12. Byrne JP, Armstrong GR, Attwood SE. Restoration of the normal squamous lining in Barrett's esophagus by argon beam plasma coagulation. Am J Gastroenterol 1998;33:1130-1134.
13. Van Laethem JL, Cremer M, Peny MO, Delhaye M, Deviere J. Eradication of Barrett's mucosa with argon plasma coagulation and acid suppression:immediate and mid-term results. Gut 1998;43:747-751.
14. Mork H, Barth T, Kreipe HH, Kraus M, Al-Zaie O, Jakob F, Scheurlen M. Reconstruction of squamous epithelium in Barrett's esophagus with endoscopic argonplasma coagulation:a prospective study. Scan J Gastroenterol 1998;33:1130-1134.
15. Schulz H, Miehlke S, Antos D, Schentke KU, et al. Ablation of Barrett's epithelium by endoscopic argon plasma coagulation in combination with high-dose omeprazole. Gastrointest Endosc 2000;51:659-663.
16. Van Laethem JL, Peny MO, Salmon I, Cremer M, Deviere J. Intramucosal adenocarcinoma arising under squamous re-epithelialisation of Barrett's oesophagus. Gut 2000;46:574-577.
17. Van Laethem JL, Jagodzinski R, Peny MO, Cremer M, Deviere J. Argon Plasma coagulation in the treatment of Barrett's high-grade dysplasia and in situ adenocarcinoma. Endoscopy 2001;33:257-261.
18. Nijhawan PK, Wang KK. Endoscopic mucosal resection for lesions with endoscopic features suggestive of malignancy and high-grade dysplasia within Barrett's esophagus. Gastrointest Endosc 2000;52:328-332.
19. Ell C, May A, Gossner L, et al. Endoscopic mucosal resection of early cancer and high-grade dysplasia in Barrett's esophagus. Gastroenterology 2000;118:670-677.
20. Overholt BF, Panjehpour M, Haydek JM. Photodynamic therapy for Barrett's esophagus: follow-up in 100 patients. Gastrointest Endosc 1999;49:1-7.

C.D. Morris, J.P. Byrne, S.E.A. Attwood (Salford)

Argon beam plasma coagulation (ABPC) is an electrocautery technique that has been used in open surgery for many years. The development of specialized probes has allowed the technique to be utilised in endoscopic surgery. Initially its use centred on the palliation of gastrointestinal tumors but with gradually increasing enthusiasm, its applications have widened to include control of haemorrhage and ablation of angiodysplatic lesions.

The principle, like that of all types of cautery is the delivery of electrical energy to the tissue to cause tissue destruction. However standard diathermy carries a significant risk of deep injury and perforation in a hollow viscus, this being greatly reduced in argon coagulation. High frequency alternating current is delivered to the tissue *via* the flow of an ionized, electrically conductive plasma of argon gas. As tissue is destroyed forming an eschar, conduction is lost preventing further damage and limiting the depth of tissue injury to 1-2 mm. For this reason it is safer in its use than techniques such as laser or conventional diathermy. It is also less expensive to purchase than laser with a purchase price of around £ 12,000, and lower running costs. An additional benefit is that energy can be applied tangentially to the tissue, which has great advantages in a narrow lumen organ such as the esophagus.

Partial regression of Barrett's esophagus has been widely reported in patients following control of gastroesophageal reflux by surgical [1] or pharmacological means [2], but complete regression is rare. Photodynamic therapy [3], laser [4] or electrocoagulation [5] have been used to destroy Barrett's tissue, and it has been shown that a neo-squamous lining will develop in its place if reflux is adequately controlled. To date studies have failed to demonstrate any difference in squamous regrowth in patients treated by surgical *versus* pharmacological control of reflux. The importance is in controlling reflux not in how it is accomplished.

In our unit patients are treated as day cases, ablation being carried out under intravenous sedation with monitoring as per standard endoscopy. As argon gas flows through the endoscope at 1-3 L/min, gaseous gastric distension occurs. This is prevented by aspiration of the gas *via* the endoscope. For this reason we prefer to use a twin-channel operating gastroscope, as the gas may be aspirated *via* the spare channel, without needing to withdraw the argon probe. The endoscope is positioned at the gastroesophageal junction (GEJ) and the argon probe advanced so that 1-cm protrudes from the endoscope. The tip is then held close to the mucosa (no-physical contact required) and the unit activated. The endoscope is pulled back at around 1 cm/sec to coagulate a longitudinal strip 3 mm across up to the squamocolumnar junction. The procedure is then repeated to coagulate another strip next to the first. The argon probe tip is withdrawn into the scope channel as the endoscope is advanced to prevent a possible perforating injury. Three areas are coagulated at the first sitting with bridges of undamaged tissue left between them as shown in *Figure 1*. At a second treatment 4-6 weeks later the remaining areas are ablated.

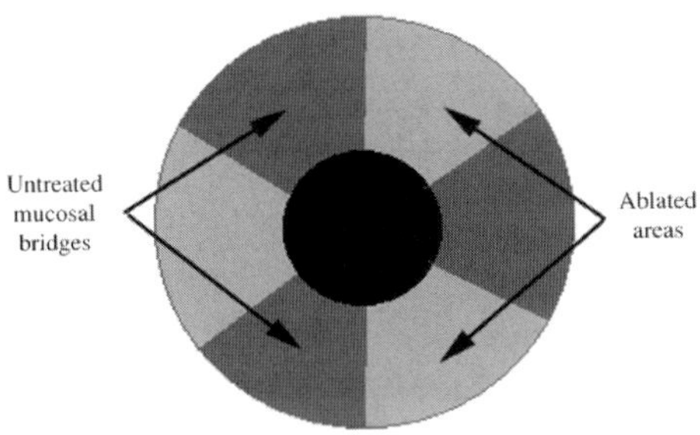

Figure 1.

Our initial experience of this technique in the ablation of Barrett's esophagus was reported in 1998 [6]. Twenty-seven patients underwent argon ablation following control of reflux (22 proton pump inhibitor, 5 antireflux surgery). Two patients had high-grade dysplasia (HGD) and four had low-grade dysplasia (LGD). Median length of the Barrett's segments was 5 cm (range 3-17). Ablation was completed when less than 3 cm of Barrett's tissue remained. All patients had regression of Barrett's with squamous regrowth to within 2 cm of the GEJ following treatment. The number of treatments ranged between 1 and 7, correlating with the pretreatment length of the Barrett's segment (3-17 cm). Minor retrosternal discomfort and odynophagia was common and was treated with simple analgesia and mucaine gel. Two perforations occurred, one managed conservatively and one surgically. Both complications occurred early in our learning experience, with no further perforations in over 300 treatments to date. We believe that deeper sedation is required to carry out therapeutic endoscopy in the esophagus, to prevent unnecessary movement, which may lead to perforation.

Other studies have had similar success in eradicating Barrett's epithelium. Mork [7] *et al.* demonstrated complete squamous regrowth in 13 of 15 patients treated with ABPC in a median of 3 treatment sessions. The study of Van Laethem *et al.* reported their experience with 31 patients in whom complete regression was seen in 81% of cases [8].

The need for acid suppression to allow squamous regrowth was emphasised in our study. Two patients with persisting reflux symptoms on omeprazole 20 mg OD initially showed no squamous regrowth after argon treatment. On doubling their dose of omeprazole squamous regrowth was achieved. The requirement for adequate acid suppression has also been documented by others [7].

A feature of the neo-squamous lining in around 30% of patients is the persistence of intestinal type glands underlying the new epithelium [6]. This has been widely reported in studies on Barrett's ablation by all methods. It is probably less common in techniques with a deeper depth of injury such as photodynamic therapy, but at the expense of greater technique complications. The fate of these buried glands is unknown. It could be postulated that by protecting the glands from further injury due to acid/duodenal juices then neoplastic progression may be halted. However there is one reported case of an intramucosal adenocarcinoma developing in a patient who had undergone ablative therapy [9]. The tumor presented as a bulge covered by squamous epithelium 18 months following argon ablation of non-dysplastic Barrett's epithelium. Though it may have originated from residual glands beneath the squamous epithelium, a pre-existing tumor could not be definitely excluded.

A further unknown is the degree of stability in the phenotype of the neosquamous epithelium. In our experience the squamous epithelium remains if reflux continues to be adequately controlled. The study by Mork documents a single cases of re-columnarization of the neosquamous epithelium in a patient who stopped acid suppression therapy of their own volition.

Two of the patients in our study had HGD and four had LGD. All 6 of these patients have histologically confirmed squamous replacement of their Barrett's metaplasia with no residual dysplasia on follow-up. This suggests that ABPC has an equally important role in the management of dysplasia. We have also treated 14 patients with localised cancer of the esophagus who were unfit for surgical resection by ABPC. To date all of these patients remain alive with a median follow-up of 21 months, 86% of the tumors showing no progression [10]. This illustrates the versatility of this technique in dealing with both dysplastic and non-dysplastic tissue in Barrett's esophagus.

In conclusion ABPC is an effective method of destroying columnar mucosa to allow squamous regrowth in the esophagus. It is simple to use and relatively cheap to purchase and maintain. It is safe in its application with minimal side effects and complications. It also has the versatility to allow debulking of advanced tumors and may have a place in the local treatment of early cancers and HGD in patients unfit for surgical resection.

References

1. Attwood SE, Barlow AP, Norris TL, Watson A. Barrett's oesophagus: effect of antireflux surgery on symptom control and development of complications. Br J Surg 1992;79(10):1050-1053.
2. Sampliner RE. Effect of up to 3 years of high-dose lansoprazole on Barrett's esophagus. Am J Gastroenterol 1994;89(10):1844-1848.
3. Overholt B, Panjehpour M. Photodynamic therapy for Barrett's esophagus:Clinical update. Am J Gastroenterol 1996;91:1719-1723.

4. Sampliner R, Hixson L, Fennerty M, Garewal H. Regression of Barrett's esophagus by laser ablation in an anacid environment. Dig Dis Sci 1993;38:365-368.
5. Sampliner R, Fennerty B, Garewal H. Reversal of Barrett's esophagus with acid suppression and multipolar electrocoagulation: preliminary results. Gastrintest Endosc 1996;44:532-535.
6. Byrne JP, Armstrong GR, Attwood SE. Restoration of the normal squamous lining in Barrett's esophagus by argon beam plasma coagulation. Am J Gastroenterol 1998;93(10):1810-1815.
7. Mork H, Barth T, Kreipe HH, Kraus M, Al Taie O, Jakob F, Scheurlen M. Reconstitution of squamous epithelium in Barrett's oesophagus with endoscopic argon plasma coagulation:a prospective study. Scand J Gastroenterol 1998;33(11):1130-1134.
8. Van Laethem JL, Cremer M, Peny MO, Delhaye M, Deviere J. Eradication of Barrett's mucosa with argon plasma coagulation and acid suppression:immediate and mid term results. Gut 1998;43(6):747-751.
9. Van Laethem J, Peny M, Salmon I, Cremer M, Deviere J. Intramucosal adenocarcinoma arising under squamous re-epithelialisation of Barrett's oesophagus. Gut 2000;46:574-577.
10. Akhtar K, Armstrong G, Byrne J, Attwood S. Argon beam plasma coagulation in the management of cancers in the oesophagus and stomach. Surg Endosc 2000;14:1127-1130.

How should areas of ectopic gastric mucosa found in the upper esophagus be treated?

A. Sibille, D. Lacremans, N. Mahy, P. Warzée (Charleroi)

Patches of ectopic gastric mucosa could be endoscopically recognized in the upper esophagus as oval salmon-pink colored patches. The reported prevalence of the so-called "inlet patch" varies widely in the literature. It is problably underdiagnosed in routine endoscopy because the examination of the upper esophagus is usually not thoroughly performed by the gastroenterologist in the absence of symptoms related to upper dysphagia. The highest prevalence rates were found in prospective studies that were specifically looking for those areas. A necropsy study in children identified the lesion in 21% of the cases [1]. Endoscopy series in adults usually reported rates of 3-5% [2] but it is worth noticing that a 10% prevalence was found by some authors [3].

The pathogenesis of ectopic gastric mucosa is a matter of debate between a congenital – embryological – and an acquired origin – consecutive to a gastroesophageal reflux (GER) like Barrett's esophagus –, the most commonly accepted theory being that these areas are embryological remnants. This hypothesis is supported by the following arguments. During fetal life the esophagus is lined by a columnar epithelium which is secondarily replaced by a squamous epithelium. The incidence of ectopic gastric mucosa seems to be higher in the childhood, particularly during the first year, and apparently declines with advancing years [1]. These patches are almost always located in the upper esophagus and other reflux associated lesions of the lower esophagus (hiatal hernia, esophagitis, Barrett's epithelium) often are not found in these patients [3]. A malignant potential of the ectopic gastric mucosa through a metaplasia-dysplasia sequence like in Barrett's esophagus has never been proven. In addition, some authors found a difference in the hormonal secretion profile measured by immunohistochemical methods between ectopic gastric mucosa of the upper esophagus and Barrett's esophagus [4, 5].

However none of these arguments rules out definitively the acid reflux hypothesis especially in relationship with some other findings reported in the litterature. Bogomoletz [6] reported that the mucin histochemistry of ectopic gastric mucosa was different from that of the heterotopic gastric mucosa found into the Meckel's diverticula, a lesion of developmental origin, but had several similarities with that of Barrett's esophagus. Jacobs [2] reported a significantly higher rate of esophagitis in the group of patients with ectopic gastric mucosa. Although this is a rare lesion, the presence of intestinal metaplasia (IM) in ectopic gastric mucosa patches has been described by Jacobs (3 cases) [2], Bogomoletz (3 cases) [6], Truong (1 case) [7] and our group (3 cases) [8]. Moreover, one case of preneoplastic lesion (adenoma with high-grade dysplasia – HGD) [9] and about fifteen cases of adenocarcinoma arising in ectopic gastric mucosa [10-12] have been reported. All these reports render a probable relationship between Barrett's esophagus and ectopic gastric mucosa relevant. Both hypothesis however are not mutually exclusive. GER can affect an underlying congenital abnormality [6].

Ectopic gastric mucosa can also be the cause of different benign symptoms or complications such as odynophagia and dysphagia [13], web and stricture [14-16], burning sensation and nausea [5], peptic ulceration and fistula [17]. The ability of the ectopic gastric mucosa to secrete acid has been demonstrated by pH monitoring [18, 19]. *Helicobacter pylori* colonization and gastritis are rare complications of the ectopic gastric mucosa but have been well established [8, 20].

Treatment of ectopic gastric mucosa has been reported only in the few symptomatic or complicated cases. Large series are lacking. H_2-antagonists and proton pump inhibitors (PPIs) were given successfully in patients with benign, acid-related symptoms [18, 19]. Endoscopic dilation or CO2-laser therapy have been performed in cases of stricturing lesions [13, 15]. In a patient with a stricturing patch, endoscopic thermal coagulation of the ectopic gastric mucosa combined with omeprazole therapy was interestingly followed by repopulation with a normal squamous epithelium [16]. Apart from the cases complicated by an adenocarcinoma, surgery was only needed in a case of HGD [9] and in a 5-year-old boy with a circumferential lesion [21]. There is no report concerning *Helicobacter pylori* eradication.

Due to the rarity of ectopic gastric mucosa in the upper esophagus and its related complications, data from the literature are scarce. For this reason the pathophysiology still remains controversial and the actual neoplastic potential is unknown. It is thus difficult to issue guidelines for surveillance and treatment. The following attitude however can reasonably be proposed. When ectopic gastric mucosa is spotted during upper endoscopy, biopsies should systematically be taken in order to detect intestinal metaplasia or dysplasia. Symptomatic patients with benign histology should be treated according to their clinical and endoscopic features. For example a stricture should be dilated and a PPI should be prescribed in case of acid-related symptoms. In this latter situation, it would be logical to eradicate *Helicobacter pylori* if present. Endoscopic surveillance should be proposed for patients with mild and moderate dysplasia. Further studies should address the question of the usefulness of a surveillance program for patients with IM. When HGD or superficial adenocarcinoma are detected in ectopic gastric mucosa, endoscopic mucosal resection or ablation therapy (Nd:YAG laser, photodynamic therapy or electrocoagulation) could be as valuable therapeutic options as they are in other similar conditions such as Barrett's esophagus or superficial esophageal cancer [22, 23]. However because these treatments have never been reported in the case of ectopic gastric mucosa, they need to be evaluated for this particular occurrence.

References

1. Variend S, Howat AJ. Upper oesphageal gastric heterotopia:a prospective necropsy study in children. J Clin Pathol 1988;41:742-745.
2. Jacobs E, Dehou MF. Heterotopic gastric mucosa in the upper esophagus:a prospective study of 33 cases and review of literature. Endoscopy 1997;29:710-715.
3. Borhan-Manesh F, Farnum JB. Incidence of heterotopic gastric mucosa in the upper oesophagus. Gut 1991;32:968-972.
4. Feurle GE, Helmstaedter V, Buerhring A, Bettendorf U, Eckardt VF. Distinct immunohistochemical findings in columnar epithelium of esophageal inlet patch and of Barrett's esophagus. Dig Dis Sci 1990;35:86-92.
5. Shah KK, DeRidder PH, Shah KK. Ectopic gastric mucosa in proximal esophagus. J Clin Gastroenterol 1986;8:509-513.
6. Bogomoletz WV, Geboes K, Feydy P, Nasca S, Ectors N, Rigaud C. Mucin histochemistry of heterotopic gastric mucosa of the upper esophagus in adults: possible pathogenic implications. Hum Pathol 1988;19:1301-1306.
7. Truong LD, Stroehlein JR, McKechnie JC. Gastric heterotopia of the proximal esophagus: a report of four cases detected by endoscopy and review of the literature. Am J Gastroenterol 1986;81:1162-1166.
8. Sibille A, Warzée P, Hérin M. Should biopsies be taken from ectopic gastric mucosa in the upper esophagus? Gastrointest Endosc 1997;45:A235.
9. Mion F, Lambert R, Partensky C, Cherkaoui M, Berger F. High-grade dysplasia in an adenoma of the upper esophagus developing on heterotopic gastric mucosa. Endoscopy 1996;28:633-635.
10. Lauwers GY, Scott GV, Vauthey JN. Adenocarcinoma of the upper esophagus arising in cervical ectopic gastric mucosa: rare evidence of malignant potential of so-called "inlet patch". Dig Dis Sci 1998;43:901-907.
11. Berkelhammer C, Bhagavan M, Templeton A, Raines R, Walloch J. Gastric inlet patch containing submucosally infiltrating adenocarcinoma. J Clin Gastroenterol 1997;25:678-681.
12. Takagi A, Ema Y, Horii S, Morishita M, Miyaishi O, Kino I. Early adenocarcinoma arising from ectopic gastric mucosa in the cervical esophagus. Gastrointest Endosc 1995;41:167-170.
13. Schroeder WW, Myer CM, Schechter GL. Ectopic gastric mucosa in the cervical esophagus. Laryngoscope 1987;97:131-135.
14. Waring JP, Wo JM. Cervical esophageal web caused by an inlet patch of gastric mucosa. South Med J 1997;90:554-555.
15. Steadman C, Kerlin P, Teague C, Stephenson P. High esophageal stricture:a complication of "inlet patch" mucosa. Gastroenterology 1988;94:521-524.
16. McBride MA, Vanagunas AA, Breshnahan JP, Barch DB. Combined endoscopic thermal electrocoagulation with high dose omeprazole therapy in complicated heterotopic gastric mucosa of the esophagus. Am J Gastroenterol 1995;90:2029-2031.
17. Kohler B, Kohler G, Riemann JF. Spontaneous esophagotracheal fistula resulting from ulcer in heterotopic gastric mucosa. Gastroenterology 1988;95:828-830.
18. Galan AR, Katzka DA, Castell DO. Acid secretion from an esophageal inlet patch demonstrated by ambulatory pH monitoring. Gastroenterology 1998;115:1574-1576.
19. Nakajima H, Munakata A, Sasaki Y, Yoshida Y. pH profile of esophagus in patients with inlet patch of heterotopic gastric mucosa after tetragastrin stimulation:an endoscopic approach. Dig Dis Sci 1993;38:1915-1919.
20. Borhan-Manesh F, Farnum JB. Study of helicobacter pylori colonization of patches of heterotopic gastric mucosa (HGM) at the upper esophagus. Dig Dis Sci 1993;38:142-146.
21. Powell RW, Luck SR. Cervical esophageal obstruction by ectopic gastric mucosa. J Pediatr Surg 1988;23:632-634.
22. Ell C, May A, Gossner L, Pech O, Günter E, Mayer G, Henrich R, Vieth M, Müller H, Seitz G, Stolte M. Endoscopic mucosal resection of early cancer and high-grade dysplasia in Barrett's esophagus. Gastroenterology 2000;118:670-677.
23. Sibille A, Lambert R, Souquet JC, Sabben G, Descos F. Long term survival after photodynamic therapy for esophageal cancer. Gastroenterology 1995;108:337-344.

Compared to the hematoporphyrin derivatives, what are the advantages of the new photosensitizers?

J. Etienne, N. Dorme (Rueil-Malmaison)

The treatment of cancers by photodynamic therapy (PDT) is based on the destruction of tumor tissues by the non-thermal photochemical effect of irradiation of a photosensitizer accumulated preferentially in the cancerous cells. The efficacy of PDT is linked to the photoefficiency of the photosensitizer. This technique has been known and used in clinical treatment with lasers since 1976 [1]. However, its development at the outset was restricted, due to the availability of photosensitizer, consisting in a not very soluble and not well defined mixture of hematoporphyrin derivatives (HPD) giving quite inconsistent results. Dougherty improved the method in 1984 [2] by the preparation of Photofrin® (Axcan, Canada). This product is also an HPD, but contains better isolated and more soluble fractions. Temoporfin (Foscan®), a chlorin molecule developed by Scotia Pharmaceuticals Ltd., is a second generation photosensitizer which has the advantage of being a pure by synthetic product. Moreover, the peak of absorption of temoporfin in the red at 652 nm improves the penetration of light through tissues compared to that of Photofrin® (630 nm). Furthermore, temoporfin has an activation peak at 514 nm, a less penetrating wavelength which is suitable for the treatment of superficial lesions in thin-walled organs like the esophagus where the risk of perforation and stenosis is high. *in vitro* and *in vivo* studies have shown that the selectivity of temoporfin, expressed as a greater affinity for cancerous cells than for healthy adjacent tissues, is much better than that of Photofrin®. Likewise, the phototoxicity of temoporfin has been found to be about 100 times higher than that of Photofrin® on account of the higher quantum yield of the temoporfin molecule. The two products have been used in man in analogous sites (esophagus, stomach, larynx, bronchi, pleura, head and neck, ovary, brain), but the studies are not equivalent: they are well-targeted, with very precise inclusion criteria for temoporfin, but sometimes less systematic for Photofrin® with often small heterogeneous series including patients treated by associated therapies.

Clinical information limited to the field of the esophagus will be presented for the two products. The side effects, particularly the risks of photosensitization and stenosis which are more reduced with Temoporfin, will also be discussed. Finally, the role of Temoporfin in tumors detected at a precancerous stage and in intramucosal cancers will be emphasized.

Structure and dose form

Temoporfin (meta-tetrahydroxyphenylchlorin-mTHPC) is a pure, synthetic chlorin molecule (*Figure 1*). The pharmaceutical form used in PDT is Foscan®, a dark purple solution for injection, containing 4 mg/ml of m-THPC. Photofrin® is presented as a mixture of purified fractions of hematoporphyrin derivatives (*Figure 2)* which are dissolved in a solvent containing dextrose. Foscan® allows for administration of a precise dose of a pure product, which guarantees more reproducible results.

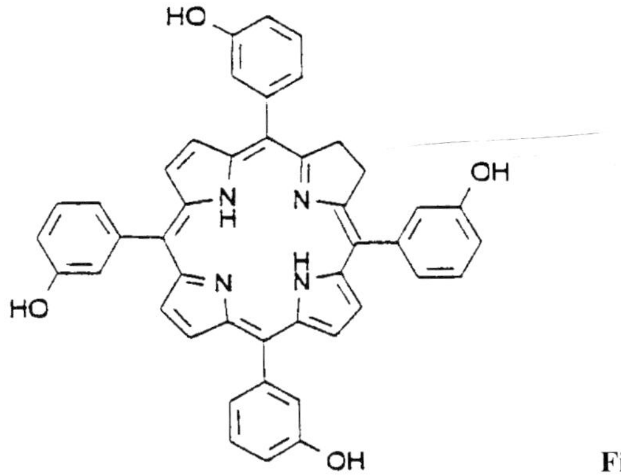

Figure 1. Temoporfin.

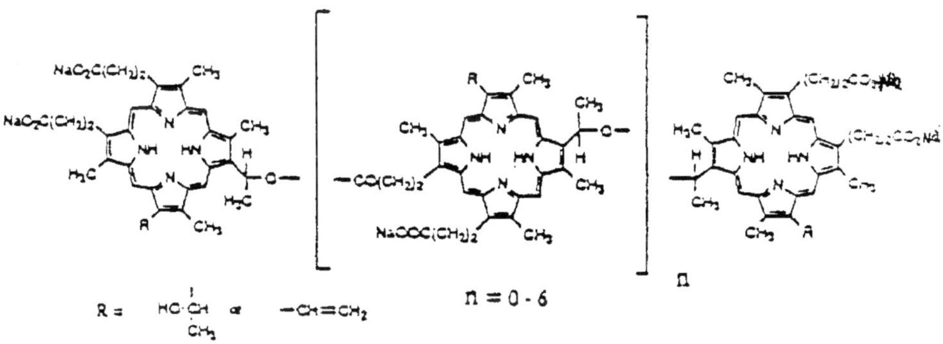

Figure 2. Photofrin.

Peaks and coefficients of absorption

The absorption spectrum of Foscan® allows for the use of PDT at two wavelengths, 652 nm in the red and 514 nm in the green. With Photofrin®, the most frequently used wavelength is 630 nm and more rarely 514 nm. At 652 nm, the coefficient of absorption of m-THPC is roughly 7 times higher than that of Photofrin® at 652 nm. The penetration of light through tissues is greater at 652 nm than at 630 nm [3]. This enhanced light penetration for Foscan® allows for tumor necrosis to a greater depth.

Selectivity

Selectivity is judged by the ratio of the photosensitizer concentration in cancerous tissues to that in adjacent healthy tissues. This has been the subject of several *in vitro* and *in vivo* studies using Foscan®: the results show a significant improvement in selectivity which varies according to the tissue, the light dose and drug-light interval, with a ratio up to 20 [4], whereas Photofrin® presents a ratio of about 1 [5].

Phototoxicity

The results of *in vitro* and *in vivo* studies in animals [4, 6-10] indicate that Foscan® has a phototoxic activity more than 100 times higher than Photofrin®. This superiority is confirmed in man and is objectively shown in clinical treatment by the light dose (fluence-joules/cm^2) and the duration of light irradiation needed, that are much lower than those required by Photofrin®.

Clinical comparisons

The use of PDT with Foscan® is characterized by the differences in the dose administered and in the parameters of irradiation applied. The active dose of m-THPC (0,15 mg/kg) is much lower than that of Photofrin® (2 mg/kg) and the ratio is close to 13. During light irradiation, the necessary fluence (joules/cm^2) is lower with Foscan® resulting in the need for a much shorter illumination time. As an example, with Foscan® in the esophagus, at 514 nm, the fluence is 75 Joules/cm^2 during 11 minutes 30 seconds, and in the bronchi, at 652 nm, the fluence is 10 Joules/cm^2 during 1 minute 7 seconds, whereas with Photofrin®: at 514 nm or at 630 nm according to the lesion, the fluence is 80-120 Joules/cm^2 and the duration can reach 20 minutes [11].

The efficacy and safety of Foscan® has been the subject of several studies in different sites according to well targeted protocols: esophagus [12-14], stomach [15], oral cavity [16, 17], bronchi [17], pleura [18], head and neck [19, 20], ovary [21], brain [22]. Photofrin® has also been used in these different sites as well as in the breast, bladder and eyes, but the protocols have often been less strict, including lesions at different stages of evolution and the use of associated therapies, which invalidate further comparisons.

Side effects

The risk of skin photosensitization, a major systemic side effect, inherent in the very principle of PDT, is less with Foscan® than with Photofrin® in terms of duration. This improvement is the result of the properties of Foscan®: a more rapid elimination and a greater phototoxicity, allowing smaller doses to be given. With Foscan® in the esophagus, the use of the wavelength of 514 nm with windowed diffusers combined with less fluence, irradiance and duration of irradiation has greatly decreased the risk of stenosis. However, in the bronchi at 652 nm the risk of stenosis and of perforation persists. With Photofrin® in the esophagus, development of stenoses (30 to 58%) [23] and fistulas is reported. In the bronchi, stenoses and fistulas have also been noted. Furthermore, in the bladder sharp pains are very frequent.

Efficacy in early esophageal cancers

In intramucosal cancers of the esophagus, Foscan® at 514 nm enables efficient curative action with greater safety on epithelioma [11] and or adenocarcinomas in Barrett's [24]. This attractive therapeutic alternative implies regular surveillance of the esophageal mucosa in high risk patients for early detection of high grade dysplasias and/or intramucosal cancers. In such indications Photofrin® has frequently given incomplete responses and several recurrences [25].

Conclusion

Temoporfin (Foscan®), a second generation photo ensitizer of the chlorin family of compounds, has considerable advantages over previous photosensitizers based on hematoporphyrin derivatives like Photofrin® and opens a new prospect of greater development of the use of PDT in precancerous and early cancerous tumors. Foscan® is a pure synthetic product and presents an absorption peak in the red at 652 nm corresponding to a better penetration of light in the tissues. It can also be used with safety at a peak of 514 nm in the green on thin-walled organs. With a better affinity for cancerous cells, a high phototoxicity, reduced drug and light dose requirements, it has already been used successfully in different sites (esophagus, stomach, larynx, bronchi, pleura, head and neck, ovary and brain). Side effects are moderate.

The low light dose requirements allows for the use of newly developed diode lasers whose cost and maintenance are cheaper than tunable dye lasers.

References

1. Kelly JF, Snell MF. Hematophorphyrine derivate a possible aid in the diagnosis and therapy of carcinoma of the bladder. J Urol 1976,;115:150-151.
2. Dougherty TJ. Photodynamic therapy (PDT) of malignant tumours. Crit Rev Hematol 1984;2:83-116.
3. Hadjur C, Lange N, Rebstein J, Monnier P, Van den Bergh H, Wagnières G. Spectroscopic studies of photobleaching and photoproduct formation of meta (tetrahydroxyphenyl) chlorin (m-THPC) used in photodynamic therapy. The production of singlet oxygen by m-THPC. J Photochem Photobiol B 1998;45:170-178.
4. Stewart JCM. Photosensitizers for photodynamic therapy. Curr Opin Invest Drugs 1993;2:1279-1289.
5. Sabben G, Lambert R. Cinétique du dérivé d'hématophorphyrine tritié dans les tumeurs digestives transplantées chez le rat Fisher. Gastroenterol Clin Biol 1984;8:74.
6. Andrejevic-Blant SA, Theumann JF, Forrer M, Wagnières G, van den Bergh H, Monnier P. Wavelength-dependent effect of tetra(m-hydroxyphenyl) chlorin for photodynamic therapy in an early squamous cell carcinoma model. Lasers Med Sci 1997;12:269-273.
7. Lofgren LA, Ronn AM, Abramson AL, et al. Photodynamic therapy using m-tetra(hydroxyphenyl) chlorin: an animal model. Arch Otolaryngol Head Neck Surg 1994;120:1355-1362.
8. Morlet L, Vonarx-Coinsmann V, Lenz P, et al. Correlation between meta(tetra hydroxyphenyl) chlorin (m-THPC) biodistribution and photodynamic effects in mice. J Photobiol Photochem B 1995;28:25-32.
9. Van Geel IP, Oppelaar H, Oussoren YG, van der Valk MA, Stewart FA. Photosensitising efficacy of mTHPC-PDT compared to photofrin-PDT in the RIFl mouse tumour and normal skin. Int J Cancer 1995;60:388-394.
10. Ansell JK, De Jode ML, Grahn MF. Characterisation of a murine model for the rapid assessment of acute photodynamic response in tumour and muscle. Lasers Med Sci 1997;12:336-341.
11. Savary JF, Grosjean P, Monnier P, Fontolliet C, Wagnieres G, Braichotte D, van den Bergh H. Photodynamic therapy of early squamous cell carcinomas of the esophagus:a review of 31 cases.Endoscopy 1998;30:258-265.
12. Savary JF, Monnier P, Wagnieres G, Braichotte D, Fontolliet C, van den Bergh H. Preliminary clinical studies of photodynamic therapy with m-tetra(hydroxyphenyl) chlorin as a photosensitising agent for treatment of early pharyngeal, oesophageal, and bronchial carcinomas. SPIE 1993;2078:330-340.
13. Grosjean P, Savary JF, Mizeret J, et al. Photodynamic therapy for cancer of the upper aerodigestive tract using tetra(m-hydroxyphenyl) chlorin. J Clin Laser Med Surg 1996;14:281-287.
14. Savary JF, Grosjean P, Monnier P, et al. Photodynamic therapy of early squamous cell carcinomas of the esophagus: a review of 31 cases. Endoscopy 1998;30:258-265.
15. Ell C, Gossner L, May A, Schneider HT, Hahn EG, Stolte M, Sroka R,.Photodynamic ablation of early cancers of the stomach by means of Foscan® (mTHPC) and laser irradiation: preliminary clinical experience. Gut 1998;43:345-349.
16. Fan KFM, Hopper C, Speight PM, Buonaccorsi GA, Bown SG. Photodynamic therapy using temoporfin for malignant disease in the oral cavity. Int J Cancer 1997;73:25-32.

17. Savary JF, Monnier P, Fontolliet C, et al. Photodynamic therapy for early squamous cell carcinomas of the esophagus, bronchi and mouth with m-tetra(hydroxyphenyl)chlorin. Arch Otolaryngol Head Neck Surg 1997;123:162-168.
18. Baas P, Murrer L, Zoetmulder FAN, et al. Photodynamic therapy as adjuvant therapy in surgically treated pleural malignancies. Br J Cancer 1997;78:819-826.
19. Dilkes MG, De Jode ML, Rowntree-Taylor A, McGilligan JA, Kenyon GS, McKelvie P. mTHPC photoclynamic therapy for head and neck cancer. Lasers Med Sci 1996;11:23-29.
20. Bing Tan I. Photodynamic therapy in the treatment of localised primary and recurrent squamous cell carcinoma of the head and neck. First International Conference on Head and Neck Oncology, Brussels 2-4 décembre 1999.
21. Wierrani F, Fiedler D, Grin W, Henry M, Dienes E, Gharehbaghi K, Krammer B, Grunberger W. Clinical effect of mesotetrahydroxyphenyl-chlorin (Foscan®) based photodynamic therapy in recurrent carcinoma of the ovary: preliminary results. Br J Obstet Gynaecol 1997;104:376-378.
22. Kostron H, Obwegeser A, Jakober R, Zimmerman A, Rueck A. Clinical results of mTHPC (Foscan®) mediated photodynamic therapy for malignant brain tumours. Int J Cancer 1997;73:230-235.
23. Overholt B, Panjehpour M. Photodynamic therapy in Barrett's oesophagus. J Clin Las Med and Surg 1996;14:245-248.
24. Etienne J, Dorme N, Bourg Heckly G, Raimbert P, Fékété F. Local curative treatment of superficial adenocarcinoma in Barrett's esophagus. First results of photodynamic therapy with a new photosensitizer. Bull Acad Natl Med 2000;184(8):1731-1747.
25. Sibille A, Lambert R, Souquet JC, Sabben G, Descos F. Long-term survival after photodynamic therapy for esophageal cancer. Gastroenterology 1995;108:337-344.

For the carrying out of the treatment, what are the advantages of spectrophorimetry?

B.F. Overholt (Knoxville)

For the purposes of the answer to this question, spectrophorimetry shall be defined as the use of light used during endoscopic therapy to induce tissue autofluorescence or tissue drug fluorescence to assist in the diagnosis and treatment of dysplastic Barrett's mucosa.

Tissue autofluorescence

Taking advantage of the biologic and physical properties of all tissues, light of specific wavelengths can be used to induce tissue autofluorescence. The induced fluorescent light can then be collected and analyzed to differentiate benign *versus* malignant tissues. Panjehpour *et al.* [1, 2] and VoDinh *et al.* [3, 4] developed a mathematical model, differentialized normal fluorescence, and using laser induced fluorescence (LIF), were able to differentiate esophageal cancer from normals in essentially 100% of cases (100% sensitivity, 98% specificity). They later reported high sensitivity and specificity in differentiating Barrett's high-grade dysplasia from normal esophagus.

In contrast to the above fiberoptic contact probe technique for LIF, Marcon [5] and Duvall [6] have described a light induced fluorescent imaging (LIFE) system that is undergoing clinical development The LIFE endoscope allows full endoscopic field illumination for evaluation of the entire mucosal surface. Using a blue light excitation wave length (437 nm), 2 images are transmitted to a monitor, one in green and one in red. These images are combined and depending on the ratio of red and green, histological differences can be detected.

Tissue drug fluorescence

Malignant tissues concentrate photosensitizers to a greater degree than normal tissues. This property allows for the measurement of fluorescent intensity as an indicator of malignancy. The higher the fluorescent intensity, the greater the likelihood of a diagnosis of cancer. Various photosensitizers can and have been used for this purpose but the most commonly studied has been 5-aminolevulinic acid (5-ALA). Gossner *et al.* [7] examined 35 patients and detected neoplasia with a sensitivity of 85% and specificity of 70%. Messmann [8] has provided an excellent review of the use of 5-ALA for detection of gastrointestinal dysplasia. Sodium porfimer (Photofrin®, Axcan, Mount Hillear, Canada) has also been used during endoscopy for fluorescent detection of Barrett's adenocarcinoma [9].

Light dosimetry during photodynamic therapy

Photosensitizer in tissue produces fluorescence when exposed to the proper excitation wavelength of light. The greater the concentration of photosensitizer, the greater the fluorescence. Studies are underway attempting to capitalize on these facts to provide guidelines for light dosimetry during photodynamic therapy (PDT). Basically, the greater the fluorescence, the lower the light dose required for PDT. Studies to date are preliminary.

Predicting results of photodynamic therapy

Measurement of photosensitizer fluorescent intensity pre- and post-PDT should allow a reasonable prediction of therapeutic effectiveness. Following PDT, the greater the reduction in fluorescent intensity, the greater the expected tissue effect. Although we have found this to be true in our studies, other than predicting a significant response, the clinical usefulness of this observation has yet to be shown.

In conclusion, spectrophorimetry for both the diagnosis of Barrett's dysplasia and for guiding or monitoring treatment is a technology in its infancy. It holds great promise.

References

1. Panjehpour M, Overholt BF, Vo-Dinh T, Haggitt RC, Edwards DH and Buckley FP III. Endoscopic flourescence detection of high grade dysplasia in Barrett's esophagus. Gastroenterology 1996;111:93-101.
2. Panjehpour M, Overholt BF, Schnidhammer JL, Farris C, Buckley PF, Vo-Dinh T. Spectroscopic diagnosis of esophageal cancer: new classification model, improved measurement system. Gastrointest Endosc 1995;41:577-581.
3. Vo-Dinh T, Panjehpour M, Overholt BF, Farris C, Buckley FP, Sneed R. In vivo cancer diagnosis of the esophagus using differential normalized fluorescence (DNF) indices. Lasers Surg Med 1995;16:41A7.
4. Vo-Dinh T, Panjehpour M, Overholt BF, Buckley P, III. Laser-induced differential fluorescence for cancer diagnosis without biopsy. Appl Spectrosc 1997;51:58-63.

5. Marcon NE, et al. The value of fluorescence techniques in gastrointestinal endoscopy-better than the endoscopists eye? II: The North American experience. Endoscopy 1998;30:419-421.
6. DuVall A, Wilson BC, Marcon N. Tissue autofluorescence. Ann Gastrointest Endosc 1997;10:25-30.
7. Gossner L, Stepp H, Sroka R, et al. Photodynamic diagnosis (PDD) of high-grade dysplasia and early cancer in Barrett's esophagus using 5-aminolevulinic acid (ALA). Gastroenterology 1998;114;A136.
8. Messmann H. 5-aminolevulinic acid-induced protoporphyrin IX for the detection of gastrointestinal dysplasia. Gastrointest Endosc Clin North Am 2000;10:497-512.
9. Von Holstein CS, Nilsson AM, Andersson-Engels S, Walther WR, Svanberg K. Detection of adenocarcinoma in Barrett's oesophagus by means of laser induced fluorescence. Gut 1996;39:711-716.

What should be said today about the potential cardiac or pleural complications following photodynamic therapy?

B.F. Overholt (Knoxville)

Complications following photodynamic therapy (PDT) occur. With 5-aminolevulinic acid PDT (ALA-PDT) no significant complications have been reported due to the superficial nature of the mucosal injury with ALA-PDT. However, with Photofrin®-PDT esophageal wall injury is considerably deeper. As expected, with deeper injury, therapeutic results are improved but at the risk of a greater incidence of complications. The question to be answered addresses 2 of those complications, pleural and cardiac.

Overholt *et al.* [1] reviewed chest X-rays in 14 patients 48 hours after Photofrin® PDT for Barrett's dysplasia. Small bilateral pleural effusions were noted in 6 patients, 4 had left effusions, 1 had a small right effusion and 3 were normal. All effusions were small and asymptomatic. The authors had previously described the need to perform thoracentesis on 2 patients who presented with hypoxia 2-3 days following Photofrin®-PDT. The effusions were transudates. Lightdale *et al.* [2] also reported small asymptomatic pleural effusions following Photofrin®-PDT for esophageal cancer. Pleural effusions following Photofrin®-PDT are common, usually small and asymptomatic and typically clear within 1-2 weeks.

Cardiac arrhythmias can also occur following Photofrin®-PDT. Overholt *et al.* [3] reported 2 patients with acute onset atrial fibrillation following Photofrin®-PDT. Both patients converted rapidly to normal rhythm with pharmacologic intervention. In a subsequent study of 12 consecutive patients treated with Photofrin®-PDT, no change was found in cardiac enzymes following PDT and no permanent electrocardiographic changes were noted [4]. Atrial fibrillation occurs in about 1% of patients following Photofrin®-PDT for Barrett's dysplasia. The arrhythmia readily responds to pharmacologic intervention if recognized and treated early. Myocardial injury has not been reported following PDT.

References

1. Overholt BF, Panjehpour M, Ayres M. Photodynamic therapy for Barrett's esophagus:cardiac effects. Laser Surg Med 1997;21:317-320.

2. Lightdale CJ, Heier SK, Marcon NE, et al. Photodynamic therapy with porfimer sodium versus thermal ablation therapy with Nd:YAG laser for palliation of esophageal cancer:a multicenter randomized trial. Gastrointest Endosc 1995;42:507-512.
3. Overholt BF, Panjehpour M. Photodynamic therapy for Barrett's esophagus:clinical update. Am J Gastroenterol 1996;91:1719-1723.
4. Overholt BF, Panjehpour M, Ayres M. Photodynamic therapy for Barrett's esophagus: cardiac effects. Laser Surg Med 1997;21:317-320.

What are the effects of low dose photodynamic therapy (hematoporphyrin and argon dye laser) on healing of Barrett's esophagus and stricture formation.

H. Barr (Gloucester)

Photodynamic therapy (PDT) is an interesting technique. Among the first uses was for the attempted selective destruction of cancers. It is based on the systemic administration of certain photosensitising agents derived often from porphyrins. These are retained in neoplastic at certain times after parenteral administration. If exposed to appropriate wavelength laser light a highly localised cytotoxic reaction occurs causing cellular destruction. The maximum differential that can be expected is approximately 2:1 and is very similar for a variety of agents. Microscopic fluorescence localisation has shown that the photosensitisers tend to accumulate in tumor stroma and the submucosal areas of the intestine [1]. *In vivo* investigation of photodynamic therapy in experimental gastrointestinal neoplasms has demonstrated important biological advantages. Full thickness intestinal damage produced by PDT unlike thermal damage does not reduce the mechanical strength of the bowel wall or cause perforation, because the sub-mucosal collagen is preserved.

There is now increasing data on the use of various derivatives of hematoporphyrin for the eradication of Barrett's esophagus. The most commonly used agent is Photofrin®. It is important to understand the background to the development of this technique.

It has been demonstrated that endoscopic photodynamic therapy for both early squamous cell carcinoma and adenocarcinoma has been followed by prolonged patient survival. Patients with T1 and T2 cancers staged using endoscopic ultrasound, who were unsuitable for surgical treatment, received endoscopic PDT. The disease specific five year survival was unaffected by the addition of chemotherapy or radiotherapy and was 74% [2]. The method of local disease control may not matter and similar results are being reported following endoscopic mucosal resection [3]. The detection of dysplasia in the esophagus is regarded by some as an indication for surgical resection if the patient is considered able to tolerate the substantial operation. This argument is justified because in the resected specimen an early invasive cancer may be found in over 40% of patients. Although some series demonstrate that with carefully biopsy the incidence may be only 11%, and some patients have died or developed serious complications following "prophylactic" esophagectomy [4].

Table I. Photodynamic therapy for dysplastic and non-dysplastic Barrett's esophagus. Data from [5, 6, 8, 9].

Prephotodynamic therapy (number of patients)			Postphotodynamic therapy (number of patients)		Follow-up (months)
HGD	LGD	Metaplasia	Residual dysplasia	Residual metaplasia	
73	14	0	16	48	19 [5]
9	32	23	5	57	25 [6, 8, 9]

HGD: high-grade dysplasia; LGD: low-grade dysplasia.

Methods

The methodology of treating large areas of Barrett's metaplasia with or without dysplasia is straightforward. Forty-eight hours after the administration of 1.5-1.75 mg/kg of hematoporphyrin derivative [5] or 2mg/kg of Photofrin® (porfimer sodium) [6], endoscopic irradiation of the esophagus is performed. The laser is tuned to deliver 630 nm light. A diffuser or a windowed centring balloon allows more accurate and even light dosimetry. The length of the light delivering device can be 3,5,7 cms. At present it is not recommended that more than 7 cms of Barrett's esophagus treated at one session [6]. The power density used is 400 mW/cm^2 to provide an energy density of 100 to 250 J/cm^2 from the diffuser to the mucosa. Treatment can be performed on an outpatient basis and patients must all received profound acid suppression with proton pump inhibitor therapy. Direct sunlight must be avoided for a period of 4-6 weeks. Some patients develop small unilateral or bilateral pleural effusions, occasionally requiring intervention

Results

The initial results of low-dose PDT showed that there was regression in the length of Barrett's esophagus and healing was followed by regeneration with neosquamous epithelium [5]. There was the concern of pseudoregression with a thin layer of squamous epithelium covering Barrett's epithelium [7]. A prospective randomized trial of low dose PDT (1.5-1.75 mg/kg hematoporphyrin derivative) clearly demonstrated that Barrett's metaplasia could be reduced with 29% of patients achieving a 4 cm decrease in the length of the metaplastic segment. The adverse events in this series were odynophagia in 25%, chest pain in 16% and minor sunburn in 30%. The incidence of esophageal strictures appeared small. In addition non-dysplastic epithelium was more susceptible to mucosal ablative therapy using this form of PDT than dysplastic tissue [8, 9].

The results of Photofrin®-PDT are also very encouraging, with 75-80% of the Barrett's mucosa being converted to neosquamous mucosa. Complete eradication of all metaplastic epithelium occurred in nearly 50% of patients. Dysplasia disappeared in most patients, although 11 developed dysplasia during follow-up and required repeat treatment. Thirteen patients were treated for early cancer (T1-12 patients; T2-1 patient), and in ten the tumor was eradicated. It is important to emphasize that the patients must remain under surveillance and repeated treatment will be necessary in some to treat residual or recurrent areas of dysplasia and metaplasia. Usually the areas are rather patchy and are best treated using thermal ablation using a potassium titanyl phosphate laser or the Argon plasma coagulator. Cutaneous photosensitivity can be a significant problem up to 2 months after photosensitization. The major concern has been the incidence of esophageal stricture. Approximately 30% of patients treated with Photofrin® developed significant stenosis that required endoscopic esophageal dilatation.

References

1. Barr H, Chatlani P, Tralau CJ, MacRobert AJ, Boulos PB, Bown SG. Local eradication of rat colon cancer with photodynamic therapy: correlation of distribution of photosensitiser with biological effects in normal and tumour tissue. Gut 1991;32:517-523.
2. Sibille A, Lambert R, Souquet JC, Sabben G, Descos F. Long-term survival after photodynamic therapy for esophageal cancer. Gastroenterology 1995;108:337-344.
3. Grosjean P, Monnier P. Photodynamic therapy and mucosectomy for early squamous cell carcinomas in the oesophagus and tracheobronchial tree. Eur J Surg Oncol 1998;24:234.
4. Cameron AJ, Carpenter HA. Barrett's oesophagus, high-grade dysplasia, and early adenocarcinoma:a pathological study. Am J Gastroenterol 1997;92:586-591.
5. Laukka MA, Wang KK. Initial results using low-dose photodynamic therapy in the treatment of Barrett's esophagus. Gastrointest Endosc 1995;42:59-63.
6. Overholt BF, Panjepour M, Haydek JM. Photodynamic therapy for Barrett's esophagus:follow-up in 100 patients. Gastrointest Endosc 1999;49:1-7.
7. Biddlestone LR, Barham CP, Wilkinson SP, Barr H, Shepherd NA. The histopathology of treated Barrett's esophagus. Am J Surg Pathol 1998;22:239-245.
8. Wang KK, WongKeeSong LM, Nourbakhsh A, Laukka M, Gutta K, Geller A, Balm R. Controlled trial of low dose photodynamic therapy for Barrett's esophagus, Gastroenterology 1997;112:A676.
9. Wang KK, WongKeeSong LM, Nijhawan P, Nourbakhsh A, Balm R. Does non-dysplastic Barrett's esophagus respond better to mucosal ablation? Gastroenterology 1998;114:A700.

Should the very variable thickness of Barrett's epithelium be considered when evaluating the results of photodynamic therapy?

P. Chandrasoma, K. Wickramasinghe (Los Angeles)

Exact anatomic measurements of the thickness of the layers of the esophagus have assumed importance recently with the emergence of new diagnostic and therapeutic modalities. Diagnostic modalities such as endoscopic ultrasound and the potential use of high wavelength acoustic microscopy, and therapeutic modalities such as mucosal ablation and endoscopic mucosal resection demand exact data on mucosal thickness in both health and disease. Such measurements are not easily available.

Routine specimens of the esophagus at autopsy and surgery are associated with artifact induced by shortening and thickening of the esophagus secondary to muscle contraction that makes measurement inaccurate. Shortening tends to be greatest in the muscle layer.

Mucosal shortening occurs to a lesser extent due to contraction of the muscularis mucosae. In addition, the range of thickness of the various layers in different individuals and disease processes complicates matters further.

Ablative techniques use different physical modalities

Multipolar electrocautery (MPEC) utilizes a standard electrocautery probe that burns the mucosa on contact. The thickness of burn achieved can be varied by changing the duration of contact [1].

Argon plasma coagulation is a form of electocoagulation which uses a probe through which a charged stream of ionized argon gas carries the electrical current to the mucosa. Contact with the mucosa is not required. Thickness of burn possible is limited by the fact that carbonization of the burnt mucosa impedes the passage of current [2].

Thermal lasers have been used for mucosal ablation. They generate heat and cause burning of tissues in a localized manner. Lasers vary according to their power output and wavelength, which determine the burning power and tissue penetrating capability. Argon lasers and potassium tytanil phosphate-YAG lasers have limited depth of penetration whereas Nd:YAG lasers permit deeper tissue penetration [3].

Photodynamic therapy depends on the selective uptake of porphyrin derivatives (hematoporphyrin derivative, Photofrin®, amino-levulinic acid) by dysplastic and neoplastic tissues. These agents cause photosensitization of the cells which make them susceptible to necrosis when exposed to light [4]. The photoradiation of the mucosa, usually with red light at 630 nm, is done *via* a special cylindrical diffusing fiber positioned in the center of the esophageal lumen. The selective uptake of the photosensitizer restricts damage to abnormal epithelial cells but the depth of penetration of the light is variable. In particular, the presence of mucosal folds results in some parts of the mucosa being shielded from the light and therefore protected from ablation.

Esophageal mucosal thickness measurements

The normal squamous epithelium is generally flat with a thin lamina propria and a thin but well defined double layered muscularis mucosae that represents the deepest mucosal layer. The submucosa separates the mucosa from the muscularis externa. Acid reflux produces significant changes in the mucosa of the esophagus. Damage to the mucosa by acid reflux may result in ulceration with associated fibrosis of the mucosa, submucosa and muscle layers with stricture formation. Both ulcerative and non-ulcerative esophagitis is associated with glandular transformation of the squamous epithelium characterized by cardiac mucosa with or without intestinal metaplasia (IM). Glandular mucosae vary from being atrophic to hyperplastic with marked reactive changes involving elongation of the foveolar region. The muscularis mucosae frequently becomes hyperplastic resulting in thickening, splitting and upward extension of muscle fibers into the lamina propria. It is not unusual to find mucosal glands, both cardiac and intestinal, entrapped in the thickened muscularis mucosae. We measured mucosal thickness in 10 patients who had esophagectomy in which Barrett's epithelium was present. Measurement in different areas were made, providing values for the least, mean, and greatest thickness of the entire mucosa and the depth of the glandular element (*Table I*). This showed a marked variation in both total mucosal thickness and glandular depth, both within different areas of the same esophagus and in different patients. The range of glandular depth varied between 0.3 mm and 1.3 mm in the entire group; in a single patient, the depth varied between 0.5 mm and 1.3 mm in two different areas of Barrett's mucosa.

Table I. Thickness of mucosa (from surface to deep aspect of muscularis mucosae) and thickness of glandular element in Barrett's esophagus, as measured in esophagectomy specimens. No attempt was made in these cases to prevent artifact resulting from postoperative muscle contraction.

Case	Gland thickness (mm)			Mucosal thickness (mm)	
	Least	Mean	Greatest	Least	Greatest
1	0.5	0.5	0.5	1.0	1.2
2	0.4	0.7	1.0	1.4	1.9
3	0.6	0.8	1.0	1.1	1.6
4	0.4	0.6	0.8	1.2	2.0
5	0.6	0.7	0.8	2.0	2.7
6	1.0	1.0	1.1	2.5	2.9
7	0.5	0.9	1.3	1.2	3.3
8	0.7	0.8	0.9*	1.7	1.9
9	0.3**	0.4	0.5	0.8	1.5
10	0.4	0.8	1.1*	1.2	2.1

* Point of measurement showed low grade dysplasia
** Point of measurement showed high grade dysplasia

At present, it is impossible to accurately gauge mucosal thickness at endoscopy from surface visualization. Endoscopic ultrasound is not sensitive enough to permit measurement of mucosal thickness and cannot be used simultaneously with ablative techniques. Endoscopic vision is limited to the surface epithelium, and the technique of ablation is blind to the vertical extent of the glandular mucosa. Once the surface has been ablated, it is very difficult to evaluate the presence or absence of residual glandular tissue in the deeper lamina propria. Ablation that is too superficial results in incomplete ablation of the glandular mucosa. Ablation that is too deep may damage the muscularis mucosae and muscularis externa and increase the risk of strictures. The variation in thickness of the glandular element and mucosa makes it impossible to develop any rules regarding the depth of ablation that is required.

Effects of ablative therapies

For these reasons, it is very likely that ablation of Barrett' mucosa is a misnomer. What is far more likely is that the ablation involves only the surface epithelium and a variable part of the superficial mucosa, leaving glands in the deeper mucosa intact. The damage is also very likely to be irregular. When ablation is coupled with antireflux treatment (surgery or effective acid suppression), the mucosa that regenerates is commonly squamous, leading to the endoscopic impression of cure [5]. However, what happens to the invisible remaining Barrett's glands in the deeper mucosa is unknown. What is clear is that if these glands remain viable, and if they already have their full complement of genetic hits that permits them to develop into neoplasms, the early recognition of such neoplasms by endoscopy will be more difficult because of the overlying squamous epithelium. Ablative techniques have been in use for too short a time for definitive conclusions to be made about these potential problems. Studies available todate suggest that it is common to have incomplete ablation of the Barrett's epithelium [1, 2, 5], and residual glands with IM are frequently present in the lamina propria overgrown by squamous epithelium on the surface [5] with all these ablative modalities. Cases have also been reported where there has been a progression from low to high-grade dysplasia after ablation [6].

References

1. Sampliner RE, Fennerty B, Garewal HS. Reversal of Barrett's esophagus with acid suppression and multipolar electrocoagulation: preliminary results. Gastrointestinal Endosc 1996;44:532-535.
2. Dumoulin FL, Terjung B, Neubrand M, Scheurlen C, Fischer HP, Sauerbruch T. Treatment of Barrett's esophagus by endoscopic argon plasma coagulation. Endoscopy 1997;29:751-753.
3. Barham CP, Jones RL, Biddlestone LR, Hardwick RH, Shepherd NA, Barr H. Photothermal laser ablation of Barrett's oesophagus: endoscopic and histological evidence of squamous re-epithelialization. Gut 1997;41:281-284.
4. Overholt BF, Panjehpour M. Photodynamic therapy for Barrett's esophagus. Gastrointestinal Endosc Clin North Am 1997;7:207-220.
5. Biddlestone LR, Barham CP, Wilkinson SP, Barr H, Shepherd NA. The histopathology of treated Barrett's esophagus: squamous reepithelialization after acid suppression and laser and photodynamic therapy. Am J Surg Pathol 1998;22:239-245.
6. Maass S, Martin WR, Spiethoff A, Riemann JF. Barrett esophagus with seveer dysplasia in argon beam therapy. Zeitsch Gastroenterol 1998;36:301-306.

Is it unequivocally necessary to combine laser ablation with acid suppression?

R. Ackroyd (Sheffield)

With our current state of knowledge, the answer to this question is unknown, and indeed it may never be known. Whilst many different ablation techniques have been employed, including electrocautery, thermal laser ablation, argon plasma coagulation (APC) and photodynamic therapy (PDT), in all published series to date these techniques have invariably been combined with some form of acid suppression, either by pharmacological or surgical means. There are no reports of ablation therapy without concurrent acid suppression or antireflux surgery.

It is known that Barrett's esophagus is due to long-standing gastroesophageal reflux (GER) (of either gastric acid and/or alkaline duodenal secretions) and therefore it is hypothesised that reducing esophageal acid exposure may lead to regression of the columnar epithelium. However, apart from isolated reports, there is little good evidence to support this hypothesis. There have been occasional reports of regression with H_2-receptor blocking agents [1], although these effects are minimal [2]. More recently some anecdotal reports of regression of Barrett's epithelium using the proton pump inhibitor omeprazole have appeared [3, 4]. Following this, several prospective but uncontrolled series have been reported, with conflicting results. Significant regression of columnar epithelium was reported using long-term omeprazole at a dose of 40 mg once daily [5], but another similar study could not confirm this finding [6]. In an open controlled study, comparing H_2-blockers with omeprazole therapy, regression was not observed in either group, although some squamous island formation was observed in the omeprazole group [7]. The only double-blind controlled trial so far reported revealed no significant regression of Barrett's esophagus following one year of lansoprazole 60 mg daily [8]. Equally there is little evidence of regression following antireflux surgery. Although, regression has been reported in 40% of patients following antireflux surgery [9], the authors' criteria for regression were based on endoscopic assessment of the level of the gastroesophageal junction before and after surgery. Alterations in the anatomy due to the operation may make such measurements difficult and cast doubt on the validity of these results. The appearance of squamous islands within the columnar mucosa has been reported following antireflux surgery [10]. However, other authors have failed to show any regression of columnar epithelium following antireflux surgery, although no objective evidence of reflux control by postoperative pH measurement was obtained [11-13].

However, there is evidence that denuded esophageal mucosa may heal with normal squamous epithelium in the absence of acid, but with columnar epithelium if acid remains. Gillen *et al.* studied the regeneration of canine esophageal mucosa under basal conditions and in the presence of GER. In normal circumstances mucosal defects healed with squamous epithelium, but in the presence of reflux of acid or acid and bile, regeneration was frequently columnar epithelium [14]. In a later study using a canine model, the same group further studied the effect of the lower esophageal milieu on the healing of a mucosal defect in 10 animals. Following stimulation of reflux, using a cardioplasty and pentagastrin injection, healing of the defect was by columnar epithelium in 7 out of 10 animals. However, 6 animals then underwent antisurgery and had their acid secretion suppressed. In these animals, healing was again by columnar epithelium, but in all 6 cases, islands of squamous epithelium were also seen [15].

In view of this, all studies of ablation therapy for Barrett's esophagus have incorporated some form of either medical acid suppression or surgical (mechanical) block. There are now many reports of the effect of combined mucosal ablation and acid suppression. As long ago as 1993, Berenson *et al.* demonstrated the feasibility of squamous re-epithelialisation using a combination of APC and high dose acid suppression [16]. Barham *et al.* used mucosal ablation by potassium titanyl phosphate (KTP) laser therapy combined with acid suppression by 40 mg omeprazole daily to treat 16 patients with dysplastic Barrett's esophagus. Ablation of all areas of glandular mucosa resulted in squamous regeneration, although in 11 patients there was evidence of buried Barrett's glands and in 9 patients squamous metaplasia was seen [17]. In a similar study, Gossner *et al.* employed KTP laser ablation with acid suppression using up to 80 mg omeprazole daily to treat 8 patients with dysplastic Barrett's esophagus and 2 with early adenocarcinoma. A complete response was obtained in all patients, with no complications, although in 2 cases, biopsies revealed specialized mucosa beneath the neo-squamous epithelium [18].

An alternative method of ablation therapy is APC. Using this form of treatment combined with omeprazole 40 mg daily, Van Laethem *et al.* treated 31 patients with

Barrett's esophagus. Complete re-epithelialisation was seen in 25 patients after a mean of 2.4 treatments, and partial re-epithelialisation in a further 3 patients. However, buried glands were again seen and, out of 17 patients with apparently complete Barrett's eradication, at one year 8 showed evidence of islands of Barrett's metaplasia despite continuous omeprazole therapy (10-40 mg daily) [19]. In a similar study, Schultz *et al.* treated 73 patients with Barrett's esophagus using a combination of APC and maximal acid suppression with omeprazole 40 mg three times daily. In 69 of 70 patients complete and lasting squamous re-epithelialisation was achieved after a median of two treatments, although three patients developed a mild stricture, necessitating bougie dilatation [20].

We have a similar experience using PDT combined with low dose (20 mg daily) omeprazole. Forty patients with dysplastic Barrett's esophagus were treated with PDT. All were given the photosensitiser aminolaevulinic acid orally at a dose of 30 mg/kg followed 4 hours later by endoscopy and administration of green laser light (514 nm). A response was seen in 33 out of 40 patients, with a median decrease in columnar epithelial area of 30% (range 0-90%). Post-treatment biopsies showed no evidence of dysplasia in 39 out of 40 patients, with low-grade dysplasia remaining in one case. No significant side effects were observed in any patient.

Whilst these results are not perfect, and many studies have demonstrated the presence of buried columnar glands under the regenerated squamous epithelium, these studies do show the potential for the use of ablation therapy in combination with acid suppression in the treatment of Barrett's esophagus. Just how important the acid suppression really is in this context remains to be seen.

References

1. Wesdorp ICE, Bartelsman J, Schipper MEI, Tytgat GN. Effect of long-term treatment with cimetidine and antacids in Barrett's esophagus. Gut 1981;22:724-727.
2. Sampliner RE, Garewal HS, Fennerty MB, Aickin M. Lack of impact of therapy on extent of Barrett's esophagus in 67 patients. Dig Dis Sci 1990;35:93-96.
3. Deviere J, Buset M, Dumonceau JM, Richaert F, Cremer M. Regression of Barrett's epithelium with omeprazole. N Engl J Med 1989;320:1497-1498.
4. Collen MJ, Strong RM. Comparison of omeprazole and ranitidine in treatment of refractory gastroesophageal reflux disease in patients with gastric acid hypersecretion. Dig Dis Sci 1992;37:897-903.
5. Gore S, Healey CJ, Sutton R, Shepherd NA, Wilkinson SP. Regression of columnar lined (Barrett's) oesophagus with continuous omeprazole therapy. Gastroenterology 1992;102:A75.
6. Bologna S, Blumenkehl M, Schubert TT, Wong D. Barrett's esophagus response to long-term omeprazole therapy. Gastrointest Endosc 1992;38:A229.
7. Igbal TH, Neumann CS, Cooper BT. Omeprazole treatment of patients with Barrett's oesophagus. Gut 1993;34:S19.
8. Sampliner RE, Mackel C, Jennings D, Greski-Rose P. Effect of 12 months of a proton pump inhibitor (lansoprazole) on Barrett's esophagus - a randomized trial. Gastroenterology 1992;102:A517.
9. Brand DL, Ylvisaker JT, Gelfand M, Pope CE. Regression of columnar esophageal (Barrett's) epithelium after antireflux surgery. N Engl J Med 1980;302:844-848.
10. Skinner DB, Walther BC, Riddell RH, Schmidt H, Iascone C, De Meester TR. Barrett's esophagus: comparison of benign and malignant cases. Ann Surg 1983;198:554-566.
11. Endo M, Kobayashi Kozu T. A case of Barrett's epithelialisation followed up for 5 years. Endoscopy 1974;6:48-51.
12. Dooner J, Cleator IG. Selective management of benign esophageal strictures. Am J Gastroenterol 1982;77:172-177.
13. Bremner CG. Barrett's oesophagus. In: Watson A, Celestin LR, eds. Disorders of the oesophagus: advances and controversies. London: Pitman, 1984:94-104.
14. Gillen P, Keeling P, Byrne PJ, West AB, Hennessy TPJ. Experimental columnar metaplasia in the canine oesophagus. Br J Surg 1988;75:113-115.
15. Li H, Walsh TN, O'Dowd G, Gillen P, Byrne PJ, Hennessy TP. Mechanisms of columnar metaplasia and squamous regeneration in experimental Barrett's esophagus. Surgery 1994;115:176-181.

16. Bereson MM, Johnson TD, Markowitz NR, Buchi KN, Samowitz WS. Restoration of squamous mucosa after ablation of Barrett's esophageal epithelium. Gastroenterology 1993;104:1689-1691.
17. Barham CP, Jones RL, Biddlestone LR, Hardwick RH, Shepherd NA, Barr H. Photothermal laser ablation of Barrett's oesophagus: endoscopic and histological evidence of squamous re-epithelialisation. Gut 1997;41:281-284.
18. Gossner L, May A, Stolte M, Seitz G, Hahn EG, Ell C. KTP laser destruction of dysplasia and early cancer in columnar-lined Barrett's esophagus. Gastrointest Endosc 1999;49:8-12.
19. Van Laethem JL, Cremer M, Peny MO, Delhaye M, Deviere J. Eradication of Barrett's mucosa with argon plasma coagulation and acid suppression:immediate and mid term results. Gut 1998;43:747-751.
20. Schulz H, Miehlke S, Antos D, Schentke KU, Vieth M, Stolte M, Bayerdorffer E. Ablation of Barrett's epithelium by endoscopic argon plasma coagulation in combination with high dose omeprazole. Gastrointest Endosc 2000;51:659-663.

Is it unequivocally necessary to combine laser ablation with antireflux surgery? What is the cost-benefit of separate or combined procedures?

E.I.T. Sihvo, J.A. Salo (Helsinki)

Laser ablation with antireflux surgery

Patients with Barrett's esophagus have a 30-125 times increased risk of developing esophageal adenocarcinoma. Due to non-regressive nature of Barrett's epithelium even under modern antireflux therapies, both medical and surgical, mucosal ablation techniques have been developed to eliminate this premalignant intestinal metaplasia (IM).

Barrett's esophagus is a complication of long-lasting reflux disease. Therefore, there is no basis to laser therapy or any other endoscopic ablation technique without long-term control of reflux. Regeneration of squamous mucosa after laser therapy of Barrett's epithelium and acid-suppression medication has been achieved with reasonable results [1]. However, unsuccessful results have also been described [2]. The reason for these failures are unclear. Recent evidence shows that failure of esophageal acid control even on high dose of proton pump inhibitor is not uncommon [3]. In addition, medical acid suppression therapy does not prevent the reflux of duodenal contents into the esophagus. On the other hand, antireflux surgery creates more physiological antireflux barrier, provides more efficient control of acid-reflux and prevents also duodeno-gastroesophageal reflux. Furthermore, a good control of reflux has been achieved in 20-year follow-up after fundoplication [4].

Therefore, antireflux surgery is better than medical treatment for long-term control of reflux and can be recommended in combination with laser ablation of Barrett's epithelium. According to our study, regenerated esophageal epithelium arising after laser ablation in reflux-free environment surgery is of squamous type [5]. Only long-term follow-up studies can prove the possible cancer-preventing results of laser therapy in a reflux-free environment. In previous studies, in which some form of mucosal ablation technique is combined to antireflux medication, areas of IM, dysplasia, and adenocarcinoma are still frequently found in follow-ups [6, 7].

Cost-benefit of separate or combined procedures

According to autopsy estimated prevalence of 376 cases per 100,000 population [8], there are about 18,800 Barrett's patients in Finland with about 5,000,000 inhabitants. In mid 1990's there has been around 140 adenocarcinomas of the esophagus and gastroesophageal junction yearly in Finland [9]. The estimated cost to treat all the Barrett's patients with laser therapy combined to antireflux surgery would be about $ 200 million equivalent to $ 1.4 million per cancer. If we could identify all the Barrett's patients on population level, limited resources and a huge number of cases would make it a too expensive way to treat these patients. At this point, it is impossible to offer surgery and ablation for all Barrett's patients.

References

1. Berenson MM, Johnson TD, Markowitz NR, et al. Restoration of squamous mucosa after ablation of Barrett's esophageal epithelium. Gastroenterology 1993;104:1686-1691.
2. Brand LJ, Kauvar DR. Laser-induced transient regression of Barrett's epithelium. Gastrointest Endosc 1992;38:365-368.
3. Fass R, Sampliner RE, Malagon IB, et al. Failure of oesophageal acid control in candidates for Barrett's oesophagus reversal on a very high dose of proton pump inhibitor. Aliment Pharmacol Ther 2000;14:597-602.
4. Luostarinen M. Nissen fundoplication for reflux esophagitis. Long-term clinical and endoscopic results in 109 of 127 consecutive patients. Ann Surg 1993;217:329-337.
5. Salo JA, Salminen JT, Kiviluoto TA, et al. Treatment of Barrett's esophagus by endoscopic laser ablation and antireflux surgery. Ann Surg 1998;227:40-44.
6. Grade AJ, Shah IA, Medlin SM, et al. The efficacy and safety of argon plasma coagulation therapy in Barrett's esophagus. Gastrointest Endosc 1999;50:18-22.
7. Overholt BF, Panjehpour M, Haydek JM. Photodynamic therapy for Barrett's esophagus:follow-up in 100 patients. Gastointest Endosc 1999;49:1-7.
8. Cameron AJ, Zinsmeister AR, Ballard DJ, Carney JA. Prevalence of columnar-lined (Barrett's) esophagus. Gastroenterology 1990;99:918-922.
9. Sihvo EIT, Salminen JT, Rämö OJ, Salo JA. The epidemiology of oesophageal adenocarcinoma: has the cancer of gastric cardia an influence on the rising incidence of oesophageal adenocarcinoma? Scand J Gastroenterol 2000;10:1082-1086.

What are the various techniques of surgical endoscopic ablation?

T. Kawano, M. Endo (Tokyo)

What is the appropriate management of Barrett's esophagus suggestive of malignancy? It is now controversial because almost all early Barrett's carcinomas show slight changes in the mucosal surface. Some cases of early Barrett's carcinoma or high-grade dysplasia (HGD) are detected by step biopsy in health check-up endoscopy. From the viewpoint of radicality, esophagectomy is the most reliable but most invasive. In general, surgical treatment for possible or definite neoplasia within Barrett's mucosa is not considered for technical reasons. Surgical approaches to the esophagus are too invasive for the perfomance of mucosal ablation alone, and there are alternatives. Some endoscopic techniques of ablation are applied for the lesions of superficial cancer and HGD in Barrett's esophagus [1-3].

Now we can choose two types of endoscopic procedure to perform tumor eradication in Barrett's esophagus. One is mucosal ablation by endoscopic mucosal resection (EMR) techniques [4, 5]. The major advantages of EMR for a lesion of malignancy or HGD are its simplicity and retrieval of the specimen [6, 7]. EMR is not only therapeutic but also can be diagnostic [1]. EMR provides a more accurate diagnosis than conventional biopsies. However, long-term studies are required to determine whether EMR can provide an alternative therapeutic approach for patients with adenocarcinoma and severe dysplasia who have comorbid illness that precludes esophagectomy.

The second procedure is ablation by mucosal destruction, such as photodynamic therapy (PDT) and electro-cauterization [8]. The Nd: Yag laser, potassium titanyl phosphate (KTP) laser, argon laser, argon plasma coagulation, and multipolar electrocoagulation are alternatives to EMR for the complete destruction of a superficial neoplasia in Barrett's esophagus. PDT is a nonthermal procedure the aim of which is the selective destruction of neoplastic tissue without altering the normal tissue. Electro-cauterization or PDT is sometimes applied with EMR as a combined therapy.

EMR is preferable for curative endoscopic treatment of a small and superficial neoplasia in Barrett's esophagus. However, EMR may be difficult if the neoplastic lesion shows poor delineation. In such cases, tumor destruction is the alternative, and PDT is currently preferred. EMR is technically possible to remove superficial neoplasia in Barrett's esophagus, but dysplasia and carcinoma in Barrett's esophagus typically present a mosaic pattern and endoscopic examination can not reliably determine whether a lesion is localized to the mucosa without metastasis. There are also some problems in destructive procedures, *e.g.* residual Barrett's islands underneath the newly formed squamous epithelium after electrocoagulation have been reported. The proof of the long-term effectiveness of these techniques is still awaited.

References

1. Kawano T, Endo M. Is there a place for endoscopic mucosectomy in early cancers of the cardia or EGJ? In: Giuli R, Galmiche JP, Jamieson GC, Scarpignato C, eds. The esophagogastric junction. Paris, John Libbey Eurotext, 1998:1204-1206.
2. Lambert R. Treatment of esophagogastric tumors. Endoscopy 2000;32:322-330.
3. Roesch T. Gastroesophageal reflux disease and Barrett's esophagus. Endoscopy 2000;32:826-835.
4. Kawano T, Miyake S, Yasuno M, et al. A new technique for endoscopic esophageal mucosectomy using a transparent overtube with intraluminal negative pressure. Dig Endosc 1991;3:159-167.
5. Inoue H, Endo M, Takeshita K, et al. Endoscopic esophageal mucosal resection using a cap-fitted panendoscope (EMRC). Gastroent Endosc 1992;34:2387-2390.
6. Makuuchi H, Kise Y, Shimada H, et al. Endoscopic mucosal resection for early gastric cancer. Semin Surg Oncol 1999;17:108-116.
7. Kawano T, Endo M. A new multipurpose tube for esophageal endoscopy. Endoscopy 1997;29:526-527.
8. Wolfsen HC. Photodynamic therapy in gastroenterology: current status in the year 2000. Endoscopy 2000;32:715-719.

What are the compared effects on esophageal layers of Cavi-pulse and other techniques for Barrett's mucosal ablation? Is Cavi-pulse technique applicable to patients?

R.M. Bremner, C.G. Bremner, H.L. Valenta (Los Angeles)

The cavitron ultrasonic surgical aspirator (CUSA) is a surgical ultrasound system that concentrates its energy very close to the tip of the transducer. This may be contrasted with diagnostic or high intensity focused ultrasound, which functions far from the transducer at a remote location in the tissue. An important characteristic of ultrasonic aspiration is its ability to fragment cellular tissue while leaving elastic connective tissue undamaged. Cavi-pulse is a function that allows more control of energy delivery through a low frequency interruption of the energy delivered. The frequency and duration of the interruption is a function of the Cavi-pulse mode. The frequency shifts from 20 to 50 Hz and the duration changes from 80 to 50% as the mode is varied from one to four. Cavi-pulse provides a vibration component, which is believed to encourage layered tissue to shear. Cavi-pulse is, then, an important feature for esophageal ablation. Its ability to separate the epithelial layer from the mucosal layers, without damage to the mucosa is a unique feature of this instrument.

Studies were performed on *in vivo* pig esophagi comparing the tissue effect of several ablation modalities: monopolar coagulation, argon beam coagulation, gold probe bipolar coagulation and CUSA. Light and polarizing microscopy were used to assess depth of tissue removal and damage to underlying tissue. Birefringence loss was used as a marker of thermal damage to sub epithelial layers. Based on the experience, the argon beam coagulator and the CUSA appeared to give the most control and most even treatment.

The CUSA was run at a Cavi-pulse setting of 2 at full stroke, which provides a low frequency modulation component of 25 Hz, a duty cycle of 75% and a stroke of 180 microns. Optimal suction and irrigation settings were found to be 13 and 8.5 respectively. Although, some slight hemorrhage and vasodilation was evident in the lamina propria, cells were not damaged as a function of the CUSA and no thermal injury was evident. Optimization of the parameters only affected the efficiency of the procedure. A principle advantage of the CUSA lies in the inherent ability to provide proper depth, which cannot be achieved by other methods without an abstract measure of penetration depth.

Table I. *In vivo* study of pig mucosa ablation.

Method	Residual islands	Thermal effects (hyalinization, compaction)	Clearcut edge	Submucosal edema	Hemorrhage
Electrosurgical	–	+++++	–	++++	Coagulation
Gold probe	++	+++	–	+++	+
Argon spray	++	+++	–	++	–
Ultracision	+	+	+	+	++
CUSA	–	–	++	+	+

Animal studies on ultrasonic epithelial ablation of the lower esophageal mucosa

Young farm pigs were used to develop the technique of applying a laparoscopic CUSA to the lower esophageal mucosa through an operating gastrostomy. Optimal settings were assessed by histological examination of the ablated esophagi. Ablated cells were aspirated through a central port and were sent for cytological examination. Adult Yakutan minipigs then underwent CUSA ablation with or without a laparoscopic Nissen fundoplication. Animals were endoscoped regularly during the healing process and were sacrificed at 6 weeks after the procedure once complete healing had occurred.

Optimal CUSA energy settings enabled complete and even ablation of the epithelium with preservation of the muscularis mucosa and submucosa. No evidence of submucosal damage or deeper damage was noted histologically. Aspirated cells preserved their integrity for cytology. Healing occurred with squamous regeneration in the absence of gross or pathologic stricture formation. The technique developed holds promise for complete ablation of the Barrett's epithelium at a single setting. The unique tissue selective nature of the ablative process allows healing to occur in the absence of stricture formation. The ability to collect the ablated cells for cytology in essence provides the "ultimate biopsy". The technique has been successfully used on a single patient without stricture formation, and more studies are planned.

Are the results of endoscopic spray cryotherapy in animal experimentation in favor of mucosal ablation in Barrett's patients?

M.H. Johnston (Bethesda)

Spray cryotherapy through an upper endoscope was independently developed by two different investigative groups: Johnston *et al.* at the Uniformed Services University of the Health Sciences (USUHS) in Bethesda, MD [1] and Pasricha *et al.* at the Johns Hopkins University Medical Center [2]. Both groups spray liquid nitrogen or nitrous oxide through an upper endoscope to freeze gastrointestinal mucosa or mucosal associated lesions. Each uses a significantly different device with potentially different clinical outcomes. The device utilized by Pasricha, utilizes the Joule-Thompson effect. In this device a gas (nitrous oxide) under pressures ranging from 450 to 750 psi is released through a specially designed catheter placed through an endoscope [3]. The release and rapid expansion of the gas at the catheter tip results in freezing. Of concern is the high pressure associated with this device. Johnston's device uses liquid nitrogen in a specially designed system that operates at a maximum of 30 psi. The catheter is multi-layered and can be electronically warmed during or after the cryo application, thus maintaining catheter pliability and the unique ability to operate at a very low pressure. Both devices use a foot pedal for control of gas release. The

Johnston device also utilizes a temperature probe for monitoring mucosal temperature during the cryo application. The degree and depth of injury is controlled by manipulating three parameters: the duration of cryo application, the extent of cryoburn (viewed endoscopically) and the temperature of the mucosa at the time of application. These parameters are monitored *via* a special software program and device that is part of the cryogenic system.

Animal data

Three separate phases of animal research have been conducted with the Johnston device at USUHS. In the first phase, twenty swine underwent cryoablation of the distal 2-3 cm of their esophagus with liquid nitrogen in either a hemicircumferential or circumferential pattern and were followed for one month post-cryotherapy [1] In the second phase of experiments 4 swine underwent endoscopic ultrasound (EUS) of their esophagus pre-cryotherapy, immediately post-cryotherapy and then at 48 hours , 7 days and 14 days to assess the effects on the esophageal wall. In the final phase, one swine was treated in different locations with Argon plasma coagulation (APC), multi-polar electrocoagulation (MPEC) and cryotherapy. The lesions were then compared both endoscopically and microscopically.

Phase I

In twenty swine liquid nitrogen was sprayed hemicircumferentially or circumferentially to the distal 2-3 cm of the esophagus. Duration of spray was varied from 10 to 60 seconds. Mucosal ablation was noted 2 to 7 days postcryotherapy in 19 of the 20 swine. Complications included 3 esophageal strictures and one aspiration pneumonia. All strictures occurred in the circumferentially treated group. Complete mucosal healing was observed in all swine by week 4. There were no deaths attributable to cryotherapy. This initial study demonstrated feasibility, efficacy in mucosal ablation and safety relative to other mucosal ablative techniques.

Phase II

Four swine underwent EUS of their distal esophagus to assess wall thickness and establish baseline anatomy. Following baseline EUS, each swine underwent a 45 second hemi-circumferential cryoburn to the distal esophagus which was followed by repeat EUS immediately and then at 2, 7 and 14 days. After EUS at 14 days the swine were euthanized and underwent esophagectomy to assess the esophagus histologically. EUS demonstrated edema of the mucosa and submucosa 5 minutes postcryo. At one week there was separation of the remaining mucosal layer from the underlying structures. Associated with this was edema throughout the other layers of the esophagus at the cryotherapy site. In most instances the wall thickness doubled. These findings resolved by day 14 post-cryotherapy. Full thickness biopsies were obtained on one of the swine to evaluate cryotherapy lesions at two different stages of evolution, one less than an hour old and one approximately

48 hours old. These revealed extravasation of RBCs into the submucosa with normal overlying epithelium at one hour, while another site 48 hours post-cryotherapy revealed complete ablation of the epithelial layer (0.5 to 1.0 mm) with mild transmural inflammation.

Phase III

In this phase one swine had three different ablative modalities applied to the distal esophagus. In the distal esophagus a cryoburn was applied in a 1-2 cm hemicircumferential pattern for 45 seconds. Proximal to this, MPEC was applied at 24 Watts *via* 10F Gold probe (Microvasive, Watertown, MA, USA) to a 1-2 cm area. Proximal to this, APC was applied at 90 Watts and 60 Watts using a flow rate of 2L/min (ERBE USA, Inc., Marietta, Ga.). The swine was then re-endoscoped at 48 hours and new lesions were applied in different areas followed by euthanasia and esophagectomy to assess both the acute and 48 hour lesions of all three modalities. The following was observed (*Tables I, II and III*) (*Figure 1*).

Table I. Comparison of argon plasma coagulation (APC), multipolar electrocoagulation (MEPC) and cryotherapy.

	APC (90 W)	APC (60 W)	Cryotherapy	MPEC
Ease of application	+++	+++	++	+
Even distribution of application	++	++	++++	+
Depth of injury	++++	++	++	+++
Inflammatory response at 1 hour	++	+	+	+
Inflammatory response at 48 hours	++++	+++	+	++
Depth of injury	++++	+++	+/++	++
Cost of device	++++	++++	+	++

Worst: + to best: ++++

Table II. Histology at 1 hour post ablative modality.

Modality	Finding
APC (90 W)	Complete epithelial ablation. Lamina propria and muscularis mucosa intact, no significant inflammation
APC (60 W)	Epithelium intact but separating from the lamina propria. No significant inflammation
MPEC	Complete epithelial ablation, lamina propria and muscularis mucosa intact, no inflammatory response
Cryotherapy	Complete epithelial ablation, no inflammatory response

Table III. Histology at 48 hours post ablative modality.

Modality	Finding
APC (90 W)	Necrosis of entire mucosal layer with significant inflammation and cellular necrosis involving the submucosa and extending to the muscularis propria
APC (60 W)	Necrosis of entire mucosal layer with significant inflammation and cellular necrosis involving the submucosa and extending to the muscularis propria < 90 Watts
MPEC	Necrosis of entire mucosal layer, transmural inflammation < APC
Cryotherapy	Complete denudation of the squamous epithelium. Transmural inflammatory response with extravasation of RBCs into the submucosa < APC

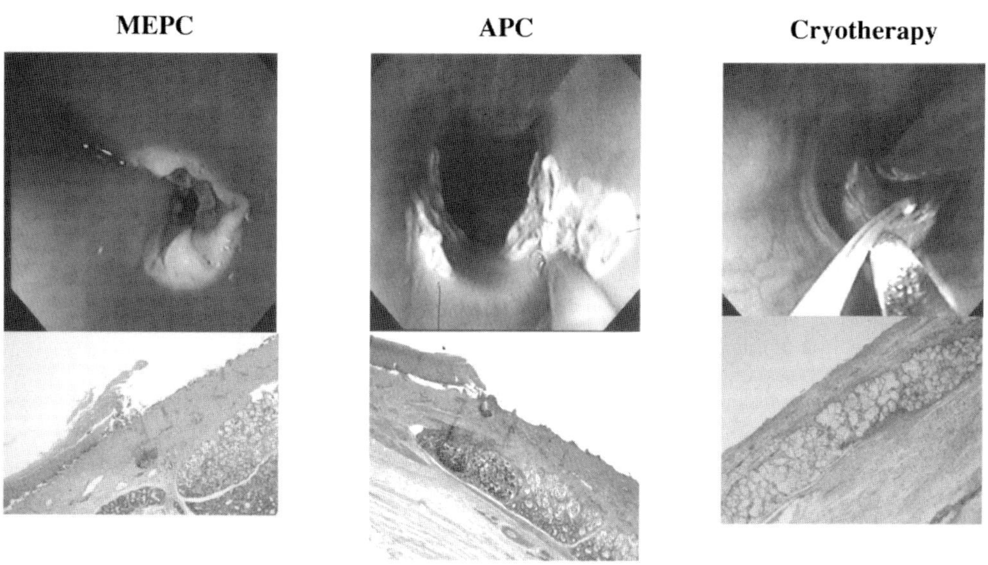

Figure 1. Endoscopy immediately and histology one hour post-ablation. In all three there is complete epithelial ablation with an intact lamina propria. (See page VI for colour figure).

Depth of injury

To understand depth of injury it is necessary to recognize that there are two stages in the process of ablation that contributes to the full depth of injury for all three modalities. There is immediate and delayed injury resulting in ablation of targeted tissue. For APC and MPEC, there is immediate ablation through cautery of the tissue contacted by the argon gas or MPEC probe and a delayed inflammatory response which results in cellular necrosis and extends the depth of injury depending on degree of inflammation. For cryo, there is immediate ablation caused by the combination of cryonecrosis due to ice-associated damage and cellular osmotic shock that follows solute concentration during the freeze-thaw process. There is also delayed ablation that occurs as a result of vascular stasis resulting in an inflammatory response and cellular necrosis [4] Epithelial ablation (0.5-1.0 mm) occurred immediately with all three modalities and was easily detected on full thickness biopsy one hour after application (*Figure 1*). The inflammatory response extends the depth of injury and is characterized by varying degrees of inflammation and cellular necrosis. The inflammatory response was greatest with APC at 90 W followed by APC at 60 W then MPEC and then cryo. Microscopically, depth of injury ranged from 4 to 1 mm and paralleled that of the inflammatory response in the same order. From phase one of the cryotherapy studies, assessed *via* endoscopy, gross injury was delayed and peaked between 2 to 7 days postcryo. Histology was not evaluated between 3 and 7 days. Consequently, it is conceivable that depth of injury from cryotherapy may have been more extensive due to the delayed inflammatory response. However, by four weeks healing was complete in all swine.

Discussion

The technique of spray cryotherapy is efficacious and safe in causing controlled mucosal ablation. The injury of cryotherapy is two phased. There is immediate cryonecrosis which is relatively superficial with an immediate depth of injury approximating 0.5 to 1.0 mm. There is a delayed inflammatory response that is often transmural and results in extension of ablation to least an additional 1 mm. Thus, the depth of injury is approximately 2 mm. The application of cryotherapy is easier and faster than that of MPEC and nearly as easy as APC. The ability to evenly distribute the cryogen compared to APC or MPEC is superior. The depth of injury is less than that of APC at 90 W but similar to APC at the currently standard setting of 60 W. Depth could be extended *via* extension of cryotherapy time but from these studies with this device, a 45 second cryotherapy burn is a reasonable target time in a human mucosal ablative trial as in Barrett's esophagus.

Conclusion

The findings from studies in animal experimentation support the use of endoscopic spray cryotherapy for mucosal ablation in patients with Barrett's esophagus. Depth of injury with a 45 second cryotherapy time should theoretically result in immediate Barrett's epithelium ablation (0.5 mm) and subsequent ablation of the remaining mucosa due to the delayed inflammatory response. Whether it is superior to the current modalities remains to be determined. It is anticipated that the device cost, the even distribution of application and the depth of ablation will be ideal.

Disclosure
The Johnston device is patented with additional patents pending. Data on file with the US Patent and Trademark Office, patent number 6,027,499. All royalties and financial entitlements to the primary inventor have been divested to a local charity in Maryland approved by the US Navy JAG Corps.

References

1. Johnston CM, Schoenfeld LP, Mysore JV, Dubois A. Endoscopic spray cryotherapy: a new technique for mucosal ablation in the esophagus. Gastrointest Endosc 1999;50(1):86-92.
2. Pasricha PJ, Hill S, Wadwa KS, Gislason GT, Okolo PI, Magee CI, Kuo WH, Baust J, Kalloo AN. Endoscopic cryotherapy: experimental results and first clinical use. Gastrointest Endosc 1999;49:627-631.
3. Data on file with the US Patent and Trademark Office, patent number 5,846,235.
4. Gage AA, Baust J. Mechanisms of tissue injury in cryosurgery. Cryobiology 1998;37:171-186.

What is the rate of esophageal stenoses observed after experimental ultrasonic ablation?

R.M. Bremner, D. Schwartz, C.G. Bremner (Los Angeles)

The last few years have seen an intense interest in ablation of the columnar lining of Barrett's esophagus in an attempt to reduce the malignant potential of this disease. The use of argon beam plasma coagulation, multipolar electrocoagulation, laser ablation, photodynamic therapy, and endoscopic mucosectomy have all been used in an attempt to convert the Barrett's columnar lining to stratified squamous epithelium[1-4]. Unfortunately all these techniques have had significant limitations including the need for multiple treatments, squamous regrowth over persistent columnar cells, and stricture formation requiring dilatation. The high incidence of stricture formation is related to the non-specific nature of these ablative processes with thermal or chemical damage invariably being caused to the underlying submucosa, and in some incidences, the muscularis propria.

We have previously shown that the Cavitron ultrasonic surgical aspirator (CUSA) exhibits a selective tissue disruption of the epithelium of the lower esophagus [5]. Tissues with a high elastin or collagen content have been found to be resistant to the ultrasound waves while tissues high in water content are susceptible to the cavitation and fragmentation effects of this energy. This allows complete epithelial ablation while leaving the muscularis mucosa and underlying submucosa undamaged. The recent development of laparoscopic CUSA instrument has allowed us to apply this technology to the lower esophageal mucosa through a modified operating gastrostomy port.

In our earlier animal models we were able to completely ablate the epithelium as evidenced by the multiple biopsies taken on the ablated areas. These biopsies were technically challenging to take as the smooth muscularis mucosa was difficult to grasp. The biopsies taken were consequently large strips of muscularis mucosa which resulted in exposure of the underlying submucosa. These animals were noted to develop ulcers at the biopsy sites with an intense histologic inflammatory reaction. These ulcers healed with fibrosis and narrowing of the lower esophagus as a result of the inflammatory reaction of the submucosa. The areas where no biopsies had been taken were noted to heal with squamous mucosa in the absence of any inflammatory response. Any ablative process that involves injury to the submucosa will probably result in a similar inflammatory process.

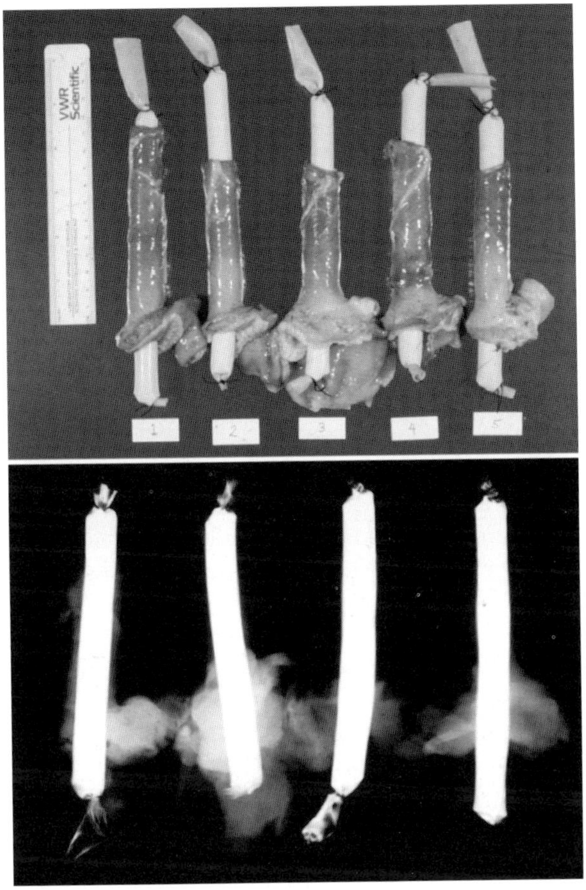

Figure 1. (See page VI for colour figure.)

Our subsequent experiments in the pig model involved complete epithelial ablation of the lower esophagus by CUSA without biopsying and disrupting the muscularis mucosa. These animal were noted to heal the ablated area with squamous epithelium in the absence of any stricture. *Figure 1* shows esophageal specimens that have undergone ultrasonic ablation and allowed to heal. They have been intubated with a penrose drain which has been filled with barium to show the absence of stricture as confirmed by the Xray of four further specimens. There was no stricture formation when an antireflux procedure was added at the time of ablation in the same animal model. Our most recent experiment has further shown that ablation after Nissen fundoplication is also possible and that, even in this setting, strictures do not form. We have now performed the ultrasonic epithelial ablation in two people without stricture formation so it appears that the healing process in humans mimics the animal model.

The tissue selective nature of ultrasonic ablation enables the epithelium to be removed without disrupting the underlying muscularis mucosa. The submucosa is subsequently undamaged which enables healing to occur in the absence of stricture formation.

References

1. Overholt BF, Panjehpour M, Haydek JM. Photodynamic therapy for Barrett's esophagus: follow-up in 100 patients. Gastrointest Endosc 1999;49:1-7.
2. Bremner CG, DeMeester TR. Proceedings from an international conference on ablation therapy for Barrett's mucosa. Brittany, France, 31 August-2 September 1997. Dis Esophagus 1998;11:1-27.
3. Johnston CM, Schoenfeld LP, Mysore JV, Dubois A. Endoscopic spray cryotherapy: a new technique for mucosal ablation in the esophagus. Gastrointest Endosc 1999;50:86-92.
4. Schulz H, Miehlke S, Antos D, Schentke KU, Vieth M, Stolte M, Bayerdorffer E. Ablation of Barrett's epithelium by endoscopic argon plasma coagulation in combination with high-dose omeprazole. Gastrointest Endosc 2000;51:659-663.

5. Bremner RM, Mason RJ, Bremner CG, DeMeester TR, Chandrasoma P, Peters JH, Hagen JA, Gadenstatter M. Ultrasonic epithelial ablation of the lower esophagus without stricture formation. A new technique for Barrett's ablation. Surg Endosc 1998;12:342-346.

With the use of centering balloons, should thermal ablation (Nd:YAG laser) be associated to photodynamic therapy in long segments of Barrett's mucosa?

M. Panjehpour (Knoxville)

We typically treat patients using a 5 or 7-cm windowed balloon. We treat a maximum of 7 cm of Barrett's mucosa in one session (one injection and laser treatment). In patients with Barrett's segments shorter than 7 cm, we typically ablate all Barrett's with one treatment session using a 7 cm balloon. In patients with longer segment of Barrett's, we treat 7 cm of the Barrett's with the worst pathology first. If the residual untreated Barrett's is longer that 1 or 2 cm in length and there is dysplasia in that area, we schedule patients for a second photodynamic therapy (PDT) treatment in 3-6 months (second injection with Photofrin®). If the residual segment is short and there is no dysplasia (or there are small islands of Barrett's mucosa), we treat them with thermal ablation using Nd:YAG laser, typically starting 3 months after initial PDT treatment. We use contact probe (rounded probe) with water cooling. After thermal ablation, a follow-up endoscopy is performed in two days to evaluate the response. Additional thermal ablation may be performed again. We use 13-15 Watts of power in CW mode using an SLT laser. Realizing that the majority of Barrett's esophagus is treated using balloon PDT, a discussion is included here on our balloon treatment.

Balloon light delivery for photodynamic therapy of Barrett's esophagus

Before development of balloons, cylindrical diffusers were used to treat a specific length of the esophagus. Initially, we [1] used a 2 cm cylindrical diffuser to treat patients with early invasive cancer in Barrett's esophagus.

Later, a balloon light delivery device was developed and tested by our group for treatment of Barrett's esophagus [2]. The balloon was constructed from a polyurethane membrane. It was determined that a windowed balloon with a diameter of 25 mm would effectively flatten the esophageal folds and would allow uniform illumination of specific length of the esophagus. Increasing the balloon diameter affected the blood flow in tissue and no PDT injury was induced even at much higher light doses [3].

This balloon with a 2 or 3 cm window was first used clinically to treat four patients [4]. A 2 cm cylindrical diffuser was used in the 2 cm windowed balloon. A 2.5 cm cylindrical diffuser was used in the 3 cm windowed balloon (3 cm diffusers were not available). Long segments were treated sequentially by repositioning of the balloon. This balloon design was used to determine the proper light dosimetry and develop the methodology [5]. The power density from the fiber was 400 mw/cm of length of diffuser. In the first patient, the position of balloon was checked using measurements on the shaft of the balloon. This technique was found to be unreliable. For all other patients, the scope was passed alongside the balloon shaft and the position of the balloon was verified using a marker on the shaft of the balloon. The marker was 3 cm proximal to the proximal edge of the balloon window. Thus, by monitoring the position of the marker using scope measurements, the position of the window was easily verified.

Treatment of long segments of Barrett's using a 2 cm or 3 cm windowed balloon required sequential treatments of the esophagus during each session. Typically, it is difficult to avoid overlapping of the treatment fields. A 5 cm long windowed balloon was developed to allow treatment of a longer segment of the Barrett's esophagus without repositioning of the balloon [6]. A flexible 5 cm cylindrical diffuser (Rare Earth Medical, Inc.) was used in the 5 cm windowed balloon. The power density from the diffuser was 400 mw/cm with a total power of 2,000 mw. In addition, the balloon design was modified for guidewire positioning of the balloon in the esophagus. Using this design, first a standard guidewire was passed into the stomach. The balloon was passed over the guidewire and positioned into the stomach. The scope was passed alongside the balloon shaft. The balloon was withdrawn until the marker on the shaft was at the desired location in the esophagus, noting that the marker is 3 cm proximal to the proximal edge of the balloon window. The guidewire was withdrawn and the balloon was inflated. The cylindrical diffuser was passed into the central channel of the balloon to a premeasured depth, aligning the diffuser with the window. The central channel of the balloon assembly was then flushed with saline through a flush-inlet to wash any contaminants inside the central channel. Contaminants can interfere with the light from diffuser causing irreversible damage to the fiber and the balloon. The laser was then activated.

Finally, balloons with a window length of 7 cm were developed that allowed a longer segment of Barrett's to be treated [7]. A 7 cm flexible cylindrical diffuser was used inside the balloon shaft as the light source (Rare Earth Medical). The power density from the diffuser was 400 mw/cm, or 2,800 mw total power for a 7 cm diffuser. Currently, a maximum of 7 cm of the esophagus is treated in one session. The light dose is 175-200 J/cm using this balloon requiring a treatment time of 438-500 seconds.

The above balloon was modified for the phase III multicenter study for treatment of high-grade dysplasia (HGD) in Barrett's esophagus (sponsored by QLT PhotoTherapeutics). The interior surface of the distal and proximal capped portions of the balloon were coated with a reflective material (Wilson-Cook Medical Inc., Winston-Salem, NC). A cylindrical diffuser 2 cm longer that the window length was used inside the central channel. The cylindrical diffuser extended 1 cm proximally and 1 cm distally beyond the window margins. Using this diffuser/balloon configuration, the uniformity of light emitted from the balloon window was improved. In addition, laboratory testing and canine studies showed that the light intensity emitted from the balloon window was 1.5 times higher using the reflective balloons design compared to that from the initial balloon design (unpublished data). This allowed using a lower power density (and power) from the diffuser while achieving the same intensity of light emitted from the balloon window. The power density of 270 mw/cm from diffuser provided a similar light intensity from the window as that provided with the original balloon [7]. Using this balloon, a light dose of 130 J/cm is used for treatment of HGD in Barrett's esophagus (phase III study). The reflective balloons are available in window lengths of 3 cm, 5 cm and 7 cm, and are currently provided by QLT PhotoTherapeutics for the phase III study. A 5 cm diffuser is used in the 3 cm windowed balloon, a 7 cm diffuser in the 5 cm windowed balloon, and a 9 cm diffuser in the 7 cm windowed balloon. The above diffusers are provided by QLT PhotoTherapeutics for Phase III study. The balloon material was changed to non-stretchable polyethylene terephthalate to achieve a balloon diameter of 25 mm even at very high balloon pressures. The original balloon was constructed from polyurethane that had the potential for membrane stretching, resulting in increased balloon diameter at higher pressures. The QLT sponsored study is closed to patient accrual.

References

1. Overholt BF, Panjehpour M, Teffteller E, et al. Photodynamic therapy for treatment of early adenocarcinoma in Barrett's esophagus. Gastrointest Endosc 1993;39:73.
2. Panjehpour M, Overholt BF, DeNovo RC, et al. Centering balloon to improve esophageal photodynamic therapy. Lasers Surg Med 1992;12:631.
3. Overholt BF, Panjehpour M, DeNovo RC, et al.Balloon photodynamic therapy of esophageal cancer: effect of increasing balloon size. Lasers Surg Med 1996;18:248.
4. Overholt BF, Panjehpour M. Barrett's esophagus: photodynamic therapy for ablation of dysplasia, reduction of specialized mucosa, and treatment of superficial esophageal cancer. Gastrointest Endosc 1995;42:64.
5. Overholt BF, Panjehpour M. Photodynamic therapy in Barrett's esophagus. J Clin Laser Med Surg 1996;14:245.
6. Overholt BF, Panjehpour M. Photodynamic therapy for Barrett's esophagus. Gastrointest Endosc Clin North Am 1997;7:207.
7. Overholt BF, Panjehpour M, Haydek JM. Photodynamic therapy for Barrett's esophagus: follow-up in 100 patients. Gastrointest Endosc 1999;49:1.

Screening and surveillance

After endoscopic therapy, how to evaluate the potential risk of dysplastic and neoplastic changes in columnar epithelium remaining beneath regenerated squamous mucosa?

H.S. Garewal (Tuckson)

Ablation therapy, *i.e.* attempts at eradicating Barrett's esophagus, is becoming increasingly popular since the fundamental approach was hypothesized several years ago. At the last symposium, I discussed the pluripotent nature of the esophageal stem cell and illustrated this by pointing out the changes that the esophageal lining goes through *in utero*. We also postulated that once intestinal metaplasia (IM) is established, by reflux, it is a stable lesion that does not go away simply by decreasing reflux. This is corroborated by the number of negative studies using long-term acid suppression, even with proton pump inhibitors (PPIs), or antireflux surgery. The most one sees is the appearance of so-called squamous islands, *i.e.* areas in which squamous epithelium appears. Currently, the approaches used for ablation combine a method for injuring the epithelium in an acid or reflux-suppressed environment. The methods differ only in the technique of re-injury, which has included photodynamic therapy, use of lasers or multipolar electrocoagulation (MPEC). With this approach, a high percentage of patients will undergo reversal of their IM back toward squamous epithelium. Nevertheless, in a significant number of cases, the reversal is incomplete with areas of IM persisting either alongside or below the squamous epithelium.

The obvious question regarding ablation is whether we are actually reducing the risk of cancer by exposing an individual to these techniques. The best approach to answering this question would clearly be a prospective trial in which the risk of cancer is assessed over time. Nevertheless, such a study is practically and logistically impossible given the number of patients that would be needed. Thus, our approach has been to study biomarkers in the reversed epithelium to assess whether they are normally or abnormally expressed.

Our initial findings suggest that complete reversal (*i.e.* only squamous epithelium is present and no residual IM) results in squamous epithelium that is indistinguishable from normal squamous epithelium. We have found that expression of p53 as well as proliferation characteristics of this epithelium are identical to normal tissue. Consequently, we postulate that this squamous epithelium will be a low risk situation. On the contrary, in the partial reversal setting, we have noticed abnormal expression of biomarkers, especially at the junction of persistent or recurrent IM and new or neo-squamous epithelium. The proliferation is increased and, in the squamous regions, occurs in multiple layers rather than the basal layer only. Similarly, proliferation in the glands on the IM side is also markedly increased. P53 expression was found to be abnormal in a number of cases, thereby raising the possibility that cancer risk may indeed be increased in this setting [1]. This is an area that needs further study fairly urgently, since ablation is becoming evermore popular for these patients. Incomplete ablation can occur in up to 30-40% of patients when carefully assessed at 6-12 months after completion of the ablation procedure. Given the difficulties with a clinical trial, use of a wide range of biomarkers needs to be assessed to guide us on this issue.

Reference

1. Garewal H, Ramsey L, Sharma P, Kraus K, Sampliner R, Fass R. Biomarker studies in reversed Barrett's esopagus. Am J Gastroenterol 1999;94:2829-2833.

Can surveillance intervals be defined?

D. Lieberman (Portland)

In order to define appropriate intervals for surveillance of patients with Barrett's esophagus we need to know the progression rates of:
- short and long segment Barrett's esophagus;
- Barrett's esophagus with no dysplasia;
- Barrett's esophagus indefinite for dysplasia;
- Barrett's esophagus with low-grade dysplasia.

We lack complete understanding of the impact of potential risk factors on progression such as:
- gender - greater risk of Barrett's esophagus and adenocarcinoma in men;
- race and ethnicity - preponderance of cancer in Caucasians;
- duration of reflux symptoms;
- control or lack of control of reflux symptoms.

The natural history of patients with no evidence of progression over time is also unknown. For example, if patients have multiple surveillance exams which show no evidence of inflammation or progression, is it safe or reasonable to stop surveillance altogether ?

In conclusion, we have no evidence upon which to base a recommendation for surveillance intervals. Studies are needed to define the natural history of Barrett's esophagus, and identify the modulating effects of various risk factors on progression to malignancy. Clinical studies which assess the risk and benefit or different surveillance intervals are needed.

Should patients with purely histologic metaplasia be on a surveillance program?

A.J. Cameron (Rochester)

A long segment Barrett's esophagus (LSBE) may be defined as 3 cm or longer of visible columnar epithelium in the esophagus, with intestinal metaplasia (IM) on biopsy. A short segment Barrett's esophagus (SSBE) may be defined as visible columnar epithelium in the esophagus of less than 3 cm length. Both LSBE and SSBE are associated with adenocarcinoma, the risk being more clearly defined and possibly greater for LSBE than for SSBE. If biopsies are taken from patients with a normally located Z-line, and no endoscopically visible Barrett's esophagus of any length, many will be found to have histologic IM of the gastric cardia. The writer will use the proposed classification of intestinal metaplasia of Sharma *et al.* [1], the 3 categories being LSBE, SSBE, and IM of the gastric cardia. This makes a distinction between the finding of IM in short tongues or segments of columnar mucosa extending into the lower esophagus, and the finding of IM on biopsies taken immediately below a normally located Z-line, which may be a different condition [2].

The following *Table I* contains information from papers [3-6] in which IM of the gastric cardia was considered separately from cases of SSBE. Biopsies were taken for research purposes in consecutive upper endoscopic examinations on patients examined for clinical indications, including those with and without reflux symptoms. These patients had a normally located Z-line seen at endoscopy.

Thus, about 15% of adults having endoscopy have IM of the gastric cardia if biopsies are taken routinely. Although this is not a true population-based sample, there is no reason to believe that the prevalence of IM of the gastric cardia found on consecutive endoscopies is much different from the general population of similar age. It is noted that the prevalence of IM of the gastric cardia increases with age and, unlike LSBE, is similar in males and in females [6].

Table I.

	Year	Intestinal metaplasia
Spechler *et al.*	1995	15%
Cameron *et al.*	1997	17%
Trudgill *et al.*	1997	17%
Voutilainen *et al.*	1999	10%

In 2 US population based studies, the annual incidence of adenocarcinoma of the cardia for males and females combined was 2.1 [7], and in our recent Olmsted County study 2.0/100,000.

There are no long term prospective follow-up studies to show the cancer risk in subjects with IM of the gastric cardia. It is possible to get an approximate estimate from combining data already available, as follows. Let us consider an area with a stable population of 100,000 persons of all ages. If the mean age at death is 80 years, 1,250 people in this population die each year from all causes. Assume that 15% of persons (over age 60) have IM of the gastric cardia, although most have never had a biopsy to show this. Therefore, about 15% of the 1,250 persons dying have IM of the gastric cardia, 188 persons. In the population of 100,000, 2 persons per year die from adenocarcinoma of the cardia. Supposing that every adenocarcinoma of the cardia begins in an area of IM of the gastric cardia, then 1 in 94 (2/188) patients with IM of the gastric cardia might develop adenocarcinoma of the cardia in their lifetime. Suppose that a typical patient is found to have IM of the gastric cardia on biopsy at age 55, with a 25-year remaining life expectancy. For each year of expected life, the risk of adenocarcinoma of the cardia is 1 in 94 times 1 in 25, that is a cancer incidence of 1 in 2,350 patient-years for this individual

The risk of adenocarcinoma of the cardia developing in IM of the gastric cardia is likely overestimated above. In 2 series, 42% of adenocarcinomas of the cardia developed in short or long segments of Barrett's esophagus [8, 9]. In some cases, no Barrett's esophagus or IM of the gastric cardia is found in cases of adenocarcinoma of the cardia.

In a decision analysis paper on cancer in Barrett's esophagus, Provenzale *et al.* [10] concluded that if the cancer incidence was less than 1 in 420 patient-years, the risks of surveillance and esophagectomy would outweigh any benefit in terms of length and quality of life.

It seems clear that the risk of adenocarcinoma of the cardia in patients with IM of the gastric cardia is very low. The writer does not recommend routine surveillance in such patients.

References

1. Sharma P, Morales TG, Sampliner RE. Short segment Barrett's esophagus-the need for standardization of the definition and of endoscopic criteria. Am J Gastroenterol 1998;93:1033-1036.
2. Nandurkar S, Talley NJ. Barrett's esophagus: the long and the short of it. Am J Gastroenterol 1999;94:30-40.
3. Spechler SJ, Zeroogian JM, Wang HH, Antonioli DA, Goyal RK. The frequency of specialized intestinal metaplasia at the squamo-columnar junction varies with the extent of columnar epithelium lining the esophagus. Gastroenterology 1995;108:A224.
4. Cameron AJ, Kamath PS, Carpenter HA. Prevalence of Barrett's esophagus and intestinal metaplasia at the esophagogastric junction. Gastroenterology 1997;112:A 82.
5. Trudgill NJ, Suvarna SK, Kapur KC, Riley SA. Intestinal metaplasia at the squamocolumnar junction in patients attending for diagnostic gastroscopy. Gut 1997;41:585-589.
6. Voutilainen M, Farkkila M, Juhola M, Nuorva K, Mauranen K, Mantynen T, Kunnamo I, Mecklin JP, Sipponen P. Specialized columnar epithelium of the esophagogastric junction: prevalence and associations. The Central Finland Endoscopy Study Group. Am J Gastroenterol 1999;94:913-918.
7. Devesa SS, Blot WJ, Fraumeni JF. Changing patterns in the incidence of esophageal and gastric carcinoma in the United States. Cancer 1998;83:2049-2053.
8. Clark GWB, Smyrk TC, Budiles P, Hoeft SF, Peters JH, Kiyabu M, Hinder RA, Bremner CG, DeMeester TR. Is Barrett's metaplasia the source of adenocarcinomas of the cardia? Arch Surg 1994;129:609-614.
9. Cameron AJ, Lomboy CT, Pera M, Carpenter HA. Adenocarcinoma of the esophagogastric junction and Barrett's esophagus. Gastroenterology 1995:109:1541-1546.
10. Provenzale D, Schmitt C, Wong JB. Barrett's esophagus: a new look at surveillance based on emerging estimates of cancer risk. Am J Gastroenterol 1999;94:2043-2053.

Are methylene blue-directed biopsies a cost-effective method for surveillance of Barrett's patients?

M.I.F. Canto (Baltimore)

Methylene blue is a vital stain taken up by actively absorbing tissues such as small intestinal and colonic epithelium. It selectively and accurately stains the intestinal-type of metaplasia or specialized columnar epithelium [1, 2], which is considered pathognomonic of Barrett's esophagus. It is also the most clinically relevant type of epithelium due to its association with adenocarcinoma of the esophagus and esophagogastric junction

Interpretation of methylene blue staining

Methylene blue staining of nondysplastic Barrett's esophagus may be either focal or diffuse (*i.e.* > 75% of Barrett's mucosa stains blue) [3]. Nearly all patients with long-segment Barrett's esophagus (LSBE) have diffuse staining because specialized columnar epithelium comprises majority of the columnar mucosa [1]. In contrast, majority of short Barrett's esophagus exhibits focal staining due to the presence of gastric-type metaplasia.

Highly dysplastic specialized columnar epithelium in long Barrett's esophagus (> 3 cm) Barrett's esophagus appears to stain differently from non-dysplastic specialized columnar epithelium [2, 3]. Nearly all areas of high-grade dysplasia (HGD) or adenocarcinoma take up less methylene blue and therefore appear unstained or light blue. In contrast, nondysplastic Barrett's esophagus usually stains dark blue. Barrett's esophagus with low-grade dysplasia stains variably [3]. The reason for this abnormal methylene blue staining is dysplastic Barrett's esophagus is possibly the decrease in goblet cells characteristic of dysplastic epithelium. The effect is similar to that seen with Lugol's iodine solution when used in early squamous cell esophageal carcinomas. Close attention should be paid to moderately or markedly heterogeneous staining or focal areas of nonstained (pink) mucosa within diffusely staining specialized columnar epithelium. This is usually observed in patients with more than 3 cm of Barrett's esophagus. This pattern has been highly associated with HGD or early adenocarcinoma [2, 3]. The endoscopist should meticulously biopsy both stained and unstained areas in the esophagus using large/"jumbo" biopsy forceps. Obtain biopsies from light blue or unstained areas first and place these in separate bottles. Increasing grade of dysplasia is significantly associated with focal areas of decreased stain intensity (from dark blue to light blue or absent stain/pink) and/or increased stain heterogeneity (*i.e.* increasing proportion of light blue or pink unstained mucosa compared to dark blue mucosa).

Methylene blue staining is cost-effective

In a prospective, controlled sequential trial [2], methylene blue staining led to a much larger proportion of specialized columnar epithelium in endoscopic biopsies compared to large particle 4-quadrant random biopsy (p = .0006), particularly in patients with limited-segment (54% *versus* 94%) and LSBE (72% *versus* 92%). Moderate to marked heterogeneity of staining (*i.e.*, decreased to absent staining within diffusely staining Barrett's esophagus) was highly associated with dysplasia or early cancer. Hence, despite fewer biopsies per patient, methylene blue directed biopsy diagnosed dysplasia or cancer in significantly more biopsies (9.2% *versus* 6.6%, p = 0.004) and more patients (46.5% *versus* 30%, p = 0.03) than random biopsy. The estimated average cost of diagnosing a cancer using methylene blue-directed biopsy was half that of 4-quadrant random biopsy.

In summary, methylene blue-directed biopsy is a more accurate and cost-effective technique than random biopsy for diagnosing specialized columnar epithelium and dysplasia/cancer, particularly in LSBE.

References

1. Canto MI, Setrakian S, Petras RE, Blades E, Chak A, Sivak MV. Methylene blue selectively stains intestinal metaplasia in Barrett's esophagus. Gastrointest Endosc 1996;44:1-7.
2. Canto M, Setrakian S, Willis J, Chak A, Petras RE, Powe NR, Sivak MV Jr. Methylene blue-directed biopsy for improved detection of intestinal metaplasia and dysplasia in Barrett's esophagus: a controlled sequential trial. Gastrointest Endosc 2000;51(5):560-568.
3. Canto M, Setrakian S, Willis J, Petras RE, Chak A, Sivak MV Jr. Methylene blue staining of dysplastic and nondysplastic Barrett's esophagus:an in vivo and ex vivo study. Gastrointest Endosc 1996;43:164.

What information can the computer cohort simulation of Barrett's patients contribute to cost-effectiveness analysis of cancer risk?

D. Provenzale (Durham)

There is an increased risk of adenocarcinoma in patients with Barrett's esophagus. The risk is estimated at 30-125 times that of the general population. Patients with high-grade dysplasia (HGD) are at greatest risk for developing adenocarcinoma. Because of their cancer risk, current recommendations are for periodic endoscopic surveillance to detect dysplasia and early cancer. Most authorities recommend esophagectomy for HGD, but because of the morbidity and mortality associated with esophagectomy, others reserve this procedure only for those with cancer. Previous reports have suggested that the incidence of cancer in patients with Barrett's ranges from 0.2% annually or 1 in 441 patient years to 2.1% annually or 1 in 48 patient years. Most recent reports, however, suggest that the incidence of cancer is in the range of 0.4% to 0.5% annually or 1 in 251 to 1 in 208 patient years. Our question for this analysis was, is surveillance of patients with Barrett's esophagus cost-effective compared to common medical practices? Because there were no controlled trials that examined the efficacy of surveillance, we created a computer cohort simulation of 50 year old patients with Barrett's esophagus and no evidence of dysplasia by biopsy. The strategies we included in our model are shown in *Table I*. We examined surveillance every 1-5 years and no surveillance in which endoscopy was performed for new or worsened dysphagia. For each of the strategies on the left, the indication for surgery that we considered was HGD. From published literature, the parameters we included in our model are shown in *Table II*. From published reports we used complications of an endoscopy of 1.3‰ procedures and an average incidence of cancer of 0.4% annually or 1 in 227 patient years. We used our measured value for quality of life after esophagectomy. On a scale from 0 to 1, with 0 equivalent to being dead, and 1 equivalent to a state of perfect health, we measured quality of life in patients who had undergone esophagectomy for HGD or cancer one year earlier at Duke University. On a scale from 0 to 1, they rated their quality of life at 0.97. Although they were symptomatic after esophagectomy, they believed that they had been cured of their cancer and this was extremely important to them [1].

The criterion, or unit of measurement for our analysis was the incremental cost-utility ratio. This is the change in cost divided by the change in quality adjusted life expectancy to move from no surveillance to surveillance or to move from less frequent surveillance to more frequent surveillance. The results are reported as dollars per quality-adjusted life year gained. We employed the standard technique of discounting in our analysis, which considers that a dollar today is worth more than a dollar in the future, and because life years are valued relative to dollars in these economic analyses, they are also discounted. The costs we included in our model are shown in *Table III*. These are direct medical costs from Duke University. They are the actual resource costs for providing these services. This is in distinction to charges which may be falsely inflated or deflated based on profit or loss to the institution. These are facility costs and medicare reimbursement for

Table I. Strategies.

Surveillance 1. Every year 2. Every 2 years 3. Every 3 years 4. Every 4 years 5. Every 5 years No surveillance Endoscopy for dysphagia	→	Esophagectomy for high-grade dysplasia

Table II. Parameters.

Risks of endoscopy*	
Complication	1.3/1,000 procedures
Incidence of cancer*	
Average	0.4% (1.227 patient-years)
Quality adjustment	
Long-term morbidity – esophagectomy	0.97

* Published data

Table III.

Endoscopy	$ 600
Endoscopy with complication	$ 3,700
Esophagectomy	$ 23,700
Perforation requiring surgery:	
- cancer	$ 23,800
- no cancer	$ 7,000
Annual F/U (post-esophagectomy)	$ 1,000
Cancer care:	
- hospice care/patient	$ 33,900

physician fees. The cost of endoscopy is $ 600. Endoscopy with complication is $ 3,700. The costs for esophagectomy and perforation requiring surgery ranging from $ 7,000 to $ 23,800. The cost for annual follow-up post esophagectomy is $ 1,000 and the cost for the care of the terminally ill patient with esophageal cancer at $ 33,900 [1].

Our results are shown in *Figure 1*. The vertical axis displays the average life time cost per patient and the horizontal axis displays the discounted quality-adjusted life expectancy in years. Each of the circles represents the results of an alternative management strategy. On the bottom left, no surveillance costs approximately $ 3,000 and is associated with living approximately 12.65 additional years after entering a surveillance program. Surveillance every 5 years costs approximately $ 12,500 and is associated with living an additional 12.74 quality-adjusted life years after entering a surveillance program. The change in cost divided by the change in life quality-adjusted expectancy to move from no surveillance to surveillance every 5 years is the incremental cost utility ratio shown on the top of the line at $ 98,000 per quality-adjusted life year gained. Focusing on the more frequent surveillance intervals every 4, 3, 2 and 1 year, the line does not connect these strategies. That is, because they are inferior to surveillance every 5 years because they cost more and yield a lower life expectancy. Costs are higher and life expectancy is lower because on average, there are more endoscopies, endoscopic complications and surgeries in these strategies. Now turn your attention to the text at the top of the slide. Compared to published incremental cost-effectiveness ratios our results show that surveillance every 5 years has an incremental cost-utility ratio of $ 98,000 per quality-adjusted life year gained. That falls somewhere in between the costs of breast cancer screening [2] and heart transplantation [3]. So, surveillance every 5 years would be considered cost-effective when compared to these other well accepted medical practices. In order to examine the cost-effectiveness of surveillance given a limited health care budget, we performed a sensitivity analysis on the willingness to pay or budget of those who make health policy and on the incidence of cancer, a critical parameter in decisions for surveillance and esophagectomy in patients with Barrett's esophagus (*Figure 2*). The vertical axis displays different levels of willingness to pay or budgets of those who make health policy, ranging from $ 25,000 to $ 300,000 per quality-adjusted life year gained. The horizontal axis displays the incidence of cancer ranging

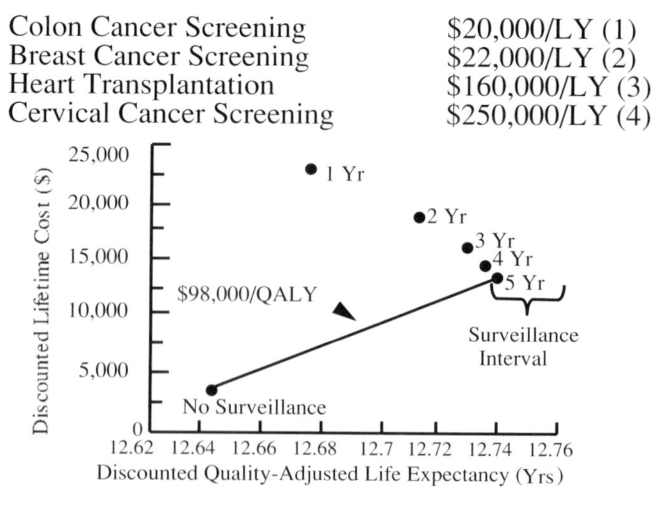

Figure 1. Results.

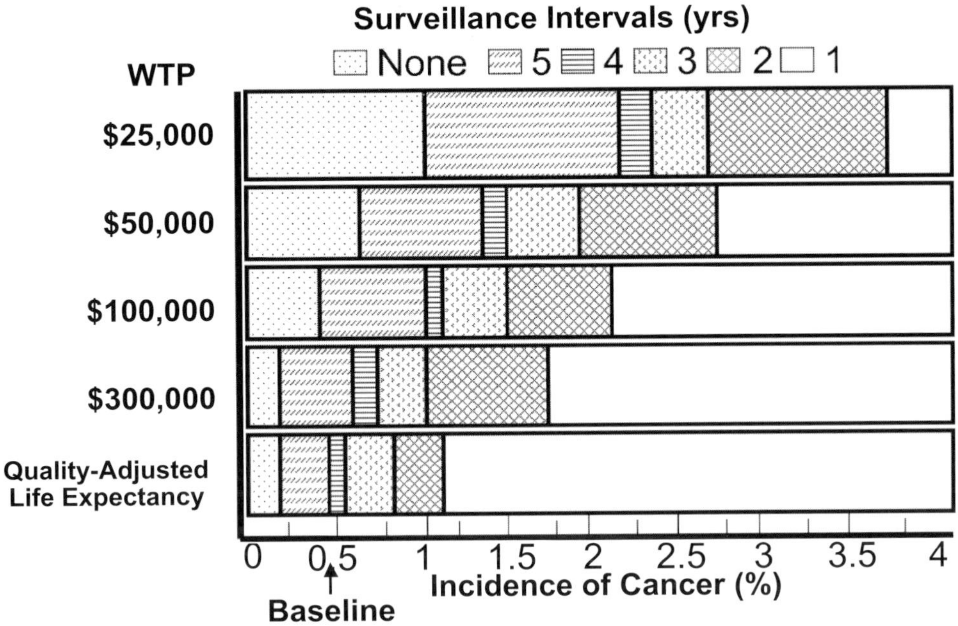

Figure 2. Sensitivity analysis-incidence of cancer.

from 0% to 4%. The baseline is at 0.4%. There are no budgetary constraints. The lower bar shows that surveillance every 5 years provides the greatest gain in quality-adjusted life expectancy. Moving up to the next horizontal bar of *Figure 2*, for the policy maker with \$ 300,000 to spend on surveillance, similar to the cost of cervical cancer screening showed earlier in *Figure 1*, it is shown that surveillance every 5 years is the only strategy that both increased life expectancy and would be within the budget of the policy maker with \$ 300,000 to spend. For the policy maker with only \$ 100,000 to spend on surveillance, similar to the cost of heart transplantation, surveillance every 5 years would increase life expectancy and would be within the budget of the policy maker with \$ 100,000 to spend. For the policy maker with only \$ 50,000 or \$ 25,000 to spend on surveillance, similar to the cost of mammography for breast cancer screening, it appears that with this limited health care budget, no surveillance is the only strategy that would not exceed the \$ 50,000 or \$ 25,000 limit.

Conclusions

- Surveillance of patients with Barrett's esophagus is effective.
- Surveillance every 5 years provides the greatest gain in quality adjusted life expectancy and has an incremental cost-utility ratio similar to those of common medical practices.
- The cost-effectiveness of surveillance is based on the budget of those who make health policy.
- Future research on the incidence of cancer and the accuracy of surveillance endoscopy are crucial for determining the most effective and cost-effective surveillance interval.

References

1. Provenzale D, Schmitt C, Wong JB. Barrett's esophagus: a new look at surveillance based on emerging estimates of cancer risk. Am J Gastroenterol 1999;94:2043-2053.
2. van der Maas PH, de Konig JG, van Ineveld BM, et al. The cost-effectiveness of breast cancer screening. Int J Cancer 1989;43:1055-1060.
3. Pennock JL, Oyer PR, Reitz BA, et al. Cardiac transplantation in perspective for the future:survival complications, rehabilitation, and cost. J Thorac Cardiovasc Surg 1982;83:168-177.

Can prostaglandin E2 be considered as involved in degeneration of Barrett's and colonic mucosa?

G. Morgan (Swansea)

The role of prostaglandin E2 (PGE2) in the degeneration of Barrett's and colonic mucosa is best illustrated by firstly considering the pharmacology of non-steroidal anti-inflammatory drugs (NSAIDs) such as aspirin.

The therapeutic and toxic properties of NSAIDs can be explained pharmacologically. In 1971 [1] it was discovered that NSAIDs inhibit the cyclo-oxygenase (COX) enzyme and thus prevent the formation of prostaglandins and thromboxanes from precursor arachidonic acid. Arachidonic acid is an essential polyunsaturated fatty acid that is derived from the diet. It is believed that the analgesic, anti-inflammatory and antipyretic effects of NSAIDs are related, at least in part, to prostaglandin inhibition. Aspirin prevention of cardiovascular disease is thought to be related to thromboxanes inhibition in platelets leading to a reduced risk of potentially dangerous blood clots forming in the heart and brain blood vessels.

Research published in 1991 and 1992 identified and characterised a second COX isoform (COX-2) [2-4]. COX-1 is expressed constitutively and produces prostaglandins and thromboxanes such that are important in many physiological processes but most notably within the stomach and kidney. In contrast with COX-1, COX-2 is not expressed in normal tissues but its expression is greatly increased (more than 20-fold) at sites of inflammation. The overexpression of COX-2 can be rapidly induced by a variety of stimuli including cytokines, growth factors and hormones.

It is believed that the therapeutic effects of NSAIDs against pain, inflammation and fever are largely related to COX-2 inhibition while the toxic effects of NSAIDs to the stomach and kidney are largely related to COX-1 inhibition. Aspirin cardiovascular protection is an important exception to this COX-1 (toxicity) and COX-2 (therapeutic) principle. Protection appears to be related to COX-1 inhibition in the platelets leading to a reduction in the synthesis of platelet thromboxanes. This appears to be related to a unique pharmacological property of aspirin over other NSAIDs. Only aspirin can irreversibly inhibit the COX-1 enzyme in platelets and thus prevent the platelet ever producing thromboxanes again.

Evidence that prostaglandin E2 is involved in degeneration

There is good evidence that NSAIDs reduce the risk of both esophageal and colorectal cancers [5-7]. It therefore follows the PGE2 inhibition is a plausible candidate for the reduced cancer risk which in turn implicates PGE2 as a potential mediator of degeneration. Esophageal and colorectal cancer development arise following a multistage process known as carcinogenesis. PGE2 is likely to play a different role at each stage of carcinogenesis although it is worth emphasizing that carcinogenesis is a complex process and a number mediators other than prostaglandins will exert effects.

With respect to esophageal carcinogenesis, there is evidence that long standing reflux disease is associated with an increase risk of esophageal adenocarcinoma [8]. PGE2 may play a role in reflux disease by driving the vicious cycle of reflux, inflammation, reduced pressure of the lower esophageal sphincter and further reflux [9]. The treatment of long standing reflux disease with NSAIDs is logical but controversial. The enzymic origin of PGE2 in reflux disease remains to be identified but COX-2 is a likely and logical source. COX-2 inhibitors such as celecoxib and rofecoxib may be helpful in the treatment long standing reflux disease in conjunction with conventional treatment agents such as acid suppressant. In addition, breaking the vicious PGE2 cycle would reduce the risk of developing Barrett's esophagus and adenocarcinoma.

Barrett's esophagus is associated with the overexpression of COX-2 [10, 11]. The pathophysiological role of COX-2 in Barrett's esophagus is not fully understood [11] although it is likely to be a marker for cancer risk. At the very least, COX-2 expression would be expected to result in a high level of PGE2 synthesis which would maintain and perpetuate the vicious cycle described earlier. At present, no clinical trials have been conducted on NSAIDs (particularly COX-2 inhibitors) in Barrett's esophagus patients and such studies are warranted.

COX-2 is also overexpressed in esophageal adenocarcinomas and esophageal squamous cell carcinomas [12, 13]. Again the role of COX-2 is not fully understood but PGE2 is known to be a potent vasodilator. It is plausible that COX-2 derived PGE2 helps to maintain carcinoma blood flow thus promoting the conditions for carcinoma survival and growth. Selective COX-2 inhibitors may thus have a therapeutic remit in the treatment of established esophageal cancers.

With respect to colorectal carcinogenesis, it is known the COX-2 is overexpressed in precancerous and cancerous tissues [5, 6]. Good evidence for the role of COX-2 in colonic degeneration has been provided by Oshima *et al.* [14]. They bred mice carrying a mutation to the adenomatous polyposis coli gene with other mice having a disrupted COX-2 gene. Mice that had 2 normal COX-2 genes developed an average of 652 polyps at 10 weeks; those with one COX-2 gene had 224 while those with no active gene had only 93 polyps. These data provide definitive data that COX-2 is an early rate limiting for precancerous adenomatous poly formation in experimental animals. COX-2 inhibitors thus hold promise as chemoprevention agents for colorectal cancer and clinical trials are in progress with celecoxib and rofecoxib in patients with the precancerous syndrome known as familial adenomatous polyposis [15].

Public health considerations

Selective COX-2 inhibitors have potential for preventing esophageal and colorectal cancer. An important, if not exclusive, mechanism of action is likely to be PGE2 inhibition. Thus PGE2 can be considered to be an important mediator of degeneration during carcinogenesis.

COX-2 inhibitors may be particularly useful as chemoprevention agents in patients with precancerous lesions such as Barrett's esophagus and familial adenomatous polyposis but there wider public health potential remains unclear. From a public health viewpoint, most patients will be without precancerous lesions and aspirin may be a more beneficial drug for cancer prevention in the general population due to the attendant risk reduction from cardiovascular disease.

Closing remarks

PGE2 can be considered to be important in degeneration of Barrett's and colonic mucosa. COX-2 inhibitors may have therapeutic remits in treating reflux disease, the chemoprevention of esophageal and colorectal cancers and treating established cancers. At the public health level, aspirin may be an optimum NSAID to use to reduce cancer risk due to additional benefits against cardiovascular disease risk.

References

1. Vane JR. Inhibition of prostaglandin synthesis as a mechanism of action for aspirin-like drugs. Nature 1971;231:232-235.
2. O'Banion MK, Sadowski HB, Winn V, Young DA. A serum- and glucocorticoid regulated 4-kilobase mRNA encodes a cyclooxygenase related protein. J Biol Chem 1991;266:23261-23267.
3. Xie W, Chipman JG, Robertson DL, Erikson RL, Simmons DL. Expression of a mitogen-responsive gene encoding prostaglandin synthase is regulated by mRNA splicing. Proc Natl Acad Sci USA 1991;88:2692-2696.
4. Sirois J, Richards JS. Purification and characterisation of a novel, distinct isoform of prostaglandin endoperoxide synthase induced by human chorionic gonadotrophin in granulosa cells of rat preovulatory follicles. J Biol Chem 1992;267:6382-6388.
5. IARC Handbooks of Cancer Prevention. Volume 1 - Non-steroidal anti-inflammatory drugs. International Agency for Research on Cancer, Lyon, 1997.
6. Morgan G. Beneficial effects of NSAIDs in the gastrointestinal tract. Eur J Gastroenterol Hepatol 1999;11:393-400.
7. Langman MJS, Cheng KK, Gilman R, Lancashire RJ. Effect of anti-inflammatory drugs on overall risk of common cancer: case-control study in general practice research database. Br Med J 2000;320:1642-1646.
8. Lagergren J, Bergstrom R, Lindgren A, Nyren O. Symptomatic gastroesophageal reflux as a risk factor for esophageal adenocarcinoma. New Engl J Med 1999;340:825-831.
9. Mason J. NSAIDs and the oesophagus. Eur J Gastroenterol Hepatol 1999;11:369-373.
10. Fu S, Ramanujam KS, Meltzer SJ, Wilson KT. Expression and localisation of inducible nitric oxide synthase and cyclooxygenase-2 in Barrett's esophagus. Gastroenterology 1997;114(2):A565.
11. Shirvani VN, Ouatu-Lascar R, Kaur BS, Omary B, Triadafilopoulos G. Cyclooxygenase 2 expression in Barrett's esophagus and adenocarcinoma: ex vivo induction by bile salts and acid exposure. Gastroenterology 2000;118:487-496.
12. Zimmerman K, Sarbia M, Weber AA, Borchard F, Gabbert HE, Schror K. Cyclooxygenase-2 expression in human esophageal carcinoma. Cancer Res 1999;59:198-204.
13. Ratnasinghe D, Tangrea J, Roth MJ, Dawsey MJ, Hu N, Anver MN, Wang QH, Taylor PR. Expression of cyclooxygenase-2 in human squamous cell carcinoma of the esophagus; an immunohistochemical study. Anticancer Res 1999;19:171-174.
14. Oshima M, Dinchuk JE, Kargman SL, Oshima H, Hancock B, Kwong E. Suppression of intestinal polyposis in Apc knockout mice by inhibition of cyclooxygenase 2 (COX-2) Cell 1996;87:803-809.
15. Gottlieb S. COX-2 inhibitors might be useful in cancer prevention. Br Med J 1999;319:1155.

Should Barrett's patients undergo colorectal screening?

J. Lagergren (Stockholm)

In several case series [1-4], Barrett's esophagus has been linked to neoplasia of the colon. A high proportion of patients with Barrett's esophagus developed colon cancer in these series. A true association between Barrett's esophagus and colon neoplasia might give reason to recommend screening for colon cancer in patients with Barrett's esophagus as proposed in some reports [1-5]. However, the clinically detected cases of Barrett's esophagus represent the "tip of an iceberg" of a much larger pool of undetected prevalent cases [6] and there is an apparent risk of selection bias in the case series since the insidious symptoms of the developing colon neoplasia could increase the likelihood that the Barrett's esophagus will be diagnosed. Due to the strong link between esophageal adenocarcinoma and Barrett's esophagus, any association between Barrett's metaplasia and colon cancer should be reflected as an association also with esophageal adenocarcinoma. A study which compared esophageal adenocarcinoma and squamous cell carcinoma patients from cancer registers with regard to their lifetime history of colorectal cancer [5], showed a significant excess in the former group (but only in men). But this study was conditional on a sufficient length of survival after the colorectal cancer to develop esophageal cancer. With the case-control design approach used, the probability of important difference in survival after colon cancer in the subpopulations that generated the esophageal adenocarcinomas and squamous cell carcinomas, respectively, would result in a spurious difference in their association with colorectal cancer.

Results from more detailed and larger studies are in conflict with the positive findings. In three controlled studies, endoscopic examinations of all subjects failed to confirm an excess risk for colorectal adenoma in patients with Barrett's esophagus [7-9]. Furthermore, in a large cohort study, no increased risk of esophageal adenocarcinoma was found among patients with colon cancer [10].

In view of the relatively weak evidence of an association between Barrett's esophagus and colorectal cancer and the negative results in several larger studies, my opinion is that there is currently no need to recommend colorectal screening in Barrett patients.

References

1. Sontag SJ, Schnell TG, Chejfec G, et al. Barrett's oesophagus and colonic tumours. Lancet 1985;1:946-949.
2. Robertson DAF, Ayres RCS, Smith CL. Screening for colonic cancer in patients with Barrett's oesophagus. Br Med J 1989;298:650.
3. Kingston RD, Kiff RS, Walsh SH. Barrett's oesophagus and colonic cancer. Lancet 1988;1:63.
4. Howden CW, Hornung CA. A systematic review of the association between Barrett's esophagus and colon neoplasms. Am J Gastroenterol 1995;90:1814-1819.
5. Vaughan TL, Kiemeney LALM, McKnight B. Colorectal cancer in patients with esophageal adenocarcinoma. Cancer Epidemiol Biomark Prev 1995;4:93-97.
6. Cameron AJ, Zinsmeister AR, Ballard DJ, Carney JA. Prevalence of columnar-lined (Barrett's) esophagus. Gastroenterology 1990;99:918-922.
7. Laitikari R, Laippala P, Isolauri J. Barrett's esophagus is not a risk factor for colonic neoplasia: a case-control study. Ann Med 1995;27:499-502.
8. Cauvin JM, Goldfain D, Le Rhun M, et al. Multicentre prospective controlled study of Barrett's oesophagus and colorectal adenomas. Lancet 1995;346:1391-1394.

9. Poorman JC, Lieberman DA, Ippoliti AF, Weber LJ, Weinstein WM. The prevalence of colonic neoplasia in patients with Barrett's esophagus: prospective assessment in patients 50-80 years old. Am J Gastroenterol 1997;92:592-596.
10. Lagergren J, Nyrén O. No association between colonic cancer and adenocarcinoma of the oesophagus. A population-based cohort study in Sweden. Gut 1999;44:819-821.

Do the current data support that an endoscopic-biopsy surveillance program prevents or does not prevent cancer in Barrett's mucosa?

H.D. Appelman (Ann Arbor)

There is little doubt that:

- Barrett's mucosa has an increased risk for esophageal carcinoma compared to the squamous mucosa it replaced;
- the survival of patients with esophageal carcinoma is directly related to the stage of the carcinoma when it is first detected;
- adenocarcinomas are detected during surveillance programs that entail endoscopy and biopsy sampling;
- the carcinomas detected during surveillance for Barrett's mucosa are, as a group, of a lower stage than are the carcinomas that occur in patients whose Barrett's mucosa was never known prior to the development of the carcinoma [1];
- dysplasias, especially high-grade dysplasias (HGD), are the precursors of invasive carcinoma, or, if not the immediate precursors, then at least markers of esophagi at great risk for cancer development.

Although the studies of dysplasias in Barrett's mucosa often supply a reference for diagnostic criteria for both HGD and low-grade dysplasias, it is obvious to experienced pathologists that the published criteria are insufficient, and not all pathologists diagnoze these dysplasias in exactly the same ways using the same sets of criteria. Neither grade of dysplasia is a single histologic diagnostic entity, but each grade contains a group of mucosal abnormalities with slightly different individual histologic criteria. As a result, all the published studies of HGD and incipient cancers developing within such dysplasias may not be talking about the same patients. This is a critical realization.

With this last limitation in mind, the following information can be accepted as helpful, but the results of the published studies must be cautiously analyzed and accepted with even more caution.

If HGD is truly the cancer precursor, then treatment of HGD theoretically prevents cancers from developing. However, when HGD is the indication for esophagectomy, invasive carcinomas are discovered in about 40% of the resection specimens. (*Table I*) [1-9]. These unsuspected cancers are detected mainly at a low stage when they are more likely to be curable, but, obviously, surveillance did not prevent their development. As a result of finding these incidental cancers, the diagnosis of HGD, not invasive carcinoma, has

Table I. Prevalence of carcinoma in resections for biopsy proven high-grade dysplasia.

Author	Year	Biopsy protocol	#CA/#HGD
Pera * [2]	1992	Not stated	9/18
Cameron* [3]	1997	4 quads q 2cm	2/19
Peters [1]	1994	4 quads q 2 cm	5/9
van Sandick [4]	1998	Not stated	1/5
Heitmiller [5]	1996	Not stated	13/30
Altorki [6]	1991	Q 1-2 cm, NFS	3/8
Edwards [7]	1996	Not stated	8/11
Rice [8]	1993	Q 2 cm, NFS	6/16
Ferguson [9]	1997	Not stated	8/15
Totals as of 8/20			55/133 (41%)

* These two studies both came from the same institution, using 2 different patient groups
The Pera paper dealt with resected cases from 1982 through 1991, whereas the Cameron paper dealt with resected cases from 1992 through 1994

become the end-point of surveillance and the usual indication for treatment in many centers, whether that treatment is resection or ablation.

Therefore, it has seemed reasonable to suggest that surveillance in Barrett's mucosa is the best way not only to detect cancer precursors, but to detect cancers when they are likely to be of low stage and curable [10, 11].

To complicate matters, in some centers, the indication for esophagectomy is not HGD, but carcinoma invading the lamina propria [12, 13]. Those cases with only HGD are continued in the surveillance programs until cancer is found in biopsies. This approach was introduced because not all HGD progressed to invasive carcinoma. In such centers, it is obvious that surveillance does not prevent cancer. Instead it demands the presence of cancer for definitive treatment.

We do not know the risk of invasive carcinoma developing in a field of HGD. We supect that this risk is high, because of the large number of cases of coexisting cancer with HGD (*Table II*) lists the most recent studies that followed patients with HGD [12-17]. The follow-up periods are short, but even in such short periods, the overall incidence of adenocarcinoma developing after HGD was first discovered is about 25%. However some cancers are detected during surveillance without a pre-existing biopsy of HGD. It is possible that this resulted from an insufficiently extensive biopsy sampling of the Barrett's segment so that a pre-existing focus of HGD was missed.

We have a great deal of data concerning the incidence of carcinoma developing in Barrett's mucosa during surveillance, invariably given as the number of patient years of follow-up needed to detect a single cancer [14, 15, 18, 19]. However, we have much less information about the incidence of the different grades of dysplasia in the same setting.

The only way to answer the question about whether surveillance prevents cancer is to conduct a controlled study of Barrett's patients. As soon as the Barrett's is identified, half the patients would be entered into an endoscopic surveillance program with a fastidious biopsy protocol, and the other half would not be surveyed but would be contacted periodically to see how they are doing. The end point of surveillance and the indication for treatment would have to be something short of carcinoma, presumably HGD. The

Table II. Incidence of carcinoma developing during surveillance after biopsy proven high-grade dysplasia.

Author	Year	Biopsy protocol	#CA/#HGD	F-U period
Levine [12]	1996	6 each 1 cm	15/58	4-89 months
Schnell* [13]	1996	Not stated	4/24 (prevalent)	7.5 years mean
			4/18 (incident)	7.5 years mean
O'Connor [14]	1999	4 quads q 2 cm	0/5	Up to 3 years
Katz [15]	1998	4 quads q 2 cm	2/5	Up to 9 years
Iftikhar [16]	1992	4 quads q 2 cm	3/3	Not stated
Weston [17]	2000	4 quads q 1 cm	4/15 definite	12-91 months
			3/15 suspicious	
Totals			32/128 (25%)	

In all biopsy protocols that were defined, not only were these routine samples taken, but multiple samples were also taken of any endoscopic suspicious areas, such as lumps, ulcers, unusual mucosa

* The cases were divided into prevalent (those with HGD on first endoscopy and during the first year) and incident (those with HGD on subsequent biopsies

difference in the cancers developing in the non-surveyed group compared with the surveyed group would give us an indication of the value of surveillance in preventing cancers. At the moment, no such studies have been published. Instituting them would require huge numbers of patients followed for many years and it would be a problem to deny half these patients access to surveillance that may prevent cancer death [11]. Since we know that Barrett's mucosa has a cancer risk, we feel bound to put all patients on surveillance.

Perhaps we can get data from Barrett's mucosa comparable to the ulcerative colitis data. Most such ulcerative colitis studies have compared survival of colitic cancer patients on surveillance with those who were not on surveillance, but none of these studies were controlled. Most such studies indicate that surveillance of long standing colitics with regular colonoscopy and extensive biopsy sampling of flat mucosa and unusual polyps may not prevent colitic cancer, but it seems to diminish colitic cancer mortality [20, 21]. There have been several studies of Barrett's patients comparing the cancer stage and patient survival of those patients whose cancers presented at the time the Barrett's was found with those whose cancers are found during surveillance. Not surprisingly, the cancers detected during surveillance were of lower stage and were associated with far better survival than were the de novo cancers. However, this comparison is different than comparing cancers that develop with or without surveillance after the nondysplastic Barrett's is first found [1, 4].

It is problematic to use the colitic model in Barrett's mucosa for several reasons. First, ulcerative colitis, although a relatively common gastrointestinal disease, is not common in the general population, so the pool of patients is small. In contrast, Barrett's mucosa seems to be a common disease in the general population, so the pool of patients may be hugs. Second, the colitics are known because of the signs and symptoms of the disease. In contrast, we do not know who has Barrett's, since there are no signs or symptoms. They have reflux symptoms, just like many other people who don't have Barrett's. Third, it is rare for colitics to present for the first time with carcinoma. In contrast, most Barrett's cancers present with signs and symptoms of the cancers; the Barrett's is discovered at the same time when biopsies are taken from mucosa next to the cancers.

This question avoids other issues pertaining to surveillance, most important of which is cost effectiveness. The pool of Barrett's patients is very large, but the true extent is unknown. The risk of cancer is also unknown, but the reported incidence figures for surveillance vary greatly from 1 in about 50 years of follow-up to 1 in about 440 years, indicating that there are likely to be population differences. Furthermore, there is some data that suggests that the cancer risk is over-estimated, especially in the studies with smaller numbers of patients and fewer patient years of follow-up.

The original question that this brief discussion attempted to answer was: do the current data support that an endoscopic biopsy program prevents or does not prevent cancer in Barrett's mucosa? The answer is that we think we are preventing cancer through surveillance, but we have no facts to support this contention. When we resect for HGD discovered during surveillance, we find unsuspected invasive carcinomas about 40% of the time, so these were not prevented by surveillance. We have no idea how many of the other 60% of esophagi resected HGD would have developed invasive carcinomas had we left them *in situ*. At the centers that don't resect until invasive carcinoma is found, then it is obvious that surveillance didn't prevent cancer; surveillance only ended when the cancers developed.

References

1. Peters JH, Clark GWB, Ireland AP, et al. Outcome of adenocarcinoma arising in Barrett's esophagus in endoscopically surveyed and nonsurveyed patients. J Thorac Cardiovasc Surg. 1994;108:813-822.
2. Pera M, Trastek VF, Carpenter HA, et al. Barrett's esophagus with high-grade dysplasia: an indication for esophagectomy? Ann Thorac Surg 1992;54:199-204.
3. Cameron AJ, Carpenter HA. Barrett's esophagus, high-grade dysplasia, and early adenocarcinoma:a pathologic study. Am J Gastroenterol 1997;92:586-591.
4. Van Sandick JW, van Lanschot JJB, Kuiken BW, et al. Impact of endoscopic biopsy surveillance of Barrett's oesophagus on pathological stage and clinical outcome of Barrett's carcinoma. Gut 1998;43:216-222.
5. Heitmiller RF, Redmond M, Hamilton SR. Barrett's esophagus with high-grade dysplasia. An indication for prophylactic esophagectomy. Ann Surg 1996;224:66-71.
6. Altorki NK, Sunagawa M, Little AG, Skinner DB. High-grade dysplasia in the columnar-lined esophagus. Am J Surg 1991;161:97-99.
7. Edwards MJ, Gable DR, Lentsch AB, Richardson JD. The rationale for esophagectomy as the optimal therapy for Barrett's esophagus. Ann Surg 1996;223:585-589.
8. Rice TW, Falk GW, Achkar E, Petras RE. Surgical management of high-grade dysplasia in Barrett's esophagus. Am J Gastroenterol 1993;88:1832-1836.
9. Ferguson MK, Naunheim KS. Resection for Barrett's mucosa with high-grade dysplasia: implications for prophylactic photodynamic therapy. J Thorac Cardiovasc Surg 1997;114:824-829.
10. Ackroyd R, Wakefield SE, Williams JL, et al. Surveillance of Barrett's esophagus:a need for guidelines. Dis Esophagus 1997;10:185-189.
11. Tytgat GNJ. Barrett's esophagus: is it all that bad? Can J Gastroenterology 1999;13:385-388.
12. Levine DS, Haggitt RC, Irvine S, Reid BJ. Natural history of high-grade dysplasia in Barrett's esophagus. Gastroenterology 1996;110:A550.
13. Schnell T, Sontag SJ, Chejfec G, et al. High grade dysplasia is not an indication for surgery in patients with Barrett's esophagus. Gastroenterology 1996;110:A590.
14. O'Connor JB, Falk, GW, Richter JE. The incidence of adenocarcinoma and dysplasia in Barrett's esophagus. Report on the Cleveland Clinic Barrett's esophagus registry. Am J Gastroenterol 1999;94:2037-2042.
15. Katz D, Rothstein R, Schned A, et al. The development of dysplasia and adenocarcinoma during endoscopic surveillance of Barrett's esophagus. Am J Gastroenterol 1998;93:536-541.
16. Iftikhar SY, James PD, Steele RJC, et al. Length of Barrett's oesophagus:an important factor in the development of dysplasia and adenocarcinoma. Gut 1992;33:1155-1158.
17. Weston AP, Sharma P, Topalovski M, et al. Long-term follow-up of Barrett's high-grade dsyplasia. Am J Gastroenterol 2000;95:1888-1893.
18. Drewitz DJ, Sampliner RE, Garewal HS. The incidence of adenocarcinoma in Barrett's esophagus:a prospective study of 170 patients followed 4.8 years. Am J Gastroenterol 1997;92:212-215.

19. Streitz JM Jr, Ellis FH Jr, Tilden RL, Erickson RV. Endoscopic surveillance of Barrett's esophagus: a cost-effective comparison with mammographic surveillance for breast cancer. Am J Gastroenterol 1998;93:911-915.
20. Choi PM, Nugent FW, Schoetz DJ Jr, et al. Colonoscopic surveillance reduces mortality from colorectal cancer in ulcerative colitis. Gastroenterology 1993;105:418-425.
21. Giardiello FM, Gurbuz AK, Bayless TM, et al. Colorectal cancer in ulcerative colitis:survival in patients with and without colorectal cancer symptoms. Inflam Bowel Dis 1996;2:6-10.

What is the cost-effectiveness of long-term surveillance of Barrett's patients after antireflux surgery?

S.R. DeMeester (Los Angeles)

Rationale for surveillance endoscopy

In contrast to screening endoscopy, surveillance endoscopy is done in patients known to have Barrett's to follow-up their Barrett's. The rationale for endoscopic surveillance in patients with Barrett's is twofold: to detect progression of disease toward cancer, and to allow early intervention while cure is still likely. Inherent in this rationale is the necessity that the surveillance will be frequent enough that rarely, if ever, does the disease progress beyond an early, curable stage during the surveillance interval, and that once disease progression is detected an intervention is performed. Continued surveillance despite disease progression may help clarify the natural history of the disease, but does little to benefit the patient. Controversy exists, however, about the point at which there has been sufficient progression to warrant intervention, and what intervention should be done.

Provenzale *et al.* used a Markov model of decision analysis to demonstrate that aggressive endoscopic surveillance combined with esophagectomy for high-grade dysplasia (HGD) would markedly reduce the incidence of cancer in patients with Barrett's esophagus, and increase both overall and quality-adjusted life expectancy [1]. The predictions of the model have now been verified in several clinical series where patients with adenocarcinoma detected within a surveillance program were found to have earlier stage tumors and a significantly improved long-term survival following esophagectomy compared to patients who presented de novo with symptoms [2, 3]. However, the most important factor in determining both the impact and the cost-effectiveness of a surveillance program for Barrett's is the risk of adenocarcinoma in an individual patient with Barrett's esophagus. This number has been difficult to pin down, but most believe it to be in the range of 0.5-1% per year. A recent meta-analysis placed the risk at 0.5% per year, but this meta-analysis included groups of patients being followed after antireflux surgery, a procedure that increasingly is being shown to decrease the incidence of cancer in Barrett's patients [4, 5]. Consequently, inclusion of these postfundoplication patients in the meta-analysis likely falsely lowered the rate from what should be expected in a group of untreated or perhaps medically treated patients with Barrett's.

Cost of surveillance for Barrett's

The cost effectiveness of surveillance endoscopy for Barrett's has recently been compared to mammography for the detection of breast cancer (*Table I*) [6]. The cost per cancer detected and the cost per patient cured was similar, but the cost per life-year saved was dramatically lower for surveillance endoscopy in Barrett's patients than mammography in women. This likely is because outside of a surveillance program esophageal cancer often presents in an advanced stage, and the clinical course is rapidly fatal. In contrast, the lag time between mammography and palpable detection of breast cancer is shorter, and the clinical course with breast cancer is often quite protracted.

Table I. Comparison of the cost of surveillance mammography for breast cancer to the cost of surveillance endoscopy for patients with Barrett's esophagus (data from [6]).

	Breast cancer/mammography	Barrett's esophagus/EGD
Cost per cancer detected	$ 54,513	$ 37,928
Cost per cure	$ 83,292	$ 83,340
Cost per life-year saved	$ 57,926	$ 4,151

Provenzale *et al.* recently reanalyzed the utility of screening in Barrett's patients again using the Markov model they had previously described [7]. They confirmed that surveillance for Barrett's had an incremental cost-utility ratio that compared favorably with other common medical practices such as mammography for breast cancer. In their analysis the two critical parameters for decisions about surveillance were the incidence of cancer and the quality of life after esophagectomy. They found that if the incidence of cancer is 1% then surveillance every 2 years provides the greatest gain in quality-adjusted life expectancy. However, the model also pointed out that the benefits of surveillance are lost if there is a high operative mortality and poor quality of life associated with esophagectomy. Consequently, it is imperative that patients with HGD and early esophageal adenocarcinoma found in Barrett's surveillance programs be treated at centers experienced with esophageal surgery in order to realize the benefits of surveillance. One last consideration is that this analysis did not take into consideration new techniques such as photodynamic therapy and endoscopic mucosal resection that may be useful for treating some patients with HGD or early malignancy. It is likely that these procedures will also impact the overall assessment of cost effectiveness for surveillance in patients with Barrett's esophagus, and new analyses should be done taking these options into consideration as more long-term efficacy data becomes available.

Surveillance frequency and risk factors for Barrett's progression

The recommended frequency for endoscopic surveillance in Barrett's patients is based upon available data about the likelihood of progression to cancer, and the risks associated with the surveillance procedure. Currently the most important identifiable risk factor for progression to cancer is the presence of dysplasia within the Barrett's mucosa. Patients with low-grade dysplasia (LGD) are one step closer to cancer, and LGD can rapidly progress to HGD and cancer in some patients. Consequently, it is recommended that patients with LGD undergo more frequent surveillance, generally every 6 months, for at least the first year [8].

An important area of investigation is focused on identifying particular risk factors for progression in patients with Barrett's to better define the population that would benefit most from surveillance endoscopy. Reid *et al.* have used flow cytometry to augment histology and further stratify the risk of progression to cancer in patients with Barrett's with and without dysplasia [9]. They found that both aneuploidy and increased 4N fractions were associated with an increased incidence of esophageal adenocarcinoma in those patients with histology showing negative, indefinite, or LGD. However, in patients with HGD the incidence of cancer was so high that flow cytometry did not further stratify patients in regards to risk of cancer. Based on their findings they suggested that in those patients without HGD and with no aneuploidy or increased 4N on flow cytometry, surveillance endoscopy intervals could be lengthened to as much as 5 years apart. Conversely, patients with flow cytometry abnormalities or HGD are at significant risk for esophageal adenocarcinoma and should be watched closely.

Recent papers by Weston *et al.* have explored the factors associated with persistence of intestinal metaplasia (IM) and a poor outcome with medical therapy for Barrett's [10, 11]. They defined a poor outcome as progression to HGD or cancer. The three factors significantly associated with progression on medical therapy were: dysplasia at diagnosis or during follow-up ($p < 0.03$), a hiatal hernia ≥ 3cm in size ($p < 0.02$), and an increasing length of Barrett's > 2 cm ($p = 0.009$). They noted that proton pump inhibitor (PPI) use was not associated with a risk for poor outcome; however, they divided patients taking PPIs into 3 groups depending on whether they took a PPI *qd, bid*, or with cisapride. Had they compared any use of a PPI to only H_2-blocker use they would have noted that 0/38 patients on H_2-blockers had a poor outcome compared to 10/70 using a PPI ($p = 0.036$ by chi-square). The obvious conclusion is that those patients on PPIs have worse disease and thus a greater risk for a poor outcome on medical therapy, and that is exactly the point. These Barrett's patients, like those with dysplasia, large hernias, and long-segments of IM, should be treated with antireflux surgery rather than acid-suppression.

Previously it was also felt that the length of IM represented a risk factor for the likelihood of progression to cancer. Intuitively it makes sense that since longer segments of IM have more mucosa at risk for progression, the incidence of cancer should be higher in these patients than it is in those with short segment Barrett's. However, a recent manuscript by Rudolph *et al.* found that there was no significant difference in the risk of developing cancer for long *versus* short segments of Barrett's [12]. Consequently, we advise our patients with any length of IM within the esophagus to undergo surveillance endoscopy, and do not alter the surveillance interval based on the length of Barrett's.

A final issue in regard to surveillance endoscopy is the safety of the procedure. Recently Levine *et al.* reviewed the University of Washington experience after 1,458 endoscopies with a total of 50,833 biopsies in 705 patients with Barrett's over a 15-year period [13]. There were no deaths, and although the overall complication rate was 1.6%, most were minor and self-limited.

Current practice in regards to surveillance for Barrett's

A recent survey of practice patterns for Barrett's surveillance among gastroenterologists in the US by Falk *et al.* found that while the concept of surveillance was widely embraced, there was considerable variation in techniques and intervals for the surveillance [14]. They reported that 98% of community physicians and 89% of academic physicians practiced surveillance for their patients with Barrett's. One concern, though, is that the response rate for the survey was only 45%. Consequently the results may have been skewed in that clinicians with an interest in Barrett's were more likely to complete the survey, and were also more likely to recommend surveillance. Evidence for this possibility comes from Patti *et al.* They questioned patients with Barrett's who were being evaluated for antireflux surgery and found that only 62% had undergone surveillance endoscopy after their diagnosis of Barrett's [15]. Gross *et al.* also reported a survey of practice patterns for Barrett's surveillance in the United States [16]. They found that most gastroenterologists (66%) agreed that surveillance was an effective way of detecting adenocarcinoma at an early, curable stage. However, they found that physicians who were reimbursed mainly on a fee-for-service basis were 2.5 times more likely to recommend aggressive surveillance than were physicians reimbursed through other mechanisms. This finding held true despite adjusting for the age of the physicians, patient volume, and perceived risk of cancer. They concluded that there could be strong non-clinical factors that influence physician management of patients with Barrett's.

It has been our practice to recommend yearly surveillance endoscopy and biopsy to all patients with Barrett's, regardless of length. We increase the frequency to every 6 months for patients with LGD, and generally recommend esophagectomy for patients with HGD. Sampliner and the Practice Parameters Committee of the American College of Gastroenterology have recently suggested that surveillance may be extended to every 2-3 years in Barrett's patients without dysplasia on biopsies from two annual endoscopies [8]. For patients with LGD they recommend that surveillance endoscopy be performed at 6-monthly intervals for the first year, and subsequently done yearly if there has been no change.

While there is increasing evidence that an antireflux operation alters the natural history of Barrett's, there is insufficient evidence to identify a point at which surveillance endoscopy no longer is necessary. Available data would certainly suggest that surveillance should be done routinely for the first 5 years, as it seems that this is the real risk period for patients with a functioning fundoplication. Additionally, the presence of recurrent symptoms or documented failure of the fundoplication would mandate continued surveillance endoscopy. Hopefully as more data become available about the risk of progression after antireflux surgery a point will be determined at which surveillance is no longer necessary in patients with a functioning fundoplication.

References

1. Provenzale D, Kemp JA, Arora S, Wong JB. A guide for surveillance of patients with Barrett's esophagus. Am J Gastroenterol 1994;89:670-680.
2. Peters JH, Clark GW, Ireland AP, Chandrasoma P, Smyrk TC, DeMeester TR. Outcome of adenocarcinoma arising in Barrett's esophagus in endoscopically surveyed and nonsurveyed patients. J Thorac Cardiovasc Surg 1994;108:813-822.

3. van Sandick JW, van Lanschot JJB, Kuiken BW, Tytgat GNJ, Offerhaus GJA, Obertop H. Impact of endoscopic biopsy surveillance of Barrett's oesophagus on pathological stage and clinical outcome of Barrett's carcinoma. Gut 1998;43:216-222.
4. Shaheen NJ, Crosby MA, Bozymski EM, Sandler RS. Is there publication bias in the reporting of cancer risk in Barrett's esophagus? Gastroenterology 2000;119(2):333-338. Comment in Gastroenterology 2000;119(2):587-589.
5. DeMeester SR, DeMeester TR. Columnar mucosa and intestinal metaplasia of the esophagus: fifty years of controversy. Ann Surg 2000;231:303-321.
6. Streitz JM Jr, Ellis FH Jr, Tilden RL, Erickson RV. Endoscopic surveillance of Barrett's esophagus: a cost-effectiveness comparison with mammographic surveillance for breast cancer. Am J Gastroenterol 1998;93:911-915.
7. Provenzale D, Schmitt C, Wong JB. Barrett's esophagus: a new look at surveillance based on emerging estimates of cancer risk. Am J Gastroenterol 1999;94(8):2043-2053.
8. Sampliner RE. Practice guidelines on the diagnosis, surveillance, and therapy of Barrett's esophagus. The Practice Parameters Committee of the American College of Gastroenterology. Am J Gastroenterol 1998;93:1028-1032.
9. Reid BJ, Levine DS, Longton G, Blount PL, Rabinovitch PS. Predictors of progression to cancer in Barrett's esophagus: baseline histology and flow cytometry identify low- and high-risk patient subsets. Am J Gastroenterol 2000;95(7):1669-1676.
10. Weston AP, Badr AS, Hassanein RS. Prospective multivariate analysis of factors predictive of complete regression of Barrett's esophagus. Am J Gastroenterol 1999;94:3420-3426. Comment in Am J Gastroenterol 1999;94(12):3395-3396.
11. Weston AP, Badr AS, Hassanein RS. Prospective multivariate analysis of clinical, endoscopic, and histological factors predictive of the development of Barrett's multifocal high-grade dysplasia or adenocarcinoma. Am J Gastroenterol 1999;94:3413-3419. Comment in Am J Gastroenterol 1999;94(12):3395-3396.
12. Rudolph RE, Vaughan TL, Storer BE, Haggitt RC, Rabinovitch PS, Levine DS, Reid BJ. Effect of segment length on risk for neoplastic progression in patients with Barrett esophagus. Ann Intern Med 2000;132(8):612-620.
13. Levine DS, Blount PL, Rudolph RE, Reid BJ. Safety of a systematic endoscopic biopsy protocol in patients with Barrett's esophagus. Am J Gastroenterol 2000;95(5),:1152-1157.
14. Falk GW, Ours TM, Richter JE. Practice patterns for surveillance of Barrett's esophagus in the united states. Gastrointest Endosc 2000;52(2):197-203.
15. Patti MG, Arcerito M, Feo CV, Worth S, De Pinto M, Gibbs VC, Gantert W, Tyrrell D, Ferrell LF, Way LW. Barrett's esophagus: a surgical disease. J Gastrointest Surg 1999;3(4):397-404.
16. Gross CP, Canto MI, Hixson J, Powe NR. Management of Barrett's esophagus: a national study of practice patterns and their cost implications.Am J Gastroenterol 1999;94(12):3440-3447.

Regression

What factors can predict progression and regression of Barrett's esophagus?

A.P. Weston (Kansas City)

The risk of malignant transformation of Barrett's esophagus has been reported to vary between 1 of 46 to 1 of 441 patient years. However, the vast majority of Barrett's patients do not undergo malignant progression, but die from unrelated diseases. Identification of simple, easily attainable, non-cumbersome clinical, endoscopic, histologic and molecular features that could accurately predict the development of Barrett's adenocarcinoma (*i.e.* risk stratification), thereby provide a guide for the timing of surveillance examinations, would be of tremendous utility in this era of medical cost containment. Likewise, understanding what features/factors of Barrett's predict complete endoscopic and histogic regression, would again provide valuable information for timing of surveillance intervals and reassurance to both the patient and health care professionals of a healthy outcome.

Barrett's progression

Factors that have been associated with esophageal adenocarcinoma and or progression of Barrett's to Barrett's adenocarcinoma include (*Table I*).

Barrett's regression and normalization: spontaneous

Barrett's has been rarely reported to undergo complete regression after successful antireflux surgery. Incomplete Barrett's regression with appearance of squamous islands and

Table I. Factors associated with esophageal adenocarcinoma and or progression of Barrett's to Barrett's adenocarcinoma

Epidemiologic	
Body mass index (BMI)	High (IV quartile)
Body somatotype	Obese
Weight gain	> 46 lbs after age 20
Diet	Lack of Vitamin C rich cruciferous vegetables Low fiber intake Decreased selenium
Smoking	Yes
Alcohol	Mixed results; possibly hard liquor
Gender	Men
Race	Caucasian
Age	Older
GERD symptoms	Duration (longer), frequency and severity
Endoscopic	
Barrett's length	Longer lengths
Hiatal hernia	Yes, especially those > 2 cm
Barrett's ulcer	Possibly
Histologic	
Dysplasia	Any dysplasia, especially high-grade at index diagnosis and anytime during surveillance
Helicobacter pylori	Absence, especially PAI/CAG +
Flow cytometry	aneuploidy, increased G2/tetraploid
Molecular genetics	p53 overexpression (IHC) and gene mutations LOH of 17p and 9p CDKN2A (p16) gene mutations

downward extension and broadening of squamous tongues is far more common occurrence and has been noted after antireflux surgery as well as with long-term continuous proton pump inhibitor treatment. The histogenesis of Barrett's esophagus has been shown to involve the replacement of damaged squamous epithelium by creeping extensions of cardiac-junctional type mucosa within which over time and with persistent inflammation, focal areas of intestinal metaplasia (IM) evolve. Progressively greater amounts of IM within the tubular esophagus develop. Barrett's regression is also a stepwise process, with specialized columnar epithelium being replaced by junctional epithelium concurrent with decreased gastric mucosa surface area within the tubular esophagus. Over prolonged periods of time the junctional epithelium is replaced by squamous tissue. Evidence for this step-wise, progressive endoscopic and histologic regression was initially reported by our center in 1997. In 50% (13 of 26) of Barrett's esophagus patients with 2 cm or less of specialized epithelium complete absence of goblet cells was noted (only junctional epithelium) during prospective follow up averaging 18.6 months. These findings have also been confirmed and expanded upon by the RK Wong and his Walter Reed Army Medical Center group with their findings updated at DDW 2000. The incidence of mucosal normalization (defined here as loss of specialized columnar epithelium) as well as decrease in Barrett's esophagus length was examined in a cohort of 71 patients, 30 with esophagogastric junction-specialized intestinal metaplasia (EGJ-SIM), 31 with short segment Barrett's esophagus (SSBE) and 10 with long segment Barrett's esophagus (LSBE). A significantly greater loss of specialized epithelium was noted for EGJ-SIM 21/30 or 70% *versus* SSBE 12/31 or 39% *versus* LSBE 1/10 or 10% ($p = 0.04$). Multivariate analysis showed that this normalization was significantly associated with shorter Barrett's lengths, lack of hiatal hernia (HH), and female gender.

Complete spontaneous Barrett's regression has recently been examined prospectively by Weston *et al.* in which 99 patients with Barrett's esophagus were followed for a minimum of 2 years (mean of 48.0 months). Overall, 7 (7.1%) of Barrett's patients had complete regression of their Barrett's esophagus. Univariate and stepwise logistic regression analysis showed that complete regression was associated with absence of HH. Re-examination of the multivariate analysis by examining only HH (present yes *versus* no) and length of Barrett's (< 6 cm *versus* > 6 cm) revealed that both HH ($p = 0.0447$) and length of Barrett's ($p = 0.0418$) were predictive of complete regression. The observed probability of complete regression was inversely related to increasing HH size: 0% probability in patients with large HH (size > 6 cm), 4.3% for small and medium sized (between 1 cm and 5 cm) and 10% with no HH.

Literature

1. Barrett MT, Sanches CA, Prevo LJ, et al. Evolution of neoplastic cell lineages in Barrett's oesophagus. Nat Genet 1999;22:106-109.
2. Reid BJ, Blount PL, Rubin CE, et al. Flow-cytometric and histological progression to malignancy in Barrett's esophagus: prospective endoscopic surveillance of a cohort. Gastroenterology 1992;102:1212-1219.
3. Weston AP, Badr AS, Hassaneni RS. Prospective multivariate anlaysis of factors predictive of complete regression of Barrett's esophagus. Am J Gastroenterol 199;94:3420-3426.
4. Lagergren J, Bergstrom R, Nyren O. Association between body mass and adenocarcinoma of the esophagus and gastric cardia. Ann Inter Med 1999;130:883-890.
5. Chow WH, Frinkle WD, McLaughlin JK, et al. The relation of gastroesophageal reflux disease and its treatment to adenocarcinomas of the esophagus and gastric cardia. JAMA 1995;274:474-477.
6. Rudolph RE, Vaughan TL, Storer BE, et al. Effect of segment length on risk for neoplastic progression in patients with Barrett's esophagus. Ann Intern Med 2000;132:612-620.
7. Weston AP, Badr AS, Hassanein RS. Prospective multivariate analysis of clinical, endoscopi and histologic factors predictive of the development of Barrett's multifocal high-grade dysplasia or adenocarcinoma. Am J Gastroenterol 1999;94:3413-3419.
8. Younes M, Ertan A, Lechago LV, et al. p53 protein accumulation is a specific marker of malignant potential in Barrett's metaoplasia. Dig Dis Sci 1997;42:697-701.
9. Weston AP, Banerjee SK, Persons DL, et al. p53 positivity in low-grade dysplasia (LGD) in Barrett's esophagus: marker predictive of progression to cancer or multifocal high-grade dysplasia. Am J Gastroenterol 1999;94(9):2603.
10. Horwhat JD, Baroni D, Maydonovitch C, et al. The incidence of regression and normalization of intestinal metaplasia in a cohort of patients with EGJ-SIM, SSBE and LSBE followed over 3 years. Gastroenterology 2000;118:A224.

What are the problems related to interpretation of "regression"?

R.E. Sampliner (Tucson)

What is regression?

Regression of Barrett's esophagus has been interpreted in many different ways: decrease in the length of Barrett's esophagus documented at endoscopy, decrease in the surface area, appearance of squamous islands in Barrett's esophagus. All of the above are approximations of what would really be desirable, *i.e.* the complete elimination of intestinal metaplasia (IM). Many assessments of the length of Barrett's esophagus in patients on standard or high dose proton pump inhibitor therapy over intervals of up to 6 years have shown little change in the length of Barrett's esophagus with the exception of a few patients who reportedly have had their Barrett's esophagus resolve [1-5]. Perhaps the methodologically strongest study evaluated 26 patients on 2 years of omeprazole 40 mg bid [4]. One of the strengths of this study is that it was controlled with 24-hour pH with a mean value of 0.1% of a 24 hour period with a pH less than 4. Even with this rigorous intraesophageal acid control, there was only an 8% decrease in the surface area of Barrett's esophagus. This measurement considered squamous islands as non-Barrett's which is not always accurate (see below). Although the 8% decrease was judged to be significant, this limited amount of regression of Barrett's esophagus from a clinical perspective is not impressive.

One of the caveats of "regression" is that it has been recognized that many patients with squamous islands have IM underlying the squamous epithelium by biopsy [6]. Although these islands have been interpreted as regression, they may represent just surface remodeling as long as there is residual IM underneath. The dilemma of regression of Barrett's as judged by squamous islands is highlighted in a case of a 58 year old man who had high-grade dysplasia and received a fundoplication. He was then subsequently treated with a proton pump inhibitor (PPI) for 4 years. He presented with respiratory failure due to herniation of his stomach into his chest. At esophagogastrectomy, intramucosal cancer was recognized to underly squamous epithelium in the area of his Barrett's esophagus [7].

Many modalities of endoscopic therapy have been used in an effort to ablate Barrett's esophagus [8]. In this context there is a clear functional definition of reversal. Endoscopically, reversal means there is no visual evidence of Barrett's esophagus. The visual sensitivity can be enhanced with Lugol's stain in the setting of a non-inflammatory esophagus [9]. Any area that fails to stain with Lugol's may represent residual IM. Additionally, reversal has to be documented histologically - at a minimum this would require 4-quadrant large capacity biopsies every 2 cm to document the lack of IM. Unfortunately, there is one patient from a multipolar electrocoagulation trial that ended up with an esophagectomy which in fact documented no residual IM in the specimen [10].

Regression with multipolar electrocoagulation

One of the modalities of endoscopic therapy that has been utilized in an effort to reverse Barrett's esophagus is multipolar electrocoagulation. Rather than reviewing all the trials, the focus will be on two large experiences.

Reversal therapy is a combination of acid reduction and endoscopic destruction of Barrett's epithelium. The acid reduction is typically accomplished with PPI therapy but can also be accomplished with fundoplication. In a multicenter trial using electrocautery plus omeprazole 40 mg bid, 58 patients with Barrett's 2-6cm in length were treated for reversal [11]. Six months after the last treatment session 85% of patients had no endoscopic evidence of Barrett's including Lugol's staining and 78% had no endoscopic nor histologic evidence of Barrett's esophagus utilizing large capacity 4-quadrant biopsies every 2 cm. In a larger trial 168 patients with Barrett's esophagus were followed a mean of 37 months after electrocautery therapy [12]. Patients were treated with lansoprazole 60 mg daily. Eighty-nine percent had short segment Barrett's esophagus and all were non-dysplastic. There was reversal of Barrett's esophagus in all patients. In 11 patients who stopped their PPI, recurrent short tongues of Barrett's were recognized. Only 3 patients in this trial had underlying IM.

In each of the above trials one patient developed a stricture requiring dilation. One patient required overnight hospitalization for chest pain management. This procedure was readily accomplished in a ambulatory setting.

The rate of squamous epithelialization of Barrett's esophagus can be over 70%. There is still a concern about standardization of the endoscopic technique as well as standardization of the documentation of reversal of Barrett's esophagus. The durability of the new epithelium is also a major issue, although in many patients the squamous epithelium is present beyond 3 years [12, 13]. IM can be recognized under squamous epithelium. Whether this represents recurrence or a sampling problem is not clear. The squamous epithelium may have been there all along but just recognized in one biopsy from an extensive biopsy protocol on a particular endoscopy.

Biologic studies have been performed in patients with reversal of Barrett's esophagus. In one trial of 11 patients, 4 with low-grade dysplasia had no residual dysplasia after therapy [14]. Ki-67, a marker of proliferation, was normally located only basally in the new squamous epithelium. By immunohistochemistry, no p53 mutations were recognized in the new Barrett's epithelium. Additionally, ornithine decarboxylase, the rate limiting step in protein metabolism, was at a lower level in the squamous epithelium as expected, in contrast to the usually elevated level in Barrett's esophagus. In contrast to the finding of the new squamous epithelium after endoscopic therapy, squamous islands after prolonged PPI therapy demonstrated multilayer Ki-67 staining in more than half of the tested patients [14].

In summary, the endoscopic and histologic criteria for reversal in the setting of endoscopic ablation can also serve to standardize and objectify the criteria for regression of Barrett's esophagus.

References

1. Malesci A, Savarino V, Ventilin P, et al. Partial regression of Barrett's esophagus by long-term therapy with high dose omeprazole. Gastrointest Endosc 1996;44:700-705.
2. Sharma P, Sampliner R, Camargo E. Normalization of esophageal pH with high dose proton pump inhibitor therapy does not result in regression of Barrett's esophagus. Am J Gastroenterol 1997;92:582-585.
3. Cooper B, Neumann C, Cox M, Iqbal T. Continuous treatment with oemprazole 20 mg daily for up to 6 years in Barrett's oesophagus. Aliment Pharmacol Ther 1998;12:893-897.
4. Peters F, Ganesh S, Kuipers E, et al. Endoscopic regression of Barrett's oesophagus during omeprazole treatment: a randomized double blind study. Gut 1999;45:489-494.
5. Wilkinson S, Biddlestone L, Gore S, Shepherd N. Regression of columnar lined (Barrett's) oesophagus with omeprazole 40mg daily: results of 5 years of continuous therapy. Aliment Pharmacol Ther 1999;13:1205-1209.
6. Sharma P, Morales T, Bhattacharyya A, Garewal H, Sampliner R. Squamous islands in Barrett's esophagus: what lies underneath? Am J Gasroenterol 1998;93:332-335.
7. Sampliner R, Fass R. Partial regression of Barrett's esophagus: an inadequate endpoint. Am J Gastroeneterol 1993;88:2092-2094.
8. Sampliner R. Ablative therapies for the columnar lined esophagus. Gastroenterol Clin North Am 1997;26:685-694.
9. Woolf G, Riddell R, Irvine E, Hunt R. A study to examine agreement between endoscopy and histology for the diagnosis of columnar lined (Barrett's) esophagus. Gastrointest Endosc 1989;35:541-544.
10. Fennerty M, Corless C, Sheppard B, Faigel D, Lieberman D, Sampliner R. Pathological documentation of complete elimination of Barrett's metaplasia following endoscopic multipolar electrocoagulation therapy. Gut 2001;49:142-144.
11. Sampliner R, Faigel D, Fennerty M, et al. Effective and safe endoscopic reversal of nondysplastic Barrett's esophagus with thermal electrocoagulation combined with high-dose acid inhibition: a multicenter study. Gastrointest Endosc 2001;53:554-558.
12. Guelrud M, Herrera I, Essenfeld H. Long term results of multipolar electrocoagulation therapy for Barrett's esophagus. Gastrointest Endosc 2001;53:AB72.
13. Sharma P, Bhattacharyya A, Garewal H, Sampliner R. Durability of new squamous epithelium following endoscopic reversal of Barrett's esophagus. Gastrointest Endosc 1999;50(2):159-164.
14. Garewal H, Ramsey L, Sharma P, Kraus K, Sampliner R, Fass R. Biomarker studies in reversed Barrett's esophagus. Am J Gastrenterol 1999;94:2829-2833.

What is the average length of follow-up necessary to document regression of Barrett's esophagus?

I.G. Martin (Auckland)

The issues surrounding the regression of Barrett's esophagus are all controversial. This section deals with one aspect of this controversy, the time scales involved. Potentially, regression can occur in two settings, firstly following effective medical or surgical treatment and secondly after ablative therapy aimed at removing the metaplastic mucosa allowing squamous regeneration in a reflux free environment. The question itself has two components. Firstly, how rapidly does regression, if it should occur, happen after antireflux therapy and secondly following ablation therapy, how long do you have to follow-up patients for, to confidently state the Barrett's has been successfully removed.

Time course of changes in the extent of Barrett's esophagus following medical therapy

It has to be stated that complete regression of Barrett's esophagus is very rarely seen after even the most effective treatment with proton pump inhibitor (PPI) treatment [1]. Very few studies have looked at the time course of changes in the extent of Barrett's esophagus. In what is probably the most detailed study in this area, Peters *et al.* demonstrated a small but significant reductions both in the area and length of Barrett's esophagus in patients on PPI therapy. There were slow and with the passage of time decreases in the total area of Barrett's mucosa, with a mean reduction of some 8% at 24 months of follow-up. In this study no patient showed complete regression. The extent of the Barrett's esophagus seemed to decrease consistently throughout the 24 months of the study and it may be that a longer period of follow-up would have shown greater decreases in the extent of the Barrett's esophagus.

However, the endoscopic finding that accounts for most of the reductions in area seen are squamous islands. If these islands are biopsied, then in around 40% of cases Barrett's mucosa will be found [2]. This "buried" glandular mucosa is susceptible to neoplastic change and therefore this finding calls into question the whole concept that regression can be quantified by macroscopic findings of squamous re-epithelialization.

It is currently impossible to give any further details regarding the time course of changes in the extent of Barrett's esophagus.

Time course of changes in the extent of Barrett's esophagus following surgical therapy

There is limited evidence that surgery can induce apparent regression in a number of patients with Barrett's esophagus. A small number of patients will have endoscopic complete regression following surgery. However the data is patchy and few if any studies have adequately looked at the issue of growth of squamous mucosa over glandular Barrett's epithelia. Published studies, recently reviewed by both Haag [1] and DeMeester [3], are very heterogenous in both quality and results. The studies followed patients for between 3 months and 12 years. On the basis of these studies it is not possible to comment on the time course of any regression after surgical treatment.

What of ablation treatments?

Ablation therapies aim to remove the Barrett's mucosa and allow regeneration of a squamous mucosa within a reflux free environment. A variety of options have been studied including:
- laser ablation,
- argon beam ablation,
- photodynamic therapy,
- multipolar electrocoagulation,
- heater probe.

Within the published studies, macroscopic complete regression has been reported in between 30 and 100% of patients. However, when biopsies have been taken from the neo-squamous epithelium, glandular Barrett's mucosa can be found in up to 50% of cases. This mucosa can also progress through to dysplasia [4] and potentially carcinoma.

There is insufficient data to answer the question, how long do you have to follow a patient to be certain that the Barrett's esophagus has remained in remission following ablative therapy. Certainly macroscopic appearances alone are insufficient to answer this question and biopsies must be taken for histological evaluation. The published studies have relatively short follow-up periods (averaging less than 12 months) and as such do not help to answer the question.

Summary

From the literature base available to us currently, we cannot with any degree of precision answer the question. Barrett's esophagus probably progresses relatively slowly in it primary state and therefore after therapies aimed at ablation we should follow our patients for at least 5 years.

References

1. Haag S, Nandurkar S, Talley NJ. Regression of Barrett's esophagus: the role of acid suppression, surgery, and ablative methods. Gastrointestinal Endosc 1999;50(2):229-240.
2. Sharma P, Morales TG, Bhattacharyya A, Garewal HS, Sampliner RE. Squamous islands in Barrett's esophagus: what lies underneath? Am J Gastroenterol 1998;93(3):332-335.
3. DeMeester SR, DeMeester TR. Columnar mucosa and intestinal metaplasia of the esophagus:fifty years of controversy. Ann Surg 2000;231(3):303-321.
4. Michopoulos S, Tsibouris P, Bouzakis H, Sotiropolou M, Kralios M. Complete regression of Barrett's oesophagus with heater probe thermocoagulation; up to three years follow-up. Gastrointestinal Endosc 1999;50:165-172.

Is regression of *short segments* Barrett's esophagus likely to occur under treatment?

R.K.H. Wong (Washington)

The prevalence of short segments Barrett's esophagus (SSBE) ranges between 5-36% depending upon how many biopsies of the columnar segment are taken, the type of histologic stain employed, and the length of the tongue biopsied. Patients accessioned into SSBE studies had upper gastrointestinal symptoms requiring endoscopy and were not normal controls. The majority of patients were on some form of acid suppressive agent, mainly H_2-receptor antagonists or proton pump inhibitors. None of the long-term studies have standard antisecretory therapy with most patients being treated symptomatically.

The term regression can be viewed in several ways:

- actual movement of columnar epithelium distally either by actual regression of specialized intestinal metaplasia (IM) or by overgrowth of squamous epithelium,
- normalization of the specialized IM to either fundic or cardiac mucosa where biopsies no longer show evidence of goblet cells.

With SSBE, proving linear regression and overgrowth with squamous epithelium is difficult, as the maximal length of a tongue is only 3 cms. Quantitating regression is only possible if:

- tattooing is performed at the upper margin of the tongue and the squamous epithelium has overgrown the tattoo,
- there are no visible tongues,
- or a 3 cm tongue regresses to less than 1 cm.

Normalization of specialized IM to mucosa without goblet cells is the more likely scenario. One can always contend that normalization does not occur in SSBE and that specialized IM was missed. Unless the entire columnar mucosa in question is completely stripped and sectioned for histologic confirmation, this criticism can never be fully addressed. On the other hand, one must remember that more biopsies are usually taken in a relatively small area of SSBE in subsequent follow-up endoscopies and hence it would be less likely to miss specialized IM.

Only 3 studies in the literature have followed SSBE patients overtime and have reported a lack of goblet cells on incident biopsy specimens. In one study by Weston *et al.* [1], 50% (13/26) of patients with SSBE who underwent multiple esophagogastric diseases and histologic sampling had no evidence of specialized IM. Of these patients, one had no specialized IM on 3 exams and 3 patients had no specialized IM on 2 exams. This was in contrast to the long segment Barrett's esophagus (LSBE) cohort in which few or non of the patients studied showed any normalization to a non-specialized IM histology.

Horwhat *et al.* [2], noted that 30% (13/44) of SSBE patients underwent normalization over a 3-4 year period. In contradistinction, none of the LSBE patients showed normalization of histology while 67% (23/43) of esophagogastric junction-specialized IM (EGJ-SIM) patients underwent normalization. There was also a slight decrement in the length of Barrett's epithelium of 0.4 cm for SSBE, 1.3 cm for LSBE and a slight increase in length in the columnar length for EGJ-SIM.

After 9 months of intensive acid suppression (pH > 4, as documented by 24 hour-pH monitoring), Hirota *et al.* [3] noted a 42% (5/12) normalization of SSBE (n = 8) and EGJ-SIM (n = 4) tissue.

These data suggest that normalization and possibly regression of SSBE may occur with treatment over time. This data is also consistent with the pathophysiology of these disease processes. With LSBE there is extensive, prolonged acid exposure in the esophagus and a higher degree of dysplasia, cancer and molecular gene alterations. In SSBE, acid exposure is not as prolonged and the prevalence of dysplasia and cancer is significantly lower. With possible fewer gene alterations in the SSBE mucosa, the specialized IM in SSBE and EGJ-SIM may be more reversible with acid suppressive therapy.

References

1. Weston AP, Krmpotich PT, Cherian R, Dixon A, Topalosvki M. Prospective long-term endoscopic and histological follow-up of short segment Barrett's esophagus: comparison with traditional long segment Barrett's esophagus. Am J Gastroenterol 1997;92:407-413.
2. Horwhat JD, Baroni D, Maydonovitch C, Osgard EM, Ormseth EJ, Rueda-Pedraza, E, Yang H, Hirota W, Wong RKH. The incidence of regression and normalization of intestinal metaplasia in a cohort of patients with EGJ-SIM, SSBE and LSBE followed over 3 years. Gastroenterology 2000;118(4):A1350.
3. Hirota WK, Loughney TM, Lazas DJ, Maydonovitch CL, Rholl V, Wong RKH. Short segment Barrett's esophagus and specialized intestinal metaplasia at the esophagogastric junction: serial endoscopic and histologic assessment after acid suppression with omeprazole. Gastroenterology 1997;112(4) A577.

Can complete regression of Barrett's mucosa and dysplasia occur under long-term treatment with proton pump inhibitors?

F.T.M. Peters, E.J. Kuipers, E.C. Klinkenberg-Knol
(Groningen, Rotterdam)

The treatment of Barrett's esophagus is aimed at several different targets which include symptom relief, healing of esophagitis, and ultimately prevention of long-term complications such as peptic stenosis. These objectives are nowadays well achieved by medical acid suppression using either H_2-blocking agents or preferentially proton pump inhibitors (PPI), and by antireflux surgery. In these aspects Barrett's esophagus is not essentially different from gastroesophageal reflux disease (GERD) in general. However, whether or not profound acid suppressive therapy also has a preventive effect on the long-term complications of Barrett's esophagus, in particular the development of dysplasia and adenocarcinoma is still under debate. The risk for esophageal adenocarcinoma in Barrett patients correlates with the severity of GERD, the length of the Barrett segment, and the local presence of dysplastic intestinal metaplasia (IM). This cancer risk might therefore be decreased by reduction of the length of the Barrett segment, preferentially leading to complete reversion of the metaplasia into normal squamous epithelium, or by decreasing the precancerous character with retention of metaplasia. As Barrett metaplasia results from chronic gastroesophageal reflux, Barrett regression can theoretically be obtained by antireflux treatment, either medical or surgical, or by mucosa ablation by *e.g.* electrocoagulation, argon plasma coagulation, laser therapy and photodynamic therapy. We will focus on the use of PPI for the prevention of neoplastic complications.

Barrett's metaplasia results from chronic exposure of the (distal) esophagus to gastric acid. For the prevention of such exposure, profound acid suppression is necessary [1-4]. Therapy with PPI also reduces the duodeno-gastroesophageal reflux and hence the exposure to bile acids [5]. The ideal endpoint for studies into the preventive effect of acid suppression with PPIs would be an objectified decrease in the incidence of esophageal adenocarcinoma, and an increase in the length of survival of patients with Barrett's esophagus [6, 7]. Such a prospective study would, however, hardly be feasible because of the required sample size [8], and thus no such prospective randomized research data on this prophylactic treatment with the absence or presence of adenocarcinoma as study endpoint are available. Therefore any conclusions are based on "surrogate" markers like regression of Barrett's metaplasia, regression of dysplasia, and normalization or improvement of biomarkers suggested to correlate with cancer risk. Several case studies into the effect of PPIs on Barrett mucosa initially described regression of the metaplastic tissue [9, 10]. These reports led to further studies using varying doses of PPIs for a more profound suppression of acid secretion and better reduction of acid reflux. These studies initially had a single arm open design [11-16], and were both retrospective and prospective. Randomized prospective studies remained rare [2, 17, 18]. More recently several papers were published with results of combined treatments, *i.e.* mucosal ablation with concomitant PPI therapy, both for treatment of IM and for (early) adenocarcinoma [19-25]. Only a few studies however checked by ambulatory 24 hour pH-metry whether or not acid suppression in their patients led to normalization of acid reflux. From these studies, it appeared that high PPI doses are necessary to achieve normalization of acid reflux, and that symptom relief is unreliable as measure for normalization. Under such circumstances endoscopic improvement was observed, but remained in most cases restricted to an increase in the number of islands of squamous epithelium, without sub-total regression of the Barrett segment [11-13, 15]. Nevertheless, statistically significant regression was observed after long-term treatment during 1 year [14], 2 years [2, 11], and 5 years [16]; although the last study showed a lack of further regression in the second half of the follow-up period. Complete regression of metaplastic tissue was rare. In a large study of reflux esophagitis patients treated with omeprazole maintenance and followed for a mean 6.5 years (range 1.4-11.2 years), neither regression nor progression of pre-existent Barrett's esophagus was observed [26]. However, new cases of Barrett's esophagus were diagnosed during follow-up. The conclusion must be that long-term normalization of acid reflux probably results in no more than a partial regression of metaplastic epithelium.

The question then is whether profound acid suppression can bring about changes for the better in the retained metaplastic epithelium. Several markers have been studied in this respect. First of all, epithelial cell proliferation, which correlates with dysplasia [27, 28], decreases during near-elimination of acid reflux [29, 30]. Villin, a marker of differentiation, is more strongly expressed after acid reflux normalization and moreover inversely proportional to proliferation rate [29]. Another marker of improvement is the reduction in sulphomucin-producing mucosa [16]. On the other hand studies in reversed Barrett's epithelium have shown that, in addition to the endoscopic difference, there is also a difference in biomarker expression between complete and partial reversal. The squamous epithelium in partially reversed Barrett's esophagus, treated with omeprazole only, differs from completely reversed epithelium (by multipolar electrocoagulation ablation with concomitant omeprazole): in case of partial reversal in more than half the patients epithelial proliferation was not confined to the basal layer and p53 protein expression was seen in more than 40% of the cases [31].

Is it necessary to suppress acid secretion with mucosa ablation? It is evident from animal studies [32] and epidemiological human studies that IM develops under acidic conditions. The chance of success to achieve reversal of metaplastic epithelium into squamous epithelium by mucosal ablation, with a lasting effect, seems to depend on adequate acid suppression during and after the endoscopic treatment. Mucosal ablation that failed during insufficient acid suppression, was successful during more profound acid suppression [22, 33]. In a short-term study, however, normalization of acid reflux did not appear to be mandatory [34]. On the other hand recurrence of metaplasia was observed after discontinuation of omeprazole maintenance [35]. Consequently, it is correct that practically all studies into the efficacy of any form of mucosal ablation have been performed during concomitant acid suppression with PPIs.

In conclusion, it is still unclear whether profound acid suppression can prevent the development of adenocarcinoma in Barrett's esophagus, but treatment with high dose PPI maintenance therapy can induce endoscopic partial reversal of Barrett's esophagus, as well as improvement in several biomarkers of cancer risk. Such therapy furthermore contributes to the success rate of mucosal ablation. Further studies are needed into the combination of PPI therapy and mucosal ablation, which might in theory enable further regression of Barrett's epithelium and prevent the development of adenocarcinoma of the distal esophagus.

References

1. Katzka DA, Paoletti V, Leite L, et al. Prolonged ambulatory pH monitoring in patients with persistent gastroesophageal reflux disease symptoms:testing while on therapy identifies the need for more aggressive antireflux therapy. Am J Gastroenterol 1996;91:2110-2113.
2. Peters FTM, Ganesh S, Kuipers EJ, et al. Endoscopic regression of Barrett's oesophagus during omeprazole therapy; a randomized double blind study. Gut 1999;45:489-494.
3. Peghini PL, Katz PO, Bracy NA, et al. Nocturnal recovery of gastric acid secretion with twice-daily dosing of proton pump inhibitors. Am J Gastroenterol 1998;93:763-767.
4. Fass R, Sampliner RE, Malagon IB, et al. Failure of oesophageal acid control in candidates for Barrett's oesophagus reversal on a very high dose of proton pump inhibitor. Aliment Pharmacol Ther 2000;14:597-602.
5. Marshall REK, Anggiansah A, Manifold DK, et al. Effect of omeprazole 20 mg twice daily on duodenogastric and gastro-oesophageal bile reflux in Barrett's oesophagus. Gut 1998;43:603-606.
6. Peters JH, Clark GWB, Ireland AP, et al. Outcome of adenocarcinoma arising in Barrett's esophagus in endoscopically surveyed and nonsurveyed patients. J Thorac Cardiovasc Surg 1994;108:813-822.
7. van Sandick JW, van Lanschot JJB, Kuiken BW, et al. Impact of endoscopic biopsy surveillance of Barrett's oesophagus on pathological stage and clinical outcome of Barrett's carcinoma. Gut 1998;43:216-222.
8. Kapadia CR. Barrett's esophagus: whom to screen? Still an unanswered question. Gastroenterology 1998;114:1101-1102.
9. Devière J, Buset M, Dumonceau J, et al. Regression of Barrett's epithelium with omeprazole. N Engl J Med 1989;320:1497-1498.
10. Ottenjann R, Heidt H. Regression der Zylinderepithel-Metaplasie bei Barrett-Oesophagus. Dtsch Med Wochenschr 1990;115:916-917.
11. Gore S, Healey CJ, Sutton R, et al. Regression of columnar lined (Barrett's) oesophagus with continuous omeprazole therapy. Aliment Pharmacol Ther 1993;7:623-628.
12. Sampliner RE. Effect of up to 3 years of high-dose lansoprazole on Barrett's esophagus. Am J Gastroenterol 1994;89:1844-1848.
13. Neumann CS, Iqbal TH, Cooper BT. Long term continuous omeprazole treatment of patients with Barrett's oesophagus. Aliment Pharmacol Ther 1995;9:451-454.
14. Malesci A, Savarino V, Zentilin P, et al. Partial regression of Barrett's esophagus by long-term therapy with high-dose omeprazole. Gastrointest Endosc 1996;44:700-705.
15. Sharma P, Sampliner RE, Camargo E. Normalization of esophageal pH with high-dose proton pump inhibitor therapy does not result in regression of Barrett's esophagus. Am J Gastroenterol 1997;92:582-585.
16. Wilkinson SP, Biddlestone LR, Gore S, et al. Regression of columnar-lined (Barrett's) oesophagus with omeprazole 40 mg daily: results of 5 years of continuous therapy. Aliment Pharmacol Ther 1999;13:1205-1209.
17. Weinstein WM, Lieberman DA, Lewin KJ, et al. Omeprazole-induced regression of Barrett's esophagus: a 2 year, randomized, controlled double blind trial. Gastroenterology 1996;110:A294.
18. Caldwell MTP, Byrne PJ, Walsh TN, et al. A randomized trial on the effect of acid suppression on regression of Barrett's oesophagus. Gastroenterology 1996;110:A74.
19. Sampliner RE, Hixson LJ, Fennerty MB, et al. Regression of Barrett's esophagus by laser ablation in an anacid environment. Dig Dis Sci 1993;38:365-368.

20. Berenson MM, Johnson TD, Markowitz NR, et al. Restoration of squamous mucosa after ablation of Barrett's esophageal epithelium. Gastroenterology 1993;104:1686-1691.
21. Barham CP, Jones RL, Biddlestone LR, et al. Photothermal laser ablation of Barrett's oesophagus: endoscopic and histological evidence of squamous re-epithelialisation. Gut 1997;41:281-284.
22. Byrne JP, Armstrong GR, Attwood SE. Restoration of the normal squamous lining in Barrett's esophagus by argon beam plasma coagulation. Am J Gastroenterol 1998;93:1810-1815.
23. Dumoulin FL, Terjung B, Neubrand M, et al. Treatment of Barrett's esophagus by endoscopic argon plasma coagulation. Endoscopy 1997;29:751-753.
24. Mörk H, Barth T, Kreipe HH, et al. Reconstitution of squamous epithelium in Barrett's oesophagus with endoscopic argon plasma coagulation:a prospective study. Scand J Gastroenterol 1998;33:1130-1134.
25. Ell C, May A, Gossner L, et al. Endoscopic mucosal resection of early cancer and high-grade dysplasia in Barrett's esophagus. Gastroenterology 2000;118:670-677.
26. Klinkenberg-Knol EC, Nelis F, Dent J, et al. Long-term omeprazole treatment in resistant gastroesophageal reflux disease: efficacy, safety, and influence on gastric mucosa. Gastroenterology 2000;118:661-669.
27. Hong MK, Laskin WB, Herman BE, et al. Expansion of the Ki-67 proliferative compartment correlates with degree of dysplasia in Barrett's esophagus. Cancer 1995;75:423-429.
28. Peters FTM, Ganesh S, Kuipers EJ, et al. Epithelial cell proliferative activity of Barrett's esophagus: methodology and correlation with traditional cancer risk markers. Dig Dis Sci 1998;43:1501-1506.
29. Ouatu-Lascar R, Fitzgerald RC, Triadafilopoulos G. Differentiation and proliferation in Barrett's esophagus and the effects of acid suppression. Gastroenterology 1999;117:327-335.
30. Peters FTM, Ganesh S, Kuipers EJ, et al. Effect of elimination of acid reflux on epithelial cell proliferative activity of Barrett's esophagus. Scand J Gastroenterol 2000;35:1238-1244.
31. Garewal H, Ramsey L, Sharma P, et al. Biomarker studies in reversed Barrett's esophagus. Am J Gastroenterol 1999;94:2829-2833.
32. Bremner CG, Lynch VP, Ellis FH. Barrett's esophagus: congenital or acquired? An experimental study of esophageal mucosal regeneration in the dog. Surgery 1970;68:209-216.
33. Brandt LJ, Blansky RL, Kauvar DR. Repeat laser therapy of recurrent Barrett's epithelium: success with anacidity. Gastrointest Endosc 1995;3:267,
34. Kovacs BJ, Chen YK, Lewis TD, et al. Successful reversal of Barrett's esophagus with multipolar electrocoagulation despite inadequate acid suppression. Gastrointest Endosc 1999;49:547-553.
35. Michopoulos S, Tsibouris P, Bouzakis H, et al. Complete regression of Barrett's esophagus with heater probe thermocoagulation; mid-term results. Gastrointest Endosc 1999;50:165-172.

What are the compared rates of regression observed after surgical or prolonged maintenance therapy?

M. France, R. Ackroyd, D.I. Watson (Adelaide, Sheffield)

It is generally accepted that Barrett's esophagus (or columnar lined esophagus) develops as a response to the reflux of both gastric and duodenal contents into the lumen of the distal esophagus, with consequent exposure of the esophageal mucosa to deleterious effects of these substances [1, 2]. It would therefore seem reasonable to hypothesise that eliminating exposure of this mucosa to gastric and duodenal fluids, either by medical or surgical intervention, might be followed by regression of Barrett's esophagus. A knowledge of whether this in fact happens is very important, as Barrett's esophagus is a premalignant condition, which can progress to adenocarcinoma of the esophagus. Furthermore, the incidence of this cancer has risen dramatically over the last three decades [3]. Fortunately, a number of studies have been published which do address the issue of whether either maintenance medical therapy or antireflux surgery is followed by regression of Barrett's esophagus, and these enable the question to be answered with some certainty.

Regression in response to prolonged medical maintenance therapy

Maintenance medical therapy using either H_2 receptor antagonists, or more recently proton pump inhibitors (PPI), aims to reduce esophageal mucosal damage by suppressing gastric acid production and the damaging effect of pepsin. Reflux continues to occur, but the gastric fluid refluxed is rendered less noxious. In addition PPI, whilst not directly preventing duodenogastric reflux, secondarily reduce duodenogastroesophageal reflux by reducing the overall volume of gastric secretions, and this reduces the total amount of fluid which reaches the esophageal lumen [4].

Initial reports following the introduction of H_2 receptor antagonists of case series of patients with Barrett's esophagus who ingested therapeutic doses of these medications, failed to demonstrate regression of Barrett's esophagus [5-7]. These reports were followed by the first prospective trial of medical therapy which was reported by Wedsorp *et al.* [8]. In this study a dose of 1.6 gm of cimetidine per day for two years failed to produce any regression in the Barrett's esophagus of 8 patients studied. A much larger study by Sampliner *et al.* [9] of 67 patients with Barrett's esophagus who used either cimetidine or ranitidine also failed to show regression.

Given that patients with Barrett's esophagus tend to have a higher gastric basal acid output [10], it would be reasonable to conclude from these initial studies that the medically treated patients may have been under treated, especially as symptom control rather than normalisation of the intraesophageal pH profile was used as the end point for treatment. It is known that Barrett's esophagus mucosa can be less sensitive to acid reflux than squamous mucosa, and for this reason clinical symptoms are not a reliable guide for the assessment of the efficacy of antireflux treatment. Furthermore it is likely that if regression is to be achieved, total elimination of intraesophageal acid might be required, and this requires either more potent medications or surgery.

Following the introduction of PPI it was hoped that with more powerful antisecretory action, regression of Barrett's esophagus might be seen, and indeed initial anecdotal reports did describe regression [11]. However, two subsequent prospective trials described mixed results. Gore *et al.* [12] showed significant regression of Barrett's esophagus in 23 patients who ingested omeprazole at a dose of 40 mg per day for 24 months. On the other hand, Sampliner [13] failed to demonstrate significant regression in length of Barrett's esophagus identified at endoscopy in a group of 27 patients who used lansoprazole at a dose of 60 mg per day, although 77% of the patients did develop islands of regenerated squamous mucosa.

If maintenance therapy is to be successful, then normalisation of pH in the distal esophagus would seem to be a prerequisite for regression. This issue was addressed in a prospective study by Malesci *et al.* [14]. Fourteen patients with histologically proven Barrett's esophagus received omeprazole 60 mg per day for 12 months. Twenty-four hour pH monitoring was performed after therapy for 10 days, 6 and 12 months, and normalisation of the distal esophageal pH profile was achieved in all but 2 patients. Endoscopy performed at 6 and 12 months showed statistically significant regression of the Barrett's esophagus in all but 3 cases compared with baseline endoscopy. However, all patients had residual Barrett's mucosa, with a mean reduction in the length of Barrett's esophagus of only 53% achieved (decreased from mean 4.5 cm to 2.1 cm length). Contrary to this study, another prospective study 15 of 27 patients with a mean follow-up of 5.7 years failed to demonstrate any significant reduction in the length of Barrett's esophagus.

In a prospective randomized controlled trial a small but significant regression of 8% was seen in 26 patients receiving a large dose of omeprazole (80 mg per day over a 2 year period) compared with 27 patients receiving standard dose ranitidine (150 mg twice daily) [16]. Again the issue of acid suppression appears to be important, as normalisation of pH was confirmed in the omeprazole treatment arm, whilst the ranitidine group continued to have abnormal 24 hour pH studies. Furthermore, the clinical significance of 8% regression could be questioned, as 92% of the original columnar lining remained following medical therapy even with high dose omeprazole. Two further randomized controlled trials comparing omeprazole with H_2 receptor antagonists showed statistically significant regression in the group using high dose omeprazole (80 mg per day for 1 year then 40 mg per day for 1 year) [17], whilst another group using only omeprazole 20 mg per day failed to show regression [18].

Given these conflicting outcomes, a failure to demonstrate even statistically significant regression in most series, and the absence of clinically significant (*i.e.* total or near total) regression in any series, it is not possible to conclude that prolonged maintenance therapy, even with high dose PPI, will lead to regression of columnar mucosa in patients with Barrett's esophagus. Even if partial regression is to be seen following medical therapy, high doses of PPI appear to be required, and the adequacy of acid suppression must be confirmed by 24-hour pH testing. This is unlikely to be worth the effort.

Regression in response to antireflux surgery

By restoring a physical barrier to gastroesophageal surgery not only prevents exposure of the esophagus to acid, but it also prevents duodenal and pancreatic secretions from refluxing into the esophageal lumen. It is thought that both acid and pancreaticobiliary secretions are required for Barrett's esophagus to develop, and then progress to cancer of the esophagus. Theoretically, therefore, we could expect a better response following antireflux surgery than acid suppression.

One of the earliest publications to examine the influence of antireflux surgery on Barrett's esophagus was reported by Brand *et al.* [19]. This suggested that fundoplication held promise for the treatment of Barrett's esophagus, with complete regression of columnar mucosa described in 4 out of 10 patients who underwent surgery. Subsequent reports, however, have been disappointing with complete regression rarely documented. In a recent review of 11 published series which incorporated a total of 340 surgically treated patients [19-29], only 4% of patients had complete regression of Barrett's esophagus, with a further 12% showing partial regression [30].

Even more disappointing was a prospective study of 152 patients who underwent conventional open surgery using either a Nissen fundoplication or Hill's posterior gastropexy [31]. Long-term mean follow-up of 8.1 years was not followed by regression of Barrett's esophagus, and even worse it was followed by the development of low-grade dysplasia in 15 patients and adenocarcinoma in a further 4 patients. Twenty-four hour pH monitoring and Bilitec™ studies both demonstrated a significant reduction in acid and duodenoesophageal reflux respectively, but values were still elevated compared to normal individuals and this might explain the progression of disease. Probably of greater importance is that progression either to dysplasia or malignancy occurred late at approximately 8 years in all cases and highlights the importance of ongoing endoscopic surveillance in these patients.

On a more favourable note, a more recent, but small series of 14 prospectively followed patients, did demonstrate partial regression with squamous re-epithelialization in 10 patients with classic long segment Barrett's esophagus (more than 3 cm length) [32]. Included in this series were 2 patients with short segment Barrett's who showed complete regression. Given that the incidence of adenocarcinoma in short segment Barrett's is probably significantly less [33] it is difficult to interpret the importance of regression until we know more about the natural history of short segment Barrett's esophagus.

One group of concern is those patients whose Barrett's esophagus progresses following antireflux surgery, either by increasing in length, or progressing to dysplasia or even carcinoma. In a series of 37 patients treated with antireflux surgery at the Lahey clinic, progression to carcinoma occurred in 3 patients despite postoperative manometry recordings which were consistent with a functioning wrap [25]. In our own department, we recently reported the outcome of 81 patients with a Barrett's esophagus who underwent a laparoscopic Nissen fundoplication for symptomatic reflux disease [34]. Four patients in this series progressed to esophagectomy for cancer or high-grade dysplasia approximately 2 years following their original fundoplication. In contrast to this, in the only published randomized trial which has compared medical *versus* surgical therapy in patients with Barrett's esophagus [29], the only patients who developed dysplasia or malignancy during follow-up, were those patients who were managed with medication, or those who had documented failed antireflux procedures. The difference between the treatment groups in this study reached statistical significance, and led the authors to conclude that there may be some advantages for surgery over standard medical maintenance therapy.

On the other hand, McEntee *et al.* [35] compared medical treatment with a H_2 receptor antagonist in 23 patients with a fundoplication in 21 patients, and demonstrated regression of Barrett's esophagus in only 1 of the patients treated with surgery. Four patients with mild dysplasia regressed to non-dysplastic epithelium following surgery, although 2 patients also progressed; 1 to mild dysplasia, and 1 from moderate dysplasia to severe dysplasia. 24-hour pH monitoring was performed in both study groups, and there was no significant reduction in acid exposure in the group receiving H_2 receptor antagonists, whilst in the surgically treated group there was a significant decrease in acid exposure in the esophagus.

From these studies we can conclude that, as with prolonged medical maintenance therapy, surgery is rarely followed by complete regression of Barrett's esophagus, and surgery at best is followed by limited partial regression in approximately 10 to 15% of patients. Nevertheless, in those patients whose Barrett's esophagus does regress, regression undoubtedly relies on a successful antireflux procedure which restores a barrier against gastroesophageal reflux.

Limitations of published studies

One of the most important issues to consider when evaluating or undertaking any study which seeks to investigate regression or regeneration of Barrett's esophagus is the potential for error when measuring the extent of the columnar lining. This can be a significant problem in patients with both Barrett's esophagus and a sliding hiatus hernia. In this situation, definition of the site of the gastroesophageal junction (GEJ), and therefore measurement of the length of Barrett's esophagus, can be particularly difficult, and errors in identification can influence study outcomes. In addition, many patients with Barrett's esophagus have no lower esophageal sphincter tone, and for this reason, locating the GEJ using manometry, is also unlikely to be helpful. In medical trials, measurement issues will probably confound treatment groups equally if a randomized and blinded study design is applied. However, in surgical trials, the identification of the GEJ is much easier once patients who have undergone fundoplication, a short length of the esophagus is compressed by the wrap (and is not visible at endoscopy), and "blinding" of the post-treatment endoscopic assessment is not feasible because an intact fundoplication is immediately obvious to any endoscopist. For all of these reasons, there may be a tendency to "measure" a shorter length of Barrett's esophagus following surgery, or even claim total regression in some patients. However, despite this, surgery can also be followed by the appearance of islands of regenerating squamous epithelium, without an overall change in the length of the columnar lining, and this does represent evidence of partial regression of the metaplastic process.

Conclusion

In the majority of patients with Barrett's esophagus, neither medical maintenance therapy nor antireflux surgery will be followed by regression of Barrett's esophagus. There are a minority of patients whose Barrett's esophagus partially regresses, and a very small number in whom complete regression appears to occur. Nevertheless, reliable regression does not occur following either antireflux surgery or prolonged medical treatment, and for this reason, mucosal ablative techniques are currently under close evaluation to determine whether they offer a better treatment which will achieve clinically significant regression for the majority of patients with Barrett's esophagus.

References

1. Vaezi MF, Richter JE. Role of acid and duodenogastroesophageal reflux in gastroesophageal reflux disease. Gastroenterology 1996;111:1192-1199.
2. Vaezi MF, Richter JE. Double reflux: double trouble. Gut 1999;44:590-592.
3. Pera M, Cameron AJ, Trastek VF, Carpenter HA, Zinsmeister AR. Increasing incidence of adenocarcinoma of the esophagus and esophagogastric junction. Gastroenterology 1993;104:510-513.
4. Marshall RE, Anggiansah A, Manifold DK, Owen WA, Owen WJ. Effect of omeprazole 20 mg twice daily on duodenogastric and gastro-oesophageal bile reflux in Barrett's oesophagus. Gut 1998;43:603-606.
5. Kothari T, Mangla JC, Kalra TM. Barrett's ulcer and treatment with cimetidine. Arch Intern Med 1980;140:475-477.
6. Humphries TJ. Effects of long-term medical treatment with cimetidine and bethanechol in patients with esophagitis and Barrett's esophagus. J Clin Gastroenterol 1987;9:28-32.
7. Cooper BT, Barbezat GO. Treatment of Barrett's esophagus with H2 blockers. J Clin Gastroenterol 1987;9:139-141.
8. Wesdorp IC, Bartelsman J, Schipper ME, Tytgat GN. Effect of long-term treatment with cimetidine and antacids in Barrett's oesophagus. Gut 1981;22:724-727.
9. Sampliner RE, Garewal HS, Fennerty MB, Aickin M. Lack of impact of therapy on extent of Barrett's esophagus in 67 patients. Dig Dis Sci 1990;35:93-96.
10. Collen MJ, Johnson DA. Correlation between basal acid output and daily ranitidine dose required. Dig Dis Sci 1992;37:570-576.
11. Deviere J, Buset M, Dumonceau JM, Rickaert F, Cremer M. Regression of Barrett's epithelium with omeprazole. N Engl J Med 1989;320:1497-1498.

12. Gore S, Healey CJ, Sutton R, Eyre-Brook IA, Gear MW, Shepherd NA, Wilkinson SP. Regression of columnar lined (Barrett's) oesophagus with continuous omeprazole therapy. Aliment Pharmacol Ther 1993;7:623-628.
13. Sampliner RE. Effect of up to 3 years of high-dose lansoprazole on Barrett's esophagus. Am J Gastroenterol 1994;89:1844-1848.
14. Malesci A, Savarino V, Zentilin P, Belicchi M, Mela GS, Lapertosa G, Bocchia P, Ronchi G, Franceschi M. Partial regression of Barrett's esophagus by long-term therapy with high-dose omeprazole. Gastrointest Endosc 1996;44:700-705.
15. Sharma P, Sampliner RE, Camargo E. Normalization of esophageal pH with high-dose proton pump inhibitor therapy does not result in regression of Barrett's esophagus. Am J Gastroenterol 1997;92:582-585.
16. Peters FT, Ganesh S, Kuipers EJ, Sluiter WJ, Klinkenberg-Knol EC, Lamers CB, Kleibeuker JH. Endoscopic regression of Barrett's oesophagus during omeprazole treatment; a randomized double blind study. Gut 1999;45:489-494.
17. Weinstein WM, Lieberman D, Lewin K, Weber L, ML B, Ippoliti A. Omeprazole-induced regression of Barrett's esophagus: a 2 year, randomized, controlled double blind trial. Gastroenterology 1996;110:A294.
18. Caldwell M, Byrne P, Walsh T, Hennessy T. A randomized trial on the effect of acid suppression on regression of Barrett's oesophagus. Gastroenterology 1996;110:A74.
19. Brand DL, Ylvisaker JT, Gelfand M, Pope CE. Regression of columnar esophageal (Barrett's) epithelium after antireflux surgery. N Engl J Med 1980;302:844-848.
20. Radigan LR, Glover JL, Shipley FE, Shoemaker RE. Barrett esophagus. Arch Surg 1977;112:486-491.
21. Ransom JM, Patel GK, Clift SA, Womble NE, Read RC. Extended and limited types of Barrett's esophagus in the adult. Ann Thorac Surg 1982;33:19-27.
22. Skinner DB, Walther BC, Riddell RH, Schmidt H, Iascone C, DeMeester TR. Barrett's esophagus. Comparison of benign and malignant cases. Ann Surg 1983;198:554-565.
23. Starnes VA, Adkins RB, Ballinger JF, Sawyers JL. Barrett's esophagus. A surgical entity. Arch Surg 1984;119:563-567.
24. DeMeester TR, Attwood SE, Smyrk TC, Therkildsen DH, Hinder RA. Surgical therapy in Barrett's esophagus. Ann Surg 1990;212:528-542.
25. Williamson WA, Ellis FH Jr, Gibb SP, Shahian DM, Aretz HT. Effect of antireflux operation on Barrett's mucosa. Ann Thorac Surg 1990;49:537-542.
26. Attwood SE, Barlow AP, Norris TL, Watson A. Barrett's oesophagus: effect of antireflux surgery on symptom control and development of complications. Br J Surg 1992;79:1050-1053.
27. Sagar PM, Ackroyd R, Hosie KB, Patterson JE, Stoddard CJ, Kingsnorth AN. Regression and progression of Barrett's oesophagus after antireflux surgery. Br J Surg 1995;82:806-810.
28. McDonald ML, Trastek VF, Allen MS, Deschamps C, Pairolero PC. Barretts's esophagus: does an antireflux procedure reduce the need for endoscopic surveillance? J Thorac Cardiovasc Surg 1996;111:11351140.
29. Ortiz A, Martinez LF, De Haro P, Parrilla G, Morales J, Molina J, Bermejo J, Liron R, Aguilar J. Conservative treatment versus antireflux surgery in Barrett's oesophagus: long-term results of a prospective study. Br J Surg 1996;83:274-278.
30. DeMeester SR, DeMeester TR. Columnar mucosa and intestinal metaplasia of the esophagus: fifty years of controversy. Ann Surg 2000;231:303-321.
31. Csendes A, Braghetto I, Burdiles P, Puente G, Korn O, Diaz JC, Maluenda F. Long-term results of classic antireflux surgery in 152 patients with Barrett's esophagus: clinical, radiologic, endoscopic, manometric, and acid reflux test analysis before and late after operation. Surgery 1998;123:645-657.
32. Low DE, Levine DS, Dail DH, Kozarek RA. Histological and anatomic changes in Barrett's esophagus after antireflux surgery. Am J Gastroenterol 1999;94:80-85.
33. Weston AP, Krmpotich PT, Cherian R, Dixon A, Topalosvki M. Prospective long-term endoscopic and histological follow-up of short segment Barrett's esophagus: comparison with traditional long segment Barrett's esophagus. Am J Gastroenterol 1997;92:407-413.
34. Yau P, Watson DI, Devitt PG, Game PA, Jamieson GG. Laparoscopic antireflux surgery in the treatment of gastroesophageal reflux in patients with Barrett esophagus. Arch Surg 2000;135:801-805.
35. McEntee GP, Stuart RC, Byrne PJ, Nolan N, Hennessy PJ. An evaluation of surgical and medical treatment of Barrett's oesophagus. Gullet 1991;1:169-172.

What is the rate of squamous re-epithelialization in Barrett's esophagus following endoscopic mucosal resection?

M. Endo (Tokyo)

Materials and methods

Twelve cases of endoscopic mucosal resection for early adenocarcinoma in Barrett's esophagus were reported in Japan [1-3]. With regard to depth of tumor invasion, mucosal cancer was observed in 9 cases and slightly invasive submucosal cancer was found in 3 cases. Vascular invasion was not observed in any of these cases. In terms of size, 6 lesions were less than 1 cm and all were within 3 cm in size. According to the Japanese macroscopic classification, all lesions were included in the 0-II type, that is, superficial and flat type. 0-IIa slightly elevated type was observed in 4 cases, reddish 0-IIb flat type in 1 case and reddish 0-IIc slightly depressed type in 7 cases.

The procedures of endoscopic mucosal resection was performed in the same way as in squamous cell carcinoma of the esophagus. Although the diagnosis was made by endoscopy and biopsy, it was difficult to recognize the contour of the lesion precisely even when using the staining technique with methylene-blue solution. Prior to endoscopic mucosal resection four marks were placed outside the lesion by electric cautery, however a larger amount of mucosa was generally resected. Piecemeal resection was performed until the target area of the mucosa has been resected. Argon plasma coagulation and laser therapy were also performed additionally when remaining of cancer tissue was suspected based on examination of the resected specimen.

Frequently the lamina propria mucosae, the muscularis mucosae and the submucosa are fibrotically thickened in Barrett's esophagus, therefore the endoscopic mucosal resection required persistence for resection. The injection of physiologic saline solution in the submucosal layer or lifting of the mucosa was not troublesome in any of the cases.

Results

Considering the postoperative complications slight stenosis was encountered in one of these cases. This case was improved easily by balloon dilatation. After endoscopic mucosal resection, proton pump inhibitors and sodium alginate were administered. Squamous re-epithelialization of mechanically induced ulcer was observed in 10 cases (83%), columnar-lined epithelium in 1 case (8%), and follow-up endoscopic examination was not performed in 1 case (8%). The longest survival period so far was 3 years and a half, with no recurrence, but multiple early adenocarcinoma were observed in 2 cases and endoscopic mucosal resection was repeated.

Summary

• Twelve cases of endoscopic mucosal resection for early adenocarcinoma in Barrett's esophagus were reported in Japan.
• Squamous re-epithelialization was observed in ten cases (83%).
• The total circumferential endoscopic mucosal resection for Barrett's esophagus at the same time has been avoided to protect postoperative stenosis.

References

1. Zeniya A, Ishioka T, Masamune O, et al. Superficial adenocarcinoma arising from Barrett's esophagus, report of a case, Stom Intest 1995;30:1445-1450.
2. Katayama O, Honda H. Endoscopic mucosal resection for superficial adenocarcinoma arising from Barrett's esophagus. Gastroenterol Endosc 1998;40:1598.
3. Hoshihara Y, Yamamoto T, Hashimoto M, et al. An adenocarcinoma in short segment Barrett's esophagus, report of a case. Stom Intest 1999;34:195-198.

How should development of squamous islands on Barrett's mucosa be interpreted?

S. Gore (Yeovil)

The incidence of adenocarcinoma of the esophagus and gastric cardia appears to be increasing more rapidly than any other cancer [1-3]. Barrett's esophagus (columnar lined esophagus - CLE) is the most important predisposing factor for esophageal adenocarcinoma, having an incidence of malignant transformation of approximately one per 100 patient years [4-6].

There has been considerable interest for many years in developing treatment strategies which could reduce the malignant potential of Barrett's esophagus by bringing about regression of the abnormal mucosa. Initial optimism was sparked by a case study reporting complete regression of 16 cm Barrett's mucosa with 18 months proton pump inhibitor (PPI) treatment [7]. These strategies have included medical [8, 9], surgical [10, 11] and photoablative [12-15] therapies and have been subject to recent review [16].

Regression of Barrett's esophagus can be measured endoscopically by reduction in the length of CLE, development of squamous islands [8, 9, 17-19] or reduction in the total area of CLE [20, 21]. The histological evidence for squamous re-epithelialization includes microscopic squamous islands, squamous encroachment at the squamocolumnar junction and apparent squamous metaplasia within Barrett's glandular mucosa [8, 17, 22, 23].

The purpose of this paper is to review the literature on the development of squamous islands within CLE and discuss their significance.

Definition

Squamous islands seen at endoscopy can be defined as patches of white and lighter coloured epithelium surrounded on all sides by columnar appearing mucosa (darker pink coloured) [24].

Microscopic squamous islands have been described in biopsy specimens from Barrett's esophagus [8, 17, 22].

Development of squamous islands

Squamous islands, both macroscopic and microscopic, may occur in untreated Barrett's esophagus [24, 25]. However, there is good evidence that their presence is greatly increased by acid suppression. In fact 50-90% of patients with Barrett's esophagus treated with PPIs develop squamous islands within the CLE. It would appear that the partial regression of Barrett's epithelium as evidenced by the development of squamous islands occurs early on with PPI therapy [8, 19].

Not only do these findings persist over 5-6 years but there appears to be further development of squamous islands with an increase in their number and size [17, 26].

There are practical difficulties in assessing the development of squamous islands endoscopically. Their size varies from 2 mm to 2 cm and with time they may coalesce to form larger islands. Thus counting numbers of squamous islands *per se* may not accurately reflect the amount of squamous re-epithelialisation within the Barrett's epithelium. Therefore, other methods to determine regression, using area of CLE, have been employed. Such a method has been used in a randomized double blind study comparing omeprazole with ranitidine in the regression of Barrett's esophagus [21]. In this study the development of squamous islands probably accounts for the small but significant partial regression of surface area of CLE (8% over 2 years) with omeprazole compared with no regression in the ranitidine group. There was no significant reduction in length of CLE in either group.

Significance of squamous islands in Barrett's esophagus

The pathological explanations for the development of squamous islands has recently been reviewed [23].

It appears likely that squamous islands both macroscopic and microscopic, derive from esophageal gland ducts [22]. Squamous re-epithelialization is more extensive with photoablative therapies where squamous metaplasia has been noted within the Barrett's glands [13, 22]. Thus, there are perhaps pluripotential cells within the Barrett's glands which may account for squamous re-epithelialization particularly in response to photoablation [12].

The key issue is: does the development of squamous islands lead to a reduction in the malignant potential of Barrett's mucosa? Sharma *et al.* [24] have found that in 38.5% of biopsies taken from macroscopic squamous islands, microscopic intestinal metaplasia (IM) was detected, concluding that the development of squamous islands does not confer any protection against future development of adenocarcinoma of the esophagus in these patients. An alternative view may be that this buried IM may be protected from the toxic stimuli within the esophageal lumen resulting in a reduced malignant potential [23]. However, an elegant study using tumor biomarkers (Ki-67 and p53 abnormalities), albeit in small numbers, has shown that completely reversed squamous epithelium following a combination of thermal injury and PPI therapy, is biologically similar to normal squamous epithelium and therefore of low cancer risk; whereas, partially reversed squamous epithelium manifest as squamous islands, is accompanied by biomarker abnormalities suggesting a continued cancer risk [27].

Conclusion

The final answer to the question as to whether the development of squamous islands confers any protection against future progression to adenocarcinoma will continue to elude us unless large, long-term, randomized trials are carried out with high-grade dysplasia or adenocarcinoma as the end point. Until then, I believe that the development of squamous islands represents, at best, a partial regression of the columnar lining of Barrett's esophagus and surveillance of these areas should continue with endoscopy and deep biopsies.

References

1. Blot WJ, Devesa S, Kneller RW, Fraumeni JF. Rising incidence of adenocarcinoma of the oesophagus and gastric cardia. JAMA 1991:265:1287-1289.
2. Pera M, Cameron AJ, Trastek VF, Carpenter HA, Zinsmeister AR. Increasing incidence of adenocarcinoma of the oesophagus and oesophagogastric junction. Gastroenterology 1993:104:510-513.
3. Cameron AJ. Epidemiology of columnar-lined oesophagus and adenocarcinoma. Gastroenterol Clin N Am 1997;26:487-494.
4. Ifthikar SY, James PD, Steele RJC, Hardcastle JD, Atkinson M. Length of Barrett's oesophagus: an important factor in the development of dysplasia and adenocarcinoma. Gut 1992;33:1155-1158.
5. Hameetman W, Tytgat GNG, Houtnoff HJ, Van den Tweel JG. Barrett's oesophagus. Development of dysplasia and adenocarcinoma. Gastroenterology 1989;96:1249-1256.
6. Wright TA, Gray MR, Morris AI, Gilmore IT, Ellis A, Smart HL, Myskow M, Nash J, Donnelly RJ, Kingsnorth AN. Cost effectiveness of detecting Barrett's cancer. Gut 1996;39:574-579.
7. Deviere J, Buset M, Dumongeau JM, Rickaert F, Cremer M. Regression of Barrett's epithelium with omeprazole. N Engl J Med 1989;320:1497-1498.
8. Gore S, Healey CJ, Sutton CJ, Eyre-Brook IA, Gear MWL, Shepherd NA, Wilkinson SP. Regression of columnar line (Barrett's oesophagus) with continuous omeprazole therapy. Aliment Pharmacol Ther 1993;7:623-628.
9. Sampliner RE. Effect up to 3 years of high-dose lansoprazole on Barrett's oesophagus. Am J Gastroenterol 1994;89:1844-1848.
10. Sagar PM, Ackroyd R, Hosie KB, Patterson JE, Stoddard CJ, Kingsnorth AN. Regression and progression of Barrett's oesophagus after antireflux surgery. Br J Surg 1995;82:806-810.
11. Ortiz A, Martinez de Haro LF, Parilla P, Morales G, Molina J, Bermejo J, Liron R, Aguilar J. Conservative treatment versus antireflux surgery in Barrett's oesophagus. Br J Surg 1996;83:274-278.
12. Berenson MM, Johnson TD, Markowitz NR, Buchi KN, Samowitz WS. Restoration of squamous mucosa after ablation of Barrett's oesophageal epithelium. Gastroenterology 1993;104:1686-1691.
13. Barr H, Shepherd NA, Dix A, Roberts DJH, Tan WC, Kransner N. Eradication of high grade dysplasia in columnar lined (Barrett's) oesophagus by photodynamic therapy with endogenously generated protoporphyrin IX. Lancet 1996;348:584-585.
14. Overholt BF, Panjehpour M, Haydek JM. Photodynamic therapy for Barrett's oesophagus: follow-up in 100 patients. Gastrointest Endosc 1999;49:1-7.
15. Barham CP, Jones RL, Biddlestone LR, Hardwick RH, Shepherd NA, Barr H. Photothermal laser ablation of Barrett's oesophagus: endoscopic and histological evidence of squamous re-epithelialisation. Gut 1997;41:281-284.
16. Haag S, Nandurkar S, Talley NJ. Regression of Barrett's oesophagus: the role of acid suppression, surgery and ablative methods. Gastrointest Endosc 1999;50:229-240.
17. Wilkinson SP, Biddlestone L, Gore S, Shepherd NA. Regression of columnar lined (Barrett's) oesophagus with omeprazole 40 mgs daily: results of 5 years of continuous therapy. Aliment Pharmacol Ther 1999;13:1205-1209.

18. Neumann CS, Iqbal TH, Cooper BT. Long term continuous omeprazole treatment of patients with Barrett's oesophagus. Aliment Pharmacol Ther 1995;9:451-454.
19. Malesci A, Savarino V, Zentilin P, Belicchi M, Mela GS, Lapertosa G, Bocchio P, Ronchi G, Franceschi M. Partial regression of Barrett's esophagus by long term therapy with high-dose omeprazole. Gastrointest Endosc 1996;44:700-705.
20. Kim R. Baggot BB, Rose S, Shar AO, Mallory DL, Kasky SS. Quantitative endoscopy: precise computerized measurement of metaplastic epithelial surface area in Barrett's oesophagus. Gastroenterology 1995;108:360-366.
21. Peters FTM, Ganesh S, Kuipers EJ, Sluiter WJ, Klinkenberg-knol EC, Lamers CBHW, Kleibenker JH. Endoscopic regression of Barrett's oesophagus during omeprazole treatment; a randomized double blind study. Gut 1999;45:489-494.
22. Biddlestone LR, Barham CP, Wilkinson SP, Barr H, Shepherd NA. The histopathology of treated Barrett's oesophagus. Squamous reepithelialisation after acid suppression and laser and photodynamic therapy. Am J Surg Pathol 1998;22:239-245.
23. Shepherd NA. Barrett's oesophagus and proton pump inhibitors: a pathological perspective. Gut 200;46:147-149.
24. Sharma P, Morales TG, Bhattacharyya A, Garewal HS, Sampliner RE. Squamous islands in Barrett's oesophagus: what lies underneath? Am J Gastroenterol 1998;93:332-335.
25. Sampliner RE, Steinbronn K, Garewal HS, Riddell RH. Squamous mucosa overlying columnar epithelium in Barrett's oesophagus in the absence of antireflux surgery. Am J Gastroenterol 1998;83:510-512.
26. Cooper BT, Neumann CS, Cox MA, Iqbal TH. Continuous treatment with omeprazole 20 mgs daily for up to 6 years in Barrett's oesophagus. Aliment Pharmacol Ther 1998;12:893-897.
27. Garewal HS, Ramsey L, Sharma P, Kraus K, Sampliner RE, Fass R. Biomarker studies in reversed Barrett's oesophagus. Am J Gastroenterol 1999;94:2829-2833.

What is the significance of persisting salivary epidermal growth factor output impairment in Barrett's patients with endoscopically healed mucosa?

C. Poplawski, M. Marcinkiewicz, T. Zbroch, J. Sarosiek
(Kansas City)

The alimentary tract mucosa is exposed to a number of injurious exogenous agents ingested almost daily as components of food, drinks, or medication. Under this continuous challenge, the mucosal integrity is maintained both through the adequate prevention of injury and quick restitution (migration of existing cells from the margin of injury) accompanied by full reconstitution (remodeling) of the mucosal architecture after any even slightest mucosal damage [1-3].

The squamous esophageal mucosa is facing a unique challenge within the alimentary tract, as it is frequently exposed to injurious components of gastric and duodenal content, especially after the meal that promotes the gastroesophageal reflux (GER) or duodeno-gastroesophageal reflux resulting in gastroesophageal reflux disease (GERD).

Among protective mechanisms balancing the duodeno-gastroesophageal refluxate injurious potential, the pre-epithelial (the mucus-buffers layer covering the mucosa) and epithelial (protection at the cellular level) defenses are instrumental in promoting the health of the squamous epithelium [3].

Peptide growth factors, ubiquitous both within the pre-epithelial and epithelial mucosal compartments, seem to play a leading role in both prevention of injury and its repair. Peptide growth factor could be categorized as:

- mucosal integrity peptides (preserving mucosal integrity),
- or luminal surveillance peptides (acting at sites of an acute injury/repair), some of which could also be considered as rapid response peptides as quick onset of restitution or reconstitution could be pivotal in prevention of chronic injury and/or complications [1-5].

Among mucosal integrity peptides transforming growth factor α (TGFα) and pancreatic secretory trypsin inhibitor (PSTI) seem to play a leading role in prevention of mucosal injury. The luminal surveillance peptides group, on the other hand is well represented by epidermal growth factor (EGF). Both trefoil peptides, such as, TFF1 (previously known as pS2), TFF2 (also called spasmolytic polypeptide) and TFF3 (also known as intestinal trefoil factor) and EGF could also be considered as rapid response peptide [1-5].

It has been recently demonstrated that patients with endoscopic reflux esophagitis exhibit impairment in the rate of secretion of salivary and esophageal EGF and that this impairment persists after healing of endoscopic changes [6-8]. Therefore, patients with GERD who develop erosive reflux esophagitis as a result of an excessive mucosal exposure to injurious factors within the refluxate, are more likely to have impaired the abluminal mucosal surveillance process and diminished rapid mucosal response to injury due to inadequate content of EGF within the pre-epithelial defense [3]. In addition, in our preliminary data we have also demonstrated that patients with Barrett's esophagus, which develops in the setting of GERD, also exhibited an impairment in EGF secretion when compared to controls [9]. This impairment in the rate of secretion of esophageal EGF could be attributed to lower expression of EGF gene at its peptide level within the esophageal submucosal mucous glands or to a lower number of submucosal mucous glands. A variation in the number of submucosal mucous glands in human esophagus from as low as 62 to as high as 741 glandular lobules has been reported by Goetsch [10].

A similar phenomenon of diminished expression of EGF peptide or a smaller size of salivary glands could also lead to decline of salivary EGF in both populations. Only approximately 1/3 of patients with reflux esophagitis exhibited low EGF in both salivary and esophageal secretion, the remaining showed decline in salivary or esophageal secretion only. The clinical importance of this phenomenon of the most severe impairment in salivary and esophageal EGF secretion requires further investigation.

These data strongly suggest that although GER is prerequisite of the development of the esophageal mucosal pathology, the quality of mucosal protective mechanisms are significant and could be decisive in determining the development of complications.

It was recently demonstrated that the rate of the luminal release of TGFα in patients with reflux esophagitis was significantly higher than in controls both in basal conditions and during mucosal challenge with HCl/pepsin, mimicking the natural GER scenario [11]. In both controls and patients with reflux esophagitis luminal release of TGFα was significantly lower during mucosal exposure to HCl or HCl/Pepsin than corresponding basal values [11]. This may indicate that enhanced secretion of TGFα in reflux esophagitis may at least partly compensate for impairment in EGF secretion, although, most likely inadequate, since patients with reflux esophagitis are still more likely to develop Barrett's esophagus and its ultimate complication: adenocarcinoma.

In patients with Barrett's esophagus an increase in expression of TGFα or EGF/TGFα receptor within columnar epithelium has been demonstrated [12]. This increase was parallel to progression from nonspecialized to specialized intestinal epithelium and even was more profound in epithelium exhibiting dysplasia and adenocarcinoma [12]. No such dynamics in EGF expression was observed in the same specimens. These changes in growth factors and its receptor expression in patients with Barrett's esophagus were accompanied by increase in proliferating cell nuclear antigen (PCNA), Ki-67 antigen, ornithine decarboxylase activity and aneuploidy indicating enhanced cell proliferation, additionally augmented by p53 gene mutation [12, 13]. Therefore, metaplastic epithelium is acquiring its own source of peptide growth factor, predominantly TGFα binding to the same EGF receptor, which may serve as a source of high proliferative activity in metaplastic epithelium, may lead to uncontrolled growth in an autocrine fashion, and finally may promote the development of dysplastic changes and perhaps adenocarcinoma.

One may assume that the normal squamous epithelium, since it exhibits a high density of EGF receptor even on the apical cell membrane, requires a steady supply of EGF from salivary glands and esophageal submucosal mucous glands which also release their content into esophageal lumen through the ducts [10, 14]. This hypothesis is supported by recently published data demonstrating esophageal squamous epithelial hyperplasia after chronic administration of EGF [15]. Deficiency of EGF hampers physiological functions of the esophageal squamous epithelium and leads to enhanced permeability of the esophageal mucosa to hydrogen ion [16, 17]. This in turn may accelerate damage to the esophageal epithelium accompanied by apoptosis or cell necrosis, depending on pH changes within the intercellular milieu in the esophageal mucosa under the impact of GER, decreasing cell-cell adhesion and adhesion of squamous cells to basement membranes hampering their migratory and firm attachment potential. This in turn may promote migration of columnar cells which are phylogenetically well equipped, within their cytoskeleton network, with all molecules necessary to maintain their integrity under the impact of gastric or gastroduodenal milieu. This may explain the receding zone of squamous epithelium and expanding columnar compartment. The borderline between these two distinct morphological compartment is probably determined by:

- the quantity and quality of duodeno-gastroesophageal refluxate,
- the intensity of esophageal propulsive primary and secondary peristalsis,
- the quantity and the quality of protective components within salivary secretion,
- the density and distribution of esophageal submucosal mucous glands and quality of their protective potential.

Since duodenal component of duodeno-gastroesophageal refluxate can be excessive, even the gastric type of metaplasia has to be supplemented or replaced by specialized intestinal epithelium which also undergoes further morphological and functional changes. This results in expression of nuclear oncogene c-myc, signal transduction oncogene ras, tumor suppressor gene rb, or fibroblast growth factor-related oncogenes hst-1 and int-2 and transformation to end point pathology manifested by the aggressive clone of transformed cells with a metastatic potential [14, 18-21].

Patients with endoscopic reflux esophagitis also exhibit impairment in secretion of esophageal glycoconjugates (mucin) and PGE_2 under the impact of luminal HCl/pepsin [22, 23]. This impairment may contribute to mucosal progression of mucosal injury under the influence of unbalanced aggressive power of the gastroesophageal refluxate.

The rate of secretion of PSTI and trefoil peptides, so important in the maintenance of mucosal integrity and in rapid response to mucosal injury, in patients with reflux esophagitis with or without Barrett's esophagus remains to be explored.

References

1. Wong WM, Playford RJ, Wright NA. Peptide gene expression in gastrointestinal mucosal ulceration: ordered sequence or redundancy. Gut 2000;46:286-292.
2. Playford RJ, Boulton R, Ghatei MA, Bloom SR, Wright NA, Goodlad RA. Comparison of the effects of transforming growth factor alpha and epidermal growth factor on gastrointestinal proliferation and hormone release. Digestion 1996;57:362-367.
3. Sarosiek J, McCallum RW. The evolving appreciation of the role of esophageal mucosal protection in the pathophysiology of gastroesophageal reflux disease. J Pract Gastroenterol 1994;18:20J-20Q.
4. Playford RJ, Marchbank T, Chinery R, Evison R, Pignatelli M, Boulton RA, Thim L, Hanby AM. Human spasmolytic polypeptide is a cytoprotective agent that stimulates cell migration. Gastroenterology 1995;108:108-116.
5. Chinery R, Playford RJ. Combined intestinal trefoil factor and epidermal growth factor is prophylactic against indomethacin-induced gastric damage in the rat. Clin Sci 1995;88:401-403.
6. Rourk RM, Namiot Z, Sarosiek J, Yu Z, McCallum RW. Diminished content of esophageal epidermal growth factor in patients with reflux esophagitis. Am J Gastroenterol 1994;89:1177-1184.
7. Rourk RM, Namiot Z, Sarosiek J, Yu Z, McCallum RW. Impairment of salivary epidermal growth factor secretory response to esophageal mechanical and chemical stimulation in patients with reflux esophagitis. Am J Gastroenterol 1994;89:237-244.
8. Edmunds MC, Namiot Z, Sarosiek J, Rourk RM, Yu Z, McCallum RW. Esophageal epidermal growth factor impairment persists depite healing of endoscopic changes in patients with reflux esophagitis. Gastroenterology 1994;106:A73.
9. Sarosiek J, Edmunds MC, Namiot Z, Marcinkiewicz M, McCallum RW. Secretory profile of Barrett's esophagus in humans: its significantly modified protective potential. Gastroenterology 1994;106:A173.
10. Goetsch E. The structure of the mammalian esophagus. Am J Anat 1910;10:1-40.
11. Marcinkiewicz M, Sarosiek J, Edmunds ME, Namiot Z, McCallum RW. Detrimental impact of acid and pepsin on the rate of luminal release of transforming growth factor alpha: its potential pathogenetic role in the development of reflux esophagitis. J Clin Gastroenterol 1996;23:261-268.
12. Filipe MI, Jankowski J. Growth factors and oncogenes in Barrett's oesophagus and gastric metaplasia. Endoscopy 1993;25:637-641.
13. Fennerty MB, Sampliner RE, Garewal HS. Barrett's esophagus-cancer risk, biology and therapeutic management. Aliment Pharmacol Ther 1993;7:339-345.
14. Jankowski J, Murphy S, Coghill G, Grant A, Wormsley KG, Sanders DS, Kerr M, Hopwood D. Epidermal growth factor receptors in the oesophagus. Gut 1992;33:439-443.
15. Juhl CO, Jensen LS, Poulsen SS, Orntoft TF, Dajani EZ. Chronic treatment with epidermal growth factor causes esophageal epithelial hyperplasia in pigs and rats. Dig Dis Sci 1995;40:2717-2723.
16. Sarosiek J, Feng T, McCallum RW. The interrelationship between salivary epidermal growth factor and the functional integrity of the esophageal mucosal barrier in the rat. Am J Med Sci 1991;302:359-363.
17. Chen MC, Chang A, Buhl T, Soll AH. Apical EGF receptors regulate tight junctions and apical barrier function of gastric monolayers via cytochalasisn D-sensitive mechanisms. Proc AGA Symp Peptide Growth Factors GI Tract, Vail, CO, 1994;25.
18. Casson AG, Mukhopadhyay T, Cleary KR, Ro JY, Levin B, Roth JA. p53 gene mutations in Barrett's epithelium and esophageal cancer. Cancer Res 1993;51:4495-4499.
19. Jankowski J, Coghill G, Hopwood D, Wormsley KG. Oncogenes and onco-suppressor gene in adenocarcinoma of the oesophagus. Gut 1992;33:1033-1038.
20. Jankowski J, McMenemin R, Hopwood D, Penston J, Wormsley KG. Abnormal expression of growth regulatory factors in Barrett's oesophagus. Clin Sci 1991;81:663-668.
21. Jankowski J, McMenemin R, Yu C, Hopwood D, Wormsley KG. Proliferating cell nuclear antigen in oesophageal diseases; correlation with transforming growth factor alpha expression. Gut 1992;33:587-591.
22. Namiot Z, Sarosiek J, Marcinkiewicz M, Edmunds MC, McCallum RW. Declined human esophageal mucin secretion in patients with severe reflux esophagitis. Dig Dis Sci 1994;39:2523-2529.
23. Marcinkiewicz M, Sarosiek J, Edmunds MC, Scheurich J, Weiss P, McCallum RW. Monophasic luminal release of prostaglandin E2 in patients with reflux esophagitis under the impact of acid and acid/pepsin solutions:Its potential pathogenetic significance. J Clin Gastroenterol 1995;21:268-274.

Is there evidence that Barrett's mucosa regresses spontaneously?

N.A. Shepherd (Gloucester)

Adenocarcinoma complicating Barrett's esophagus (columnar-lined esophagus, CLE) is rapidly becoming a major health problem for western communities. Its almost exponential rise in incidence in the last 20 years has ensured that cancer of the esophagus is now the cancer with the fifth highest mortality in UK males. Therefore there is currently much interest in regression of CLE, either spontaneously or in response to the various therapeutic modalities, in an attempt to halt the disquieting increase in the incidence of esophageal adenocarcinoma in the Western World.

Definitions: regression, reversal or what?

The term regression, when applied to CLE, has undoubtedly become tainted with confusion and misunderstanding. The Oxford Dictionary defines regression as "the action of returning to or toward a place or point of departure". Thus regression does not, necessarily, imply that the CLE has disappeared or been ablated entirely. Nevertheless many have, seemingly, used the term in this way and this has led to confusion. Perhaps it is best defined as "the total loss of columnar mucosa from an area previously occupied by columnar mucosa". However, pathological studies have demonstrated that various therapeutic modalities, including acid suppressive therapy afforded by proton pump inhibitors (PPIs) [1, 2], laser therapy [3, 4], photodynamic therapy (PDT) [5] and various electrocoagulation therapies [6-8] can induce squamous re-epithelialisation on the surface whilst CLE-type epithelium remains below [9, 10]. Some have designated such changes as pseudo-regression (Appelman, personal communication). It is certainly the case that the demonstration of such pseudo-regression requires the histopathologist's interpretation of biopsies as the endoscopist is unable to determine whether such CLE remains below [10].

Regression can be subclassified as complete, partial or focal. The latter two patterns have been described following all the therapeutic manoeuvres previously mentioned. Whilst complete regression is the ultimate goal, evidence of partial regression may also be important for reducing the cancer risk [11, 12]. Some have preferred the term "reversal" rather than regression for the phenomenon of squamous re-epithelialization [6, 13]. This is because of a belief that the term "regression" is both ambiguous and has been tainted with misunderstanding when applied to CLE. Reversal still does not imply that the CLE has entirely been replaced by squamous mucosa or destroyed completely; such remaining CLE epithelium may still have important implications for neoplastic potential [10].

How do we assess regression/reversal?

Regression/reversal can be defined by both endoscopic and histopathological means. Simple endoscopic imaging and measurement of segment length and surface area provide some evidence for regression [2, 14]. Measuring the length of Barrett's mucosa will indicate the amount of squamous over-riding that has occurred at the squamocolumnar junction [14] whilst measurement of the surface area will assess not only the squamous overriding, but also the extent of squamous islands within the Barrett's mucosa [2]. However quantitative endoscopic imaging using computerized image analysis is probably the most accurate means [15]. This will more accurately assess both the length of the segment and the presence and extent of squamous islands [15].

Pathologically, regression (or pseudo-regression) is characterized by the squamous overriding at the squamocolumnar junction and by the presence of macroscopic and microscopic squamous islands [9]. There is good evidence to suggest that these squamous islands arise from native structures within the esophagus, the esophageal gland ducts, and this relationship is often demonstrated in the microscopic squamous islands [9, 16]. Such an association may not be demonstrated in larger macroscopically (and endoscopically) visible squamous islands but it is presumed that such larger squamous islands evolve from these microscopic squamous islands, themselves evolving from metaplasia from native esophageal gland ducts [9].

Evidence for regression: spontaneous and therapeutic

In answer to the question "Is there evidence of spontaneous regression of CLE?", the answer appears to be critically dependent on the CLE type. There is some evidence that short segment CLE (SSCLE) can regress with the total disappearance of all tongues and patches of Barrett's mucosa in conjunction with only squamous mucosa on biopsy [17]. It would appear that the most important determinant of regression is the absence of an associated hiatus hernia rather than concurrent therapy: patients with SSCLE showing complete regression may not be on PPIs [17]. For long segment/traditional/classical CLE, there is no compelling evidence for spontaneous complete regression. Most cases of complete regression of CLE have occurred after therapy particularly aimed at achieving such complete regression, most notably laser and PDT [3-5]. Spontaneous complete regression of long segment CLE has not, to this author's knowledge, been demonstrated in a scientifically rigorous manner. The situation is very much complicated by the fact that many patients, at the time of diagnosis of CLE, are already on acid suppressive therapy because of symptomatology [18]. Any evidence for regression is more likely to be a response to PPI therapy and it is becoming increasingly difficult to demonstrate any evidence of "spontaneous regression".

Microscopic squamous islands have been described in untreated CLE [19]. Could these represent foci of regression? Given that the number, size and extent of squamous islands increases in patients on acid-lowering therapy [1, 14], it could be that these microscopic squamous islands, in untreated CLE patients, may represent areas of reduced refluxate exposure and thus microscopic areas of "regression". There is no compelling evidence for this: it is just as likely that these microscopic squamous islands represent remaining, and undamaged, foci of pre-existing squamous mucosa.

There remains controversy concerning the extent of regression that occurs after PPI therapy: some have shown partial regression with reduction in CLE length [1, 14, 20] and an increase in squamous islands and thus decrease in surface area [1, 14, 21, 22]. One double blind controlled trial reported has also demonstrated regression in both of these parameters [2]. However, other studies have not been able to show evidence of regression in PPI-treated patients [23, 24].

There are also controversies as to whether surgical techniques induce any regression of CLE: most workers believe they do not result in significant regression [11, 25]. However partial regression has been described, especially in children [26, 27]. One conundrum here is the fact that CLE mucosa itself produces acid from the fundic-type mucosa: reducing acid reflux from the stomach may not induce regression if the CLE mucosa itself is maintaining an acidic environment. Many studies of the effects of reflux surgery on CLE have predated the use of powerful acid suppressive drugs. The combination of reflux surgery and PPI therapy could theoretically induce squamous re-epithelialization and partial regression of CLE in a similar way, but perhaps more prominently, than PPI therapy alone. There is as yet no direct evidence that such regression occurs in many patients.

It is not intended to dwell on the various ablative methodologies that have been used to induce "regression" of CLE, as these are described in much more detail elsewhere. Success has been demonstrated in ablation of CLE and replacement by squamous mucosa using lasers [3, 4], PDT [5], and various electrocoagulation methods [6-8]. All of these may be associated with the phenomenon of covert CLE epithelium beneath surface squamous mucosa [9].

Heresy: do we really need complete regression/reversal of columnar-lined esophagus?

The critical question, in terms of reducing the cancer risk, is not whether complete or partial regression is consistently achievable, but what promotes the progression of the dysplasia-carcinoma sequence in CLE. If it is acid, then it may be controlled by acid suppressive therapy. This, of course, assumes that high acid levels in the esophagus are the only important factor in inducing neoplastic change. There is, however, some evidence to implicate duodeno-gastroesophageal reflux (DGER), particularly bile in this sequence [28, 29]. Thus acid-lowering therapy may not be the whole answer: however, there is also evidence to suggest that reduction of acid in the stomach reduces DGER and thus reduces the amount of bile exposure in CLE [30].

Is there current evidence to suggest that acid-lowering drugs, such as PPIs, not only lead to partial regression of CLE [1, 2], but also cause epithelial stability of the remaining CLE mucosa [12]? There is as yet little. We have demonstrated a reduction in the amount of unstable sulphomucin-positive mucopolysaccharide after 5 years of PPI therapy [1] whilst there is also a reduction in cyclin-D1, essentially a proliferation marker, in patients with CLE treated with PPIs [31]. Furthermore there is evidence that effective intraesophageal acid suppression leads to a reduction in CLE proliferation and to differentiation [32]. These data would suggest that effective control of acid in the esophagus may indeed lead to epithelial stability which itself could reduce the neoplastic potential. Thus insistence that the only means of ensuring a reduction in neoplastic potential is the production of complete regression/reversal, as has been implied [33], may not necessarily be essential [12]. An interesting counterbalance of these studies of the remaining CLE mucosa is a recent study demonstrating continued biomarker abnormality in the squamous epithelium in squamous islands in treated CLE [13]. However, it could be that these changes merely reflect the inevitable cellular proliferative activity in this regenerative mucosa.

Covert columnar-lined esophagus mucosa: does it matter?

Given that many therapeutic modalities can induce squamous re-epithelialization both at the squamocolumnar junction and as a result of induction of squamous islands which themselves enlarge and coalesce, what are the implications for any remaining CLE mucosa that remains below [10]? Some have suggested that this retains neoplastic potential and there are cases of neoplasia, both dysplasia and carcinoma, in this concealed mucosa beneath re-epithelialized squamous mucosa after therapeutic ablation of CLE [33-35]. These cases could represent de novo neoplastic change in such clandestine Barrett's mucosa; equally they could represent dysplastic or carcinomatous mucosa that was pre-existing before therapy and has simply become buried by squamous re-epithelialization. This author believes that covert but non-neoplastic CLE mucosa, beneath squamous mucosa, may not have the same neoplastic potential as surface CLE mucosa as it is not being exposed to the noxious intraluminal agents, be they acid, bile or other agent [12].

Conclusions

Complete regression of CLE currently remains our goal in attempts to reduce the neoplastic potential of CLE. However, it may be that indicators of partial regression, such as reduction in length and squamous area, squamous re-epithelialization in the form of encroachment at the squamocolumnar junction and squamous islands, may merely be surrogate markers for a profound stabilisation of the mucosa of the CLE when not exposed to the noxious agents, particularly acid and bile, that have been implicated in the neoplastic sequence of CLE. We require further studies of the CLE mucosa, most notably molecular studies of cell cycle and apoptosis genes and proteins and the genetic abnormalities implicated in the neoplastic sequence, to determine whether there is such epithelial stability.

Complete regression of CLE may not be the Holy Grail for the management of this enigmatic disease. We live quite happily with metaplastic epithelia, particularly that with a mature phenotype, at many sites in the body and it is often further injurious agents that induce neoplastic change in such metaplastic epithelium. Could it not be that CLE might survive and yet mature under appropriate conditions and may not necessarily have the neoplastic potential of untreated CLE?

References

1. Wilkinson SP, Biddlestone L, Gore S, Shepherd NA. Regression of columnar-lined (Barrett's) oesophagus with omeprazole 40 mg daily: results of 5 years of continuous therapy. Aliment Pharmacol Ther 1999;13:1205-1209.
2. Peters FT, Ganesh S, Kuipers EJ, Sluiter WJ, Klinkenberg-Knol EC, Lamers, et al. Endoscopic regression of Barrett's oesophagus during omeprazole treatment;a randomized double blind study. Gut 1999;45:489-494.
3. Sampliner RE, Hixson LJ, Fennerty MB, Garewal HS. Regression of Barrett's esophagus by laser ablation in an anacid environment. Dig Dis Sci 1993;38:365-368.
4. Barham CP, Jones RL, Biddlestone LR, Hardwick RH, Shepherd NA, Barr H. Photothermal laser ablation of Barrett's oesophagus: endoscopic and histological evidence of squamous re-epithelialisation. Gut 1997;41:281-284.
5. Overholt BF, Panjehpour M. Photodynamic therapy in Barrett's esophagus. J Clin Laser Med Surg 1996;14:245-249.
6. Sampliner RE, Fennerty B, Garewal HS. Reversal of Barrett's esophagus with acid suppression and multipolar electrocoagulation: preliminary results. Gastrointest Endosc. 1996;44:532-535.
7. Dumoulin FL, Terjung B, Neubrand M, Scheurlen C, Fischer HP, Sauerbruch, et al. Treatment of Barrett's esophagus by endoscopic argon plasma coagulation. Endoscopy 1997;29:751-753.

8. Grade AJ, Shah IA, Medlin SM, Ramirez FC. The efficacy and safety of argon plasma coagulation therapy in Barrett's esophagus. Gastrointest Endosc 1999;50:18-22.
9. Biddlestone LR, Barham CP, Wilkinson SP, Barr H, Shepherd NA. The histopathology of treated Barrett's esophagus: squamous reepithelialization after acid suppression and laser and photodynamic therapy. Am J Surg Pathol 1998;22:239-245.
10. Sharma P, Morales TG, Bhattacharyya A, Garewal HS, Sampliner RE. Squamous islands in Barrett's esophagus: what lies underneath? Am J Gastroenterol 1998;93:332-335.
11. Attwood SE. Barrett's esophagus. Curr Opin Gen Surg 1993;180-188.
12. Shepherd NA. Barrett's oesophagus and proton pump inhibitors: a pathological perspective. Gut 2000;46:147-149.
13. Garewal H, Ramsey L, Sharma P, Kraus K, Sampliner R, Fass R. Biomarker studies in reversed Barrett's esophagus. Am J Gastroenterol 1999;94:2829-2833.
14. Gore S, Healey CJ, Sutton R, Eyre-Brook IA, Gear MW, Shepherd NA, et al. Regression of columnar lined (Barrett's) oesophagus with continuous omeprazole therapy. Aliment Pharmacol Ther 1993;7:623-628.
15. Kim R, Rose S, Shar AO, Weiner M, Reynolds JC. Extent of Barrett's metaplasia: a prospective study of the serial change in area of Barrett's measured by quantitative endoscopic imaging. Gastrointest Endosc 1997;45:456-462.
16. Berenson MM, Johnson TD, Markowitz NR, Buchi KN, Samowitz WS. Restoration of squamous mucosa after ablation of Barrett's esophageal epithelium. Gastroenterology 1993;104:1686-1691.
17. Weston AP, Badr AS, Hassanein RS. Prospective multivariate analysis of factors predictive of complete regression of Barrett's esophagus. Am J Gastroenterol 1999;94:3420-3426.
18. Krueger KJ, DiPalma JA. Omeprazole and Barrett's regression: is asymptomatic good enough? Am J Gastroenterol 1997;92:177-178.
19. Sampliner RE, Steinbronn K, Garewal HS, Riddell RH. Squamous mucosa overlying columnar epithelium in Barrett's esophagus in the absence of antireflux surgery. Am J Gastroenterol 1988;83:510-512.
20. Malesci A, Savarino V, Zentilin P, Belicchi M, Mela GS, Lapertosa G, et al. Partial regression of Barrett's esophagus by long-term therapy with high-dose omeprazole. Gastrointest Endosc 1996;44:700-705.
21. Neumann CS, Iqbal TH, Cooper BT. Long term continuous omeprazole treatment of patients with Barrett's oesophagus. Aliment Pharmacol Ther 1995;9:451-454.
22. Cooper BT, Neumann CS, Cox MA, Iqbal TH. Continuous treatment with omeprazole 20 mg daily for up to 6 years in Barrett's oesophagus. Aliment Pharmacol Ther 1998;12:893-897.
23. Bozymski EM, Shaheen NJ. Barrett's esophagus: acid suppression, but no regression. Am J Gastroenterol 1997;92:556-558.
24. Sharma P, Sampliner RE, Camargo E. Normalization of esophageal pH with high-dose proton pump inhibitor therapy does not result in regression of Barrett's esophagus. Am J Gastroenterol. 1997;92:582-585.
25. Spencer J. Surgery in Barrett's oesophagus. Eur J Cancer Prev 1992;1:331-335.
26. Hassall E, Weinstein WM. Partial regression of childhood Barrett's esophagus after fundoplication.Am J Gastroenterol 1992;87:1506-1512.
27. Sagar PM, Ackroyd R, Hosie KB, Patterson JE, Stoddard CJ, Kingsnorth AN. Regression and progression of Barrett's oesophagus after antireflux surgery. Br J Surg 1995;82:806-810.
28. Vaezi MF, Richter JE. Role of acid and duodenogastroesophageal reflux in gastroesophageal reflux disease. Gastroenterology 1996;111:1192-1199.
29. Stein HJ, Kauer WK, Feussner H, Siewert JR. Bile reflux in benign and malignant Barrett's esophagus: effect of medical acid suppression and Nissen fundoplication. J Gastrointest Surg 1998;2:333-341.
30. Marshall RE, Anggiansah A, Manifold DK, Owen WA, Owen WJ. Effect of omeprazole 20 mg twice daily on duodenogastric and gastro-oesophageal bile reflux in Barrett's oesophagus. Gut 1998;43:603-606.
31. Arber N, Lightdale C, Rotterdam H, Han KH, Sgambato A, Yap E, et al. Increased expression of the cyclin D1 gene in Barrett's esophagus. Cancer Epidemiol Biomark Prev 1996;5:457-459.
32. Ouatu LR, Fitzgerald RC, Triadafilopoulos G. Differentiation and proliferation in Barrett's esophagus and the effects of acid suppression. Gastroenterology 1999;117:327-335.
33. Sampliner RE, Fass R. Partial regression of Barrett's esophagus - an inadequate endpoint. Am J Gastroenterol 1993;88:2092-2094.
34. Barr H, Shepherd NA, Dix A, Roberts DJ, Tan WC, Krasner N. Eradication of high-grade dysplasia in columnar-lined (Barrett's) oesophagus by photodynamic therapy with endogenously generated protoporphyrin IX. Lancet 1996;348:584-585.
35. Van Laethem JL, Cremer M, Deviere J, et al. Intramucosal adenocarcinoma arising under squamous re-epithelialisation of Barrett's oesophagus. Gut 2000;46:574-577.

Adenocarcinomas

Is the diagnosis of adenocarcinoma in Barrett mucosa the same worldwide?

M. Vieth, M. Stolte (Bayreuth)

No, the diagnosis of adenocarcinoma in Barrett's mucosa is not the same worldwide. Especially in United States, for various reasons, very often the diagnosis of high-grade dysplasia (HGD) instead of adenocarcinoma (that is limited to the mucosa) is made.

But fortunately there is a key to the question what is still HGD and what is already adenocarcinoma in Barrett's mucosa.

The key seems to be the publication of Takahashi and Iwama 1985. The authors analyzed the microstructure of well differentiated tubular gastric adenocarcinomas with a 3-dimensional reconstruction. It could be shown that the carcinomatous tubuli invaded the lamina propria and anastomosed with neighbouring tubuli. The result is described as a skeleton network (*Figure 1*) of invasive tubuli.

The analysis of the 3-dimensional microstructure showed definitive differences between normal gastric mucosa, adenoma and G1-adenocarcinoma. This pattern can easily be adapted to Barrett's adenocarcinoma.

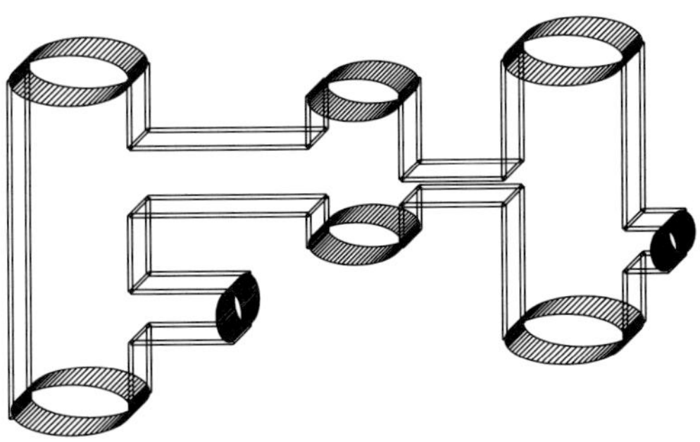

Figure 1. Network-skeleton in early Barrett's adenocarcinoma (modified from [1]).

In conclusion, the so called pattern-recognition of skeleton network in combination with cytologic criteria of malignancy suffices very well for the diagnosis of Barrett's adenocarcinoma and thus represents the most minimal signs for invasion and might explain why many HGD in biopsies turn out to be already adenocarcinoma in the operation specimen.

Reference

1. Takahashi T, Iwama N. Three-dimensional microstructure of gastrointestinal tumors. Gland pattern and its diagnostic significance. Pathol Annu 1985;20:419-440.

What is the acceptable definition of cardiac carcinoma?

H.D. Appelman (Ann Arbor)

Four adenocarcinomas arise in the vicinity of the esophagogastric junction (EGJ). Immediately above the junction, the carcinomas develop in dysplastic Barrett's mucosa. Immediately below the junction are the carcinomas that arise in the most proximal stomach, the cardia. The third group contains carcinomas that straddle the junction, and have no Barrett's mucosa in the lower esophagus above the tumor and no dysplasia below it in the proximal stomach to indicate a site of origin there. These are presumably a mixture of cancers arising in minute dysplastic foci both in ultra-short segment Barrett's mucosa and in the cardia. The fourth group includes large carcinomas arising in the gastric fundus or proximal body that extend to or even across the gastroesophageal junction (GEJ). The definitions of Barrett's carcinomas are much the same from study to study, and they usually include location predominantly within the tubular esophagus accompanied by adjacent Barrett's mucosa. If the Barrett's epithelium is dysplastic, that solidifies the diagnosis. In contrast, the definition of the cardiac carcinoma is not as clear as is the definition of the Barrett's carcinoma. Why is this the case?

The following facts are irrefutable

• Study after study has reported an increase in the prevalence of proximal gastric cancers, commonly designated as cardiac, with a concomitant decrease in more distal gastric cancers [1-4].
• A literature devoted to carcinoma of the gastric cardia exists, and it has been expanding rapidly [1-34].
• There are many recent studies that deal with inflammation of the cardia (carditis), goblet cells at the cardia, and their causes.

These facts indicate that there must be a specific, well-established anatomic site in the proximal stomach called the cardia, and that it has both inflammatory and neoplastic diseases. Therefore, the definition of this cardia must be well-established and uniformly accepted, but is it?

What is the gastric cardia?

A major problem in evaluating studies dealing with cardiac cancers lies in the definition of the cardia itself as an established anatomic entity. Is the cardia a specific gross anatomic area, or is it only a microscopic area, that is, the part of the proximal gut lined by a distinctive cardiac mucosa. Here are some such definitions of the cardia that have been published, many in prestigious textbooks and journals. Unfortunately, these definitions are for the gross cardiac region or the microscopic cardiac mucosa, but usually not both.

• In the 31st edition of *Gray's Anatomy* published in 1954, a classic in exquisitely detailed anatomic description, mention is made of a cardiac orifice, a cardiac notch and cardiac glands, the latter identified as "occurring close to the cardiac orifice", but there is no region of the stomach specifically identified or defined as the cardia, although there is a microscopic drawing of the "cardiac part of the stomach". The 1987 version of the same classic tome lists the cardiac orifice and glands, changes the name "notch" to "incisura cardiaca", and adds a cardiac antrum (a dilated portion), but there is still no specific statement indicating exactly where the cardia is and how big it is [5].

• In the 1997 edition of the AJCC *Cancer Staging Manual*, there is a statement that "its (the stomach's) first part is the esophagogastric junction which is located immediately below the diaphragm and is often called the cardia" [6]. In this definition, a gross definition, the cardia is synonymous with the junction. It is even given its own site code, C16.0.

• In one well-known textbook of gastrointestinal pathology, the gross cardia is defined as the "narrow, approximately 1.0 cm long portion of the stomach immediately distal to the gastroesophageal junction" [7].

• In another reference text, *Histology for Pathologists*, published in 1997, the gross or anatomic cardia is described in this way: "The cardia is found just distal to the lower end of the esophagus. It is a small and ill defined area extending 1 to 3 cm from the esophagogastric junction". The author then discusses the histologic cardiac mucosa as "extending distally from the gastroesophageal junction, approximately 1 to 2 cm" [8]. Thus, in this author's opinion, there may be a small difference in the length between the gross and microscopic cardias.

• In a well-known 1996 pathology text devoted to tumors of the esophagus and stomach, the gross "cardia region has no macroscopic visible landmarks; it refers to a short zone measuring several centimeters where the stomach immediately adjoins the esophagus" [9].

• Another gastrointestinal pathology text mentions that "on endoscopy (in other words grossly), cardiac type mucosa starts abruptly at the esophageal squamocolumnar junction and extends into the stomach for 0.5-4 cm" [10].

• In an epidemiologic study of gastric cancers in Olmstead County Minnesota, the home of the Mayo Clinic, the cardia was considered to be "all gastric mucosa within 5 cm of the EGJ", presumably a microscopic definition, thus virtually doubling the size of the cardia compared to other definitions [11].

• In a detailed analysis utilizing endoscopic examinations on patients without hiatal hernias and gross examination of resected specimens, the authors found that the histologic cardiac gland area "was found to straddle the esophagogastric disease at a range of about 1 cm proximal and 2 cm distal to the junction" [12]. Using this definition, microscopic cardiac mucosa normally is not just confined to the stomach, but it is also normal in the distal 1 cm of the esophagus. This takes into consideration the frequent occurrence of normal cardiac mucosa, if there is such a thing as normal cardiac mucosa, in the distal most 1-2 cm of the tubular esophagus, roughly coinciding with the length of the lower esophageal sphincter [13, 14].

• In a publication from Germany, there is a statement that "the region of the cardia is in fact a narrow zone between the esophagus and stomach proper" [15]. This gross definition actually takes the cardia out of the stomach all together.

If we were going to study the cardia *in vivo*, based upon the above definitions, we would have trouble deciding where to take the biopsies. Since the cardia seems to be a very small zone, biopsies of it should be very close to the squamocolumnar junction. There are such biopsy studies supposedly of the cardia, and the biopsy sites are usually within 5 mm below the normal-appearing squamocolumnar junction or from the Z-line [16, 17]. However, in some studies, biopsies said to come from the cardia are taken as much as 3 cm below the junction, which in other studies would be considered to be well within the stomach proper [18].

In spite of these inconsistencies, it appears that the gross cardia, if it exists as a distinct entity, is very small, no more than a small number of millimeters at the most proximal end of the stomach, although in some people, the microscopic cardiac mucosa also extends into the distal 1-2 cm of the tubular esophagus. This raises a critical question, namely how can such a tiny zone measured in millimeters give rise to an increasing number of cancers?

What are cardiac carcinomas?

Since the definition of the cardia is not clear cut, it should come as no surprise that there is no uniform definition of cardiac carcinoma. In many studies, cardiac carcinomas are included with those arising at the cardioesophageal junction. Here are some published examples of how cardiac carcinoma has been defined:

• In a study from the US analyzing the role of *H. pylori* in cardiac disease, cardiac carcinomas were those that were limited to the cardia in the absence of gastroesophageal reflux disease (GERD) symptoms or Barrett's esophagus, but no more specific details as to location were given [19].

• In a Belgian study of molecular markers, cardiac cancers were those that were "clearly localized in the proximal stomach" [20].

• In the 1996 *AFIP Fascicle on Tumors of the Esophagus and Stomach*, cardiac carcinomas were defined as being "normally located within 1 cm proximal and 2 cm distal to the esophagogastric junction, provided that there is no Barrett's mucosa above it" [9]. This definition fails to account for the fact that tumors located within 1 cm proximal to the junction may arise in short segment Barrett's mucosa and obliterate it, so that there may be no Barrett's left proximal to the tumor.

• In a Swedish study comparing Barrett's and cardiac cancers, a tumor was classified as cardiac if its center was within 2 cm proximal, or 3 cm distal, to the GEJ [21]. This increases the range by one cm on both sides compared to definition #3 above.

• In still other studies cardiac carcinomas were equated with or defined as those arising at the cardioesophageal junction or "when the epicenter is located at the GEJ" [22-24]. When this definition was used, there was a high association between these "cardiac" carcinomas and Barrett's mucosa. This suggests that some studies of cardiac carcinomas really include distal Barrett's cancers.

• In one study from the University of Michigan, cardiac carcinomas were defined as "tumors occurring within or immediately below the GEJ with replacement of all or a significant part of the cardiac mucosa, and sparing of the distal stomach" [2].
• The same group modified this definition within a year when they defined cardiac carcinomas as those arising in the proximal one to two centimeters of the stomach [25].
• In a Dutch study in which the authors decided that cardiac and Barrett's cancers were a single clinical entity, cardiac cancers were those whose epicenter was at and immediately below the GEJ, extending approximately 2 cm downward [26].
• In a Japanese study of early cancer, that is, cancer invading no deeper than the submucosa, early cardiac carcinomas were defined as those whose central point was located within 2 cm of the cardioesophageal junction [27].
• In another study from the US analyzing molecular markers, cardiac carcinomas were identified as those arising within 3 cm of the GEJ [28].
• In a study from China, cardiac carcinoma is defined as that originating from "cardial glands 3 cm distal to the GEJ" [29]. This definition not only identifies a site but a precursor, cardiac glands, which no other study has implicated as being precancerous.
• A report from Germany and another from Japan considered a cardiac carcinoma to be a carcinoma occurring at the EGJ or of the fundus which has reached the cardia or has crossed over to the distal esophagus [30, 31]. This definition seems to include carcinomas that arise in the proximal stomach as long as they involve the cardia, although they need not actually arise in the cardia.
• In a British study, if a carcinoma affected the cardia (which was not defined) and the lower esophagus, the tumor was included as a cardiac carcinoma [3].
• A Dutch study used the term "proximal third gastric carcinomas" as synonymous with cardiac carcinomas. (Heidl) However, that is a large area, and many such tumors are likely to be primary in the fundus and proximal body, in other words, not really cardiac cancers at all.
• Some publications on cardiac carcinomas don't even include a definition of the entity [1, 32, 33].

As is seen from the definitions above, in some studies, all proximal gastric carcinomas are equated with cardiac carcinomas, but that may be inappropriate, since carcinomas arising in the proximal body or fundus can invade the cardia, yet they are not cardiac carcinomas [30, 34, 35]. To complicate this situation, Barrett's carcinomas sometimes extend below the junction into the cardia, while some cardiac cancers grow upward to involve the distal esophagus.

The question that this discussion was to answer is "what is the acceptable definition of cardiac carcinoma?" The answer is obvious; there is no such definition. It is time we produce one, but that can only be accomplished when we produce a universally acceptable definition of the cardia, and so far, that definition also does not exist. As soon as we determine the extent and location of the cardia, only then can we define the ideal cardiac carcinoma as one that arises in the cardia from cardiac mucosa.

One critical issue is raised by this discussion. There is almost complete agreement by the experts in the field of gastric and esophageal cancer epidemiology that adenocarcinomas of the cardia are rapidly increasing in frequency in Western societies, especially among white men. However, if the definition of cardiac carcinoma is so unsettled, then we must pose the obvious question: what are the carcinomas that are supposed to be increasing so greatly in frequency? Until we decide on the unambiguous definition of cardiac carcinoma, then in truth, we have absolutely no idea what the answer is to that question.

References

1. Devesa SS, Blot WJ. Fraumeni JF JR. Changing patterns in the incidence of esophageal and gastric carcinoma in the United States. Cancer 1998;83:2049-2053.
2. Kalish RJ, Clancy PE, Orringer MB, Appelman HD. Clinical, epidemiologic, and morphologic comparison between adenocarcinomas arising in Barrett's esophageal mucosa and in the gastric cardia. Gastroenterology 1984;86:461-467.
3. Rios-Castellanos E, Sitas F, Shepherd NA, Jewell DP. Changing pattern of gastric cancer in Oxfordshire. Gut 1992;33:1312-1317.
4. Wang HH, Antonioli DA, Goldman H. Comparative features of esophageal and gastric adenocarcinomas: recent changes in type and frequency. Hum Pathol 1986;17:482-487.
5. Johnston TB, Whillis J. Gray's anatomy. Descriptive and applies, 31st ed. London: Longmans, Green and Co., 1954:1388-1396.
6. American Joint Committee on Cancer. AJCC cancer staging manual, 5th ed. Philadelphia: Lippincott-Raven, 1997:71.
7. Antonioli DA, Madara JL. Functional anatomy of the gastrointestinal tract. In: Ming SC, Goldman H, eds. Pathology of the gastrointestinal tract. Baltimore: Williams & Wilkins, 1998:16-18.
8. Owen DA. Stomach. In: Sternberg SS, ed. Histology for pathologists. New York: Lippincott-Raven Publishers, 1997:481-483.
9. Lewin KJ, Appelman HD. Tumors of the esophagus and stomach, Fascicle 18, 3rd series. Washington: Armed Forces Institute of Pathology, 1996:317
10. Toner PG, Cameron CHS. The gastric mucosa. In: Whitehead R, ed. Gastrointestinal and oesophageal pathology. New York: Churchill Livingstone, 1995:16.
11. Locke GR, Talley NJ, Carpenter HA, et al. Changes in the site- and histology-specific incidence of gastric cancer during a 50-year period. Gastroenterology 1995;109:1750-1756.
12. Misumi A, Murakami A, Harada K, et al. Definition of carcinoma of the gastric cardia. Langenbecks Arch Chir 1989;374:221-226.
13. Geisinger KR. Is the lower esophagus lined by columnar epithelium always Barrett's mucosa? In: Giuli R, Tytgat GNJ, DeMeester TR, Galmiche JP, eds. The esophageal mucosa. Amsterdam: Elsevier, 1994:798-803.
14. Haggitt RC. Barrett's esophagus, dysplasia, and adenocarcinoma. Hum Pathol 1994;25:982-993.
15. Heidl G, Langhans P, Krieg V, et al. Comparative studies of cardia carcinoma and infracardial carcinoma. J Cancer Res Clin Oncol 1993;120:91-94.
16. Genta RM, Huberman RM, Graham DY. The gastric cardia in Helicobacter pylori infection. Hum Pathol 1994;25:915-919.
17. Goldblum JR, Vicari JJ, Falk GW, et al. Inflammation and intestinal metaplasia of the gastric cardia: the role of gastroesophageal reflux and H pylori infection. Gastroenterology 1998;114:633-639.
18. Byrne JP, Bhatnagar S, Hamid B, et al. Comparative study of intestinal metaplasia and mucin staining at the cardia and esophagogastric junction in 225 symptomatic patients presenting for diagnostic open-access gastroscopy. Am J Gastroenterol 1999;94:98-103.
19. Peek RM Jr, Vaezi MF, Falk GW, et al. Role of Helicobacter pylori cagA+ strains and specific host immune responses on the development of premalignant and malignant lesions in the gastric cardia. Int J Cancer 1999;82:520-524.
20. van Decken H, Gelen E, Dinjens WN, et al. Comparative genomic hybridization of cancer of the gastroesophageal junction: deletion of 14Q31-32.1 discriminates between esophageal (Barrett's) and gastric cardia adenocarcinomas. Cancer Res 1999;59:748-752.
21. Lagergren J, Bergstrom R, Lindgren A, Nyren O. Symptomatic gastroesophageal reflux as a risk factor for esophageal adenocarcinoma. N Engl J Med 1999;340:825-831.
22. Blot WJ, Devesa SS, Kneller RW, Fraumeni JF Jr. Rising incidence of adenocarcinoma of the esophagus and gastric cardia. JAMA 1991;265:1287-1289.
23. Cameron AJ, Lomboy CT, Pera M, Carpenter HA. Adenocarcinoma of the esophagogastric junction and Barrett's esophagus. Gastroenterology 1995;109:1541-1546.
24. Clark GWB, Smyrk TC, Burdiles P, et al. Is Barrett's metaplasia the source of adenocarcinomas of the cardia? Arch Surg 1994;129:609-624.
25. Appelman HD, Kalish RJ, Clancy PE, Orringer MB. Distinguishing features of adenocarcinoma in Barrett's esophagus and in the gastric cardia. In: Spechler SJ, Goyal RK, E-eds. Barrett's esophagus: pathophysiology, diagnosis and management. New York: Elsevier Science Publishing Co Inc, 1985:167-187.
26. Wijnhoven BPL, Siersema PD, Hop WCJ, et al. Adenocarcinoma of the distal oesophagus and gastric cardia are one clinical entity. Br J Surg 1999;86:529-535.
27. Mori M, Kitagawa S, Iida M, et al. Early carcinoma of the gastric cardia. A clinicopathologic study of 21 cases. Cancer 1987;59:1758-1766.

28. Iannettoni MD, Lee, SS, Bonnell MR, et al. Detection of Barrett's adenocarcinoma of the gastric cardia with sucrase isomaltase and p53. Ann Thorac Surg 1996;62:1460-1466.
29. Guanrei Y, Sunglian Q. Incidence of adenocarcinoma of the gastric cardia, and endoscopic classification of early cardial carcinoma in Henan Province, the People's Republic of China. Endoscopy 1987;19:7-10.
30. Husemann B. Cardia carcinoma considered as a distinct clinical entity. Br J Surg 1989;76:136-139.
31. Wang LS, Wu CW, Hsieh MJ, et al. Lymph node metastasis in patients with adenocarcinoma of the gastric cardia. Cancer 1993;71:1948-1953.
32. Ellis FH Jr, Watkins E Jr, Krasna MJ, et al. Staging of carcinoma of the esophagus and cardia:a comparison of different staging criteria. J Surg Oncol 1993;52:231-235.
33. Palli D, Bianchi S, Decarli A, et al. A case-controlled study of cancers of the gastric cardia in Italy. Br J Cancer 1992;65:263-266.
34. Maehara Y, Takahashi I, Okuyama T, et al. Diagnostic factors in gastric cardia cancer invading the esophagus. Cancer 1993;71:302-305.
35. Okamura T, Korenaga D, Saito A, et al. Reactive changes in the esophageal epithelium and predictability of survival for patients with adenocarcinoma of the upper third of the stomach. Cancer 1989;63:769-773.

What are the histologic criteria for the diagnosis of incipient invasion in Barrett's mucosa with high-grade dysplasia?

H.D. Appelman (Ann Arbor)

From a pathologist's perspective, there are three recurrent annoying diagnostic problems that are inherent in Barrett's. First, the diagnosis of low-grade dysplasia in Barrett's mucosa is often difficult, since regenerative or reparative epithelium shares features with dysplastic epithelium, including primitive cytoplasm, large nuclei and mitoses. Because of this the category of "indefinite for dysplasia" was invented. In contrast, the diagnosis of high-grade dysplasia (HGD) is somewhat easier, because it has a much greater degree of cellular and architectural disorganization and more profound nuclear changes of hyperchromatism, crowding, pleomorphism and mitoses. However, the second diagnostic problem, although less common than the other two, relates to those dysplastic epithelia that are mainly low-grade, but they have some features that suggest that the transition to high-grade is occurring. There are no tightly defined histologic guidelines for determining at exactly what point HGD is present. The third major problem is determining if there incipient invasion of carcinoma cells into the lamina propria within a field of HGD. The issue of whether there is incipient invasion usually arises when a biopsy with HGD contains dysplastic tubules that are crowded and/or have strange shapes or in which single cells or strands of cells seem to be disengaged from the adjacent dysplastic tubules. Pathologists try to make the diagnosis of incipient invasion, but what are the criteria they use to do so? Considering the importance of the diagnosis of invasive carcinoma in Barrett's mucosa, there is amazingly little in the way of published criteria, not just for incipient invasion, but for supposedly obvious or clear-cut invasion.

In the new Vienna classification of epithelial neoplasia for the entire gastroenteric tract, the term noninvasive carcinoma "stands for absence of evident invasion" while the term intramucosal carcinoma "stands for invasive into the lamina propria or muscularis mucosae" [1-3]. These definitions were agreed upon by an international group of gastrointestinal pathologists, some of the current giants in the field, but, unfortunately, they neglected to offer us specific criteria for applying those definitions. So, what about the rest of the world's literature; does it offer diagnostic help?

In some studies, the definition of incipient invasion is given as "invasion beyond (or through) the epithelial basement membrane", but this has little meaning unless the term is explained in great detail [4, 5]. Does this mean that the basement membrane is incomplete and any dysplastic cells adjacent to the defect in the basement membrane are invasive? Basement membranes beneath dysplastic epithelium are likely to be attenuated or even absent in small patches, yet we do not usually conclude that such defects indicate that invasion has occurred. Does invasion through the basement membrane mean that cells actually stick out from the dysplastic tubules through defects in the basement membrane into the lamina propria? We don't know, because details are rarely given. Furthermore, the basement membrane is not visible in routine H & E sections. It can only be visualized in special stains for basement membrane components, such as type IV collagen or laminen, and pathologists do not routinely stain biopsies for basement membrane components in order to prove that such defects occurs. In addition, some carcinomas actually synthesize basement membrane material, so that invasive structures may actually be encased in basement membrane.

A more detailed set of criteria for intramucosal carcinoma in gastric mucosa that should be applicable to Barrett's mucosa uses "irregularity of pit outlines with irregular infiltration into the lamina propria" as something that is used operationally, but the strict definition of "irregular infiltration into the lamina propria" is not given [2]. In the paper in which this is discussed the authors mention that separating small glands that are attached to larger tubules can be difficult to distinguish from lamina propria invasion, but no specific criteria for lamina propria invasion were given.

One criterion that seems to be used commonly for invasion is the presence of single dysplastic cells or small clumps of them, within the lamina propria, separated from the tubules of the background dysplasia [6, 7]. The problem with this criterion is that it requires serial sections to ensure that the cells are truly separated from the adjacent tubules.

In another study the authors mentioned different criteria for invasion in discussing three specific cases. The diagnosis of intramucosal carcinoma in biopsies in these cases was based on "glandular crowding or intraluminal necrosis, but actual invasion was not demonstrated". Furthermore, more traditional evidence of invasion, namely "single-cell invasion, proliferation of irregular shaped glands, and sheets of neoplastic cells or stromal desmoplasia were not seen". As it turned out, when these three esophagi were resected, no invasive carcinoma was found, so the criteria used to identify invasion, namely glandular crowing or necrosis, may not have been the right ones [8].

Desmoplasia, that is, fibroblastic stromal proliferation usually including collagen and mucopolysaccharides, has been mentioned as a helpful hint in identifying invasion. There is one basic problem with desmoplasia. It virtually never occurs when the carcinoma is limited to the mucosa, but it develops when the carcinoma reaches the submucosa. Thus it is of no use in identifying incipient invasion of the lamina propria.

There is one indirect but very powerful histologic hint that an invasive carcinoma is present when the biopsy only contains HGD. That is an ulcer appearing either as granulation tissue from the ulcer bed or as a separate fragment of exudate in the biopsy [9, 10]. Dysplasias virtually never ulcerate, while carcinomas commonly do so.

If the criteria for invasion are so unsettled, how then do we pathologists make that diagnosis. The answer given at the OESO Congress four years ago by Riddell has not changed [11]. He said that "the only criterion for the confident or unequivocal diagnosis of invasive carcinoma in the lamina propria is the pathologists own subjective and personal interpretation that invasion may or may not be present. If in many instances minimal invasion is not based on objective criteria but on hunches, experience, and the fear of missing an underlying carcinoma, then there are no minimal criteria for" such invasion. What this says is that experienced pathologists have developed subjective criteria for detecting incipient invasion in biopsies, and such criteria appear to correlate with the finding of invasion once the esophagus has been resected. They try to create objective descriptions of these subjective criteria, but they often fail in these attempts. I have been using such a subjective approach for years, and I suspect that so have virtually every other pathologist who deals with intraepithelial neoplasia in the columnar gastrointestinal tract. It is likely that this unsettled bit of reality explains why the literature on this subject is also so unsettled.

References

1. Schlemper RJ, Riddell RH, Kato Y, et al. The Vienna classification of gastrointestinal epithelial neoplasia. Gut 2000;47:251-255.
2. Lauwers GY, Riddell RH. Gastric epithelial dysplasia. Gut 1999;45:784-790.
3. Geboes K, Van Eyken P. The diagnosis of dysplasia and malignancy in Barrett's oesophagus. Histopathology 2000;37:99-107.
4. Peters JH, Clark GWB, Ireland AP, et al. Outcome of adenocarcinoma arising in Barrett's esophagus in endoscopically surveyed and nonsurveyed patients. J Thorac Cardiovasc Surg 1994;108:813-822.
5. Van Sandick JW, van Lanschot JJB, Kuiken BW, et al. Impact of endoscopic biopsy surveillance of Barrett's oesophagus on pathological stage and clinical outcome of Barrett's carcinoma. Gut 1998;43:216-222.
6. Haggitt, RC. Barrett's esophagus, dysplasia, and adenocarcinoma. Hum Pathol 1994;25:982-993.
7. Lewin KJ, Appelman HD. Tumors of the esophagus and stomach. Fascicle 18, 3rd series. Atlas of tumor pathology. Washington: Armed Forces Institute of Pathology, 1996:135.
8. Cameron AJ, Carpenter HA. Barrett's esophagus, high-grade dysplasia, and early adenocarcinoma: a pathological study. Am J Gastroenterol 1992;92:586-591.
9. Burke AP, Sobin LH, Shekitka KM, Helwig EB. Dysplasia of the stomach and Barrett's esophagus: a follow-up study. Mod Pathol 1991;4:336-341.
10. Montgomery EA. Unpublished data, September, 2000.
11. Riddell RH. Are there minimal criteria for the confident or unequivocal diagnosis of invasive carcinoma in the lamina propria both in Barrett's mucosa and in squamous mucosa? In: Giuli R, Galmiche JP, Jamieson GC, Scarpignato C, eds. The esophagogastric junction. Paris: John Libby Eurotext, 1998:1171-1172.

What are the epidemiologic similarities and differences between carcinomas arising in Barrett's mucosa and in the gastric cardia?

L. Bernstein (Los Angeles)

This effort was supported by NIH grants CA59636 and CA17054 as well as contract N01-CN-67010 from the National Cancer Institute. The Los Angeles County cancer incidence data were collected, in part, under Subcontract 050K-8709 with the Public Health Institute.

Incidence

The incidence rates for esophageal adenocarcinomas have increased dramatically over the past two decades in the United States and Europe [1-8]. Similar, but smaller increases have occurred in the incidence rates of adenocarcinomas of the gastric cardia.

We have evaluated the patterns of incidence of esophageal adenocarcinomas and adenocarcinomas of the gastric cardia in detail, using data from the Los Angeles County Cancer Surveillance Program, the population-based cancer registry that covers this ethnically diverse population of more than 9.5 million people. Overall, incidence rates of esophageal adenocarcinomas and adenocarcinomas of the gastric cardia vary substantially by race and gender (*Table I*). Non-Hispanic and Hispanic white men have the highest rates

Table I. Age-adjusted incidence rates of adenocarcinomas of the esophagus (EAC) and gastric cardia (GCA) per 100,000 population by race/ethnicity. Los Angeles County, 1972-1997. Number of cases given in parentheses.

Racial/ethnic group	Esophagus	Gastric cardia	Ratio (GCA/EAC)
Males			
Non-Hispanic white	1.7 (1,008)	3.1 (1,865)	1.8
Hispanic white	1.7 (180)	2.6 (280)	1.5
Black	0.5 (45)	1.4 (109)	2.8
Chinese	0.6 (9)	2.0 (31)	3.3
Japanese	0.9 (14)	3.1 (49)	3.4
Filipino	0.3 (5)	1.1 (18)	3.7
Korean	– (1)	2.1 (19)	–
All races	1.5 (1,263)	2.7 (2,391)	1.8
Females			
Non-Hispanic white	0.2 (213)	0.6 (503)	3.0
Hispanic white	0.2 (23)	0.7 (95)	3.5
Black	0.2 (22)	0.4 (45)	2.0
Chinese	– (1)	0.6 (11)	–
Japanese	– (2)	0.3 (5)	–
Filipino	– (1)	0.7 (11)	–
Korean	– (0)	1.1 (13)	–
All races	0.2 (263)	0.6 (690)	

Note: rates not presented if fewer than 5 cases

of esophageal adenocarcinomas, rates that are more than 3 times those of blacks. Asians also have lower rates of esophageal adenocarcinomas than whites. Rates of adenocarcinomas of the gastric cardia are also higher for whites than for blacks, but the 2-fold difference in incidence is smaller than is observed for esophageal adenocarcinomas. Esophageal adenocarcinomas and adenocarcinomas of the gastric cardia are substantially less likely to be diagnosed among women with male-to-female rate ratios ranging from 8 for esophageal adenocarcinomas to 5 for adenocarcinomas of the gastric cardia among non-Hispanic whites. As shown in *Figure 1*, rates of esophageal adenocarcinomas have surpassed those for adenocarcinomas of the gastric cardia among non-Hispanic white men in Los Angeles County. The same is true for Hispanic white men (data not shown). This crossover has not been observed among white women, blacks or Asians. The rates of adenocarcinomas of the gastric cardia among non-Hispanic white men (as well as Hispanic white men) increased somewhat in the early to mid-1970s, but have remained relatively constant since that time (*Figure 1*). This contrasts with reports from other areas of the US that show a steady increase in incidence [1]. Among white women and among blacks and Asians in Los Angeles County, esophageal adenocarcinomas rates increased, but adenocarcinomas of the gastric cardia rates remained fairly constant throughout the period of study (data not shown). Socioeconomic status (based on the median household income and education level of residents Los Angeles County census tracts) is predictive of risk of squamous cell carcinoma of the esophagus (SCCE) in Los Angeles County (data not shown) with rates lowest among those with the highest socioeconomic status ranking as would be expected for a cancer that is strongly related to smoking and alcohol intake; both esophageal adenocarcinomas and adenocarcinomas of the gastric cardia appear to be unrelated to socioeconomic status in Los Angeles County (*Figure 2*).

One of the issues that may mask more extreme epidemiologic differences in incidence between esophageal adenocarcinomas and adenocarcinomas of the gastric cardia is the lack of a consistent description of what constitutes the cardia. In general, cancer registries throughout the world rely on the pathologist's attribution of site. Yet, as noted by Appleman [9], no clear definitions that separate cardiac cancers from distal Barrett's cancers of the esophagus have been uniformly accepted in the pathology literature. Cancer statistics are based on the International Classification of Diseases for Oncology [10], which includes tumors originating at the gastroesophageal junction (GEJ) with cardia primaries.

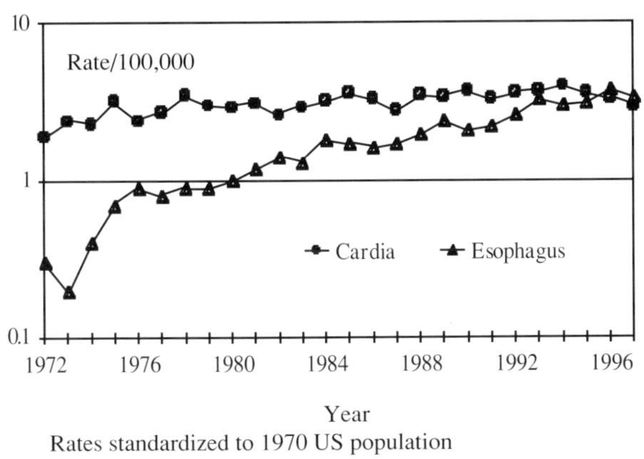

Figure 1. Secular trends in the age-adjusted incidence rates of carcinomas of the esophagus and gastric cardia of non-Latino white males in Los Angeles County 1972-1997. Incidence rates adjusted to the 1970 US population.

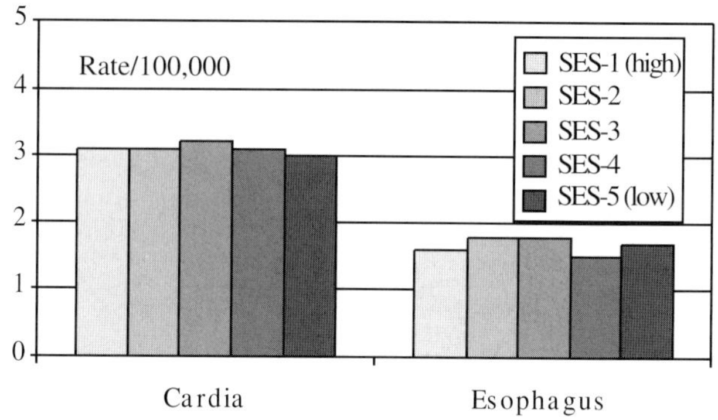

Figure 2. Age-adjusted incidence rates of carcinomas of the esophagus and gastric cardia in non-Hispanic white males according to socioeconomic status at the time of diagnosis, Los Angeles County 1972-1997. Incidence rates adjusted to the 1970 US population.

Potential risk factors

The rapid rise in incidence of esophageal adenocarcinomas and adenocarcinomas of the gastric cardia observed throughout US and Europe suggests that environmental risk factors are important in the development of these cancers. Risk factors currently being considered as possible explanations for these emerging patterns of incidence are tobacco and alcohol consumption, body mass index, the use of drugs that affect gastroesophageal function or treat gastroesophageal conditions, and the existence of these conditions themselves. Because these types of cancer are still relatively rare and because their descriptive epidemiologies are similar, early studies of risk factors combined the two types of cancer, preventing a direct comparison of risk factors.

Here we contrast the findings from the two major epidemiologic studies where the two cancer sites have been individually studied in the same population: a Swedish case-control study [11-13] and a US case-control study [14-18]. The Swedish study recruited patients diagnosed at one of 195 hospitals and used a carefully prescribed protocol for serial biopsies collected from the proximal stomach through the lower esophagus to a location where normal squamous-cell epithelium was encountered to define subsite. Cancer of the cardia was restricted to lesions within 2 cm proximal or 3 cm distal to the GEJ. This study included 189 patients with esophageal adenocarcinomas, 262 patients with adenocarcinomas of the gastric cardia and 820 control subjects The US study collected cases from cancer registries in 3 areas of the US (New Jersey, Connecticut and western Washington state); histologic material and surgical, endoscopic and radiology reports were reviewed by a panel of pathologists to confirm subsite attribution. This study included 293 patients with esophageal adenocarcinomas, 261 patients with adenocarcinomas of the gastric cardia and 695 control subjects.

Tobacco and alcohol

Cigarette smoking and alcohol abuse are known risk factors for SCCE [19] and evidence is accumulating to show that cigarette smoking is a risk factor for gastric cancer [20]. Tobacco smoking and alcohol consumption may cause esophagitis and increase episodes of gastric reflux. Tobacco smoking also may slow gastric emptying, alter acid secretion, or serve as a source of N-nitroso compounds. Condensation products from tobacco smoke may have an irritant effect on the esophagus and gastric mucosa. Tobacco smoke also has a wide range of effects on gastrointestinal physiology which include slowing gastric emptying, altering acid secretion, inducing duodenogastric and gastroesophageal reflux, and impairing the healing and increasing rates of recurrence of duodenal ulcer [21-24]. All of these effects may in turn contribute to an increase in risk of esophageal adenocarcinomas and adenocarcinomas of the gastric cardia.

In the US case-control study, smoking was associated with increased risk of esophageal adenocarcinomas and adenocarcinomas of the gastric cardia with risk estimates similar for both subsites [14] whereas the risk estimates obtained in the Swedish study showed a much stronger effect for adenocarcinomas of the gastric cardia than for esophageal adenocarcinomas [13] (*Table II*). These risk estimates are lower than those observed for SCCE [13, 14]. One of the more interesting findings in both studies is that the risk of ex-smokers is not substantially lower than that of current smokers as is usually observed for smoking-related cancers including SCCE. In fact, the risk among ex-smokers appears to be relatively stable for at least 25 to 30 years after smoking cessation.

Table II. Multivariate relative risk (odds ratio = OR and 95% confidence interval = 95% CI) of adenocarcinomas of the esophagus (EAC) and gastric cardia (GCA) associated with cigarette smoking.

Characteristic		EAC OR 95% CI	GCA OR 95% CI
Gammon *et al.* [14]			
Smoking status	Never smoker	1.0	1.0
	Ex-smoker	2.0 (1.4-2.9)	1.9 (1.3-2.9)
	Current smoker	2.2 (1.4-3.3)	2.6 (1.7-4.0)
Ex smokers: stopped smoking	< 11 years ago	2.7 (1.6-4.4)	2.9 (1.8-4.8)
	11-20 years ago	2.3 (1.4-3.8)	1.6 (0.9-2.8)
	21-30 years ago	1.9 (1.1-3.2)	2.2 (1.3-3.7)
	> 30 years ago	1.2 (0.7-2.2)	1.1 (0.6-2.0)
Ever smokers: duration	< 20 years	1.4 (0.9-2.2)	1.6 (1.0-2.6)
	20-31 years	1.7 (1.0-2.8)	1.8 (1.1-2.9)
	32-42 years	2.9 (1.8-4.4)	2.7 (1.7-4.2)
	> 42 years	2.4 (1.5-3.7)	2.9 (1.8-4.7)
Lagergren *et al.* [13]			
Smoking status	Never smoker	1.0	1.0
	Ex-smoker	1.9 (1.2-2.9)	3.4 (2.2-5.2)
	Current smoker	1.6 (0.9-2.7)	4.5 (2.9-7.1)
Recency of smoking: smoked	0-2 years ago*	1.7 (1.0-3.0)	5.0 (3.2-8.0)
	3-10 years ago	2.4 (1.2-4.8)	4.9 (2.8-8.7)
	11-25 years ago	1.6 (0.9-2.5)	4.2 (2.6-7.0)
	> 25 years ago	1.6 (0.9-2.8)	2.1 (1.2-3.6)
Ever smokers: duration	< 21 years	1.8 (1.1-3.1)	2.1 (1.2-3.4)
	21-35 years	1.5 (0.9-2.6)	3.9 (2.4-6.2)
	> 35 years	2.0 (1.2-3.3)	5.7 (3.6-9.1)

* Includes current smokers

In both studies, alcohol consumption was unrelated to the risk of esophageal adenocarcinomas and adenocarcinomas of the gastric cardia, with multivariate relative risk estimates generally below 1.0 [13, 14]. In three previous studies that combined esophageal adenocarcinomas and adenocarcinomas of the gastric cardia patients, consumption of large amounts of alcoholic beverages, especially regular consumption of hard liquor, was associated with increased risk [25-27]. These risk estimates were lower than is generally observed for SCCE [25].

Obesity

Both the Swedish study and the US study have published results examining the relationship between body mass index (measured as weight in kg divided by height in meters-squared) and risk of esophageal adenocarcinomas and adenocarcinomas of the gastric cardia [12, 17]. The Swedish study obtained measures of height and weight 20 years before the interview (and diagnosis of cancer), whereas the US study based analyses on body mass index one year before interview (or diagnosis). Obesity appears to be related to greater risk of both esophageal adenocarcinomas and adenocarcinomas of the gastric cardia [12, 17]; however, the magnitude of risk varies in these two studies and it appears that the effect is stronger for esophageal adenocarcinomas than adenocarcinomas of the gastric cardia (*Table III*). The prevalence of obesity is increasing dramatically in the western world; between 1976-1980 and 1988-1994, the proportion of the adult US population with a body mass index of 30 or greater increased 8% [28]. In the Swedish study, among persons with a body mass index greater than 30, the risk of esophageal adenocarcinomas was 19.7 and of

Table III. Multivariate relative risk (odds ratio = OR and 95% confidence interval = 95% CI) of adenocarcinomas of the esophagus (EAC) and gastric cardia (GCA) associated with Body mass index.

Characteristic		EAC OR 95% CI	GCA OR 95% CI
Chow *et al.* [17]			
Body mass index 1 year before interview/diagnosis			
Men	Quartile 1 - low	1.0	1.0
	Quartile 2	1.5 (0.8-2.5)	0.9 (0.6-1.6)
	Quartile 3	2.0 (1.2-3.5)	1.3 (0.8-2.2)
	Quartile 4	3.0 (1.7-5.0)	1.8 (1.1-2.9)
Women			
	Quartile 1 - low	1.0	1.0
	Quartile 2	0.8 (0.2-3.4)	0.9 (0.2-3.2)
	Quartile 3	2.1 (0.6-7.4)	2.2 (0.7-7.1)
	Quartile 4	2.6 (0.8-8.5)	1.3 (0.4-4.2)
Lagergren *et al.* [12]			
Body mass index 20 years before interview/diagnosis (sex-specific quartiles developed)			
	Quartile 1- low	1.0	1.0
	Quartile 2	2.2 (1.0-4.7)	0.9 (0.6-1.5)
	Quartile 3	3.8 (1.9-7.7)	1.4 (0.9-2.2)
	Quartile 4	7.6 (3.8-15.2)	2.3 (1.5-3.6)

adenocarcinomas of the gastric cardia was 4.8 relative to study participants in the lowest quartile of body mass index.

Obesity is related to risk of gastroesophageal reflux disease (GERD). A recent study of participants in the US National Health and Nutrition Examination Survey (NHANES-I) who were hospitalized for GERD showed that body mass index was a predictor of the risk of being hospitalized with GERD [29]. However, it is uncertain whether weight loss reduces symptoms of GERD [30].

Medical conditions

Barrett's esophagus is considered the major risk factor for esophageal adenocarcinomas and for lesions occurring at the GEJ. Barrett's esophagus is a relatively common disorder, diagnosed in 0.8 to 3.9% of all upper endoscopies [4]. Not all Barrett's esophagus is associated with symptomatology, however, and, the reported prevalence on autopsy is more than 20 times greater than that seen clinically [31].

A number of medical conditions and symptoms, including a history of chronic esophageal reflux, esophagitis or esophageal ulcer, hiatal hernia and difficulty swallowing are associated with increased risk of esophageal adenocarcinomas and adenocarcinomas of the gastric cardia [32]. These epidemiologic results confirm clinical observations showing that these conditions and symptoms are more prevalent among patients with esophageal adenocarcinomas and adenocarcinomas of the gastric cardia than among patients with more distal gastric tumors or SCCE. Lagergren *et al.* directly compared the effects of reflux symptoms on risk of esophageal adenocarcinomas and adenocarcinomas of the gastric cardia in the Swedish case-control study [11]. They included only symptoms that occurred five or more years before interview (or diagnosis) and showed that persons who experienced reflux symptoms at least weekly had 7.7-fold greater risk of esophageal adenocarcinomas than persons without such symptoms. A much weaker effect was noted for adenocarcinomas of the gastric cardia where the relative risk was about 2. Frequency, duration and intensity of reflux symptoms were all predictors of risk, with marked dose-response effects observed for esophageal adenocarcinomas.

In the US case-control study, greater frequency and duration of GERD symptoms predicted greater risk of esophageal adenocarcinomas, but not adenocarcinomas of the gastric cardia [18]. Hiatal hernia and esophagitis or esophageal ulcer were associated with significant increased risk of esophageal adenocarcinomas; however, gastric ulcer and duodenal ulcer were unrelated to risk. None of these conditions were related to risk of adenocarcinomas of the gastric cardia.

Drugs

Histamine (H_2) receptor antagonists (blockers) have become widely used in the US since the late 1970s as a preferred treatment for duodenal and gastric ulcers, esophageal reflux and other benign conditions of the stomach, esophagus and duodenum. The rationale for considering their use as a potential risk factor for esophageal adenocarcinomas is based on some clinical survey data [33, 34], animal studies showing that alkaline reflux causes esophageal adenocarcinomas [35], and the fact that Barrett's esophagus is thought to result from alkaline reflux [4].

Other mechanisms are possible. Use of H_2-blockers could result in higher amounts of gastric colonization by nitrate-reducing bacteria, thereby increasing intragastric levels of carcinogenic nitrosamines. Furthermore, two H_2-blockers, cimetidine and ranitidine, are themselves nitrosated under acidic conditions [36, 37].

The issues involved in assessing the risk associated with use of H_2-blockers and other antacids are complex. Conditions for which these drugs may be prescribed are also potential risk or predisposing factors for esophageal adenocarcinomas and possibly adenocarcinomas of the gastric cardia. Lagergren *et al.* have carefully evaluated this issue in their case-control study by comparing the risk of esophageal adenocarcinomas among persons who used medications for reflux symptoms at least 5 years prior to study to the risk among person with symptoms who did not use any medication [11]. They report that risk was nearly 3-fold higher among those using medications for symptoms than among those who took no medication. Results for adenocarcinomas of the gastric cardia were not reported.

Farrow *et al.* also evaluated the risk of esophageal adenocarcinomas and adenocarcinomas of the gastric cardia in association with the use of H_2-blockers [18]. They noted an increased risk of esophageal adenocarcinomas only among those persons who did not experience GERD symptoms regularly (at least monthly) in direct contrast to the results of the Swedish study [11]. The US study also observed an increase in risk of both esophageal adenocarcinomas and adenocarcinomas of the gastric cardia associated with use of over-the-counter antacid products.

Drugs that promote GER by their own action or by relaxing the lower esophageal sphincter may also affect risk of esophageal adenocarcinomas and adenocarcinomas of the gastric cardia. Calcium channel blockers, tricyclic antidepressants, and some asthma medications are known to have these effects. The US case-control study examined the effects of such drugs on risk of esophageal adenocarcinomas and adenocarcinomas of the gastric cardia, and found that risk of esophageal adenocarcinomas but not adenocarcinomas of the gastric cardia was elevated among persons who used asthma drugs containing theophylline or b agonists (odds ratios of 2.5 and 1.7 respectively) [15]. Use of calcium channel blockers and tricyclic antidepressants did not increase the risk of cancer at either site.

Non-steroidal anti-inflammatory drugs (NSAIDs) appear to reduce the risk of colon and several other cancers, possibly by inhibiting prostaglandin synthesis, reducing prostaglandin-induced immunosuppression, and inducing apoptosis [38, 39]. These effects would suggest that use of NSAIDs should reduce esophageal adenocarcinomas and adenocarcinomas of the gastric cardia risk. However, NSAIDS also have been associated with benign esophageal stricture and may act as irritants to the gastric mucosa. In this case, increased cell division might occur during the process of repair of the damaged tissue resulting eventually in neoplastic transformation [40]. There is also some evidence that the continued use of NSAIDs impairs the healing of gastric ulcers by H_2-blockers [41]. Evaluation of the relationship of NSAIDs to esophageal adenocarcinomas and adenocarcinomas of the gastric cardia risk is problematic since patients with chronic gastrointestinal symptoms are less likely to use these compounds and are at increased risk of these cancers. The US case-control study showed a lower risk of esophageal adenocarcinomas among current users of NSAIDs, but no effect on risk of adenocarcinomas of the gastric cardia [16].

Summary

Epidemiologic studies of esophageal adenocarcinomas and adenocarcinomas of the gastric cardia are difficult to conduct because of the relatively short survival of many patients. Two major studies have now provided some results on possible risk factors that might account for the rapid increase in incidence of esophageal adenocarcinomas over the past 2 decades. During this time frame, endoscopy has become a standard diagnostic tool and new drugs have been introduced to treat gastrointestinal conditions. In addition, the prevalence of obesity has increased dramatically. Cigarette smoking appears to have some effect on risk of esophageal adenocarcinomas and adenocarcinomas of the gastric cardia, although the strength of these effects is far less than is observed for SCCE where the relationship between these two risk factors and disease development is considered to be causal. It is possible that the effects of smoking are stronger for adenocarcinomas of the gastric cardia than for esophageal adenocarcinomas. Obesity is predictive of risk at both cancer sites, with effects possibly stronger for esophageal adenocarcinomas. GERD symptoms are more strongly predictive of risk of esophageal adenocarcinomas than of adenocarcinomas of the gastric cardia. Still unresolved is whether H_2-blockers or other antacid preparations are related to risk or simply reflective of the intensity of GERD symptoms.

References

1. Blot WJ, Devesa SS, Kneller RW, et al. Rising incidence of adenocarcinoma of the esophagus and gastric cardia. JAMA 1991;265:1287-1289.
2. Pera M, Cameron AJ, Trastek VF, et al. Increasing incidence of adenocarcinoma of the esophagus and esophagogastric junction. Gastroenterology 1993;104:510-513.
3. Zheng T, Mayne ST, Holford TR, et al. Time trend and age-period-cohort effects on incidence of esophageal cancer in Connecticut, 1935-89. Cancer Cause Control 1992;3:481-492.
4. Kim R, Weissfeld JL, Reynolds JC, et al. Etiology of Barrett's metaplasia and esophageal adenocarcinoma. Cancer Epidemiol Biomarkers Prev 1997;6:369-377.
5. Powell J, McConkey CC. Increasing incidence of adenocarcinoma of the gastric cardia and adjacent sites. Br J Cancer 1990;59:440-443.
6. Tuyns AJ. Oesophageal cancer in France and Switzerland: recent time trends. Eur J Cancer Prev 1992;1:275-278.
7. Moller H. Incidence of cancer of the oesphagus, cardia and stomach in Denmark. Eur J Cancer Prev 1992;1:159-164.
8. Hansson LE, Sparen P, Nyrén O. Increasing incidence of both major histologic types of esophageal carcinomas among men in Sweden. Int J Cancer 1993;54:402-407.
9. Appleman HD. Do all adenocarcinomas at or near the esophagogastric junction have the same epidemiologic characteristics? In: Guili R, Galmiche JP, Jamieson GG, Scarpignato C, eds. The esophagogastric junction. Paris: John Libbey Eurotext, 1998:1155-1158.
10. Percy C, Van Holten V, Muir C. International classification of diseases for oncology, 2nd edition. Geneva: World Health Organization, 1990.
11. Lagergren J, Bergström R, Lindgren A, Nyrén O. Symptomatic gastroesophageal reflux as a risk factor for esophageal adenocarcinoma. N Engl J Med 1999;340;825-831.
12. Lagergren J, Bergström R, Nyrén O. Association between body mass and adenocarcinoma of the esophagus and gastric cardia. Ann Intern Med 1999;130:883-890.
13. Lagergren J, Bergström R, Lindgren A, Nyrén O. The role of tobacco, snuff and alcohol use in the aetiology of cancer of the oesophagus and gastric cardia. Int J Cancer 2000;85:340-346.
14. Gammon MD, Schoenberg JB, Ahsan H, et al. Tobacco, alcohol and socioeconomic status and adenocarcinomas of the esophagus and gastric cardia. J Natl Cancer Inst 1997;89:1277-1284.
15. Vaughan T, Farrow D, Hansten PD, et al. Risk of esophageal and gastric adenocarcinomas in relation to use of calcium channel blockers, asthma drugs and other medications that promote gastroesophageal reflux. Cancer Epidemiol Biomarkers Prev 1998;7:749-745.
16. Farrow DC, Vaughan TL, Hansten PD, et al. Use of aspirin and other nonsteroidal anti-inflammatory drugs and risk of esophageal and gastric cancer. Cancer Epidemiol Biomarkers Prev 1998;7:97-102.

17. Chow WH, Blot WJ, Vaughan TL, et al. Body mass index and risk of adenocarcinomas of the esophagus and gastric cardia. J Natl Cancer Inst 1998;90:150-155.
18. Farrow DC, Vaughan TL, Sweeney C, et al. Gastroesophageal reflux disease, use of H2 receptor antagonists, and risk of esophageal and gastric cancer. Cancer Causes Control 2000;11:231-239.
19. International Agency for Research on Cancer. Monographs on the evaluation of the carcinogenic risk of chemicals to humans. Tobacco smoking. Vol 38. Lyon: IARC, 1986.
20. Trédaniel J, Boffetta P, Buiatti E, et al. Tobacco smoking and gastric cancer:Review and meta-analysis. Int J Cancer 1997;72:565-573.
21. Johnson RD, Horowitz M, Maddox AF, et al. Cigarette smoking and rate of gastric emptying: effect on alcohol absorption. Br Med J 1991;302:20-23.
22. Murthy SNS, Dinoso VP, Clearfield HR, et al. Simultaneous measurement of basal pancreatic, gastric acid secretion, plasma gastrin and secretion during smoking. Gastroenterology 1977;73:758-761.
23. Muller-Lissner SA. Bile reflux is increased in cigarette smokers. Gastroenterology 1986;90:1205-1209.
24. McCarthy DM. Smoking ulcers - time to quit. N Engl J Med 1984;311;726-728.
25. Kabat GC, Ng SKC, Wynder EL. Tobacco, alcohol intake, and diet in relation to adenocarcinoma of the esophagus and gastric cardia. Cancer Cause Control 1993;4:123-132.
26. Vaughan TL, Davis S, Kristal A, et al. Obesity, alcohol and tobacco as risk factors for cancers of the esophagus and gastric cardia: adenocarcinoma versus squamous cell carcinoma. Cancer Epidemiol Biomarkers Prev 1995;4:85-92.
27. Brown LM, Silverman DT, Pottern SM, et al. Adenocarcinoma of the esophagus and esophagogastric junction in White men in the United States:alcohol, tobacco and socioeconomic factors. Cancer Causes Control 1994;5:333-340.
28. Flegal KM, Troiano RP. Changes in the distribution of body mass index of adults and children in the US population. Int J Obesity 2000;24:807-818.
29. Ruhl CE, Everhart JE. Overweight, but not high dietary fat intake, increases risk of gastroesophageal reflux disease hospitalization: the NHANES I epidemiologic followup study. Ann Epidemiol 1999;9:424-435.
30. Li SD, Mobarhan S. Association between body mass index and adenocarcinoma of the esophagus and gastric cardia. Nutr Rev 2000;58:54-56.
31. Cameron AJ, Zinsmeister AR, Ballard DJ, et al. Prevalence of columnar-lined (Barrett's) esophagus. Comparison of population-based and autopsy findings. Gastroenterology 1990;99:918-922.
32. Chow WH, Finkle WD, McLaughlin JK, et al. The relation of gastroesophageal reflux disease and its treatment to adenocarcinomas of the esophagus and gastric cardia. JAMA 1995;27:474-477.
33. Elder JB, Ganguli PC, Gillespie IE. Cimetidine and gastric cancer. Lancet 1979;1:1005-1006.
34. Reed PI, Cassell PG, Walters CL. Gastric cancer in patients who have taken cimetidine. Lancet 1979;1:1234-1235.
35. Attwood SE, Smyrk TC, DeMeester TR, et al. Duodenoesophageal reflux and the development of esophageal adenocarcinoma in rats. Surgery 1992;111:502-510.
36. Ichinotsubo D, MacKinnon EA, Liu C, et al. Mutagenicity of nitrosated cimetidines. Carcinogenesis 1981;2:261-264.
37. De Flora S, Bennicelli C, Camoirano A, et al. Genotoxicity of nitrosated ranitidine. Carcinogenesis 1983;4:255-260.
38. Berkl HJ, Holcombe RF, Middlebrooks M, et al. Nonsteroidal antiinflammatory drugs and colorectal cancer. Epidemiol Rev 1996;18:205-217.
39. Morgan G. Non-steroidal anti-inflammatory drugs and the chemoprevention of colorectal and oesophageal cancers. Gut 1996;38;646-648.
40. Preston-Martin S, Pike MC, Ross RK, et al. Increased cell division as a cause of human cancer. Cancer Res 1990;50:7415-7421.
41. Walan A, Bader JP, Classen M, et al. Effect of omeprazole and ranitidine on ulcer healing and relapse rates in patients with benign gastric ulcer. N Engl J Med 1989;320:69-75.

J. Lagergren (Stockholm)

The close anatomical locations, without distinct borders, and the similarities in incidence trends and risk factor profiles in previous epidemiological studies have led to the suspicion that adenocarcinomas of the esophagus and gastric cardia are actually the same disease [1].

A nationwide case-control study in Sweden, however, indicates that the risk factor profile is different for esophageal and cardia adenocarcinoma. The comparison of risk factor profiles of the esophageal and cardia adenocarcinomas of this study is presented.

Methods

A nationwide case-control study in Sweden was conducted during the period 1995-1997 with the aim to identify risk factors for adenocarcinoma of the esophagus and gastric cardia. It was an interview study of prospectively recruited cases and 820 population-based control subjects. The 189 patients with a diagnosis of esophageal adenocarcinoma and the 262 patients with cardia adenocarcinoma that were interviewed represented 85% of all eligible cases. The tumor classification was very thorough with the aim to strictly separate adenocarcinomas arising in the esophagus and in the gastric cardia. The details of the classification and methodology has been presented elsewhere [2].

Results

Gastroesophageal reflux, as measured by reflux symptoms, was a very strong risk factor for adenocarcinoma of the esophagus, but only a moderately strong risk factor for adenocarcinoma of the gastric cardia [2]. The risk estimates increased with increases in the frequency of symptoms, the symptom score, and the duration of symptoms. Among persons with both long-standing and severe symptoms, the odds ratio (OR) for esophageal adenocarcinoma was 43.5 (95% confidence interval (CI), 18.3-103.5), and 4.4 (95% CI, 1.7-11.0) for cardia adenocarcinoma as compared with asymptomatic persons.

Similarly, a strong association was found between increasing body mass and the risk of esophageal adenocarcinoma, while the association with gastric cardia adenocarcinoma was weaker [3]. Obese persons (BMI > 30) had an OR of 16.2 (95% CI, 6.3-41.4) for esophageal adenocarcinoma and 4.3 (95% CI, 2.1-8.7) for cardia adenocarcinoma, compared with the leanest (BMI < 22).

Table I. Schematic summary of the present findings concerning risk factor profiles for esophageal adenocarcinoma and gastric cardia adenocarcinoma.

Risk factor	Esophageal adenocarcinoma	Gastric cardia adenocarcinoma
Reflux	+++	+
Obesity	+++	+
Tobacco smoking	–	++
Alcohol use	–	–
Use of medications that relax the lower esophageal sphincter	++	–
Low dietary intake of antioxidants	++	–
Low dietary intake of fiber	–	++
Heredity	–	+

+ denotes a weak positive association, ++ a moderately strong association, +++ a strong association, and – absence of a statistically significant association

We found no significant associations between tobacco smoking and esophageal adenocarcinoma. Gastric cardia adenocarcinoma, on the other hand, was dose-dependently associated with smoking [4]. The OR was 1.1 (95% CI, 0.6-2.2) for esophageal adenocarcinoma and 4.2 (95% CI, 2.5-7.0) for cardia adenocarcinoma among those who had smoked more than 20 cigarettes per day during more than 35 years compared with never smokers. There was no positive association between the use of alcohol and the risk of any of the two studied locations of adenocarcinoma [4].

Past use of medications that can relax the lower esophageal sphincter was significantly associated with the risk of esophageal adenocarcinoma, but cardia adenocarcinoma was not associated with these medications [5]. Among daily, long-term users (> 5 years) of any of these medications (nitroglycerin, aminophyllines, beta-receptor agonists, anticholinergics, benzodiazepines), OR of esophageal adenocarcinoma was 3.8 (95% CI, 2.2-6.4) compared with never-users.

We found that higher intake of antioxidants were associated with a decreased risk of esophageal adenocarcinoma, but not with cardia adenocarcinoma [6]. Among persons in the highest quartile of the parallel intake of vitamin C, alpha-tocopherol and beta-carotene the risk of esophageal adenocarcinoma was 50% reduced (95% CI, 0.3-0.9). There was a strong dose-dependent inverse association between dietary fiber intake and risk of gastric cardia adenocarcinoma, but no association was found with adenocarcinoma of the esophagus (unpublished data). The OR of esophageal adenocarcinoma among persons in the highest quartile of cereal fiber intake compared with the lowest was 0.3 (95% CI, 0.2-0.5).

Hereditary factors seem to play minor role in the etiology of esophageal adenocarcinoma, while such factors might be more important for cardia cancer [7]. The occurrence of esophageal cancer among first-degree relatives did not increase the risk of adenocarcinoma of the esophagus. Nor were there any significant associations with familial occurrence of gastric cancer or other gastrointestinal tumors. The risk of cardia adenocarcinoma was increased among persons with first-degree relatives with gastric cancer (OR 1.6; 95% CI, 1.0-2.6), however.

Conclusions

Our large-scale case-control study has revealed that the risk factor profiles of adenocarcinomas arising in the esophagus and in the gastric cardia are different and these tumors should be regarded as distinct disease entities in further research of the etiology.

References

1. Zhang ZF, Kurtz RC, Sun M, Karpeh M Jr, Yu GP, Gargon N, et al. Adenocarcinomas of the esophagus and gastric cardia: medical conditions, tobacco, alcohol, and socioeconomic factors. Cancer Epidemiol Biomark Prev 1996;5:761-768.
2. Lagergren J, Bergström R, Lindgren A, Nyrén O. Symptomatic gastroesophageal reflux is a strong risk factor for esophageal adenocarcinoma. N Engl J Med 1999;340:825-831.
3. Lagergren J, Bergström R, Nyrén O. Body mass as a risk factor for esophageal and gastric cardia adenocarcinoma. Ann Intern Med 1999;130:883-890.
4. Lagergren J, Bergström R, Lindgren A, Nyrén O. The role of tobacco, alcohol and snuff use in the aetiology of oesophageal and gastric cardia cancer. Int J Cancer 2000;85:340-346.

5. Lagergren J, Bergström R, Adami HO, Nyrén O. Association between medications that relax the lower esophageal sphincter and risk of esophageal adenocarcinoma. Ann Intern Med 2000;133:165-175.
6. Terry P, Lagergren J, Ye W, Wolk A, Nyrén O. Antioxidants and cancers of the esophagus and gastric cardia. Int J Cancer 2000;1:750-754.
7. Lagergren J, Ye W, Lindgren A, Nyrén O. Heredity and cancer of the esophagus and gastric cardia. Cancer Epidemiol Biomark Prev 2000;9:757-760.

In experimental esophageal cancer development, what is the relationship between the type of neoplastic epithelium and the type of reflux material?

C.D. Morris, S.E.A. Attwood (Salford)

A relationship between reflux disease and esophageal carcinoma development has been suspected for many years and the recent study by Lagergren [1] provides conclusive proof of the relationship of reflux disease and esophageal adenocarcinoma. They found no such relationship with squamous cell carcinoma. The changing epidemiology of esophageal cancer, with the rapid increase of adenocarcinoma and gradually decreasing squamous cell carcinoma also points to differences in their aetiology. These findings are supported by studies carried out in animal models examining the role of refluxed agents in esophageal carcinogenesis.

The initial work on reflux injury carried out in rabbit models, such as that of Johnson and Harmon [2] demonstrated esophageal injury by both acid and duodenal juices in short term studies, with duodenal juices leading to greater tissue injury than acid alone. Due to the short duration of these studies however, no malignant potential was suspected. When rats are exposed to nitrosamine carcinogens such as 2,6-di-methyl-nitrosomorpholine (DMNM) or methyl-N-amyl nitrosamine (MNAN) they reliably develop diffuse esophageal papillomatosis in up to 85-100% and squamous cell carcinomas in 25-65% with maximal carcinogen doses [3]. Using lower, less toxic doses of carcinogens, cancers can be produced in around 25% of animals with minimal morbidity, however adenocarcinomas are not seen [4]. With the accumulating evidence that duodenal juices may have a role in the development of esophageal and gastric stump carcinomas following partial gastrectomy, Pera *et al.* investigated the effect of surgically induced reflux of gastroduodenal juice on esophageal carcinoma formation, and found a shift towards adenocarcinoma formation [5]. This work was extended by Attwood *et al.* who compared the effects of esophagogastroplasty (reflux of gastric juice) with duodenoesophageal anastomosis (reflux of gastric and duodenal juice) on the development of carcinoma [4]. The results are shown in *Table I*.

With the compelling evidence for the role of duodenal juices in adenocarcinoma development, the requirement for gastric juice was questioned. Further studies from the same laboratory demonstrated that in carcinogen treated rats subjected to duodenal reflux, the incidence of esophageal adenocarcinoma was significantly elevated from 30% to 87%

Table I. Influence of reflux of gastric juice or gastroduodenal juice on the differentiation of esophageal carcinoma (modified from [4]).

Animal group	Number	SCC	ADC	Diffuse polyposis
No reflux	16	0	0	0
No reflux + DMNM	12	3 (25%)	0	3 (25%)
Gastric reflux	9	0	0	0
Gastric reflux + DMNM	10	2 (20%)	0	3 (30%)
Duodenal reflux	14	0	1 (7%)	7 (50%)
Duodenal reflux + DMNM	20	9 (45%)	7 (35%)	13 (65%)

when gastric juice was excluded from the refluxed juice by gastrectomy or downstream diversion [6]. However the different reflux models had no influence on the development of squamous carcinomas. This study suggests that gastric juice may actually protect the esophagus from adenocarcinoma induction by duodenal content.

An interesting finding in the study of Attwood *et al.* was the development of an adenocarcinoma in a rat with reflux of duodenal juice without the administration of carcinogen. This has been studied further in gastrectomized rats subjected to diversion of duodenal juice into the esophagus without exogenous carcinogen [7]. This study had two important findings. Firstly that adenocarcinoma could be induced in around half the rats exposed to duodenal juice without carcinogen, and secondly that addition of acid to the drinking water tended to reduce the yield of cancers confirming the apparent protection by acid described by Ireland *et al.* It is interesting to note that this model also demonstrated columnization of the esophagus in 87% of animals subjected to reflux.

The question of which component of the refluxed duodenal juice causes the increase in adenocarcinoma is controversial. Pera *et al.* investigated the role of pancreatic and biliary reflux on carcinogen induced esophageal carcinoma development [8]. Animals exposed to reflux of pancreatic juices only, developed adenocarcinoma in 2/22 rats, while those exposed to pancreatic and bile reflux developed adenocarciona in 5/27 rats. They concluded that pancreatic secretions were needed for tumor induction and bile reflux had a promoting role. Trypsin, the major component of pancreatic juice has been shown to injure the esophagus and may therefore promote cancer development. However no studies have shown it or other pancreatic enzymes to be carcinogenic.

Bile acids alone have not been shown to be carcinogenic in mutagenesis assays either [9], though they have been implicated as tumor promoters in studies on colon cancer [10]. Bile acids are however a rich source of amides and can, under the action of certain bacteria, react with nitrites in the stomach to form N-nitroso compounds such as N-nitrosotaurocholic acid and N-nitrosoglycocholic acid which have been shown to act as carcinogens [11]. This latter fact may also tie in the protecting effect of acid, as loss of acid may lead to bacterial overgrowth with nitrite formation, which under bacterial action then reacts with refluxed bile to produce carcinogenic N-nitroso compounds. The bile acids deoxycholate and chenodeoxycholate have been shown to induce expression of the enzyme COX-2 [12], which is becoming increasingly implicated in gastrointestinal malignancy including esophageal adenocarcinoma. Our own data has shown an increased COX-2 expression in the progression to high-grade dysplasia and adenocarcinoma in Barrett's metaplasia in the human [13]. Once induced COX-2 leads to a number of cellular changes including a reduced capacity for apoptosis, increased proliferation, altered cell adhesion and increased invasive potential, all of which may contribute to neoplastic progression.

Dietary factors may also influence cancer development, particularly the fat content. High intakes of dietary fat have been widely implicated in colon carcinogenesis [14] and indeed the rise in esophageal adenocarcinoma appears to be in higher social groups with a tendency towards obesity [15]. Experimental studies in the rat have also demonstrated promotion of tumor formation in animals fed diets with a high fat content [16]. It is likely that at least part of the effect of specific fats is via alterations in the production and secretion of bile [17].

Iron supplementation has also been implicated in experimental esophageal adenocarcinoma formation. It was noted that surgically treated rats became anaemic and iron supplements given to prevent this lead to an increase in tumor formation [18]. This may be *via* increased tissue damage due to oxidative stress, as iron is a potent inducer of reactive oxygen species which have been implicated in the esophageal tissue damage caused by gastroduodenal juices [19].

In summary, studies from a number of centres have shown a consistent relationship between the reflux of duodenal juices into the esophagus and subsequent development of columnar metaplasia and adenocarcinoma. Dietary fat and also iron supplementation appear to enhance tumor formation. Gastric acid alone does not appear to share this adenocarcinoma producing effect and indeed may even be protective against the effect of duodenal juices. This has obvious implications for our management of reflux disease, implying that abolition of the reflux of duodenal juices into the esophagus is at least as important if not more important than acid suppression, in cancer prevention.

References

1. Lagergren J, Bergstrom R, Lindgren A, Nyren O. Symptomatic gastroesophageal reflux as a risk factor for esophageal adenocarcinoma. N Engl J Med 1999;340(11):825-831.
2. Johnson LF, Harmon JW. Experimental esophagitis in a rabbit model. Clinical relevance. J Clin Gastroenterol 1986;8:26-44.
3. Bulay O, Mirvish S. Carcinogenesis in rat esophagus by intraperitoneal injection of different doses of Methyl-n-amylnitrosamine. Cancer Res 1979;39:3644-3646.
4. Attwood SE, Smyrk TC, DeMeester TR, Mirvish SS, Stein HJ, Hinder RA. Duodenoesophageal reflux and the development of esophageal adenocarcinoma in rats. Surgery 1992;111(5):503-510.
5. Pera M, Cardesa A, Bombi JA, Ernst H, Pera C, Mohr U. Influence of esophagojejunostomy on the induction of adenocarcinoma of the distal esophagus in Sprague-Dawley rats by subcutaneous injection of 2,6-dimethylnitrosomorpholine. Cancer Res 1989;49(23):6803-6808.
6. Ireland AP, Peters JH, Smyrk TC, DeMeester TR, Clark GW, Mirvish SS, Adrian TE. Gastric juice protects against the development of esophageal adenocarcinoma in the rat. Ann Surg 1996;224(3):358-370.
7. Fein M, Peters JH, Chandrasoma P, Ireland AP, Oberg S, Ritter MP, Bremner CG, Hagen JA, DeMeester TR. Duodenoesophageal reflux induces esophageal adenocarcinoma without exogenous carcinogen. J Gastrointest Surg 1998;2(3):260-268.
8. Pera M, Trastek VF, Carpenter HA, Fernandez PL, Cardesa A, Mohr U, Pairolero PC. Influence of pancreatic and biliary reflux on the development of esophageal carcinoma. Ann Thorac Surg 1993;55(6):1386-1392.
9. Silverman S, Andrews A. Bile acids:comutagenic activity in the salmonella-mammalian-microsome mutagenicity test. J Natl Cancer Inst 1977;59:1557-1559.
10. Stadler J, Yeung KS, Furrer R, Marcon N, Himal HS, Bruce WR. Proliferative activity of rectal mucosa and soluble fecal bile acids in patients with normal colons and in patients with colonic polyps or cancer. Cancer Lett 1988;38(3):315-320.
11. Busby W, Shuker D, Charnley G, Newberne P, Tanenbaum S, Wogan G. Carcinogenicity in rats of the nitrosated bile acid conjugates N-nitrosoglycocholic acid and N-nitrosotaurocholic acid. Cancer Res 1985;45:1367-1371.

12. Zhang F, Subbaramaiah K, Altorki N, Dannenberg AJ. Dihydroxy bile acids activate the transcription of cyclooxygenase-2. J Biol Chem 1998;273(4):2424-2428.
13. Morris C, Bigley G, Armstrong G, Attwood S. Expression of cyclo-oxygenase 2 (COX-2) in Barrett's esophagus, dysplasia and adenocarcinoma. Gastroenterology 2000;118(4):A685.
14. Boutron M, Wilpart M, Faivre J. Diet and colorectal cancer. Eur J Cancer Prev 1991;1:13-20.
15. Brown L, Swanson C, Gridley G, Swanson G, Schoenberg J, Greenberg R, Silverman D, Pottern L, Hayes R, Schwartz A, Liff J, Fraumeni J, Hoover R. Adenocarcinoma of the esophagus: role of obesity and diet. J Natl Cancer Inst 1995;87:104-109.
16. Clark G, Smyrk T, Mirvish S, Anselmino M, Yamashita Y, Hinder R, Demeester T, Birt D. Effect of gastroduodenal juice and dietary fat on the development of Barrett's esophagus and esophageal neoplasia: an experimental rat model. Ann Surg Oncol 1994;1(3):252-261.
17. McLaughlin J, Grazia Luca M, Jones MN, D'Amato M, Dockray GJ, Thompson DG. Fatty acid chain length determines cholecystokinin secretion and effect on human gastric motility. Gastroenterology 1999;116(1):46-53.
18. Goldstein SR, Yang GY, Curtis SK, Reuhl KR, Liu BC, Mirvish SS, Newmark HL, Yang CS. Development of esophageal metaplasia and adenocarcinoma in a rat surgical model without the use of a carcinogen. Carcinogenesis 1997;18(11):2265-2270.
19. Naya MJ, Pereboom D, Ortego J, Alda JO, Lanas A. Superoxide anions produced by inflammatory cells play an important part in the pathogenesis of acid and pepsin induced esophagitis in rabbits. Gut 1997;40(2):175-181.

What is the relationship between symptomatic reflux and adenocarcinoma?

J. Lagergren (Stockholm)

There is a paucity of epidemiological data on the association between reflux and the risk of adenocarcinoma of the esophagus or gastric cardia. A case-control study based on medical records of patients with adenocarcinoma of the esophagus or cardia found a 2-fold increased risk for adenocarcinoma among patients whose records indicated that they had reflux disease [1].

Methods

We conducted a large-scale case-control study to identify risk factors for adenocarcinomas of the esophagus and gastric cardia [2]. The study encompassed the whole population of Sweden during 1995-1997. All newly diagnosed cases of adenocarcinoma of the esophagus or gastric cardia and half the newly diagnosed cases of esophageal squamous-cell carcinoma were eligible. A comprehensive organization, with contact persons at all 195 relevant hospital in Sweden ensured that all cases were identified shortly after diagnosis. Uniform routines for the documentation of the tumors were introduced in all participating sites. At endoscopy, the distances between the gastroesophageal junction and the upper and lower borders of the tumor were measured and serial biopsy specimens were obtained. Surgeons and pathologists gave standardized, detailed descriptions of the location of the cancer in resected cases. A single pathologist reviewed the biopsy samples or surgical specimens. All cases and controls underwent computer-aided personal interviews by professional interviewers. Among several others, questions were asked about recurrent heartburn and regurgitation. To avoid reversed causality, we disregarded symptoms that had occurred less than five years before the interview. Information was collected about several potential confounders. Altogether, 189 cases of adenocarcinoma of the esophagus and 262 with cardia cancer together constituted 85% of all eligible adenocarcinoma cases in Sweden during the study period. The 820 controls and 167 esophageal squamous-cell carcinoma cases represented 73% of all eligible.

Results

The risk of esophageal adenocarcinoma was almost 8 times as high among persons in whom heartburn, regurgitation, or both occurred at least once a week as among persons without these symptoms (*Table I*). Symptoms of reflux at night were associated with a risk nearly 11 times as high. The frequency of symptoms of reflux was strongly linked to the risk: the more frequent the symptoms, the higher the risk. Similarly, increasing severity of symptoms entailed increasing risk estimates. The risk of esophageal adenocarcinoma also increased with an increasing duration of symptoms. Among persons with both long-standing symptoms (> 20 years) and severe symptoms, the odds ratio for esophageal adenocarcinoma was 43.5 (95% confidence interval (CI) = 18.3-103.5), as compared with asymptomatic persons. Reflux symptoms were moderately strongly associated with the risk of adenocarcinoma of the gastric cardia (*Table I*). The risk among individuals with symptoms of reflux was approximately 2 times as high as among those without symptoms. Persons who reported both long-standing and severe reflux symptoms had an odds ratio of 4.4 (95% CI = 1.7-11.0). Esophageal squamous-cell carcinoma was not associated with symptoms of reflux, irrespective of the frequency, severity, or duration of the symptoms (*Table I*).

Is Barrett's esophagus precarcinogenic?

In 118 (62%) of the 189 esophageal adenocarcinoma cases, Barrett's esophagus was detected. The strength of the association with symptoms of reflux was identical for patients with esophageal adenocarcinomas who had Barrett's esophagus and those who did not. Barrett's esophagus appears not to be a necessary step in the evolution of esophageal adenocarcinoma [3]. The excess risk of adenocarcinoma among patients with Barrett's esophagus has been estimated to be 30-60 times that of the general population in large studies [4-7]. Because the risk among subjects in our study with the most severe and long-standing symptoms of reflux was of the same magnitude, and because the association was equally strong among esophageal adenocarcinoma with Barrett's esophagus and those without it, we hypothesize that gastroesophageal reflux, may be the crucial factor. Therefore, it may be necessary to reappraise the critical role of Barrett's esophagus in the carcinogenic pathway.

Table I. Reflux symptoms and risk of esophageal adenocarcinoma, gastric cardia adenocarcinoma, and esophageal squamous cell carcinoma. Multivariately adjusted odds ratios (OR) and 95% confidence intervals (CI).

Reflux symptoms	Esophageal adenocarcinoma OR (95% CI)	Cardia adenocarcinoma OR (95% CI)	Esophageal squamous-cell carcinoma OR (95% CI)
At least once a week			
No	1.0 (referent)	1.0 (referent)	1.0 (referent)
Yes	7.7 (5.3-11.4)	2.0 (1.4-2.9)	1.1 (0.7-1.9)
At night			
No	1.0 (referent)	1.0 (referent)	1.0 (referent)
Yes	10.8 (7.0-16.7)	2.4 (1.5-3.8)	0.9 (0.4-2.0)
Frequency			
No symptoms	1.0 (referent)	1.0 (referent)	1.0 (referent)
1 per week	5.1 (2.8-9.4)	2.0 (1.1-3.6)	0.9 (0.4-2.4)
2-3 per week	6.3 (3.8-10.3)	1.9 (1.2-3.1)	1.2 (0.6-2.5)
>3 per week	16.7 (8.7-28.3)	2.3 (1.2-4.3)	1.4 (0.5-3.7)
Severity score			
No symptoms	1.0 (referent)	1.0 (referent)	1.0 (referent)
1-2 points	1.4 (0.7-3.0)	1.7 (1.0-2.9)	1.7 (0.8-3.5)
2.5-4 points	8.1 (4.7-16.1)	1.8 (1.0-3.2)	0.6 (0.2-1.7)
4.5-6.5 points	20.0 (11.6-34.6)	2.8 (1.6-5.0)	1.1 (0.4-3.0)
Duration			
No symptoms	1.0 (referent)	1.0 (referent)	1.0 (referent)
< 12 years	7.5 (4.2-13.5)	1.6 (0.9-2.9)	1.6 (0.7-3.7)
13-20 years	5.2 (3.1-8.6)	1.8 (1.1-2.9)	0.9 (0.4-1.9)
> 20 years	16.4 (8.3-28.4)	3.3 (1.8-6.3)	1.2 (0.4-3.7)

* In the multivariate logistic model adjustments were made for: age, gender, socio-economic status, body mass index, tobacco smoking, alcohol use, intake of fruit and vegetables, energy intake, working in a stooping posture, and physical activity at work, and physical activity during leisure time

Can antireflux therapy prevent adenocarcinoma development among reflux patients?

Antireflux medication

We compared the risk of esophageal adenocarcinoma among persons who used medication for symptoms of reflux at least 5 years before the interview with that among symptomatic persons who did not use such medication. The odds ratio was 3.0 (95% CI = 2.0-4.6) without adjustment for the severity of symptoms and 2.9 (95% CI = 1.9-4.6) with this adjustment. Hence, we found no indication that treatment of reflux reduced the risk of esophageal cancer, but rather the contrary. Although we adjusted our data for the severity of symptoms, residual confounding by severity of reflux may have affected our estimates.

Moreover, the subjects in our survey had almost invariably received sporadic short-term courses of medical treatment. The advent of increasingly potent inhibitors of acid production in the past 20 years does not seem to have affected the rising incidence curve for esophageal adenocarcinoma. Pleas for more active treatment to prevent esophageal adenocarcinoma can be based on speculation only. Further studies are needed.

Antireflux surgery

Among the 14 subjects with esophageal adenocarcinoma and the 6 control subjects who had been surgically treated for reflux, the risk estimates were similar to those for the total group of patients with symptoms of reflux. Although small numbers hampered this analysis, no dramatic protective effect was found. Further studies are needed.

Can reflux explain the increasing incidence of adenocarcinomas?

There are no firm data to substantiate the idea that reflux is becoming more common. Hence, the role of reflux as a cause of the rapid rise in incidence of adenocarcinoma of the esophagus and cardia is uncertain. Studies are needed to evaluate the incidence of gastroesophageal disease. The strong 7:1 male predominance among cases with esophageal and cardia adenocarcinoma [8] is not explained by reflux disease, a condition with more even sex distribution.

References

1. Chow WH, Finkle WD, McLaughlin JK, Frankl H, Ziel HK, Fraumeni JF Jr. The relation of gastroesophageal reflux disease and its treatment to adenocarcinomas of the esophagus and gastric cardia. JAMA 1995;274:474-477.
2. Lagergren J, Bergström R, Lindgren A, Nyrén O. Symptomatic gastroesophageal reflux is a strong risk factor for esophageal adenocarcinoma. N Engl J Med 1999;340:825-831.
3. Kim R, Weissfeld JL, Reynolds JC, Kuller LH. Etiology of Barrett's esophagus and esophageal adenocarcinoma. Cancer Epidemiol Biomark Prev 1997;6:369-377.
4. Spechler SJ, Robbins AH, Rubins HB, Vincent ME, Heeren T, Doos WG, et al. Adenocarcinoma and Barrett's esophagus. An overrated risk. Gastroenterology 1984;87:927-933.
5. Cameron AJ, Ott BJ, Payne WS. The incidence of adenocarcinoma in columnar-lined (Barrett's) esophagus. N Engl J Med 1985;314:857-858.
6. Van Der Veen AH, Dees J, Blankenstein JD, Blankenstein M. Adenocarcinoma in Barrett's esophagus: an overrated risk. Gut 1989;10:16-18.
7. Drewitz DJ, Sampliner RE, Garewal HS. The incidence of adenocarcinoma in Barrett's esophagus: a prospective study of 170 patients followed 4.8 years. Am J Gastroenterol 1997;92:214-215.
8. Blot WJ, Devesa SS, Kneller RW, Fraumeni JF. Rising incidence of adenocarcinoma of the esophagus and gastric cardia. JAMA 1991;265:1587-1589.

What is the annual incidence of adenocarcinoma in patients with endoscopically evident Barrett's esophagus?

S.J. Spechler (Dallas)

A recent study by Shaheen *et al.* has suggested that the cancer risk in Barrett's esophagus had been overestimated for years because of publication bias, the selective reporting of studies that have positive or extreme results [1]. The investigators used the premise that cancer risk estimates derived from small studies should be less accurate than those from large studies, because sampling error is inversely related to sample size. Compared to a group of large studies, therefore, a group of small studies should describe a wider range of risk estimates, and those estimates should be symmetrically distributed around the mid-point value (similar in pattern to a bell-shaped curve). If there is publication bias, however, small studies that find low risks either will not be submitted to journals at all, or the submitted manuscripts will be rejected by editors who deem the reports uninteresting. In this situation, the preponderance of small studies published will describe high risks. To seek evidence of publication bias in the reporting of cancer risk in Barrett's esophagus, Shaheen *et al.* searched the available literature on this subject and identified 24 informative studies. The annual incidence of cancer in Barrett's esophagus described in those reports ranged from 0.2% to 2.9%. As would be expected in the case of publication bias, the investigators found a strong, inverse correlation between the magnitude of the cancer risk and the size of the study population. No significant associations were found between cancer risk and a number of factors other than study size that might have influenced the observed outcome (*e.g.* country of origin, retrospective study design, year of publication).

Some authors have pooled data from published studies to derive a composite estimate of cancer risk in Barrett's esophagus [2, 3]. Using such pooled data, one widely quoted report has estimated the cancer risk at 1% per year [2]. However, data pooling does not obviate the problem of publication bias, because the derived estimates are based on data that are skewed to exaggerate the incidence of cancer. Furthermore, available studies on cancer risk in Barrett's esophagus are comprised largely of patients referred to tertiary care centers. The incidence of cancer for such patients may exceed that for patients treated in primary care practices. With these biases in the published studies, it is likely that the risk of esophageal cancer for patients with Barrett's esophagus in the general population is substantially lower than the pooled literature would suggest. Although the precise risk remains unclear, Shaheen *et al.* suggest that an esophageal cancer incidence rate of 0.5% per year might be a reasonable estimate [1]. This estimate is in keeping with the results of three modern, large, prospective studies on cancer incidence in Barrett's esophagus [2-4].

It seems paradoxical that the risk of adenocarcinoma in Barrett's esophagus appears to have been overestimated for the past several decades, a period during which the frequency of this tumor has increased dramatically in the United States [5]. However, it is important to put this trend into perspective. The overall incidence of esophageal cancer in this country has not changed substantially over the past 25 years [6]. What has changed during this period is the proportion of esophageal cancers that are adenocarcinomas. For most of the twentieth century, squamous cell carcinoma was the major histologic type of esophageal cancer, and adenocarcinoma of the esophagus was rare [7]. The incidence of esophageal adenocarcinoma has nearly quadrupled over the past 25 years, but 25 years ago the incidence of this tumor was extremely low (< 1 case per 100,000) [5-8]. Despite the impressive relative rise in the frequency of esophageal adenocarcinoma, the total number of new cases remains low. In 1997, there were an estimated 12,500 new cases of esophageal cancer in the United States, of which approximately 5,750 (46%) were adenocarcinomas [8]. For comparison, there were an estimated 131,200 new cases of colorectal cancer that same year [6]. Further supporting the notion that the risk of cancer in Barrett's esophagus has been exaggerated are data from studies showing that Barrett's esophagus does not adversely influence long-term survival [9].

The data discussed above primarily pertain to patients who have Barrett's esophagus without dysplasia. Dysplasia in Barrett's esophagus can be an ominous finding. For patients with high-grade dysplasia, the risk of developing esophageal adenocarcinoma may be orders of magnitude greater than that for patients who have no dysplasia. For the latter, however, the risk of developing esophageal cancer appears to have been exaggerated for years. A reasonable estimate of adenocarcinoma incidence in patients with endoscopically-evident Barrett's esophagus is 0.5% per year.

References

1. Shaheen NJ, Crosby MA, Bozymski EM, Sandler RS. Is there publication bias in the reporting of cancer risk in Barrett's esophagus? Gastroenterology 2000;119:333-338.
2. Drewitz DJ, Sampliner RE, Garewal HS. The incidence of adenocarcinoma in Barrett's esophagus: a prospective study of 170 patients followed 4.8 years. Am J Gastroenterol 1997;92:212-215.
3. O'Connor JB, Falk GW, Richter JE. The incidence of adenocarcinoma and dysplasia in Barrett's esophagus. Report on the Cleveland Clinic Barrett's esophagus registry. Am J Gastroenterol 1999;94:2037-2042.
4. Spechler SJ, Lee E, Ahnen D, Goyal RK, Hirano I, Ramirez F, Raufman JP, Sampliner R, Schnell T, Sontag S, Vlahcevic ZR, Young R, Williford W. Long-term outcome of medical and surgical treatments for gastroesophageal reflux disease. Follow-up of a randomized controlled trial. JAMA 2001;285:2331-2338.
5. Devesa SS, Blot WJ, Fraumeni JF Jr. Changing patterns in the incidence of esophageal and gastric carcinoma in the United States. Cancer 1998;15;83:2049-2053.
6. Ries LAG, Eisner MP, Kosary CL, Hankey BF, Miller BA, Clegg L, Edwards BK. SEER cancer statistics review, 1973-1997. Bethesda: National Cancer Institute, 2000.
7. Hesketh PJ, Clapp RW, Doos WG, Spechler SJ. The increasing frequency of adenocarcinoma of the esophagus. Cancer 1989;64:526-530.
8. Data provided by SEER Program, National Cancer Institute, Bethesda, MD, August 1999 submission.
9. Eckardt VF, Kanzler G, Bernhard G. Life expectancy and cancer risk in patients with Barrett's esophagus:a prospective controlled investigation. Am J Med 2001;111:33-37.

Can the rate of degeneration of short segment Barrett's esophagus be evaluated?

P. Sharma (Kansas City)

The recent rapid rise in the incidence of adenocarcinoma of the distal esophagus and the gastric cardia has generated significant interest in the premalignant lesion - Barrett's esophagus [1-3]. The traditional definition of Barrett's esophagus included > 3 cm of columnar mucosa in the distal esophagus. Recent studies have suggested that dysplasia and adenocarcinoma can also be associated with short segment Barrett's esophagus (SSBE) *i.e.* < 3 cm of columnar mucosa [4]. Barrett's esophagus has now come to be defined by the histological presence of intestinal metaplasia (IM) within esophageal columnar mucosa.

The diagnosis of SSBE requires a combination of endoscopic and histologic criteria. At the time of upper endoscopy, there must be evidence of columnar-appearing mucosa in the distal esophagus which is < 3 cm in length and biopsies from the columnar mucosa must reveal IM [4].

Dysplasia and cancer in short segment Barrett's esophagus

The prevalence of dysplasia in patients with SSBE is approximately 8-10% [5, 6]. Three prospective series have reported the incidence of dysplasia and cancer in patients with SSBE. Sharma *et al.* studied 59 patients with SSBE (dysplasia prevalence 8.5%) with 32 patients followed for a mean of 36 months [6]. Dysplasia developed in 5 patients, 3 with low-grade dysplasia (LGD) and 2 with high-grade dysplasia (HGD) (dysplasia incidence 5.7% per year). One patient with HGD developed adenocarcinoma of the esophagus during follow-up. Weston *et al.* reported a dysplasia incidence of 6.1% per year in 26 patients followed for 10.6 + 7.8 months – no cancers developed in this group during follow-up [5]. The incidence of cancer in patients with SSBE (without HGD at index diagnosis) was 0.4% in 69 patients followed for a mean of 3.7 years. This incidence rate was lower, but not significantly different compared to cancer incidence in patients with long segment Barrett's esophagus [7].

Hamilton *et al.* reported the association of SSBE with esophageal cancer; 64% of adenocarcinomas of the distal esophagus and esophagogastric junction (EGJ) were associated with Barrett's and 34% of esophageal adenocarcinomas were detected in short segments of IM [8]. In one series of 31 cardia adenocarcinomas, 13 were related to Barrett's and 6 of 13 had a Barrett's length of 2.7 ± 1.8 cm [9]. In an autopsy study from the Mayo Clinic of 24 specimens of the EGJ cancers, half of the Barrett's associated tumors had a mucosa length of 1-2.5 cm [10]. Recently, investigators from the Hines VAMC reported that more than 40% of prevalence and incidence esophageal adenocarcinomas in a large population of patients with Barrett's esophagus, were associated with SSBE [11].

Given the potential of SSBE patients to develop dysplasia and cancer, it is prudent to enroll such patients in a surveillance program for the detection of cancer at an early stage. Currently available dysplasia and cancer rates are based on relatively short follow-up periods and additional data are, however, needed regarding the actual incidence of adenocarcinoma in patients with SSBE. This is important before appropriate management strategies and surveillance intervals can be developed.

References

1. Blot WJ, Devesa SS, Kneller RW, et al. Rising incidence of adenocarcinoma of the esophagus and gastric cardia. JAMA 1991;265:1287-1289.
2. Pera M, Cameron AJ, Trastek VF, et al. Increasing incidence of adenocarcinoma of the esophagus and esophagogastric junction. Gastroenterology 1993;104:510-513.
3. Blot WJ, Devesa SS, Fraumeni JF Jr. Continuing climb in rates of esophageal adenocarcinoma:An update. JAMA 1993;270:1320.
4. Sharma P, Morales TG, Sampliner RE. Short-segment Barrett's esophagus. The need for standardization of the definition and of endoscopic criteria. Am J Gastroenterol 1998;93:1033-1036.
5. Weston AP, Krmpotich P, Makdisi WF, et al. Short segment Barrett's esophagus: clinical and histological features, associated endoscopic findings, and association with gastric intestinal metaplasia. Am J Gastroenterol 1996;91:981-986.
6. Sharma P, Morales TG, Bhattacharyya A, et al. Dysplasia in short-segment Barrett's esophagus:A prospective 3-year follow-up. Am J Gastroenterol 1997;92:2012-2016.
7. Rudolph RE, Vaughan TL, Storer BE, et al. Effect of segment length on risk for neoplastic progression in patients with Barrett esophagus. Ann Intern Med 2000;132:612-620.
8. Hamilton SR, Smith R, Cameron JL. Prevalence and characteristics of Barrett esophagus in patients with adenocarcinoma of the esophagus or esophagogastric junction. Hum Pathol 1988;19:942-948.
9. Clark G, Smyrk TC, Burdiles P, et al. Is Barrett's metaplasia the source of adenocarcinomas of the cardia? Arch Surg 1994;129:609-614.
10. Cameron AJ, Lomboy CT, Pera M, et al. Adenocarcinoma of the esophagogastric junction and Barrett's esophagus. Gastroenterology 1995;109:1541-1546.
11. Schnell T, Sontag SJ, Chejfec G, et al. Does more Barrett's really mean more cancer? Comparison of incidence rates of adenocarcinoma in prospectively followed patient cohorts with short and long segments of Barrett's esophagus. Gastroenterology 1998;114:G2783.

What is the expectable rate of Barrett's adenocarcinoma arising after incomplete resection of the Barrett's epithelium?

M. Pera (Barcelona)

The major clinical importance of Barrett's esophagus is that it is a premalignant condition, with Barrett's esophagus patients having an increase risk of developing an esophageal adenocarcinoma through a multistep sequence of events that leads to dysplasia, and finally to adenocarcinoma. The overall incidence of adenocarcinoma arising in long segments of Barrett's esophagus ranges from 1 in 187 to 1 in 208 patient-years observation [1, 2]. Biopsy sampling error during endoscopic surveillance due to the multifocal distribution of dysplasia in Barrett's esophagus make the assessment of the natural history of dysplasia very difficult. Despite these limitations, Katz *et al.* [2] assessed 97 patients with Barrett's esophagus without any dysplasia or adenocarcinoma at baseline and, by 3 years of follow-up, approximately 8% of these patients had developed dysplasia (low-grade or higher). They observed that a significant fraction (7%) of patients with nondysplastic Barrett's esophagus developed low-grade dysplasia (LGD) within the first 2 years of follow-up. In contrast to the relatively short latency period observed for LGD, patients with nondysplastic Barrett's esophagus did not develop high-grade dysplasia (HGD) or adenocarcinoma until > 2 years had elapsed after the initial diagnosis. The University of Washington group, using an intensive biopsy protocol [3], examined the natural history of HGD in 70 patients and found early carcinoma on prompt follow-up endoscopy within two months in 12 (17%) patients, while early stage carcinoma developed in 15/58 (26%) other patients during a median follow-up of 24 months. The remaining patients either continued to have HGD (47%) or regressed to lesser lesions on follow-up (27%). In patients with Barrett's esophagus, especially those with HGD and adenocarcinoma, who require esophagectomy or any type of endoscopic ablative therapy every attempt should be made to resect the entire Barrett's esophagus in order to remove all mucosa at risk for adenocarcinoma.

Arguments in favor of complete resection of dysplastic Barrett's esophagus

The distribution of dysplasia and early adenocarcinoma in Barrett's specialized epithelium is usually patchy and irregular [4]. Cameron and Carpenter [5] mapped 30 esophagectomy specimens and found that HGD showed three different patterns of distribution: eleven patients (three with invasive carcinoma) had large areas or bands of HGD, occupying almost all of the Barrett's esophagus in one; eleven more patients (one with carcinoma) had scattered multiple foci of HGD and eigth patients (three with carcinoma) had a single focus of HGD. Of interest they also found that microscopic areas of different grades of dysplasia were commonly intermingled. These findings, therefore, clearly suggest that incomplete eradication of Barrett's esophagus leaving residual areas of dysplastic specialized intestinal metaplasia (IM) does not eliminate the potential risk for the development of adenocarcinoma.

Risk of adenocarcinoma in residual Barrett's esophagus after esophageal resection

The goals of esophageal resection in patients with HGD or Barrett's adenocarcinoma are to completely remove all areas of Barrett's metaplasia. Complete removal must be emphasized because adenocarcinoma arising in residual Barrett's esophagus after esophagectomy has been reported within months or years of surgery [6-8].

Risk of adenocarcinoma after incomplete endoscopic ablation of Barrett's esophagus

It has been shown that destruction of Barrett's epithelium is followed by squamous reepithelialization in an anacid environment [9]. Based on this observation enthusiasm has developed for eradication of Barrett's esophagus, especially those cases with dysplasia and early adenocarcinoma. Eradication of Barrett's esophagus by means of photodynamic therapy (PDT) or thermal coagulation combined with intense acid suppression accomplished by fundoplication or pharmacologic means has been developed in recent years. The goal of ablative treatment in patients with nondysplastic Barrett's esophagus is to reduce the risk for the development of adenocarcinoma and to decrease the need for lifelong endoscopic surveillance. In patients with dysplastic Barrett's esophagus the main goal of these endoscopic techniques would be to eliminate all dysplastic areas and to prevent progression toward adenocarcinoma. The outcome of these therapeutic modalities will clearly depend on the complete destruction of the specialized epithelium with subsequent persistent squamous reepithelialization without leaving any focus of IM beneath the new squamous epithelium [10]. When the natural course of HGD in Barrett's esophagus is examined, the probability of carcinoma developing during the subsequent few years appears to be greater than 30% [11]. Therefore, incomplete eradication of dysplastic Barrett's esophagus would perpetuate the potential risk of malignant transformation. This is the reason why partial reversal of Barrett's esophagus would be considered an inadequate end point. Complete elimination of Barrett's esophagus after application of PDT or thermal ablation is achieved in only one third of patients. Current technology for PDT, including the laser wavelength, the photosensitizer, and the laser diffusion system is not perfect, and so underpenetration is a problem in some areas. The result is incomplete and irregular destruction of Barrett's esophagus, thereby creating a potential for persistance of Barrett's mucosa or the occurrence of dysplasia or cancer in mucosa that remain beneath the new squamous epithelium. To date, there is lack of information about the expectable rate of adenocarcinoma after incomplete eradication of Barrett's esophagus. However, the existence of this potential risk is supported by different reports showing HGD and adenocarcinoma arising in islands of residual IM after the use of different modalities of endoscopic ablative therapy [8, 12]. The largest PDT study was carried out by Overholt *et al.* on 100 patients with dysplasia or superficial carcinoma [8]. After Porfimer PDT and having a mean follow-up of 19 months, 43 patients had complete disappearance of Barrett's mucosa. Nd:YAG laser ablation was additionally used in 35 of these patients to destroy small areas of residual Barrett's esophagus. Dysplasia was eliminated in 69 of the 87 (79%) non cancer patients. However, dysplasia developed in untreated Barrett's areas in 11 of 48 patients (23%). Of great concern is that 2 patients each developed a small island of metaplastic mucosa with HGD under areas completely covered with squamous epithelium 18 and 22 months after treatment [8]. Another patient develop a subsquamous 2x4 mm adenocarcinoma 6 months after PDT. A high recurrence rate of HGD was observed in those patients with intractable gastroesophageal reflux. This observation confirms that control of reflux is paramount to the success of these techniques. Preliminary results of the multicenter international controlled trial assessing Photofrin-PDT for Barrett's HGD have recently been reported [13]. Two hundred eight patients were randomized between PDT plus omeprazole *versus* omeprazole alone. After a mean follow-up of nearly 12 months, the incidence of cancer was 10% in the first arm and 19% in the second one. Future prospective studies are also needed in order to know the potential risk of cancer progression after ablative therapy in Barrett's esophagus patients with lesser degree of dysplasia. Recent data suggest that real-time imaging modalities allowing visualization of dysplastic areas would make it possible to target ablative treatment toward all these areas and to assess the adequacy of therapy [14]. Future studies should determine whether these new endoscopic modalities may help to reduce the prevalence of residual islands of dysplastic IM and to detect the reappearance of dysplastic lesions or adenocarcinoma after endoscopic ablative treatment.

References

1. Drewitz DJ, Sampliner RE, Garewal HS. The incidence of adenocarcinoma in Barrett's esophagus: a prospective study of 170 patients followed 4.8 years. Am J Gastroenterol 1997;92:212-215.
2. Katz D, Rothstein R, Schned A, Dunn J, Seaver K, Antonioli DA. The development of dysplasia and adenocarcinoma during endoscopic surveillance of Barrett's esophagus. Am J Gastroenterol 1998;93:536-541.
3. Levine DS, Haggitt RC, Irvine S, Reid BJ. Natural history of high-grade dysplasia in Barrett's esophagus. Gastroenterology 1996;110:A550.
4. McArdle JE, Lewin KJ, Randall G, Weinstein WM. Distribution of dysplasias and early invasive carcinoma in Barrett's esophagus. Hum Pathol 1992;23:479-482.
5. Cameron AJ, Carpenter HA. Barrett's esophagus, high-grade dysplasia and early adenocarcinoma: a pathological study. Am J Gastroenterol 1997;92:586-591.
6. Hamilton SR, Hutcheon DF, Ravich WJ, Cameron JL, Paulson M. Adenocarcinoma in Barrett's esophagus after elimination of gastroesophageal reflux. Gastroenterology 1984;86:356-360.
7. Berenson MM, Riddell RH, Skinner DB, Freston JW. Malignant transformation of esophageal columnar epithelium. Cancer 1978;41:554-561.
8. Overholt BF, Panjehpour M, Haydek JM. Photodynamic therapy for Barrett's esophagus: follow-up in 100 patients. Gastrointest Endosc 1999;49:1-7.
9. Berenson MM, Johnson TD, Markowitz NR, Buchi KN, Samowitz WS. Restoration of squamous mucosa after ablation of Barrett's esophageal epithelium. Gastroenterology 1993;104:1686-1691.
10. Wang KK. Current status of photodynamic therapy of Barrett's esophagus. Gastrointest Endosc 1999;49:S20-S23.
11. Sampliner RE. Practice guidelines on the diagnosis, surveillance, and therapy of Barrett's esophagus. Am J Gastroenterol 1998;93:1028-1032.
12. Bonavina L, Carazzone S, Ferrero S, Buffa R, Peracchia A. Ablation of Barrett's epithelium with Nd-YAG laser followed by antireflux surgery: late results of a pilot clinical trial. In: Peracchia A, Bonavina L, ed. Barrett's esophagus: an up-to-date. Milano: Edra, 1999:99-105.
13. Overholt BF. Porfimer PDT for Barrett's high grade dysplasia. Preliminary results of the multi-center international controlled trial. Barrett 2000. 6th OESO Meeting, Paris, 2000.
14. Mallery S, Van Dam J. Endoscopic practice at the start of the New Millenium. Gastroenterology 2000;118:S129-S147.

Can we thwart death or the development of adenocarcinoma in Barrett's patients?

S.J. Sontag (Hines)

In an attempt to thwart the development of esophageal adenocarcinoma in patients with Barrett's esophagus, numerous strategies by participants in almost every discipline in medicine have been suggested and tried. We present data from our 20-year database that supports some therapeutic attempts and rejects others as a means to prevent the development of esophageal cancer or prevent death from esophageal cancer. The four modalities we present are as follows:
- antireflux surgery,
- medical therapy,
- spiritual therapy,
- mucosal ablation.

The Hines veterans affairs hospital database

We selected from our database the following small groups:
- antireflux surgery patients who subsequently developed adenocarcinoma (n = 3);
- antireflux surgery patients who subsequently developed high-grade dysplasia (HGD) (n = 5);
- patients with early adenocarcinoma and ablative therapy (n = 2);
- patient with early adenocarcinoma and high-dose, narrow beam radiation therapy (n = 1);
- patient with early adenocarcinoma and spiritual therapy (n = 1).

The patients in the small groups were compared with the following larger groups:
- antireflux surgeries outside Hines VA (n = 28);
- antireflux surgeries at Hines VA (n = 93);
- patients who developed adenocarcinoma without previous antireflux surgery (n = 92).

Results: antireflux surgery

Of the 93 patients who had previously received antireflux surgery at Hines VA:
- 0 (0%) were subsequently diagnosed with Barrett's adenocarcinoma;
- 5 (5.4%) were subsequently diagnosed with Barrett's HGD;
- 44 (47.3%) were subsequently diagnosed with Barrett's low-grade dysplasia (LGD);

Of the 28 patients who had previously received antireflux surgery at outside hospitals:
- 3 (10.7%) were diagnosed years later with Barrett's adenocarcinoma;
- 1 (3.6%) was diagnosed years later with Barrett's HGD;
- 10 (36.7%) were diagnosed years later with Barrett's LGD.

Results: medical therapy

Of 18 patients who developed Barrett's adenocarcinoma during the surveillance program:
- 14 patients had few gastroesophageal reflux symptoms and had taken no proton pump inhibitors (PPIs);
- 1 patient had taken 600 mg PPI over a 1-month period;
- 1 patient had taken 1,200 mg PPI over a 2-month period;
- 1 patient had taken 1,800 mg PPI over a 3-month period;
- 1 patient had taken 4,800 mg PPI over a 24-month period.

Results: mucosal ablation/radiation therapy

- 1 patient died of heart failure, free of adenocarcinoma, 4.1 years after ablation therapy;
- 1 patient remains alive 5.1 years after ablation therapy;
- 1 patient died peacefully with heart failure, free of adenocarcinoma, 9 months after radiation therapy.

Results: spiritual therapy

One ultra-religious patient with early Barrett's adenocarcinoma decided on surgical resection 15 months after the diagnosis of adenocarcinoma. During the 15 months, he prayed regularly and attended church almost daily. The lesion was determined to be T1NoMo (Stage 1) by endoscopic ultrasound and was confirmed as such at surgery.

Summary

Antireflux surgery

Almost 11% of the patients who were endoscoped at Hines and who had received antireflux surgery at another hospital were diagnosed with Barrett's adenocarcinoma. No patients receiving antireflux surgery at Hines VA have yet to develop adenocarcinoma. It is likely that the difference in incidence is due to the difference in time between the surgery and the presentation for endoscopy. The 3 patients with outside antireflux surgery had their procedures done from 15 to 40 years before diagnosis of adenocarcinoma. At Hines VA, the longest time interval is 20 years. It is possible that, in time, adenocarcinoma may yet develop in the Hines group.

Ablation and radiation

Electrocoagulation ablation therapy and high-dose, narrow-beam radiation therapy in 3 patients were effective – and probably curative – in obviating the need for esophageal resection. Two patients died peacefully of heart failure 9 months and 4.1 years after such therapy, and one remains alive and well.

Spiritual

Spiritual therapy did not appear to reverse Stage 1 adenocarcinoma, but did not appear to encourage progression.

Conclusion

The absence of data in the literature allows for either of the following absurd statements:
- antireflux surgery protects against Barrett's adenocarcinoma;
- antireflux surgery causes Barrett's adenocarcinoma.

The small database of patients at Hines VA may suggest the following:
- antireflux surgery does not protect against development of Barrett's adenocarcinoma;
- electrocoagulation ablation therapy of early tumors might be a worthwhile cooperative research project;
- radiation therapy of early Barrett's adenocarcinoma might be something to think about.

Can a possible iatrogenic role of widespread proton pump inhibitor usage in the etiology of gastric cardia and esophageal adenocarcinoma be envisaged?

A.C. Svoboda (Santa Barbara)

Adenocarcinoma of the tubular esophagus over the past two to three decades increased in incidence in the US and Western Europe more rapidly than any other tumor. In white males, the incidence of esophageal adenocarcinoma rose from 0.7/100,000 to 3.2 between 1974-1976 and 1992-1994, an increase of over 350%. In those ages 65 - 74, the incidence was 4.5/100,000. In some countries in Western Europe that figure is 8 or greater. Similar increases in adenocarcinoma of the gastric cardia were observed although less dramatic.

There is an established etiologic relationship to both gastroesophageal reflux and Barrett's specialized columnar epithelium and adenocarcinoma of the esophagus. Between 700,000 and one million persons in the United States have Barrett's esophagus. From 0.5 to 1% of these die with cancer each year.

Surveillance of patients with Barrett's columnar epithelium is recommended and vigorously pursued by most gastrointestinal endoscopists. However, in the United States and Western Europe only 1.5-7.0% of those diagnosed with esophageal adenocarcinoma had preceding knowledge of the presence of Barrett's. Fewer than 10% of adenocarcinoma patients survive five years and fewer than 25% who are candidates for surgery. The obvious approach must be prevention and successful prevention is dependent on elucidating etiologic factors.

Among the proposed explanations for this "epidemic" have been:

- cigarette smoking;
- alcohol consumption;
- increased obesity;
- increased use of lower esophageal sphincter pressure lowering drugs;
- increased use of nonsteroidal anti-inflammatory drugs (NSAIDs) and salicylates;
- dietary changes (low fruits and vegetables, high red meat, fat calories);
- an aging population;
- a decrease in the prevalence of *Helicobacter pylori*.

Whatever the explanation, it should also explain gender and racial differences. While there is some merit to several of the above suggestions, I would like to focus on the role of acid suppressing medications, especially proton pump inhibitors (PPIs)

The increasing popularity of PPIs is well deserved. They have been a significant improvement in controlling patient symptoms, healing or improving serious inflammatory damage due to acid reflux and preventing relapse. However, there are several lines of evidence implicating the increasing use of these drugs.

Evidence at the primitive level of clinical experience is suggestive.

There is a parallelism between the introduction and increasing sales of potent acid suppressing medications and adenocarcinoma of the cardia and distal esophagus. The sales of other medications such as NSAIDs and those lowering the lower esophageal sphincter pressure showed similar dramatic increase in usage but it was the high dose H_2 receptor antagonists and PPIs that were prescribed particularly for reflux symptoms.

It has been observed that those with specialized columnar epithelium show a rapid increase in the occurrence of dysplasia above levels present at diagnosis (when usually acid suppressing drugs are initiated). There is a wide variation in duration of symptoms prior to diagnosis and yet a relatively narrow range in the prevalence of dysplasia (8-10%) in those not on prior treatment. I would contend that if the diagnosis (and use of medications) were delayed by a year or two that the prevalence of dysplasia would still be 8-10% rather than displaying the 5-10% increase a year seen on therapy.

Gastric non-neoplastic polyps (hyperplastic or fundal gland) can occur during prolonged PPI therapy in patients with Barrett's. There is a high risk (83%) of developing dysplasia in patients with long segment Barrett's who develop such polyps.

The polyps will regress or disappear on discontinuation of PPIs but it is not known whether dysplasia regresses.

Patients who have effective antireflux surgery and are able to discontinue their medications show a decrease and even a disappearance of dysplasia and a regression and even disappearance of intestinal metaplasia (IM). There is even the suggestion that the adenocarcinoma risk is decreased and may not occur late after effective procedures.

Finally, results from "the International Comparative Study of Intestinal Metaplasia/Dysplasia at the Gastroesophageal Junction" of which I am the principal investigator, has enrolled large numbers of patients from countries where the reported incidence of adenocarcinoma is low. Preliminary figures show that the incidence of IM is as high or higher than in the US or Western Europe but that dysplasia either does not or rarely will occur. In these countries in Eastern Europe the Eastern Mediterranean, South American and the Caribbean and Vietnam PPIs, until recently, have rarely, if ever, been used because they are unavailable or cost precludes their use. The lack of dysplasia is highly statistically significant.

How do PPIs potentially contribute to carcinogenesis? Mechanisms include:

- a direct drug effect on biochemical mechanisms,
- effects secondary to lowered gastric acidity,
- effects of secondary serum gastrin elevations,
- potentiation of above when *Helicobacter pylori* is present.

PPIs by decreasing gastric acid production (increasing gastric pH for prolonged periods) allow increased colonization by bacteria which can synthesize carcinogenic N-nitroso compounds from nitrites. Nitrite levels in gastric juice increase because of bacterial generation from dietary nitrates, and nitrites are stable or remain in solution in the presence of hypochlorhydria. Omeprazole delays gastric emptying increasing time for nitrosation. All these changes are accentuated by *Helicobacter pylori* as is the depletion of gastric juice vitamin C. The removal of nitrite from gastric juice by converting it to nitrous oxide depends on the presence of ascorbic acid in the gastric juice as well as the acidity of the gastric juice.

H. pylori positive patients receiving omeprazole develop moderate to severe corpus atrophy. Increased serum gastrins and interleukin-8 are associated with a higher degree of chronic atrophic gastritis. Serum B12 levels decrease with the gastritis. Serum B12 levels decrease with the degree of PPI use, in part due to decreased absorption.

Omeprazole causes gastric ECL cell hyperplasia and hypergastrinemia. Over 80% of gastroesophageal reflux disease patients on long-term omeprazole therapy develop hypergastrinemia. Gastrin is a trophic hormone and acts as a mediator inducing a state of hyperproliferation with normal and neoplastic tissue.

PPIs increase cytokines and peptide growth factors. They increase PGE_2, epidermal growth factor and transforming growth factors. These may promote a metaplastic and dysplastic phenotype. Oncogenes, which are excited (cyclins D1 and E), may predispose the epithelium to malignant transformation.

Finally, in animals, gastric acid blockade with omeprazole promotes gastric carcinogenesis induced by duodenogastric reflux.

Many developing lines of evidence should increase our concern about the use, particularly indiscriminate, of these potent agents (the PPIs). Particularly without endoscopic and biopsy evidence as to the health of the gastroesophageal mucosa.

If this concern about carcinogenesis related to PPIs is justified, do current recommendations for evaluation and treatment of reflux symptoms warrant special concern? In this era of cost containment in the United States, guidelines frequently recommend a therapeutic trial of a PPI once or twice daily. These medicines are very likely to control most or all of the patient's symptoms. The very busy practitioner will frequently find it easier to renew such medications rather than find the time to extensively review the medical record and recommend a diagnostic endoscopy, especially if the patient is symptom free. Further, the medications are going over the counter and even consultation with a physician may be delayed. Finally the endoscopic diagnosis of malignant or premalignant esophageal or gastric changes is more difficult and occurs less often in patients on full medication. If the axiom "Before all else, do not harm" applies, a re-evaluation of potential long term risks with PPIs is indicated.

Are the data obtained from ambulatory 24-hour fiberoptic monitoring of bilirubin reliable enough to support the role of bile reflux in degeneration of Barrett's mucosa?

W.K.H. Kauer, H.J. Stein, J.R. Siewert (Munich)

Reflux of alkaline duodenal contents into the stomach and up into the esophagus is increasingly recognized as an important pathophysiologic factor in gastroesophageal reflux disease (GERD). About one quarter of patients with gastroesophageal reflux (GER) develop recurrent progressive disease manifested by complications that advance from erosive esophagitis to stricture, ulceration, and/or Barrett's esophagus despite medical therapy [1]. Evidence is accumulating that the composition of the refluxed gastric juice has an important role in the development of this progressive mucosal injury [2, 3] Animal studies have shown that the presence of components of duodenal juice is associated with marked augmentation of acid induced mucosal injury [4, 5]. Clinical observations in patients with GERD have shown that esophagitis, stricture, and Barrett's esophagus are more prevalent when there is increased esophageal exposure to either acidity or alkalinity [6]. These complications are more severe in patients with acid/alkaline reflux than in those with acid reflux alone [6]. Prolonged esophageal aspiration studies have documented an increase in bile acids in patients with severe esophagitis and Barrett's esophagus [7]. These observations strongly suggest a noxious and synergistic role of components of duodenal juice in the refluxed gastric juice. Bilitec™, an ambulatory monitoring system, allows spectrophotometric measurement of luminal bilirubin concentration [8, 9]. Using bilirubin as a marker, the time of esophageal exposure to duodenal contents can be measured. This study reports the *in vitro* validation of this spectrophotometric probe together with measurements made in normal volunteers and patients with GERD.

Materials and methods

In vitro validation studies

A dependable system for the detection of intraluminal bilirubin must meet four criteria. It should offer specificity for the measurement of bilirubin, accurate detection of bilirubin at and above normal physiological concentrations, consistency in its measurements despite pH changes due to environment or food intake, and a reliable absorbance threshold for the detection of intraluminal bilirubin.

Studies performed by Bechi *et al.* [9] confirmed that spectrophotometry based on absorption at a wavelength of 453 nm is specific for bilirubin and that the absorbance spectrum is sufficient to detect bilirubin throughout human physiological ranges. Additional studies were performed in our laboratory to evaluate the third and fourth criteria.

All *in vitro* studies were performed in a lightproof black container to avoid interference by external light. A water bath provided a constant temperature of 37°C. Concentration/absorbance curves were constructed by using prediluted solutions containing 0.2 to 33.2 mg/dL of bilirubin in a bovine serum base (Sigma Chemical Co., St Louis, Missouri). Prior to testing, the probes were calibrated for zero absorption with Ringer's lactate solution. The bilirubin absorbance in six increasing concentrations was measured with the Bilitec™ system. Measurements in each concentration series were repeated five times. To assess the effect of pH on the absorbance readings a solution with a bilirubin concentration of 32 mg/dL was diluted to 3.2, 1.6, and 0.8 mg/dL in a pH environment of 7.7 and 1.4 by adding Ringer's lactate and HCl, respectively. Bilirubin absorbance was measured with the Bilitec™ system in each solution for 15 minutes. For all pH measurements a standard pH meter (Radiometer America, Cleveland, Ohio) was utilized.

Absorbance measurements were made from samples of foods used in the standard diet for 24-hour esophageal pH monitoring or diets recommended by the manufacturer of the Bilitec™. Each food sample was blenderized into a liquid phase to prevent large particles from interfering with the measurements. To resemble postprandial GER, the blenderized food was diluted with 0.1 mol/L HCl in a ratio of one part food to four parts HCl. Absorbance of the commercially available liquid diet (Nutren 1.5, Clinitec, Deerfield, Illinois) was measured in a similar fashion.

Clinical studies

Twenty normal subjects (male:female ratio 16:4; median age 27 years, range 19 to 42) and 21 patients with GERD (male:female ratio 14:7; median age 48, range 31 to 76) volunteered to have 24-hour esophageal monitoring for bilirubin exposure using the Bilitec™ 2000 apparatus. In all volunteers the absence of GER was confirmed by a normal DeMeester score on simultaneous esophageal pH monitoring. The presence of GER was proven by an abnormal DeMeester score on simultaneous pH monitoring in 11 patients and prior pH monitoring in 10. On endoscopy, 4 patients had no mucosal injury, 5 had erosive esophagitis, and 12 had Barrett's metaplasia confirmed by the presence of specialized intestinal metaplasia on biopsy.

Esophageal manometry was performed to identify the location of the lower esophageal sphincter (LES). The motility catheter consisted of an assembly of five fluid-filled, perfused polyvinyl tubes bonded together with five 0.8 mm lateral openings placed 5 cm apart and radially oriented. The catheter was continuously perfused with distilled water by way of a low compliance pneumohydraulic capillary infusion pump (Amdorfer, Greendale, Wisconsin) at a rate of 0.5 mL/min [10]. Each tube was connected to an external pressure transducer (Model P2306 Statham transducer, Gould, Cleveland, Ohio) positioned at the midaxillary level. Before each test, the pressure transducers were calibrated using a mercury-filled manometer. The pressure wave forms generated were printed by a 16 channel recorder (Model ESIOOO, Gould) on paper running at a speed of 5 mm/s. Manometry was performed in the supine position after an overnight fast. All medications were discontinued 48 hours prior to the test. The catheter was passed transnasally into the stomach, then withdrawn back into the esophagus in 1-cm increments every 20 seconds. Tracings were analyzed by hand and the LES pressure, overall length, and abdominal length were measured in a manner previously described. A pH spectrophotometer probe and esophageal pH probes were passed transnasally and positioned 5 cm above the upper border of the LES as located by manometry.

Esophageal pH was monitored with a glass electrode and a portable digital data recorder. Medications were discontinued 48 hours prior to the test except for omeprazole which was discontinued at least 2 weeks beforehand. The probes were calibrated in buffer solutions at pH 7 and pH 1 before and after monitoring. Electrode drift < 0.3 pH units was considered satisfactory. No patient was eliminated because of excessive drift.

The patient was sent home and instructed to remain in the upright or sitting position until retiring for the night and to follow a special solid or liquid diet composed of food with a pH between 5 and 7. Patients were required to eat three meals at intervals of no less than 4 hours, and to wait at least 4 hours from the last meal before laying down to steep. All meals had to be eaten at one sitting over a 20 to 30 minute period. Patients kept diaries of food and fluid intake, symptoms, the time they assumed the supine position in preparation for sleep, and the time they resumed the upright position in the morning.

The data were analyzed using a commercial software program (Gastrosoft, Dallas, Texas). Esophageal acid exposure was scored using previously published criteria [11]. Patients were considered to have abnormal esophageal exposure if their composite score exceeded by more than two standard deviations the mean score previously published for 50 control subjects [11]. The absorbance threshold chosen to measure esophageal exposure to bilirubin in the patient population was determined by calculating the percentage of time during which the esophagus was exposed to bilirubin. Thresholds between 0 and

0.4 absorbance were analyzed in the 20 normal subjects to determine the optimal thresholds for clinical studies. In the 11 patients who had simultaneous pH monitoring, a customized software program allowed a comparison of the pH exposure with the bilirubin exposure.

Results

In vitro validation studies

Concentration/response relationship

Figure 1 shows the relationship of absorbance measurements and increasing bilirubin concentrations. The readings were highly reproducible for the five measurements made at each dilution. The first portion of the curve showed a linear relationship between the measured absorbance and bilirubin concentration up to 3 mg/dL. At higher concentrations the sensitivity declines and large changes in concentration result in small changes in absorbance.

Influence of environmental changes

Figure 2 demonstrates the effect of pH on the absorbance measurements. In both acid and alkaline environments there was a linear relationship between absorbance and bilirubin concentration in the physiologic range of 0 to 3 mg/dL. There was approximately 35% lower absorbance in an acid environment.

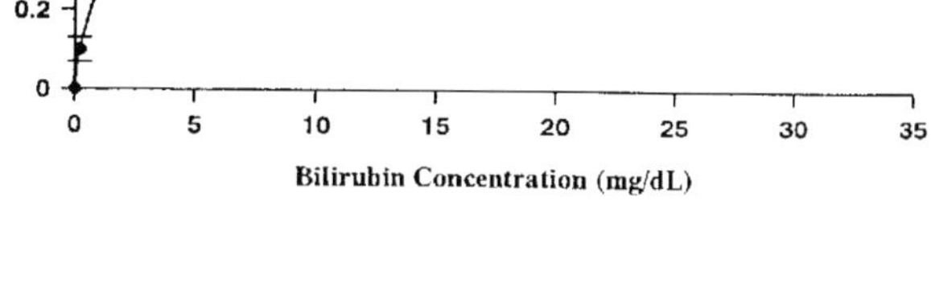

Figure 1. Absorbance/concentration curve established in prediluted solutions containing 0.2 to 33.2 mg/dL bilirubin. Data represent 5 measurements plotted as median with 25th and 75th percentiles.

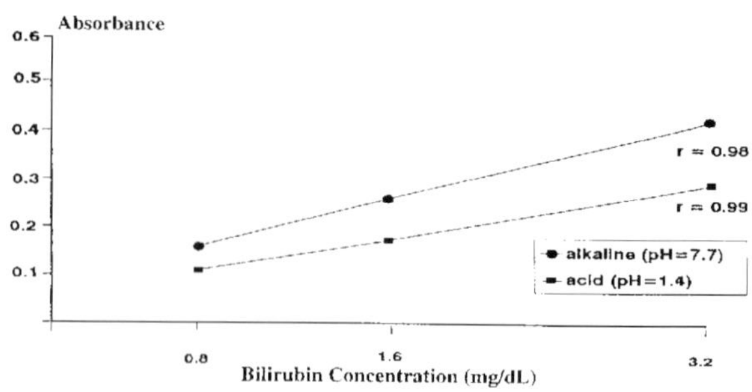

Figure 2. Absorbance/concentration curve established in an acid and alkaline environment with bilirubin concentrations of 0.8, 1.6, and 3.2 mg/dL.

Figure 3 shows the absorbance of blenderized food. All food tested gave values consistently below 0.1. Beverages such as coffee, tea, and cola gave absorbance measurements between 0.3 and 0.5 and were excluded from the diet during 24-hour measurement of esophageal bilirubin exposure.

Clinical studies

Figure 4 shows the median percentage of time of esophageal bilirubin exposure using various absorbance thresholds in 20 healthy normal subjects. Esophageal bilirubin exposure was negligible above an absorbance threshold of 0.14. This value was chosen as the threshold for clinical studies.

Figure 5 shows the percentage of total monitored time that the esophagus was exposed to bilirubin in the patients with GERD. The mean esophageal bilirubin exposure between patients with erosive esophagitis and those with Barrett's esophagus was similar. The highest individual values were found in patients with Barrett's esophagus. Both groups had significantly higher exposure than normal subjects. *Figure 6* shows the median percentage of time that the esophagus was exposed to bilirubin when the esophageal pH was < 4, 4 to 7, and > 7 in patients with Barrett's esophagus. There was a significantly higher bilirubin exposure when the pH was < 4 or between 4 and 7 compared to controls.

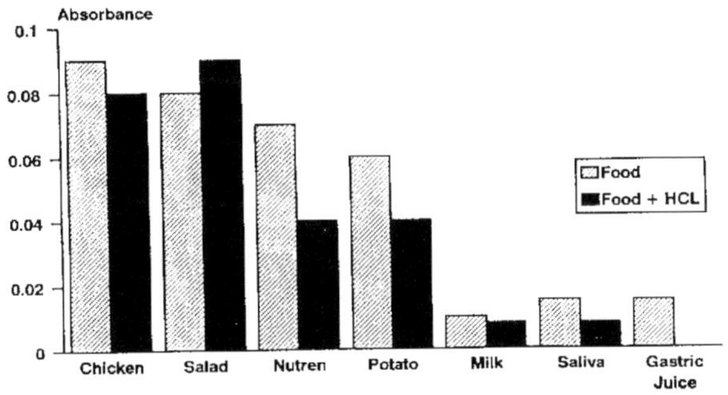

Figure 3. Bilirubin absorbance of different blenderized food samples, a commercialy available liquid diet, and physiological fluids. To resemble the gastric environment, the tests were repeated after dilution of each sample with 0.1 mmol/L HCl, in the ratio of 1 part food to 4 parts HCl.

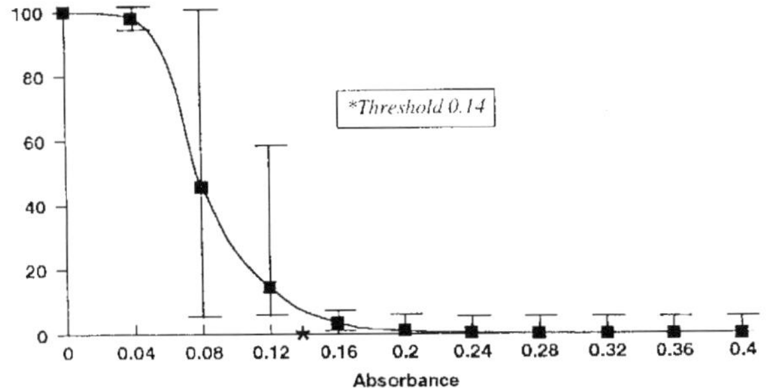

Figure 4. Cumulative descending frequency distribution graph of total study time above different absorbance thresholds in 20 controls. Data are plotted as medians with the 25th and 75th percentiles.

Figure 5. Percentage of total study period during which the esophageal mucosa of each subject was exposed to bilirubin (*i.e.* absorbance exceeded 0.14). Values of each subject are plotted and the median of each group is denoted by the horizontal line. Patients with mucosal injury and Barrett's esophagus had a significantly highler bilirubin absorbance compared to controls ($p < 0.004$, Mann-Whitney).

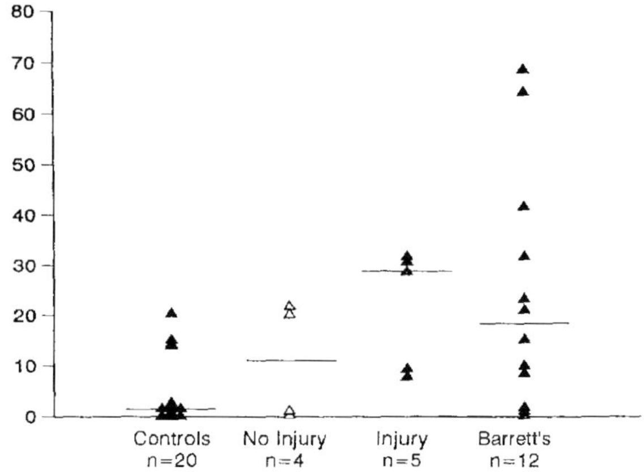

Figure 6. Percentage of time in the indicated pH intervals that the esophagus was exposed to bilirubin in controls and Barrett's. Values are represented as medians.
* Barrett's *versus* controls ($p < 0.01$, Mann-Whitney).

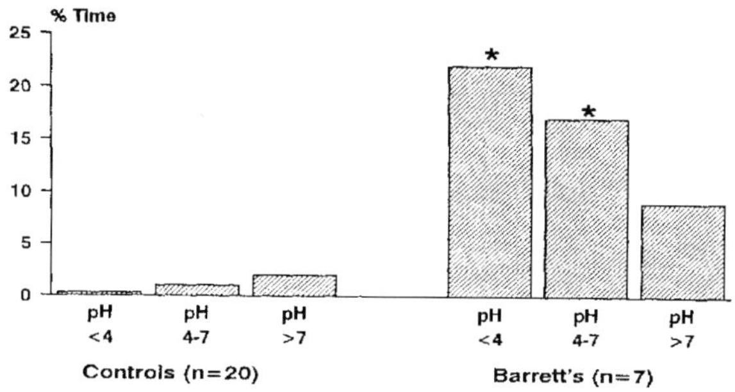

Comments

The relationship of duodenogastric reflux to Barrett's esophagus has been investigated for several years. Injury to the esophageal mucosa of animals by bile was studied extensively in the early eighties by Hannon *et al.* [12], Salo and Kivilaakso [13], and Kivilaakso *et al.* [14]. These investigations show that bile, especially conjugated bile salts, causes changes in esophageal mucosal potential differences and increases hydrogen permeability. Early clinical studies utilized the percentage of time the pH was above 7 on ambulatory esophageal pH monitoring as an indirect method of identifying esophageal exposure to duodenal contents. They measured only the most severe episodes of duodenogastric and GER and found an increased esophageal exposure to pH > 7 in patients with severe mucosal injury and Barrett's esophagus.

The obstacle to defining the role of duodenogastric reflux in Barrett's esophagus has been the lack of a method to confidently identify the presence of duodenal juice in the esophagus. An enzyme probe was developed which was highly sensitive to bile salts [15], but interference by changes in pH made the technique unsuitable for use in the stomach or esophagus. The infusion of radiolabeled bile salts and their detection with an intraesophageal gamma probe allowed only a qualitative measurement of bile reflux over a short time course while the patient was immobilized [16]. Prolonged esophageal aspiration studies, utilizing direct ambulatory aspiration of the refluxate in the esophagus, confirmed the presence of bile salts and thus duodenal juice in the esophagus. However, they required pooling of the aspirate, and hence did not allow correlation between the exposure and esophageal pH [7].

The Bilitec™ 2000 introduces a new technique for long-term ambulatory detection of duodeno-gastroesophageal reflux (DGER). Using bilirubin as a naturally occurring marker for duodenal juice, the fiberoptic system eliminates the need for patients to consume radioactive material and allows the measurement of esophageal exposure to bilirubin over a long-term period while the patient is ambulatory and during sleep. The ability to transfer the data to computer makes correlation with simultaneous pH monitoring easier. An important advantage of ambulatory testing is that the study can be done in a physiologic environment while patients eat, sleep, and go about their daily routines. Only a limited variety of food can be eaten, however, without altering the photometric absorbance spectrum of the probe. Careful studies were done to find food with absorbance threshold below 0.1 so that an alteration of the optimal absorbance range could be excluded and still provide enough variety to allow three meals during the test period. A liquid diet avoids food interference completely, but also compromises physiologic conditions. In addition, it decreases the extent of GER, and so under-reflects the actual degree of disease. Consequently, we preferred to use a solid diet and were pleased to observe no relevant disturbances in the absorbance tracings.

The optimal absorbance range for the Bilitec™ 2000 is 0.14 to 0.5 [8]. We found using an absorbance threshold of 0.1 that normal volunteers on a strict diet had minimal esophageal exposure to bilirubin. This left a wide range of higher absorbance values open for detecting gradations of increased esophageal exposure to duodenal juice.

Patients with GERD and erosive esophagitis or Barrett's esophagus have increased esophageal bilirubin exposure, indicating that the gastric content refluxed is a mixture of gastric and duodenal juice [17, 18]. Attwood *et al.* in 1989 [19] and Stein *et al.* in 1992 [6] pointed out the importance of a mixed acid and alkaline reflux in causing mucosal injury. By performing simultaneous bilirubin and pH monitoring, we were able to show that exposure to bilirubin can occur when the esophageal pH is below 4 or between 4 and 7, out of the range in which the pH probe can detect reflux. These studies suggest that reflux of mixed gastric and duodenal juice into the esophagus can cause esophageal mucosal injury. They also indicate that these reflux events may be asymptomatic, or may become asymptomatic when acid suppression therapy reduces the acid component of the mixed refluxate.

These findings may bear particularly strongly on the medical treatment of reflux esophagitis. Overall, medical treatment heals 75% of patients with reflux esophagitis. The remaining patients experience persistent esophagitis despite prolonged treatment with standard doses of acid suppression. They are likely to have a mechanically defective LES and DGER. Under these conditions, acid suppression therapy reduces acid exposure and relieves the symptom of heartburn while exposure to duodenal juice and less acidic gastric juice continues unabated. The resulting esophageal pH of 4 to 7 may provide the environment for continued mucosal damage from components in the refluxed gastric juice while the patient experiences symptomatic relief. An antireflux procedure prevents the reflux of both gastric and duodenal juice, and should be the treatment of choice in this situation.

In conclusion, the Bilitec™ 2000 is a very useful and reliable complementary tool to esophageal pH monitoring in the investigation of patients with foregut symptoms. Our results show that reflux of duodenal juice in addition to gastric juice does occur in patients with severe GERD, that GER can occur at normal esophageal pH levels, and in some patients may go unnoticed when esophageal pH monitoring is performed in isolation. The combination of pH and bilirubin esophageal monitoring will further our understanding and improve our care of patients with GERD.

References

1. Ollyo JB, Monnier P, Fontolliet C, Savary M. The natural history and incidence of reflux esophagitis. Gullet 1993;3:3-10.
2. Iascone C, DeMeester TR, Little AG, Skinner DB. Barrett's esophagus. Functional assessment, proposed pathogenesis and surgical therapy. Arch Surg 1983;118:543-549.
3. Gillen P, Keeling P, Bryne PJ, Hennessy TPJ. Barrett's esophagus: pH profile. Br J Surg 1987;74:774-776.
4. Attwood SEA, Smyrk TC, DeMeester TR, et al. Duodenoesophageal reflux and development of esophageal adenocarcinoma in rats. Surgery 1992;111:503-510.
5. Clark GWB, Smyrk TC, Mirvish SS, et al. Effect of gastroduodenal juice and dietary fat on the development of Barrett's esophagus and esophageal neoplasia: an experimental rat-model. Ann Surg Oncol 1994;1(3):252-261.
6. Stein HJ, Barlow AP, DeMeester TR, Hinder RA. Complications of gastroesophageal reflux disease. The role of the lower esophageal sphincter, esophageal acid/alkaline exposure, and duodenogastric reflux. Ann Surg 1992;216:35-43.
7. Stein HJ, Feussner H, Kauer W, et al. "Alkaline" gastroesophageal reflux: assessment by ambulatory esophageal aspiration and pH monitoring. Am J Surg 1994;1 67:163-168.
8. Bechi P, Falciai R, Baldini F, et al. A new fiber optic sensor for ambulatory entero-gastric reflux detection. In: Katzir A, ed. Fiber optic medical and fluorescent sensors and applications. Bellingha, Washington: SPIE;1992,1648:130-135.
9. Bechi P, Pucciani F, Baldini F, et al. Long-term ambulatory enterogastric reflux monitoring. Validation of a new fiberoptic technique. Dig Dis Sci 1993;38:1297-1306.
10. Zaninotto G, DeMeester TR, Schwizer W, et al. The lower esophageal sphincter in health and disease. Am J Surg 1988;155:104-111.
11. Jamieson JR, Stein HJ, DeMeester TR, et al. Ambulatory 24h esophageal pH monitoring:normal values, optimal thresholds, specificity, sensitivity, and reproducibility. Am J Gastroenterol 1992;87(9):1102-1111.
12. Harmon J, Johnson L, Maydonovitch C, Effects of acid and bile salts on the rabbit esophageal mucosa. Dig Dis Sci 1981;26:65-72.
13. Salo JA. Kivilaakso E. Role of bile salts and trypsin in the pathogenesis of experimental alkaline esophagitis. Surgery 1982;92:61-68.
14. Kivilaakso E, Fromm D, Silen W. Effect of bile salts and related compounds on isolated esophageal mucosa. Surgery 1980;87:280-285.
15. Armstrong D, Lennox B, Albery J, et al. Is continuous ambulatory monitoring of duodenogastric reflux feasible? In vitro assessment of an enzymatic amperometric bile acid electrode. Gut 1987;28:AI395.
16. Stoker DL, Williams JG, MacCleod MA, et al. The evaluation of a gastric bile probe. Nuc Med Comm 1990;1 1:777-790.
17. Gotley DC, Morgan AP, Cooper MJ. Bile acid concentrations in the refluxate of patients with reflux esophagitis. Br J Surg 1988;75:587-590.
18. Iftikhar SY, Ledingham S, Steele RJC, et al. Bile reflux in the columnar-lined esophagus. Ann R Coll Surg Engl 1993;75:411-416.
19. Attwood SE, DeMeester TR, Bremner CG, et al. Alkaline gastroesophageal reflux: implications in the development of complications in Barrett's columnar-lined lower esophagus Surgery 1989;106:763-770.
20. Sontag SJ, Hirschowitz BI, Holt S, et al. Two doses of omeprazole versus placebo in symptomatic erosive esophagitis: the US multicenter study. Gastroenterology 1992;102-.119-118.

What is the role of bacterial overgrowth in the rising incidence of adenocarcinoma?

C.D. Morris, S.E.A. Attwood (Salford)

There are two areas where we can currently find clues about the contribution of bacteria in the pathogenesis of esophageal adenocarcinoma. These are the roles of *Helicobacter pylori* and bacterial overgrowth secondary to acid suppression.

Helicobacter pylori

Since *Helicobacter pylori* colonisation of Barrett's epithelium was first described in 1985, much interest has surrounded its possible contribution to the rising incidence of Barrett's adenocarcinoma. A recent review of the incidence of *Helicobacter pylori* colonisation of Barrett's epithelium found a 24% colonisation rate [1] of the Barrett's epithelium, which was not significantly different from the incidence of gastric infection in the same patients. However the incidence of gastric infection in controls was higher at 41% suggesting a lower rate of *Helicobacter pylori* infection in patients with Barrett's esophagus.

Despite initial fears that this *Helicobacter pylori* colonisation may contribute to esophageal carcinogenesis, the converse appears to be true. Chow *et al.* [2] found odds ratios for esophageal/gastric cardia adenocarcinoma of 0.4 (CI 0.2-0.8) in patients carrying cagA+ strains of *Helicobacter pylori*. This apparent protective effect not only applies to adenocarcinoma but also to other complications of reflux as the review by Bowrey suggests. In the study of Weston *et al.* [3] the prevalence of cagA+ strains was decreased in a stepwise manner in patients with gastroesophageal reflux disease (44.2%), Barrett's esophagus (35.1%) / low-grade dysplasia (36.2%) and high-grade dysplasia (14.3%) / adenocarcinoma (15.1%).

The controversy regarding the association between reflux and *Helicobacter pylori* infection may be explained by the pattern of gastric colonisation. Gastric antral infection tends to lead to increased acid production *via* hypergastrinaemia [4]. These patients will be at risk of duodenal ulceration and reflux disease, which would both improve on *Helicobacter pylori* eradication. However in the corpus predominant gastritis, glandular atrophy leads to hypochlorhydria [5] and these patients are therefore protected from reflux. These patients would have increased reflux on *Helicobacter pylori* eradication, and indeed there is evidence that severity of reflux increases in patients who have undergone *Helicobacter pylori* eradication as part of the management of conditions such as duodenal ulceration [6]. The nature of colonisation depends on a number of factors including CagA status, with cagA+ strains leading to greater Corpus gastritis. This would explain the apparent protective role for these organisms in reflux disease and adenocarcinoma. There is also some evidence that *Helicobacter pylori* colonisation increases the efficacy of acid suppression by H_2 receptor antagonists or proton pump inhibitors (PPIs) leading to superior control of reflux [7].

In view of the accumulating evidence for a protective effect of *Helicobacter pylori* in reflux disease and esophageal adenocarcinoma, and the lack of data supporting

Helicobacter pylori eradication in reducing gastric cancer, the policy of blanket *Helicobacter pylori* eradication in any patient found to be a carrier may turn out to be expensive both financially and medically.

Bacterial overgrowth

The ability for bacteria to colonize the stomach is largely dependent on the pH of the gastric content, with bacterial overgrowth frequently occurring in conditions with diminished acid output such as atrophic gastritis. As the pH rises to above 4, salivary organisms are able to survive, and once the pH reaches 5 a large flora develops including faecal organisms [8]. This can lead to diarrhoea, malabsorption [9] and the formation of potentially carcinogenic compounds [10]. Initial reports of the bacterial changes occurring during acid suppression therapy with H_2 receptor antagonists were controversial with some but not all demonstrating elevations in bacteria levels on treatment [11]. However with the more profound acid suppression seen with PPIs there is little doubt that bacterial overgrowth of salivary and faecal organisms occurs, both in the stomach and duodenum [11]. These changes are reversed following the normalisation of acid levels.

Whether this bacterial overgrowth contributes to the rising incidence of adenocarcinoma of the esophagus and gastroesophageal junction is unknown, though there are a number of mechanisms by which it could promote carcinogenesis. Firstly many of the bacteria present in the stomach of acid suppressed patients, such as Enterococcus and Bacteroides are able to deconjugate bile acids [12]. Studies have demonstrated clear increases in deconjugated bile acids secondary to bacterial overgrowth in patients on PPI [12] and H_2 receptor antagonist therapy [13]. These deconjugated bile acids are most damaging to the foregut mucosa at more neutral pH when they are unionized and are able to gain access into the cells. These pH changes are obviously encouraged by acid suppression therapy. The bile acids may cause cellular injury by disrupting cell membranes or accumulating within cells and disturbing cellular processes [14, 15].

A further possible damaging mechanism is the metabolism of salivary and dietary nitrates to nitrites by the bacteria. These can react with amides and amines to form carcinogens. Bile acids are a rich source of amides which react with nitrites in the stomach under the action of bacteria to form N-nitroso compounds such as N-nitrosotaurocholic acid and N-nitrosoglycocholic acid which have been shown to be carcinogenic [16]. Some studies have been able to demonstrate an elevation in the levels of nitrite and N-nitrosamine, associated with a fall in nitrate in gastric juice as bacterial levels increase due to profound acid suppression, these changes reverting to normal on discontinuing therapy [10]. Other studies however have been unable to confirm such changes in nitrosamines due to the overgrowth [11], and an element of doubt therefore remains concerning the production and contribution of these endogenous nitrosamines.

In summary, the mechanisms described above may be important in explaining the rising incidence of esophageal adenocarcinoma, and links bacterial overgrowth, bile reflux and N-nitroso carcinogens, all of which have been implicated in this disease. The rise in adenocarcinoma incidence has also occurred along a similar time scale to the rising use of acid suppression, though this may be a coincidental finding, due to treating an increasing prevalence of reflux disease.

References

1. Bowrey D, Williams G, Clark G. Interactions between Helicobacter pylori and gastrooesophageal reflux disease. Dis Esophagus 1998;11:203-209.
2. Chow WH, Blaser MJ, Blot WJ, Gammon MD, Vaughan TL, Risch HA, Perez Perez GI, Schoenberg JB, Stanford JL, Rotterdam H, West AB, Fraumeni JF Jr. An inverse relation between cagA+ strains of Helicobacter pylori infection and risk of esophageal and gastric cardia adenocarcinoma. Cancer Res 1998;58(4):588-590.
3. Weston AP, Badr AS, Topalovski M, Cherian R, Dixon A, Hassanein RS. Prospective evaluation of the prevalence of gastric Helicobacter pylori infection in patients with GERD, Barrett's esophagus, Barrett's dysplasia, and Barrett's adenocarcinoma. Am J Gastroenterol 2000;95(2):387-394.
4. Moss S, Legon S, Bishop A, et al. Effect of Helicobacter pylori on gastric somatostatin in duodenal ulcer disease. Lancet 1992;340:930-932.
5. El-Omar E, Oien K, El-Nujumi A, et al. Helicobacter pylori infection and chronic gastric acid hyposecretion. Gastroenterology 1997;113:15-24.
6. Labenz J, Blum A, Bayerdorffer E, et al. Curing Helicobacter pylori in patients with duodenal ulcer may provoke reflux esophagitis. Gastroenterology 1997;112:1442-1447.
7. Koster E. Adverse events of HP eradication:long term negative consequences of HP eradication. Acta Gastroenterol-Belg 1998;61(3):350-351.
8. Stockbruegger R. Bacterial overgrowth as a consequence of reduced gastric acidity. Scand J Gastroenterol 1985;19:355-364.
9. Saltzman J, Russell R. Nutritional consequences of intestinal bacterial overgrowth. Compr Ther 1994. 20(9):523-530.
10. Sharma B, Santana I, Wood E, Walt R, Pereira M, Noone P, Smith P, Walters C, Pounder R. Intragastric bacterial activity and nitrosation before, during and after treatment with omeprazole. Br Med J 1984;289:717-719.
11. Thorens J, Froehlich F, Schwizer W, Saraga E, Bille J, Gyr K, Duroux P, Nicolet M, Pignatelli B, Blum A, Gonvers J, Fried M. Bacterial overgrowth during treatment with omeprazole compared with cimetidine:a prospective randomized double blind study. Gut 1996;39(1):54-59.
12. Shindo K, Machida M, Fukumura M, Koide K, Yamazaki R. Omeprazole induces altered bile acid metabolism. Gut 1998;42(2):266-271.
13. Shindo K, Yamazaki R, Koide K, Fukumura M, Hirai Y. Alteration of bile acid metabolism by cimetidine in healthy humans. J Investig Med 1996;44(8):462-469.
14. Batzri S, Harmon JW, Schweitzer EJ, Toles R. Bile acid accumulation in gastric mucosal cells. Proc Soc Exp Biol Med 1991;197(4):393-399.
15. Thomas AJ, Nahrwold DL, Rose RC. Detergent action of sodium taurocholate on rat gastric mucosa. Biochim Biophys Acta 1972;282(1):210-213.
16. Busby W, Shuker D, Charnley G, Newberne P, Tanenbaum S, Wogan G. Carcinogenicity in rats of the nitrosated bile acid conjugates N-nitrosoglycocholic acid and N-nitrosotaurocholic acid. Cancer Res 1985;45:1367-1371.

What is the role of cellular proliferation and apoptosis?

C.D. Morris, S.E.A. Attwood (Salford)

Increased epithelial proliferation is known to precede the development of esophageal neoplasia in experimental models. This is likely to be due to a greater proportion of cells in the replication cycle where they are particularly susceptible to mutagens. Much interest has been directed at the degree of proliferation in Barrett's metaplasia and changes that occur in the progression to dysplasia and adenocarcinoma. Increased proportions of proliferating cells have been shown in benign Barrett's epithelium compared to normal gastric mucosa, but with the proliferating cells remaining in a similar arrangement to the naturally occurring proliferative zones [1]. Gray *et al.* demonstrated variable proliferation rates between different cell types within the Barrett's epithelium by proliferating cell nuclear antigen

(PCNA) labelling, proliferation being greater in specialized cells compared to junctional or gastric type metaplasia [2]. Gulizia *et al.* showed this increased proliferation also occurred in microscopic specialized intestinal metaplasia (IM) at the gastroesophageal junction [3]. How the rate of proliferation varies with the progression to dysplasia is controversial with some authors finding no differences as dysplasia developed. However others have shown clear changes as histological abnormalities progress. Gillen *et al.* used immunostaining for PCNA to show increasing proliferation during the progression from benign metaplasia to dysplasia to adenocarcinoma [4]. Hong *et al.* demonstrated an increasing size of the proliferating zone along with a shift away from the normal crypt zones to more superficial layers as the grade of dysplasia increases by Ki-67 detection [1]. Interestingly the study by Gillen also suggested elevated levels of proliferation in benign metaplasia adjacent to adenocarcinomas compared to metaplasia from cases without cancer.

The degree of proliferation in the Barrett's epithelium appears to be partly controlled by the presence and timing of reflux episodes. Fitzgerald *et al.* used a tissue culture model to show that continuous acid exposure led to decreased cell proliferation and an increased Villin expression suggesting a differentiated cell type [5]. In contrast, pulsed acid led to increased cell proliferation with no effect on cell differentiation. These effects may be mediated *via* changes in the intracellular pH mediated by the Na^+/H^+ exchanger, and blocking this exchanger could abolish that the proliferation induced by acid pulses. How the changes in intracellular pH lead to increased proliferation is not fully understood. It is suggested that on recovery from the cell acidification caused by an acid pulse there is a period of "alkaline overshoot", which may stimulate cells to move from G0/G1 to the S phase of the cell cycle, leading to proliferation. This could certainly be one mechanism by which reflux disease contributes to carcinogenesis.

The degree of cellular proliferation can also be influenced by growth factors and hormones. Decreased levels of salivary epidermal growth factor (EGF) have been demonstrated in patients with Barrett's esophagus compared to esophagitis and control groups [6] but with no differences in tissue EGF levels between Barrett's metaplasia and adenocarcinoma [7]. Transforming growth factor α is part of the same family as EGF and has been shown to be elevated in intestinal-type compared to gastric-type metaplasia with further increases in dysplasia and adenocarcinoma [8]. Interestingly EGF receptor expression has also been shown to be elevated in Barrett's dysplasia and adenocarcinoma [8] and may be involved in elevating rates of proliferation. This receptor bears considerable sequence homology with the C-erbB-2 proto-oncogene, which has been implicated in esophageal carcinogenesis.

Intermittent pH elevations of the gastric antrum, as occurs in reflux of duodenal juices can lead to elevated gastrin secretion by the parietal G cells. Gastrin has a number of effects on the gastrointestinal tract and has been implicated in the development of intestinal neoplasia [9]. As Barrett's mucosa contains areas of IM, then it may behave in a similar fashion in response to gastrin. However to date gastrin has only been shown to be mitogenic and not mutagenic, that is it stimulates proliferation [10] but has not been shown to induce carcinogenesis, and is therefore most likely to act as a growth promoter.

In addition to proliferation changes, alterations in the degree of apoptosis have been suggested in Barrett's metaplasia. Low rates of apoptosis have been found in Barrett's tissue compared to adjacent squamous epithelium [11], though this low apoptosis may be due to decreased cell injury, as the cell type is more resistant to the reflux insult. Some have argued that the progression to dysplasia may be a result of a failure of apoptosis [12], though others have documented increasing apoptosis in higher degrees of dysplasia [13]. However, differences in bcl-2, bcl-x and bax, proteins that regulate apoptosis have been found in varying degrees of dysplasia [12, 13] suggesting that the control of apoptosis is likely to be altered in dysplastic progression, though their exact roles and control mechanisms remain to be elucidated. Elevated levels of COX-2, the rate limiting enzyme in the production of prostaglandins have been found in Barrett's esophagus [14] and data from our own institution shows significant further elevations in dysplasia and adenocarcinoma [15]. COX-2 expression can be induced by exposure of the esophageal epithelium to acid and bile acids [16], and once induced leads to a decreased capacity for apoptosis and elevated cellular proliferation [17].

References

1. Hong MK, Laskin WB, Herman BE, Johnston MH, Vargo JJ, Steinberg SM, Allegra CJ, Johnston PG. Expansion of the Ki-67 proliferative compartment correlates with degree of dysplasia in Barrett's esophagus. Cancer 1995;75(2):423-429.
2. Gray MR, Hall PA, Nash J, Ansari B, Lane DP, Kingsnorth AN. Epithelial proliferation in Barrett's esophagus by proliferating cell nuclear antigen immunolocalization. Gastroenterology 1992;103(6):1769-1776.
3. Gulizia JM, Wang H, Antonioli D, Spechler SJ, Zeroogian J, Goyal R, Shahsafaei A, Chen YY, Odze RD. Proliferative characteristics of intestinalized mucosa in the distal esophagus and gastroesophageal junction (short-segment Barrett's esophagus): a case control study. Hum Pathol 1999;30(4):412-418.
4. Gillen P, McDermott M, Grehan D, Hourihane DB, Hennessy T. Proliferating cell nuclear antigen in the assessment of Barrett's mucosa. Br J Surg 1994;81:1766-1768.
5. Fitzgerald RC, Omary MB, Triadafilopoulos G. Altered sodium-hydrogen exchange activity is a mechanism for acid-induced hyperproliferation in Barrett's esophagus. Am J Physiol 1998;275:G47-55.
6. Gray MR, Donnelly RJ, Kingsnorth AN. Role of salivary epidermal growth factor in the pathogenesis of Barrett's columnar lined esophagus. Br J Surg 1991;78(12):1461-1466.
7. Jankowski J, McMenemin R, Hopwood D, Penston J, Wormsley KG. Abnormal expression of growth regulatory factors in Barrett's esophagus. Clin Sci Colch 1991;81(5):663-668.
8. Jankowski J, Hopwood D, Wormsley KG. Flow-cytometric analysis of growth-regulatory peptides and their receptors in Barrett's esophagus and esophageal adenocarcinoma. Scand J Gastroenterol 1992;27(2):147-154.
9. Thorburn CM, Friedman GD, Dickinson CJ, Vogelman JH, Orentreich N, Parsonnet J. Gastrin and colorectal cancer: a prospective study. Gastroenterology 1998;115(2):275-280.
10. Karaki Y, Shimazaki K, Okamoto M, Ookami H, Fujimaki M. Effect of endogenous hypergastrinemia on carcinogenesis in the rat esophagus. Surg Today 1996;26(1):5-11.
11. Wetscher GJ, Schwelberger H, Unger A, Offner FA, Profanter C, Glaser K, Klingler A, Gadenstaetter M, Klinger P. Reflux-induced apoptosis of the esophageal mucosa is inhibited in Barrett's epithelium. Am J Surg 1998;176(6):569-573.
12. Katada N, Hinder RA, Smyrk TC, Hiki Y, Kakita A. Duodenoesophageal reflux induces apoptosis in rat esophageal epithelium. Dig Dis Sci 1999;44(2):301-310.
13. Soslow RA, Remotti H, Baergen RN, Altorki NK. Suppression of apoptosis does not foster neoplastic growth in Barrett's esophagus. Mod Pathol 1999;12(3):239-250.
14. Wilson KT, Fu S, Ramanujam KS, Meltzer SJ. Increased expression of inducible nitric oxide synthase and cyclooxygenase-2 in Barrett's esophagus and associated adenocarcinomas. Cancer Res 1998;58(14):2929-2934.
15. Morris C, Bigley G, Armstrong G, Attwood S. Expression of cyclo-oxygenase 2 (COX-2) in Barrett's esophagus, dysplasia and adenocarcinoma. Gastroenterology 2000;118(4):A685.
16. Zhang F, Subbaramaiah K, Altorki N, Dannenberg AJ. Dihydroxy bile acids activate the transcription of cyclooxygenase-2. J Biol Chem 1998;273(4):2424-2428.
17. Tsujii M, DuBois RN. Alterations in cellular adhesion and apoptosis in epithelial cells overexpressing prostaglandin endoperoxide synthase 2. Cell 1995;83(3):493-501.

May carcinogenic process be induced by diet particularities?

S.A. Wajed, C.G. Bremner (Los Angeles)

The rapid and consistent rise in the incidence of adenocarcinoma of the distal esophagus and cardia over the recent decades has become a focus of serious concern [1, 2]. Other than the fact that this is a disease predominantly of white males within affluent and industrialised nations [3], very little is understood about specific risk factors for the disease. Esophageal adenocarcinoma markedly contrasts with the now declining squamous cell cancer of the esophagus in its epidemiology and etiological factors, and it does not appear to share risk factors with distal stomach cancers either. The presence of Barrett's metaplastic epithelium within the distal esophagus represents a precursor lesion, which has malignant potential, and is the only convincing and reliable established risk factor for the subsequent development of cancer. Approximately one in ten patients with Barrett's metaplasia will go on develop adenocarcinoma [4].

Barrett's metaplasia forms on a background of gastroesophageal reflux disease (GERD), and possibly duodeno-gastroesophageal reflux (DGER) [5, 6]. Gastric and possibly duodenal secretions bathe the lower esophageal cells, and in a form of protective response to this mucosal injury, the cells undergo the transformation from squamous to specialized columnar type epithelium. While reflux disease and the subsequent presence of Barrett's metaplasia represent the first steps in carcinogenesis, it is unclear as to how this process is initiated, and what other factors might be involved in accelerating or attenuating the disease process. Quantitative and qualitative variations in dietary pattern may be a possible key element in this puzzle, and the experimental and epidemiological evidence for this hypothesis is discussed.

Can diet induce the carcinogenic progression in esophageal adenocarcinoma?

Although there are some reports of "familial" type Barrett's esophagus, this seems to be related to an inherited predisposition to reflux disease rather than genetic susceptibility to neoplasia [7]. Worldwide, Barrett's metaplasia is rare in non-Caucasian ethnic groups. In an analysis of 212 patients with Barrett's in South Africa, where the Black African population exceeds that of the White by some five fold, less than 5% of lesions were in Black African patients [8]. Since these groups differ substantially in their dietary patterns, this kind of discrepancy may relate to either qualitative difference in the diet between each ethnic group or their inherent susceptibility to GERD and its consequences. There is some evidence from experimental models of carcinogenesis and large epidemiological studies which suggest that dietary variations could be influential in determining disease progression.

Experimental models

In rats, treatment with carcinogenic chemicals such as N-nitroso compounds methyl-n-amylnitrosomine (MNAN) and 2,6-dimethylnitrosomorpholine (DMNM) can induce the formation of squamous cell cancers [9, 10]. If these rats are subjected to increased duodeno-esophageal reflux through the formation of an esophagoduodenal anastomosis, then not only is the number and rate of formation of tumors increased, but many of these now develop an adenocarcinoma [11]. This switching of phenotype is not observed if isolated gastroesophageal acid reflux alone is present following the formation of a surgical gastroesophagoplasty [12].

Extending these observations further, Clark *et al.* [13] investigated the possibility that dietary fat might act as a proliferative factor in the presence of DGER. They performed esophagoduodenostomy in rats, artificially creating severe DGER, and postoperatively treated some of the rats with the carcinogen MNAN. The rats were further subdivided into groups and fed diets with differing fat and calorific contents for 20 weeks. In the absence of carcinogen, specialized columnar epithelium (*i.e.* Barrett's) or dysplasia occurred in 7 of 39 rats (18%) that had surgery alone. Squamous cell carcinoma occurred in a further one (3%), but diet in this group appeared to have no influence on the course of disease. However, in the presence of carcinogen, tumors arose in 63 of 111 operated rats, and of these, 42% were adenocarcinoma. The incidence of this lesion was significantly higher in the group fed with a semi-purified, high fat diet (83%) as compared to the other groups fed with semi-purified control diet (45%); semi-purified calorie restricted diet (55%) or a chow diet (42%). Thus in these models, a premalignant lesion can be induced by gastroduodenal reflux alone, and in the presence of a carcinogen, a high fat content diet can enhance tumor growth. Restriction of calories alone did not protect against carcinogenesis.

Epidemiological studies

Highly specific geographical locations, even within the same regions, have been recognized as hotspots for squamous cell cancer incidence. This is often attributable to the presence of certain environmental agents with carcinogenic properties [14]. A natural assumption would be the possibility of the existence of similar agents responsible for esophageal adenocarcinoma. Epidemiological studies have attempted to identify both exogenous factors, which are specific to the etiology of esophageal adenocarcinoma, as well as the relationship with established risk factors from other, anatomically local lesions such as esophageal squamous cell carcinoma and distal stomach cancers.

Tobacco smoking and excessive alcohol consumption are the usual suspects in many cancers and have been well established as risk factors in esophageal squamous cell carcinoma [15]. Kabat examined the possibility that these may also be implicated in esophageal adenocarcinoma using data from 28 hospitals in eight US cities [16]. An analysis of the smoking, drinking and dietary habits of 173 hospitalized patients with esophageal adenocarcinoma was made, and this was compared with 4,544 hospitalized men who had been admitted for non-smoking or non gastrointestinal tract diseases. A further 136 patients with esophageal squamous cell carcinoma and 122 patients with distal gastric cancers provided additional control subjects. The odds ratio of a current smoker and esophageal adenocarcinoma was 2.3 (1.0 defined by "never smoked" patients) for men, and 4.8 for women. This compared with odds ratios of 4.5 and 6.8 for men and women respectively with esophageal squamous cell carcinoma, and values of 1.7 and 3.2 for distal stomach cancers. Smoking therefore was a risk factor, though this association is weaker in esophageal adenocarcinoma as compared to squamous cell carcinoma, and more significant in women than men. Similarly there was also an association with heavy alcohol consumption (defined as greater than four or more whiskey equivalents per day) and again the relationship was stronger in women with an odds ratio of 3.8 compared to 2.3 in men, but these figures were approximately a fifth of the values for squamous cell carcinoma. These associations were not affected by adjustments for dietary factors or other co-variates. Analysis of dietary intake indicated that a high total fat intake represented a significant risk factor with an odds ratio of 2.9, thus more significant than smoking or drinking in men. Additionally, there was found to be a greater risk with increased vitamin A intake from animal sources, but this trend was reversed for vitamin A intake from plant sources. A negative association with high fiber intake was also established, but body mass index (BMI) did not relate to esophageal adenocarcinoma. Thus the data from this large study suggest a that there is a weak link between esophageal adenocarcinoma and smoking and drinking, and that this disease is also related to high fat intake, foods from animal as opposed to plant sources and low fiber intake.

Brown *et al.* [17] reported on the results of a case-control interview study carried out from the National Cancer Institute Bethesda on the diet of 174 white men with esophageal adenocarcinoma against 750 controls living in three separate regions of the United States. In this study, no significant correlation could be established between intake of fatty foods or a high calorific diet and esophageal adenocarcinoma. However, obese patients, that is with a BMI in the upper quartile or greater were shown to have an increased risk with an odds ratio of 3.1. Obesity as quantified by the BMI may arise as a secondary effect of high dietary fat or calorific intake, but neither of these variables were significant for risk. The consumption of raw fruit and vegetables appeared to confer a protective effect against cancer.

The lack of dietary fruit and vegetables as a risk factor was also confirmed in another hospital based case control study at the Memorial Sloan-Kettering Cancer Center in New York [18]. Ninety-five cases of esophageal adenocarcinoma were matched with cancer free control subjects, and a statistical analysis of nutritional and dietary factors was evaluated. In this study, both high calorific intake and dietary fat did in fact prove to be significant risk factors for disease. The presence of several other dietary factors was also found to be protective against cancer risk, and these include high fiber intake, lutein and niacin, vitamin B6 and minerals iron and zinc. High intake of other trace elements including phosphorus and potassium vitamins A and E, beta-carotene and folate were also associated with lower cancer risk, but they were not statistically significant in this particular study.

The main conclusions with regards to BMI, calorie fat and fiber intake from these studies is summarized in the *Table I*.

Table I. Odds ratio of diet related risk factors with esophageal adenocarcinoma.

Author	Year	High BMI	High calorie intake	High fat intake	High fiber intake
Kabat *et al.* [16]	1992	NS	-	2.9	0.3
Brown *et al* [17]	1995	3.1	NS	NS	0.4
Zhang *et al.* [18]	1997	-	2.8	2.4	0.3

NS = not significant

Mechanisms of diet induced carcinogenesis

From these preliminary studies, the dietary risk factors for esophageal adenocarcinoma as distinct from other foregut malignancies, appear to be an increased association with a high fat and calorific intake, which may in turn give rise to obesity. The ingestion of fiber, raw fruit and vegetables and certain vitamins, minerals and trace elements may infer a protective effect.

Hiatal hernia, associated with obesity, may compromise the function of the lower esophageal sphincter, which can then lead to GERD, therefore exposing the individual to the risk of the development of Barrett's metaplasia and its consequences [19]. It is interesting to note that there has been a rise in the number of men classified as being overweight between 1976 and 1991 in the United States as derived from national survey data, a trend which is similar to that of esophageal adenocarcinoma. [20]

High calorific intake and dietary fat may induce obesity, but could also have a direct carcinogenic effect through oxidative DNA damage [21] or through up regulation of protein kinase C in stem cells, and this latter effect could be increased by alterations in the intake level of certain minerals [22]. High sodium, and low levels of potassium, magnesium and phosphorus can induce a "PCK syndrome" which may promote fat related tumorigenesis. Fatty foods can also delay gastric emptying time and gastric distension which then exacerbates GERD, as well as stimulating increased pancreatic and biliary secretions. Any pre-existing DGER is then potentiated. Dietary intake of fat has actually fallen in the United States over the last two decades, so in broad terms, this does not support an obvious explanation to the rising levels of esophageal adenocarcinoma [23].

Raw vegetables and fruit appear to be protective against this disease. The abundance of natural fiber, vitamins and minerals within these foods could have several beneficial effects. Non-degradable fiber can simply clear the lower esophagus and upper gastrointestinal tract of residual food and partly digested materials and secretion by a direct mechanical action. Certain carcinogens are able to bind to components of dietary fiber which itself remains undigested [24]. Mucosal exposure to potentially harmful factors is therefore limited and likely to cause less damage. Potentially carcinogenic DNA damage my also arise as a result of the action of free radicals and these effect may be counterbalanced by certain foods [25]. Natural anti-oxidants within fresh fruit and vegetables, such as vitamin C, vitamin E, lutein, selenium may limit this damage and hence prevent carcinogenesis. Vitamin B6, niacin and folate are also involved in DNA repair mechanisms, and so deficiency in these components may increase the effect of potential carcinogens. The ability of the body to mount an immune response may also be important in resistance to the development of cancer, and so mineral deficiency such as zinc and iron which normally contribute to this action may impact the disease process.

Conclusion

A clear explanation for the rise in the incidence of esophageal adenocarcinoma is not yet forthcoming. Certain dietary factors may play a role in stimulating or promoting the formation of early metaplastic lesions and then fuelling their progression to more advanced and eventually invasive disease. Fatty foods, high calorie diet and obesity which may all be inter-related seem to bear an increased risk of cancer. Raw fruit, vegetables, and dietary fiber on the other hand may exert a protective effect. These food groups can potentially influence the course of disease through both direct and indirect means, and may eventually play a role in designing cancer prevention strategies.

References

1. Blot WJ, Devesa SS, Kneller RW, Fraumeni JFJ. Rising incidence of adenocarcinoma of the esophagus and gastric cardia. JAMA 1991;265:1287-1289.
2. Pera M, Cameron AJ, Trastek VF, Carpenter HA, Zinsmeister AR. Increasing incidence of adenocarcinoma of the esophagus and esophagogastric junction. Gastroenterology 1993;104:510-513.
3. Rogers EL, Goldkind SF, Iseri OA, et al. Adenocarcinoma of the lower esophagus. A disease primarily of white men with Barrett's esophagus. J Clin Gastroenterol 1986;8:613-618.
4. Sarr MG, Hamilton SR, Marrone GC, Cameron JL. Barrett's esophagus: its prevalence and association with adenocarcinoma in patients with symptoms of gastroesophageal reflux. Am J Surg 1985;149:187-193.
5. Iascone C, DeMeester TR, Little AG, Skinner DB. Barrett's esophagus. Functional assessment, proposed pathogenesis, and surgical therapy. Arch Surg 1983;118:543-549.
6. Attwood SE, DeMeester TR, Bremner CG, Barlow AP, Hinder RA. Alkaline gastroesophageal reflux: implications in the development of complications in Barrett's columnar-lined lower esophagus. Surgery 1989;106:764-770.
7. Romero Y, Cameron AJ, Locke GR, et al. Familial aggregation of gastroesophageal reflux in patients with Barrett's esophagus and esophageal adenocarcinoma. Gastroenterology 1997;113:1449-1456.
8. Mason RJ, Bremner CG. The columnar-lined (Barrett's) esophagus in black patients. South Afr J Surg 1998;36:61-62.
9. Bulay O, Mirvish SS. Carcinogenesis in rat esophagus by intraperitoneal injection of different doses of methyl-n-amylnitrosamine. Cancer Res 1979;39:3644-3646.
10. Ovelar MY, Cardesa A, Mohr U. Carcinogenic effect of chronic subcutaneous injections of 2,6-dimethylnitrosomorpholine in Sprague-Dawley rats. Cancer Lett 1981;13:159-163.
11. Pera M, Cardesa A, Bombi JA, Ernst H, Pera C, Mohr U. Influence of esophagojejunostomy on the induction of adenocarcinoma of the distal esophagus in Sprague-Dawley rats by subcutaneous injection of 2,6-dimethylnitrosomorpholine. Cancer Res 1989;49:6803-6808.
12. Attwood SE, Smyrk TC, DeMeester TR, Mirvish SS, Stein HJ, Hinder RA. Duodenoesophageal reflux and the development of esophageal adenocarcinoma in rats. Surgery 1992;111:503-510.
13. Clark GW, Smyrk TC, Mirvish SS, et al. Effect of gastroduodenal juice and dietary fat on the development of Barrett's esophagus and esophageal neoplasia:an experimental rat model. Ann Surg Oncol 1994;1:252-261.
14. Ribeiro UJ, Posner MC, Safatle-Ribeiro AV, Reynolds JC. Risk factors for squamous cell carcinoma of the esophagus. Br J Surg 1996;83:1174-1185.
15. Pottern LM, Morris LE, Blot WJ, Ziegler RG, Fraumeni JFJ. Esophageal cancer among black men in Washington, D.C. I. Alcohol, tobacco, and other risk factors. J Natl Cancer Inst 1981;67:777-783.
16. Kabat GC, Ng SK, Wynder EL. Tobacco, alcohol intake, and diet in relation to adenocarcinoma of the esophagus and gastric cardia. Cancer Caus Control 1993;4:123-132.
17. Brown LM, Swanson CA, Gridley G, et al. Adenocarcinoma of the esophagus:role of obesity and diet. J Natl Cancer Inst 1995;87:104-109.
18. Zhang ZF, Kurtz RC, Yu GP, et al. Adenocarcinomas of the esophagus and gastric cardia: the role of diet. Nutr Cancer 1997;27:298-309.
19. Stene-Larsen G, Weberg R, Froyshov L, Bjortuft O, Hoel B, Berstad A. Relationship of overweight to hiatus hernia and reflux esophagitis. Scand J Gastroenterol 1988;23:427-432.
20. Kuczmarski RJ, Flegal KM, Campbell SM, Johnson CL. Increasing prevalence of overweight among US adults. The National Health and Nutrition Examination Surveys, 1960 to 1991. JAMA 1994;272:205-211.
21. Djuric Z, Kritschevsky D. Modulation of oxidative DNA damage levels by dietary fat and calories. Mut Res 1993;295:181-190.
22. McCarty MF. Up-regulation of intracellular signalling pathways may play a central pathogenic role in hypertension, atherogenesis, insulin resistance, and cancer promotion; the "PKC syndrome". Medi Hypoth 1996;46:191-221.
23. Byers T. Dietary trends in the United States. Relevance to cancer prevention. Cancer 1993;72:1015-1018
24. Harris PJ, Ferguson LR. Dietary fibre: its composition and role in protection against colorectal cancer. Mut Res 1993;290:97-110.
25. Stavric B. Role of chemopreventers in human diet. Clin Biochem 1994;27:319-332.

How can the continuous rise in rates of adenocarcinomas at the gastric cardia be explained?

S.J. Spechler (Dallas)

There is no universally accepted means to identify the gastric cardia. This fundamental problem confounds any discussion on cardiac tumors. When reading literature on this topic, one must ask: What specifically do the authors mean when they use the term "cancer of the gastric cardia"? Does the term refer merely to the anatomic location of the tumor, or does it imply that the cancer arose from cardiac epithelium? Authors frequently are not clear on this issue, perhaps because they have mistakenly assumed that tumors of the proximal stomach must have arisen from cardiac epithelium. Recent studies have shown that the proximal stomach normally is lined predominantly, if not exclusively, by oxyntic (acid-producing) epithelium [1-5]. Therefore, even a tumor that is unquestionably "cardiac" in anatomic location may not have arisen from cardiac epithelium. Conversely, a tumor that clearly is located in the distal esophagus conceivably could have arisen from esophageal cardiac epithelium.

In most published studies, the anatomic location of the epicenter or predominant mass of the tumor is used to determine whether a neoplasm involving the gastroesophageal junction is esophageal or gastric in origin. These criteria are arbitrary, and it is not clear that the predominant location of the tumor is a useful predictor of the cell of origin. Conceivably, a cancer of the distal esophagus might exhibit a predominantly distal pattern of growth (into the stomach), whereas a tumor of gastric origin might grow proximally to involve the esophagus predominantly. The use of these arbitrary classification systems virtually guarantees that the patient population in studies on cancers of the gastric cardia will be heterogeneous, including some patients with gastric tumors and others with tumors of esophageal origin. I would contend that misclassification of esophageal adenocarcinomas as tumors of the "gastric cardia" has contributed substantially to the alleged rise in the frequency of cardiac tumors.

The factors underlying the rising frequency of adenocarcinomas of the esophagus and esophagogastric junction remain unknown, but perhaps the most plausible hypothesis has been proposed by Labenz *et al.* [6]. Those researchers found that patients with duodenal ulcers frequently developed reflux esophagitis after receiving antibiotic treatment that eradicated their *H. pylori* infections. This observation suggested that *H. pylori* infection might protect some individuals against the development of gastroesophageal reflux disease (GERD). The increase in the incidence of adenocarcinoma in Barrett's esophagus over the past 20 years has been accompanied by a decrease in the prevalence of *H. pylori* infection in the Western countries. Labenz *et al.* have speculated that these phenomena may be related. Without *H. pylori* infection to prevent GERD, they contend, more individuals may be predisposed to develop Barrett's esophagus and malignancy. Graham *et al.* have proposed that *H. pylori* infections which cause severe pangastritis decrease gastric acid secretion, thereby protecting against GERD, Barrett's esophagus, and esophageal adenocarcinoma [7].

References

1. Kilgore SP, Ormsby AH, Gramlich TL, Rice TW, Richter JE, Falk GW, Goldblum JR. The gastric cardia:fact or fiction? Am J Gastroenterol 2000;95:921-924.
2. Chandrasoma PT, Der R, Ma Y, Dalton P, Taira M. Histology of the gastroesophageal junction: an autopsy study. Am J Surg Pathol 2000;24:402-409.
3. Öberg S, Peters JH, DeMeester TR, Chandrasoma P, Hagen JA, Ireland AP, Ritter MP, Mason RJ, Crookes P, Bremner CG. Inflammation and specialized intestinal metaplasia of cardiac mucosa is a manifestation of gastroesophageal reflux disease. Ann Surg 1997;226;522-532.
4. Chandrasoma P. Pathophysiology of Barrett's esophagus. Semin Thorac Cardiovasc Surg 1997;9:270-278.
5. Chandrasoma PT, Lokuhetty DM, DeMeester TR, Bremner CG, Peters JH, Oberg S, Groshen S. Definition of histopathologic changes in gastroesophageal reflux disease. Am J Surg Pathol 2000;24:344-351.
6. Labenz J, Blum AL, Bayerdörffer E, Meining A, Stolte M, Börsch G. Curing Helicobacter pylori infection in patients with duodenal ulcer may provoke reflux esophagitis. Gastroenterology 1997;112:1442-1447.
7. Graham DY, Yamaoka Y. H. pylori and cagA: relationships with gastric cancer, duodenal ulcer, and reflux esophagitis and its complications. Helicobacter 1998;3:145-150.

J. Lagergren (Stockholm)

A few risk factors for adenocarcinoma located near the gastroesophageal junction have been identified, but the reasons for the rapidly increasing incidence of these tumors are uncertain.

Symptomatic gastroesophageal reflux (GER) has been established as a major risk factor for adenocarcinoma of the esophagus and gastric cardia [1]. If GER is the main reason for the increasing incidence of the adenocarcinomas, the incidence of reflux disease should have risen during recent decades. There is unfortunately a lack of data on the incidence of gastroesophageal reflux disease. If this incidence is rising, this increase in turn must be caused by some other environmental or hereditary factor. Such potential environmental factors are the use of medications that relax the lower esophageal sphincter (LES) and thereby facilitate reflux. Some groups of LES-inhibiting drugs that were widely introduced before the start of the epidemic of esophageal adenocarcinoma are nitroglycerin, anticholinergics, beta-adrenergic agonists, aminophyllines, and benzodiazepines. Results of the analyses of medication data from a large case-control study indicate that the use of such medications may be of importance [2]. A positive association between previous use of such medications and the risk of esophageal adenocarcinoma was identified. Another study showed conflicting results, however [3]. Furthermore, although there seems to be a male predominance for GER [4], one concern about the hypothesis that reflux is the main reason for the rising incidence is that this sex imbalance is far less pronounced than that for adenocarcinoma of the esophagus and gastric cardia [5]. The influence of GER on the incidence of the adenocarcinomas remains to be further evaluated before any firm conclusions can be made.

Obesity seems to be an important risk factor for adenocarcinoma of the esophagus and cardia [6, 7]. It would be tempting to attribute the increase in the incidence of esophageal and cardia adenocarcinoma to the increase in average body mass index (BMI) observed in Western populations [8], especially in men. Furthermore, the incidence of esophageal adenocarcinoma has increased to a greater extent than that of cardia adenocarcinoma, which is well compatible with the difference in magnitude of the association between BMI and the risk of these two cancers in our study. However, the apparently sudden deflection of the incidence curve for esophageal adenocarcinoma, [9], the rapidity of the increase, [5], and the marked, 6-8 fold, male predominance, [5] are observations not entirely consistent with this interpretation. These inconsistencies remain to be solved before obesity can be considered the main reason for the increasing incidence of adenocarcinoma of the esophagus and gastric cardia.

Tobacco smoking has been proposed to be a risk factor contributing to the rising incidence of adenocarcinoma of the esophagus and gastric cardia in a US case-control study [10]. The association between smoking and squamous cell carcinoma of the esophagus was stronger than that with adenocarcinoma, however. Furthermore, smoking has declined markedly among men, as reflected by a decreasing incidence of lung cancer [11]; the increasing incidence of esophageal adenocarcinoma has been practically confined to men [5]. A recent population-based case-control study in Sweden did not find any association between smoking and risk of esophageal adenocarcinoma, but a moderate association with cardia adenocarcinoma [12]. Taken together, tobacco smoking does not seem to be the main reason for the increasing incidence of these tumors.

In conclusion, GER, the use of medications that might cause such reflux, and obesity might be key factors to explain the increasing incidence of adenocarcinoma of the esophagus and gastric cardia, but several inconsistencies need to be resolved before this suspicion can be established.

References

1. Lagergren J, Bergström R, Lindgren A, Nyrén O. Symptomatic gastroesophageal reflux is a strong risk factor for esophageal adenocarcinoma. N Engl J Med 1999;340:825-831.
2. Lagergren J, Bergström R, Adami HO, Nyrén O. Association between medications that relax the lower esophageal sphincter and risk of esophageal adenocarcinoma. Ann Intern Med 2000;133:165-175.
3. Vaughan TL, Farrow DC, Hansten PD, Chow WH, Gammon MD, Risch HA, et al. Risk of esophageal and gastric adenocarcinomas in relation to use of calcium channel blockers, asthma drugs, and other medications that promote gastroesophageal reflux. Cancer Epidemiol Biomark Prev. 1998;7:749-756.
4. Ter RB, Castell DO. Gastroesophageal reflux disease in patients with columnar-lined esophagus. Gastroenterol Clin North Am 1997;26:549-563.
5. Blot WJ, Devesa SS, Kneller RW, Fraumeni JF. Rising incidence of adenocarcinoma of the esophagus and gastric cardia. JAMA 1991;265:1287-1289.
6. Chow WH, Blot WJ, Vaughan TL, Risch HA, Gammon MD, Stanford JL, et al. Body mass index and risk of adenocarcinoma of the esophagus and gastric cardia. J Natl Cancer Inst 1998;90:150-155.
7. Lagergren J, Bergström R, Nyrén O. Body mass as a risk factor for esophageal and gastric cardia adenocarcinoma. Ann Intern Med 1999;130:883-890.
8. Seidell JC, Flegal KM. Assessing obesity:classification and epidemiology. Br Med Bull 1997;53:238-252.
9. Pera M, Cameron AJ, Trastek VF, Carpenter HA, Zinsmeister AR. Increasing incidence of adenocarcinoma of the esophagus and esophagogastric junction. Gastroenterology 1993;104:510-513.
10. Gammon MD, Schoenberg JB, Ahsan H, Risch HA, Vaughan TL, Chow WH, et al. Tobacco, alcohol, and socioeconomic status and adenocarcinomas of the esophagus and gastric cardia. J Natl Cancer Inst 1997;89:1277-1284.
11. Cancer Registry. Cancer incidence in Sweden 1993, 1994 and 1995. National Board of Health and Welfare, Stockholm 1996, 1997 and 1998.
12. Lagergren J, Bergström R, Lindgren A, Nyrén O. The role of tobacco, alcohol and snuff use in the aetiology of esophageal and gastric cardia cancer. Int J Cancer 2000;85:340-346.

In the delineation framework of a preventive strategy, should screening endoscopy be indicated in all patients with gastroesophageal reflux symptoms?

J. Lagergren (Stockholm)

Since the poor survival rates for adenocarcinoma of the esophagus and gastric cardia [1] are improved only by early tumor detection [2], it is important to identify high-risk persons in whom endoscopic surveillance might be warranted. Recently, symptomatic reflux and obesity were identified as strong independent risk factors for these tumors, particularly for esophageal adenocarcinoma [3, 4]. Since reflux symptoms are common [5] and adenocarcinomas are still rare diseases, endoscopic surveillance in reflux patients would rapidly overtax available health care resources [3]. The possible benefits of endoscopic surveillance should exceed the costs and inconveniences for patients and health care systems. Symptoms severe enough to be associated with a risk of esophageal adenocarcinoma eight times as high as normal were reported by 9% of our control subjects. If endoscopic surveillance were restricted to men older than 40 who had symptoms of reflux that were so severe as to entail a risk 20 times as high as normal, our calculations revealed that a Swedish physician would need to follow more than 1,400 such patients for one year to encounter a single case of esophageal adenocarcinoma; such a policy would surely overtax the available health care resources [3].

In a re-analysis of Swedish nationwide case-control data, we estimated the number of endoscopies needed to identify one esophageal or cardia adenocarcinoma in persons with various combinations of both obesity and reflux [6]. Based on the prevalence of reflux and obesity among the control subjects, we estimated the sizes of risk strata in the Swedish population. Our complete and nationwide case ascertainment allowed calculations of incidence rates in each strata. The number needed to survey annually to identify one adenocarcinoma was calculated as 1/(incidence rate). Risk of both esophageal and cardia adenocarcinoma increased dose-dependently with increasing body mass index (BMI) and reflux severity (*Table I*). The risks combined in a multiplicative manner. Among obese persons (BMI > 30 kg/m^2) with reflux symptoms, odds ratio (OR) was 184 (95% CI, 36-949) for esophageal adenocarcinoma and 12.5 (95% CI, 3.0-51) for cardia adenocarcinoma compared with lean persons (BMI < 22 kg/m^2) without reflux. Among persons with BMI ≥ 25 kg/m^2 and severe (severity score > 4) and long-standing (> 20 years) reflux symptoms, OR was 103 (95%CI, 21.5-492) for esophageal adenocarcinoma and 16.6 (95%CI, 3.4-82) for cardia adenocarcinoma. We then estimated the number needed to detect one esophageal or cardia adenocarcinoma. Given the marked male (8:1) predominance, the rarity of tumors in younger persons, and the demanding curative surgery, surveillance is not justified in women or persons younger than 50 or older than 79 years. Thus, the group to evaluate is men of ages 50-79 with high BMI and reflux symptoms. *Table II* shows the prevalence of various constellations of BMI and reflux symptomatology among our male control subjects aged 50-79 years, the estimated adenocarcinoma incidence in the strata exhibiting these constellations in the Swedish population, and the number needed to survey to detect one esophageal or cardia adenocarcinoma per year. Six percent had the combination of BMI ≥ 25 kg/m^2 and reflux symptoms, but only 0.3% of persons with reflux had BMI > 30 kg/m^2.

Table I. Reflux symptoms and body mass index (BMI) and risk of esophageal and gastric cardia adenocarcinoma*.

				Esophageal adenocarcinoma		Cardia adenocarcinoma	
			Number of controls	Number of cases	Adjusted* odds ratio (95% CI)	Number of cases	Adjusted* odds ratio (95% CI)
BMI < 22[1] (lean)	Reflux symptoms	No	180	4	1.0 (referent)	37	1.0 (referent)
		Yes	27	6	10.7 (2.8-41.3)	10	1.9 (0.8-4.5)
BMI 22-24.9 (average)	Reflux symptoms	No	299	27	3.9 (1.3-11.4)	70	1.2 (0.8-2.0)
		Yes	67	41	28.5 (9.7-83.7)	30	2.6 (1.4-4.7)
BMI 25-30 (overweight)	Reflux symptoms	No	180	35	8.2 (2.8-24.0)	64	2.2 (1.4-3.6)
		Yes	38	54	61.4 (20.5-184.0)	27	3.9 (2.0-7.5)
BMI > 30 (obesity)	Reflux symptoms	No	22	10	17.4 (4.9-62.1)	16	3.8 (1.7-8.4)
		Yes	3	12	179.2 (34.8-922.7)	8	12.2 (3.0-50.3)
No reflux symptoms	BMI < 25[1]		479	31	1.0 (referent)	107	1.0 (referent)
	BMI ≥ 25		202	45	3.3 (2.0-5.5)	80	2.1 (1.5-3.0)
Reflux severity score[2] > 4 p.	BMI < 25		25	29	19.9 (10.2-39.2)	12	2.3 (1.1-5.0)
	BMI ≥ 25		9	35	59.6 (25.6-139.1)	15	7.3 (3.0-17.7)
Duration of reflux symptoms > 20 years	BMI < 25		18	21	23.0 (10.7-49.5)	13	4.4 (2.0-9.9)
	BMI ≥ 25		9	19	30.1 (12.1-75.0)	9	4.8 (1.8-13.0)
Reflux severity score > 4 p. and duration of reflux >20 years	BMI < 25		8	18	44.8 (17.3-116.6)	5	3.4 (1.0-11.6)
	BMI ≥ 25		2	13	100.2 (21.0-479.4)	8	16.4 (3.3-81.2)

* In the multivariate logistic model adjustments were made for: age, sex, socioeconomic status, tobacco smoking, alcohol use, intake of fruit and vegetables, energy intake, and physical activity
1. This variable constitutes the referent category in the point estimates beneath
2. The severity score included symptom characteristics (heartburn only = 1 point, regurgitation only = 1 point, heartburn and regurgitation combined = 1.5 points), nightly symptoms (no = 0 points, yes = 2 points), and symptom frequency (once a week = 0 points, 2-6 times a week = 1 point, 7-15 times a week = 2 points, > 15 times a week = 3 points)

Table II. Efforts needed to identify esophageal or gastric cardia adenocarcinoma among men aged 50-79 years at different levels of body mass index (BMI) and reflux symptoms.

BMI (kg/m^2)	Reflux	Percent of all men 50-79 years*	Estimated incidence per 10^5/year[1]	Number of persons needed to survey for one year to detect one case (95% confidence interval)
BMI ≥ 25	Yes	5.6	45.7	2,189 (1,796-2,698)
	Severe[2]	2.0	73.1	1,367 (1,054-1,807)
BMI ≥ 26	Yes	3.3	61.3	1,631 (1,304-2,068)
	Severe[2]	0.9	118.9	841 (623-1,165)
BMI ≥ 27	Yes	2.4	62.1	1,611 (1,239-2,136)
	Severe[2]	0.8	91.1	1,097 (755-1,664)
BMI ≥ 28	Yes	1.7	63.0	1,587 (1,170-2,209)
	Severe[2]	0.6	84.2	1,188 (769-1,944)
BMI ≥ 29	Yes	0.8	87.2	1,147 (782-1,758)
	Severe[2]	0.3	99.0	1,010 (575-1,968)
BMI ≥ 30	Yes	0.3	168.4	594 (385-972)

* Derived from the control group in the case-control study

1. Derived from the nationwide case ascertainment effort in Sweden 1995 through 1997

2. Severity score > 2 points and duration > 11 years

The number of persons needed to survey to detect one adenocarcinoma varied from 2,189 in the former stratum, to 594 in the latter. Thus, if 60 obese men aged 50-79 with reflux symptoms, are followed for 10 years, one esophageal or cardia adenocarcinoma will be observed. The size of this latter high-risk group, 0.3% of the male population between 50 and 79 years, is seemingly manageable, but the number of patients included in surveillance programs tends to accumulate with time.

In conclusion, we have identified a limited group with a relative risk that greatly exceeds that of the general population. Endoscopic surveillance for esophageal or cardia adenocarcinoma in this group would, however, consumes considerable health care resources. Given the poor results of treatment of the cancer when it occurs, surveillance may still be considered, especially if the incidence of these tumors continues to increase. Importantly, from our data we conclude that screening endoscopy can not be recommended in other groups of persons with reflux symptoms.

References

1. Boring CC, Squires TS, Tong T. Cancer statistics, 1993. CA-Cancer J Clinicians 1993;43:7-26.
2. Altorki NK, Skinner DB. Adenocarcinoma in Barrett's esophagus. Semin Surg Oncol 1990;6:274-278.
3. Lagergren J, Bergström R, Lindgren A, Nyrén O. Symptomatic gastroesophageal reflux as a risk factor for esophageal adenocarcinoma. N Engl J Med 1999;340:825-831.
4. Lagergren J, Bergström R, Nyrén O. The association between body mass and adenocarcinoma of the esophagus and gastric cardia. Ann Int Med 1999;130:883-890.
5. Locke GR, Talley NJ, Fett SL, Zinsmeister AR, Melton LJ. Prevalence and clinical spectrum of gastroesophageal reflux: a population-based study in Olmsted County, Minnesota. Gastroenterology 1997;112:1448-1456.
6. Lagergren J, Ye W, Bergström R, Nyrén O. The combination of symptomatic gastroesophageal reflux and obesity as an indicator of the need for endoscopic surveillance for adenocarcinoma of the esophagus and gastric cardia. JAMA, in press.

What is the accuracy of endosonographic staging of adenocarcinomas of the esophagus and esophagogastric junction?

I. Waxman (Galveston)

Presently, Barrett's esophagus has been identified as the single most important risk factor for adenocarcinoma of the esophagus and gastric cardia [1, 2]. Over the past two decades, the incidence of adenocarcinoma of the esophagus increased at a rate exceeding that for any other cancer to the point that today, 50% of all esophageal cancers in white American men are adenocarcinomas. Patients with Barrett's esophagus develop adenocarcinoma of the esophagus at a rate of 1/125 patient-years, an incidence that is 30-125 times that of the general population. For every 100,000 patients with Barrett's esophagus, 800 will develop an adenocarcinoma each year [3]. The prognosis of adenocarcinoma in Barrett's esophagus is related to the stage at diagnosis [4]. The timely identification and surgical resection of intramucosal adenocarcinoma, or an early submucosal cancer within Barrett's esophagus offers an 80-100% chance of cure [5-7].

Prognosis and staging

Once adenocarcinoma of the esophagus becomes symptomatic, it carries a poor prognosis, with a 5-year survival of approximately 17% after complete resection of tumor, and less than 1% for unresectable lesions [8-11]. Esophageal adenocarcinoma tends to metastasize to the lymph nodes early in the disease process. In patients undergoing en bloc esophagectomy with extended abdominal and mediastinal lymphadenectomy for intramucosal adenocarcinoma for example, 33% had lymph node metastases. The prevalence of nodal metastases rose to 66% for those whose tumor had spread into the muscularis propria and to 89% in those with transmural tumors [12]. Only 50% of patients with lymph node metastases will be alive two years after resection, and about 15% survive more than 5 years [13].

Depth of esophageal wall invasion, in particular the distinction between partial and full thickness penetration, has major prognostic implications regarding lymph node status, long-term survival and local recurrence [14-16].

Therefore accurate staging has important clinical implications. The American Joint Committee on Cancer published their classification for staging esophageal cancer in 1987 and has so far remained unchanged [17]. This classification is based on the TNM staging system, which defines the anatomical extent of the disease. T indicates the depth of primary tumor invasion into the gastrointestinal tract wall; N indicates the spread of cancer to specified regional lymph nodes. In the case of adenocarcinoma of the esophagus, any regional lymph node metastasis is considered N1. M indicates distant metastases to lymph nodes outside specific regional lymph nodes, or to organs not in direct contact with the primary tumor. Metastatic celiac axis nodes are considered M1 for adenocarcinomas located mainly on the esophageal side of the esophagogastric junction (EGJ) and N2 (distant regional lymph nodes) when most of the tumor involves the gastric side of the EGJ [18].

Endosonographic evaluation

Over the last decade, endoscopic ultrasonography (EUS) has become a powerful tool for gastrointestinal cancer staging. EUS provides high resolution imaging of the layered structure of the gastrointestinal wall and surrounding structures [19]. At the conventional echoendoscope frequencies of 7.5 and 12 MHz, the gastrointestinal tract wall is imaged as a five acoustic layered structure, which corresponds with mural histology. In a recent review on esophageal cancer staging by EUS, Rosch reported an average accuracy for EUS of 84% and 77% in preoperative T and N staging, compared to surgical pathology results [20].

For patients with cancer of the esophagus and EGJ, EUS has been shown to be far superior to CT-scan in determining the depth and the presence of regional lymph node involvement [21, 22]. Reported overall EUS accuracy in assessing the depth of invasion in esophageal cancer range from 76% to 92% when compared to 49% to 59% for CT-scan, and for nodal status, 72% to 80% and 46% to 51% for EUS and CT-scan respectively [22-25]. For M staging, EUS is limited due to it's inability to image distant metastases, making this an area where CT-scan should be used in a complementary fashion.

Clinical impact of endosonography

In addition to accurate staging information, preoperative EUS findings have been shown to correlate with survival and predict surgical outcome. Hiele *et al.* analyzed survival data in 86 patients who underwent EUS staging of tumors of the esophagus and the EGJ. The authors found a median survival of 28 months for patients with tumors staged as T2 compared to a 19 months for those staged as T3. Patients whose tumors where staged as T4 had the worst prognosis with a median survival of 8 months. Regarding lymph node status, patients staged N0 by EUS had a median survival of 28 months as compared with 8 months for patients in whom malignant nodes where suspected. In patients with EGJ cancers in particular, involvement of celiac axis nodes had a significant correlation with survival. Median survival was 30 months and 3 months in the absence and presence of positive celiac axis nodes on EUS. Finally, in patients with stage II (absence of pathological lymph nodes) tumors, over 90% had a curative resection [26].

EUS has also been shown in a retrospective study to predict poor outcome in patients staged as T4 (invasion of adjacent structures). The study also suggested no difference in survival between patients who underwent surgical and non-surgical palliation, providing important information that could impact management by avoiding surgical interventions in this subset of patients [27].

As preoperative treatment decisions get influenced by the presence or absence of lymphadenopathy, adjuvant therapy (N1) and/or surgical resection (M1 a: celiac lymph node), EUS-guided FNA may play an important role in preoperative staging of patients with esophageal carcinoma. Preliminary studies suggest that EUS FNA is more accurate and sensitive than EUS alone in assessing nodal disease, improving the sensitivity from 63% to 93% and the accuracy from 70% to 93% [28].

Endosonography in Barrett's esophagus with high-grade dysplasia

For patients with cancer in Barrett's esophagus, EUS appears to have a role in staging the tumor, and some authors have suggested that the technique may be useful in determining when to operate on patients with high-grade dysplasia (HGD) who have no endoscopic evidence of carcinoma [29]. Srivastava *et al.* reported their preliminary experience with EUS in the evaluation of Barrett's esophagus [30]. Esophageal wall thickening was found by endosonography in patients with Barrett's esophagus (n = 15, six with dysplasia) when compared to a control group (n = 10) without esophageal disease. No significant difference in thickness was noted in the patients with dysplasia as compared to those with non-dysplastic Barrett's esophagus. Two of the patients had thickening of the submucosal layer, which proved to be submucosal cancer after surgical resection. Falk *et al.* looked specifically at the role of endosonography in patients with Barrett's esophagus and HGD [31]. Nine patients who were candidates for esophagectomy and who had HGD in the absence of carcinoma were studied. Endosonography was able to identify only one out of three cancers found at surgery and overstaged it as invasive carcinoma (T2, N1 *versus* T1s). In two patients without intramucosal carcinoma furthermore, endosonography predicted invasive carcinoma (T2, N0). In all cases of overstaging, mucosal nodularity was noted. The authors concluded that current endosonography techniques cannot consistently predict the presence of intramucosal carcinoma and that the finding of mucosal nodularity should be interpreted with caution.

High frequency ultrasound probe sonography (HFUPS) with a 20 MHz ultrasound catheter probe provides finer resolution of the esophageal wall and is able to define up to nine layers of the gastrointestinal wall in contrast to the five layers detected by the conventional endoscope. Waxman *et al.* studied prospectively the utility of HFUPS in predicting the presence of carcinoma in patients with Barrett's esophagus and HGD [32]. A total of nine patients with Barrett's esophagus and HGD who were candidates for esophagectomy were enrolled. In all patients, HFUPS found diffuse thickening of the superficial hyperechoic and deep hypoechoic sonographic layers of the Barrett's esophagus mucosa. Four of the nine patients were suspected to have invasive carcinoma. Of the four, one was over-staged, one was under-staged, one was pathologically negative for carcinoma and one was correctly staged. Two patients with carcinoma went undiagnosed. The authors concluded that even high frequency ultrasonography was inaccurate at detecting or monitoring HGD, carcinoma *in situ* or early adenocarcinoma in patients with Barrett's esophagus.

Similar experience was reported by Parent *et al.* [33] in 13 patients with HGD. Thickening of layer two was noted in all patients studied but HFUPS could not detect adenocarcinomas in patients with HGD in the absence of endoscopically visible lesions. Furthermore, in patients with biopsy proven intramucosal carcinoma where studied, a normal sonographic examination could not exclude the presence of submucosal carcinoma [33].

To date, the data addressing the role of endosonography in patients with dysplasia in Barrett's epithelium are few, and suggests that the technique is not sufficiently accurate in predicting tumor at an early stage [35].

Limitations of endosonography

Limitations of EUS accuracy in staging involve overstaging (especially T1 and T2) due to peritumoral fibrotic or inflammatory changes and understaging, due to microscopic tumor invasion below the resolution of the scanning device with the majority of cases in T3 lesions. High-grade malignant strictures prevent adequate tumor evaluation by preventing passage of the endoscope in 20 to 38% of patients with esophageal carcinoma. This finding has been associated with an advanced carcinoma usually stage III or IV in up to 91% of patients. Attempts at EUS staging of these tumors from the region proximal to the stenosis have a poor accuracy [36]. At the present time, most endosonographers agree that esophageal dilatation solely for the purpose of passing the echoendoscope for staging does not outweigh the 24% risk of perforation reported [36]. The role of through the endoscope catheter probes is still being studied at the present time [25, 37]. The accuracy for detection of lymph node metastases is increasing due to the introduction of the curved linear array echoendoscope, which permits ultrasound scanning parallel to the long axis of the endoscope, allowing us-guided tissue sampling [38]. In spite of these technological advances, nodal micrometastases below the resolution of current EUS devices will continue to present a challenge in the staging of this disease [39].

References

1. Spechler SJ. Barrett's esophagus. Semin Oncol 1994;21:431-437.
2. Haggitt RC. Adenocarcinoma in Barrett's esophagus: a new epidemic? Hum Pathol 1992;23:475-476.
3. Spechler SJ. Endoscopic surveillance for patients with Barrett's esophagus: does the cancer risk justify the practice? Ann Intern Med 1987;106:902-904.
4. Streitz JM, Andrews CW, Ellis FH. Endoscopic surveillance of Barrett's esophagus: does it help? J Thorac Cardiovasc Surg 1994;105:383-388.
5. Altorki NK, Sunagawa M, Little AG, Skinner DB. High-grade dysplasia in the columnar-lined esophagus. Am J Surg 1991;161:97-100.
6. Rusch VW, Levine DS, Haggitt RC, Reid BJ. The management of high-grade dysplasia and early cancer in Barrett's esophagus. A multidisciplinary problem. Cancer 1994;74:1225-1229.
7. Pera M, Trastek VF, Carpenter HA, Allen MS, Deschamps C, Pairolero PC. Barrett's esophagus with high-grade dysplasia: an indication for esophagectomy? Ann Thorac Surg 1994;54:199-204.
8. Skinner DB. En block resection for neoplasms of the esophagus and cardia. J Thorac Cardiovasc Surg 1983;85:59-71.
9. Ellis FH, Gibb SP, Watkins E. Esophagogastrectomy, a safe, widely applicable and expeditious form of palliation for patients with carcinoma of the esophagus and cardia. Ann Surg 1983;198:531-540.
10. Galandiuk S, Hermann RE, Gassman JJ, et al. Cancer of the esophagus. The Cleveland Clinic experience. Ann Surg 1983;198:101-108.
11. DeMeester TR, Zaninotto G, Johansson KE. Selective therapeutic approach to cancer of the lower esophagus and cardia. J Thorac Cardiovasc Surg 1988;95:42-54.
12. Clark GW, Peters JH, Ireland AP, Ehsan A, Hagen JA, Kiyabu MT, Bremner CG, DeMeester TR. Nodal metastasis and sites of recurrence after en block esophagectomy for adenocarcinoma. Ann Thorac Surg 1994;58:646-653.
13. Akiyama H, Tsurumaru M, Kawamura T, Ono Y. Principles of surgical treatment for carcinoma of the esophagus: analysis of lymph node involvement. Ann Surg 1981;194:438-446.
14. Rice TW, Zuccaro G, Adelstein DJ, Rybicki LA, Blackstone EH, Goldblum JR. Esophageal carcinoma: depth of tumor invasion is predictive of regional lymph node status. Ann Thorac Surg 1998;65:787-792.
15. Skinner DB, Little AG, Ferguson MK, Soriano A, Staszak VM. Selection of operation for esophageal cancer based on staging. Ann Surg 1986;204:391-401.
16. Sagar PM, Johnston D, McMahon MJ, Dixon MF, Quirke P. Significance of circumferential resection margin involvement after esophagectomy for cancer. Br J Surg 1993;80:1386-1388.
17. Beahrs OH, Henson DE, Hutter RVP, Kennedy BJ, eds. Manual for staging of cancer, 4th ed. Philadelphia: JB Lippincott, 1992.
18. Hermanek P, Henson DE, Hutter RVP, Sobin LH. TNM supplement 1993 A commentary on uniform use. New York: Springer-Verlag, 1993.

19. Tio TL, Tytgat GNJ. Endoscopic ultrasonography of normal and pathologic gastrointestinal wall structure. Comparison of studies in vivo and in vitro with histology. Scan J Gastroenterol 1986;21(suppl 123):27-33.
20. Rosch T, Endosonographic staging of esophageal cancer: a review of literature results. Gastrointest Endosc Clin North Am 1995;5:537-547.
21. Tio TL, Cohen P, Coene PP, Udding J, den Hartog Jager FCA, Tytgat GNJ. Endosonography and computed tomography of esophageal carcinoma. Preoperative classification compared to the new (1987) TNM system. Gastroenterology 1989;96:1478-1486.
22. Botet JF, Lightdale CJ, Zauber AG, Gerdes H, Urmacher C, Brennan MF. Preoperative staging of esophageal cancer:comparison of endoscopic US and dynamic CT. Radiology 1991;181:419-425.
23. Tio TL, Coene PP, den Hartog Jager FCA, Tytgat GNJ. Preoperative TNM classification of esophageal carcinoma by endosonography. Hepatogastroenterology 1990;37:376-381.
24. Murata Y, Muroi M, Yoshida M, Ide H, Hanyu F. Endoscopic ultrasonography in the diagnosis of esophageal carcinoma. Surg Endosc 1987;1:11-16.
25. Van Dam J. Endosonographic evaluation of the patient with esophageal cancer. Chest 1997;112:184S-190S.
26. Hiele M, De Leyn P, Schurmans P, et al. Relation between endoscopic ultrasound findings and outcome of patients with tumors of the esophagus or esophagogastric junction. Gastrointest Endosc 1997;45:381-386.
27. Chak A, Canto M, Gerdes H, et al. Prognosis of esophageal cancers preoperatively staged to be locally invasive (T4) by endoscopic ultrasound (EUS): a multicenter retrospective cohort study. Gastrointest Endosc 1995;42:501-506.
28. Vazquez-Sequeiros E, Norton ID, Clain JE, Wang KK, Affi A, et al. Impact on endosonography guided fine needle aspiration biopsy (EUS FNA) on lymph node staging in patients with esophageal carcinoma. Endoscopy 2000;32:A22.
29. Hameeteman W, Tytgat GNJ, Houthoff HJ, Van Den Tweel JG. Barrett's esophagus: development of dysplasia and adenocarcinoma. Gastroenterology 1989;96:1249-1256.
30. Srivastava AK, Vanagunas A, Kamel P, Cooper R. Endoscopic ultrasound in the evaluation of Barrett's esophagus: a preliminary report. Am J Gastroenterol 1994;89:2192-2195.
31. Falk GW, Catalano MF, Sivak MV Jr, Rice TW, Van Dam J. Endosonography in the evaluation of patients with Barrett's esophagus and high-grade dysplasia. Gastrointest Endosc 1994;40:207-212.
32. Waxman I, Raju G, Critchlow J, Lahoti S, Spechler SJ. Can high frequency ultrasound probe sonography identify invasive adenocarcinoma in patients with Barrett's esophagus and high-grade dysplasia? A prospective study. Am J Gastroenterol 1999;94:A101.
33. Parent J, Levine DS, Haggitt RC, Reid BJ, Kimmey MB. Role of endoscopic ultrasound in patients with Barrett's esophagus and high grade dysplasia. Gastrointest Endosc 1997;45:A76.
34. Parent J, Levine DS, Haggitt RC, Wood DE, Reid BJ, Kimmey MB. Accuracy of endoscopic ultrasound staging in patients with Barrett's esophagus and intramucosal carcinoma. Gastrointest Endosc 1997;45:A76.
35. Waxman I. Endosonography in columnar-lined esophagus. Gastroenterol Clin North Am 1997;26:607-612.
36. Van Dam J, Rice TW, Catalano MF, Kirby T, Sivak MV Jr. High-grade malignant stricture is predictive of esophageal tumor stage: risks of endosonographic evaluation. Cancer 1993;71:2910-2917.
37. Waxman I. Clinical impact of high-frequency ultrasound probe sonography during diagnostic endoscopy. A prospective study. Endoscopy 1998;30:S166-S168.
38. Carr-Locke DL, Branch MS, Byrne WJ, et al. Technology assessment committee of the ASGE. Technology assessment status evaluation: tissue sampling during endosonography. Gastrointest Endosc 1998;47:576-578.
39. Izbicki JR, Hosch SB, Pichlmeier U, et al. Prognostic value of immunohistochemically identifiable tumor cells in lymph nodes of patients with completely resected esophageal cancer. N Engl J Med 1997;337:1188-1194.

Endoscopic ultrasonography using Sonoprobe for early esophageal carcinoma

T. Kawano, M. Ohshima, T. Iwai (Tokyo)

Endoscopic ultrasonography (EUS) has been assessed as an appropriate examination modality with which to obtain information on the esophageal wall and adjacent organs in terms of ultrasonic tomograms, and good studies on the diagnosis of the depth of tumor invasion in esophageal carcinoma have been reported [1, 2].

Although a conventional ultrasound scope has played an important role in the staging of advanced cancer and lymph node metastasis in the mediastinum, the fact that it has a transducer in the distal tip has been used for the diagnosis of superficial esophageal carcinoma by detecting rather rough changes in the layered-structure. Due to its inability to scan the area of interest under simultaneous endoscopic observation when diagnosing superficial esophageal carcinoma with a less rugged surface than that of advanced cancer, the correlation between the lesion and its ultrasound tomogram is often uncertain, and furthermore, the tumor itself can not be always visualized as an image.

In contrast, the high frequency ultrasound diagnostic equipment (hereinafter referred to thin ultrasound probe) can be delivered through the instrument channel of an endoscope to obtain ultrasound images under direct endoscopic observation of the lesion of interest. The Sonoprobe System™, which drives the thin ultrasound probe at higher frequency of 20 MHz, provides a remarkable improvement in the axial resolution. In addition, it is equipped with multi modes of linear and radial scanning and so is considered to have an advantage over the conventional ultrasound scope for the diagnosis of superficial esophageal carcinoma.

Recently MRI examination using an intraluminal coil has been introduced as a method for the tomographic examination of the gastrointestinal tract [3]. However, at present, EUS by a thin ultrasound probe is the most suitable method for the diagnosis of superficial esophageal carcinoma. We have reported initial experiences of EUS by the thin ultrasound probe in superficial esophageal tumors in Japanese [4-6]. In this paper, we report our experience with the diagnosis of superficial esophageal carcinoma using the thin ultrasound probe.

Patients and methods

Eighty-five patients with superficial esophageal carcinoma initially diagnosed by endoscopy between 1990 and 1999 were enrolled in the study. Multiple primary esophageal lesions were examined in 8 patients, and the total numbers of EUS was 96. Accuracy of diagnosis in terms of the depth of tumor invasion was evaluated histopathologically after surgical or endoscopic resection.

EUS with the Sonoprobe System™ (SP-101 and SP-501, Fujinon, Japan: hereinafter referred to Sonoprobe) was performed by the over-tube method in 18 patients, the soft-balloon method in 39, and the water repletion method in 28 [5] (*Figure 1*). Although the initial endoscopies were performed by several endoscopists, EUS with the Sonoprobe was carried out by one examiner. Interpretations of the depth of tumor invasion were based on our fundamental studies of ultrasonograms taken with the 20 MHz probe [4] (*Figure 2, Table I*).

Results

Since slight abnormalities were visualized in the ultrasound images of superficial esophageal carcinomas, it was rather difficult to diagnose mucosal cancer that peculiarly showed no changes in thickness. Because of this, it was necessary to proceed with diagnosis by comparing the sonograms with those taken at a normal portion adjacent to the lesion of

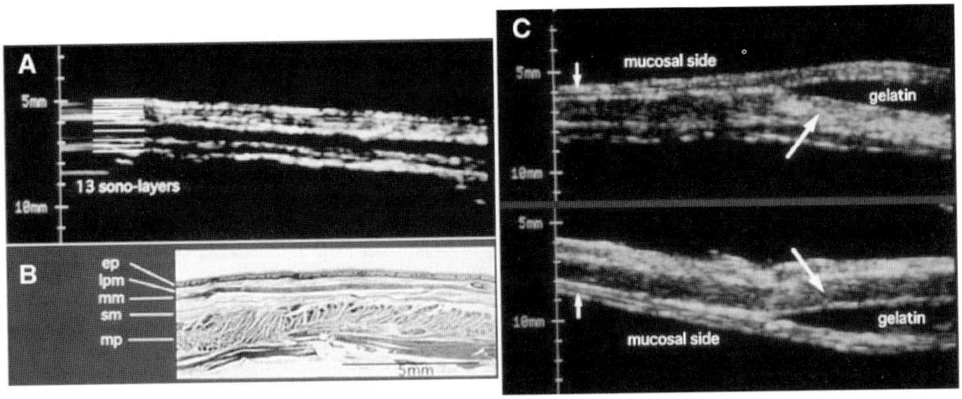

Figure 1. A. Thirteen sonolayers obtained by the 20 MHz Sonoprobe and the corresponding histological structure in a normal part of the resected esophagus (cited from [4] with permission). **B.** Various appearances of sonolayers (from 13 to 7 layers) in intact esophagus (cited from [5] with permission). **C.** Ultrasonograms obtained after submucosal gelatin injection *in vitro*. Head shows ultrasound radiation from the mucosal side and bottom shows it from the adventitia side. Note that the gelatin affects the echo level in the layer below the gelatin (circular muscle, large arrows). The large and small arrows indicate the same echo layer (cited from [5] with permission).

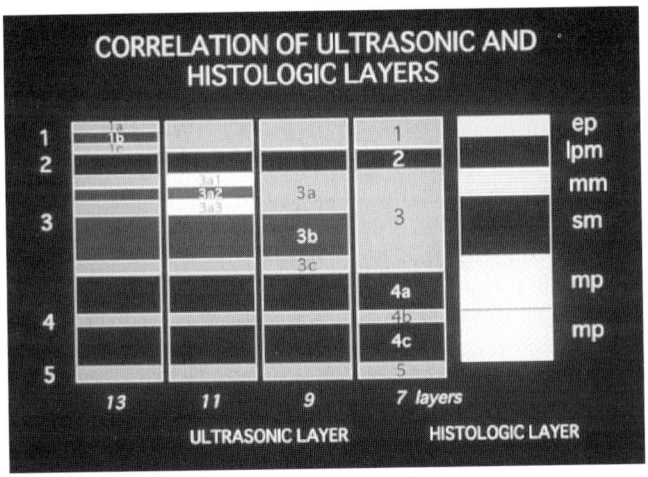

Figure 2 Correlation between an ultrasonogram and the histologic structure (cited from [5] with permission).

Table I. Guidelines for the diagnosis of superficial esophageal cancers by the 20 MHz ultrasonography.

• Direct finding: hypoechoic shadow of a tumor mass • Indirect findings: interruption, obscurity, or thickening of sonolayers • Superficial mucosal tumor: intact third sonolayer • Deep mucosal tumor: thickening or obscurity of the 3a sonolayer* • Submucosal tumor: interruption of the 3a sonolayer
*sometimes this means lymphoid hyperplasia in the deep mucosa

interest, and it was also important to take pictures of the esophageal wall surrounding the lesion as a background. During examination, the lesion was to be identified through endoscopic observation and radial scanning was performed along the axis of the esophagus by comparison with a normal portion to capture the total image of the lesion. Linear scanning was performed when a detailed investigation was required. Trials to visualize the area where endoscopy detected no abnormality and the side of the wall opposite to the area of the interest were encouraged. Lymphoid hyperplasia, an occasional problem in superficial esophageal carinoma, was visualized as a thickened layer; furthermore, since it tended to be visualized as a hypoechoic area like a tumor, lymph tissue infiltration was often estimated as carcinoma and the assessment of the degree of invasion was deeper than in fact. Although a clear assessment of micro-invasion and lymphoid hyperplasia surrounding the tumor of interest remains speculative, the accuracy of diagnosis for 96 lesions of superficial esophageal carcinoma was 93% in terms of differentiating between mucosal and submucosal carcinoma (*Table II*).

Table II. Accuracy of diagnosis in examination with 20 MHz Sonoprobe

EUS Dg	Histological Dg mucosal	submucosal
Mucosal	56	4
Submucosal	3	33
	59	37

Discussion

We use the Sonoprobe, Ultrasound Probe for Endoscopy™ (UM-3R, Olympus, Japan) and Intraluminal Ultrasound Diagnostic Equipment™ (SSD-550, Aloka, Japan) in usual EUS examinations of superficial esophageal cancer [5]. Although the concepts for the development of these systems appear to differ only slightly, the systems show rather large differences in resolution, capability of visualization, characteristics of the images generated, scanning procedures, and durability of the probe. In this paper, we chose a high resolution Sonoprobe with two kinds of linear and radial scanning, of which the former mode provides easier comparison with the histological findings. This is because EUS with the thin ultrasound probe is not always easy, and the examinations with the Sonoprobe were all carried out by one examiner.

Until thin probes driven at high frequency were developed, the infiltration of superficial esophageal cancers into the wall was mainly diagnosed by X-ray and endoscopy, with the diagnosis based on surface information [6-9]. Therefore, the thin ultrasound probe was expected to allow the visualization of the extent of tumor infiltration as live images [4,10].

When the thin probe was first used clinically, however, there had been insufficient basic investigations into its diagnostic capability, and the images were not yet understood well enough to establish its efficacy [11]. To date, histopathological investigations of the resected esophageal specimens in many research institutes are implemented along the longitudinal axis. In this situation, it is impossible to compare exactly a tomogram scanned transversally in the esophagus with the histopathological image. Even with the same sectioning direction, corroboration of the images between *in vivo* and *in vitro* conditions is often inaccurate due to probable changes in the resected tissue. Therefore, we first thought it important to compare images linearly scanned with histopathological images taken using the resected and fixed specimens, in order to obtain an accurate corroboration between the two images [4].

When a 20 MHz probe is used, the normal esophageal wall of a resected specimen under the best conditions can be visualized as multi-layers of 13 consecutive high-low-high layers [4] (*Figure 1a*). However, the gray scale images merely represent the echo levels of the area of interest, and this means that an adjacent echo band is relatively higher or lower than the next one. Since the image quality of an echo tomogram is varies widely according to the equipment set-up, scanning conditions, and the situation of the esophagus to be examined, attention should be paid to these points when taking and interpreting images using the 20 MHz probe.

We have made various investigations under the best conditions using resected esophageal specimens to obtain a correlation between the images taken through the 20 MHz probe and esophageal tissues. Our investigations verify that some tomograms at 20 MHz show echo layer structures corresponding to those of anatomically different tissues having each boundary echo layer and its proper echo layer. It was believed that not only the conditions of the examination, but also changes in the anatomical structure of the esophageal wall are reflected on an ultrasound image. The healthy esophagus with its well-developed muscularis mucosae is visualized as having the maximum 13-layer structure in some cases, but only a 7-layer structure in others [4] (*Figure 1b*).

When an image with a multi-layered structure is interpreted, artifacts such as multiple echoes should be taken into consideration. However, since investigations made by scanning the specimen from the innermost layer of the mucosa to the outermost layer of the adventitia showed that both ultrasonographic structures are visualized in the same way, the multiple echo layers are proved not to be caused by artifacts (*Figure 1c*). This figure also, shows that the boundary echo layer is generated opposite to the incident direction of ultrasound waves, as verified by Aibe *et al.* and Kimmey *et al.* [12, 13], and shows that the far field echoes are affected by changes in the conditions on the incident side.

The linear scanning mode of the Sonoprobe is suitable for visualizing the layer structure in more detail than the radial scanning mode. Twenty-six resected and fixed specimens of healthy esophageal wall were subjected to a total 250 linear scannings. The visualization rate was 3 % for 13 layers, 19% for 11 layers, 74% for 9 layers, and 4% for 7 layers. The esophageal wall proved to be visualized as having nine layers in most cases [4]. It is significant for diagnosis to determine to which portion of the tissue these layers correspond *in vitro*, or which echoes are derived from what kinds of tissue. We compared sonograms of resected esophagus with the histological findings after injecting gelatin into the submucosal layer. Stereomicroscopic observation of the end surface was made posterior to a scan of the same area from the surface. The assessment made by comparing the sonograms with the histological findings showed that such lesions as esophageal leiomyoma and intramural metastasis are easily differentiated due to their histologically eccentric location. From these results, the correspondence between the ultrasound images and esophageal tissue was estimated (*Figure 2*). A conventional ultrasound endoscope visualizes the esophageal wall as having a five-layer structure. It has been reported that the second low echoic layer corresponds to the lamina propria and the third hyperechoic layer is derived from the submucosal layer [12]. However, a clearer visualization of the mucosal and submucosal layers, which bears significant meaning for the diagnosis of superficial esophageal carcinoma, is obtained using the thin ultrasound probe, which can visualize the boundary echo more clearly under optimal scanning conditions. The layer with a higher echo than that of the proper layer proved to be derived from the muscularis mucosae, although it is relatively a hyperechoic rather than boundary echo. Although it was thought that the muscularis mucosae would be visualized as segregated from the upper boundary of the conventional third layer (hyperechoic layer, 3a), in many cases it was instead visualized in the same way as the boundary echo from the lamina propria-muscularis mucosae and muscularis mucosae-submucosa, that is, as existing in a single hyperechoic layer. It was rare for the muscularis mucosae to be visualized as a hypoechoic layer like the muscularis propria. It was recognized that the muscularis mucosae in the esophagus are flat with a thickness of 0.2 mm and are not always clearly visualized in clinical cases. Taking the criteria established by the conventional ultrasound endoscope into consideration, the diagnostic basics of the Sonoprobe were established in compliance with the histopathological findings (*Figure 2*).

In EUS for superficial esophageal carcinoma using the Sonoprobe, when the same scanning conditions used to scan surgical specimens were applied, it was occasionally possible to obtain similar images to those obtained histologically with such characteristics as a subtle uneven surface and the shape of the tumor itself apparent while the tumor is growing expansively. However, it is often difficult to visualize a morphological tomogram of such mucosal lesions as an intraepithelial tumor with a smooth surface growing infiltratively in the lamina propria and submucosa (*Figure 3*).

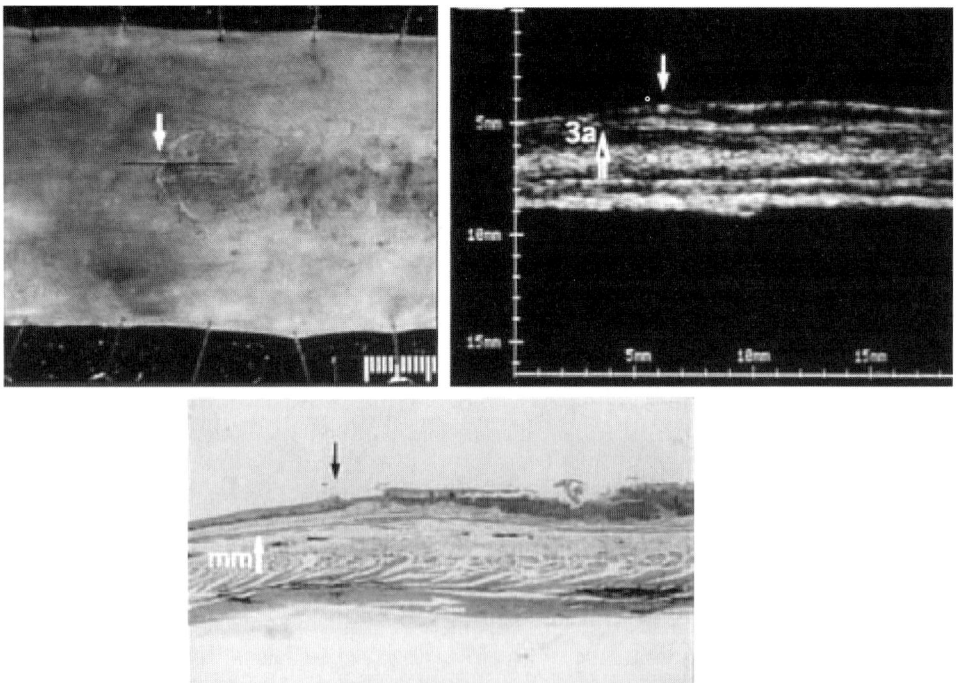

Figure 3. Ultrasonograms obtained by a 20MHz Sonoprobe in a resected specimen (cited from [5] with permission).

In EUS using the Sonoprobe for superficial esophageal carcinoma, by applying the same scanning conditions as obtained from scanning on the surgical specimens, it was occasionally possible to obtain relatively similar images to those of histology which had such characteristics as subtle uneven surface and the shape of the tumor itself when it is growing expansively. However, it is often difficult to clearly visualize a morphological tomogram of such mucosal lesions as intraepithelial tumor with a smooth surface and infiltratively growing in the lamina propria and submucosa (*Figure 3*).

In addition, one of the merits of EUS is its ability to measure the depth of tumor invasion. It is difficult to illustrate protrusion, tumor depression, or tumor thickness by X-ray examination and endoscopy. Occasionally, the same lesion can be clinically recognized as oppositely protruded or depressed. This is caused by the fact that protrusion or depression cannot be described as objective images due to different recognition of morphology or criterion even with the same recognition. Considering these points, we thought EUS by the thin ultrasound probe might affect the criteria of the clinical staging classification because it is capable of visualizing the ruggedness and thickness of each layer.

In the case of minutely progressive tumors, it is impossible at present to discriminate between infiltration of the carcinoma and an increase in lymphatic tissue, and the proper esophageal gland can not be identified. However, hypoechoic layers suggested to be the vein or occupying a small area have occasionally been observed, and the growth of lymph follicles and enlarged esophageal glands can be sometimes identified. This will lead to better diagnostic judgment brought about by an accumulation of clinical cases leading to the further development of diagnostic equipment.

There are certain conditions needed for examiners to obtain good images with the 20 MHz probe, the most important being the perpendicular emission of ultrasound waves toward the area of interest using a good acoustic medium and optimum set-ups for observation and recording. The probe has to be placed at a given distance from the area of interest in order to obtain better images. It is very important to visualize the normal layer structure of the esophagus as a reference for interpreting the lesion of interest.

Real time imaging is available in the radial scanning mode, but due to the likelihood that the probe will shift from the center of the esophagus and the difficulty in pinpointing the area of interest perpendicularly by the ultrasound waves, it is not always easy to obtain good images.

The main examining techniques reported so far are shown (*Figure 4*). De-aerated water is usually used as the acoustic medium. Continuous irrigation with water or the application of a balloon at the anal, oral or both sides for scanning are ways to retain water in the esophagus. With each method, procedures must be performed rapidly to obtain good images.

In EUS using the thin ultrasound probe, the surface structure can be observed endoscopically, and therefore, theoretically, it is more accurate than conventional EUS in which information about the region of interest is obtained by collating data from an endoscopic image and its tomogram. However, in actual practice, it is not easy to scan the legion of interest optimally under endoscopy, because movement of the esophageal wall due to peristalsis, extrinsic heartbeat, and respiration make it difficult to maintain the probe in an optimal position. When abnormal images are obtained, it is a usual to move the probe closer to the area of interest. However, since no obvious marking on the ultrasound image is available, it is sometimes difficult to collate a tomogram with that taken during

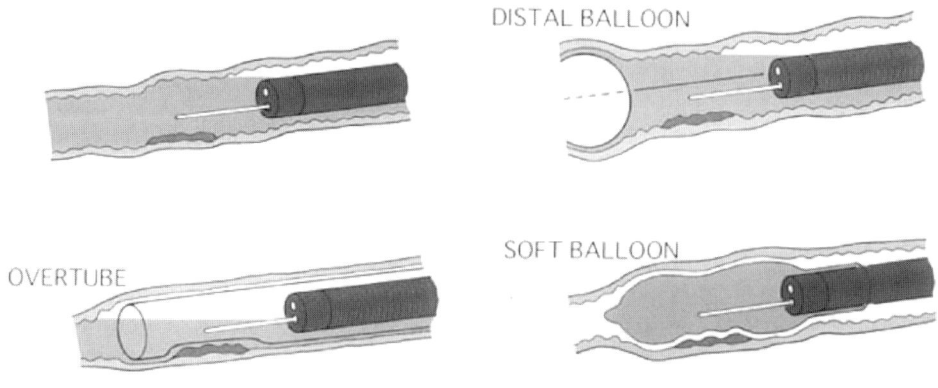

Figure 4. Schema of scanning techniques using a thin probe (cited from [21] with permission).

simultaneous endoscopy and that of microscopic images of the resected specimen. In this sense, when the transparent over-tube is used together with the Sonoprobe, since the window for both linear and radial scanning is limited to the lateral slit provided on the over-tube, there is a surer correlation between the endoscopic and ultrasound images [4] (*Figure 5a*).

We have been performing EUS using an anal side balloon or transparent over-tube to retain water [4, 14], and at present we use a soft balloon applied to the distal end of the endoscope and fill it with water during scanning [5, 15] (*Figure 5b*). Through this method, the water retention allows for a satisfactory examination. Unlike the conventional balloon technique, this method does not over-compress the lesion and allows the esophagogastric junction and cervical esophagus to be visualized easily using a panendoscope [5]. Problems peculiar to the soft balloon method, such as a small decrease in the field of view, missing a slight ruggedness on the surface of a 0-IIc lesion, or inability to carry out treatment during examination remain. However, the method has made examinations simpler and causes less discomfort to patients; it is especially useful for lesions that are elevated.

In this study, we used three EUS techniques with the Sonoprobe, *i.e.* over-tube method, soft-balloon method, Water repletion method. We chose these techniques to be applied to each patient at random, and no comparison between the three methods was performed. Each technique has advantages and disadvantages [5]. It is easiest to obtain good ultrasound images using the soft-balloon method.

Several methods for EMR have been reported [16]. We usually use the np-EEM (Endoscopic esophageal mucosectomy using a transparent over-tube with intraluminal negative pressure) [17] or EMRC (Endoscopic mucosal resection using a cap-fitted panendoscope) technique [18]. In our department, we have performed EMR on more than 300 patients with esophageal tumors. The depth of tumor invasion determines the indication for EMR. At present, mucosal tumors are good indicators for EMR; superficial submucosal tumors without clinical metastasis are also indicators for EMR in terms of step-up therapy [19-21]. Therefore, the most important use of EUS with a thin ultrasound probe is for assessing the depth of tumor invasion. During endoscopic esophageal

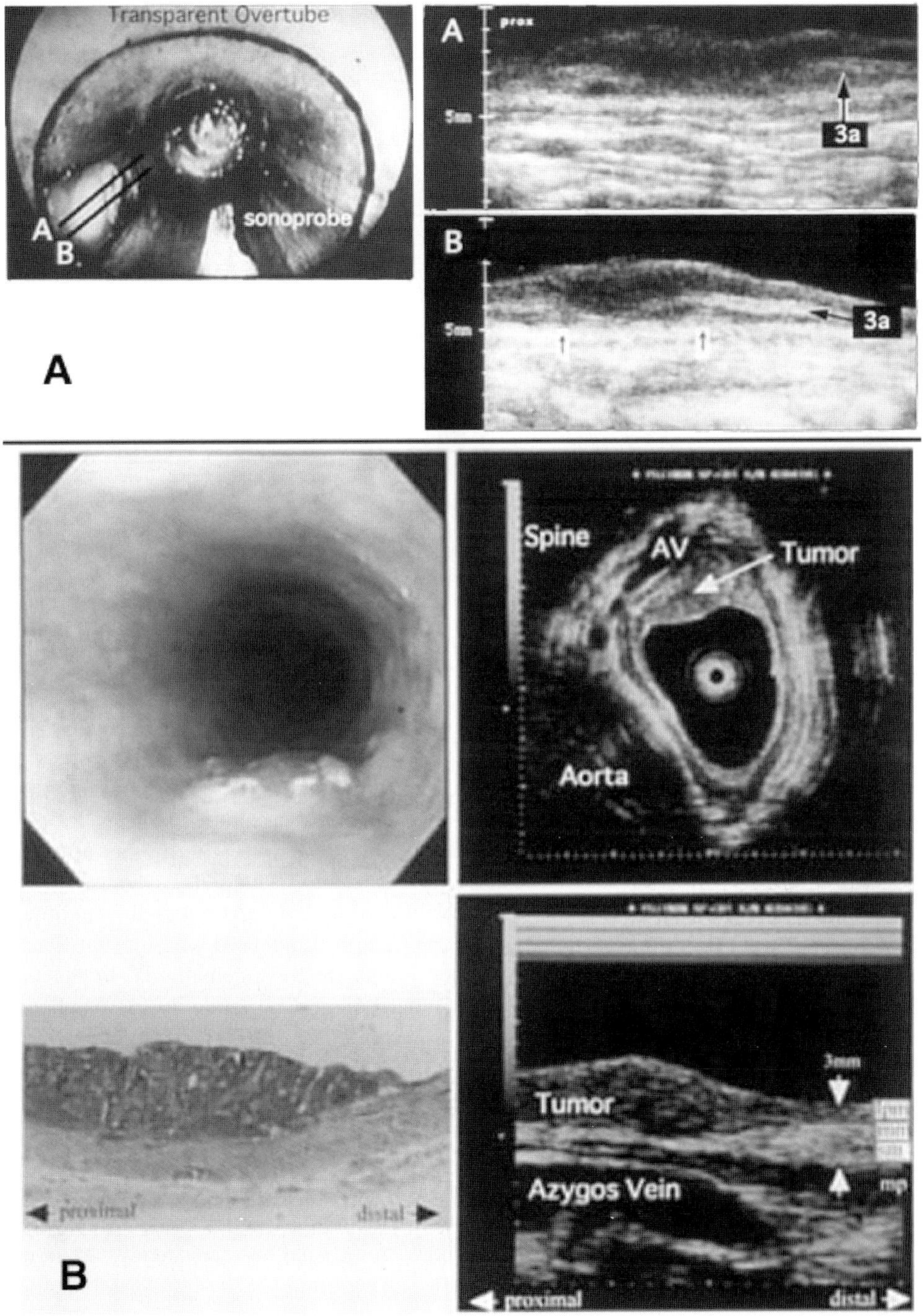

Figure 5. A. Ultrasonograms obtained by the overtube method (cited from [4] with permission). **B.** Ultrasonograms obtained by the soft balloon method (cited from [5] with permission). (See page VII for colour figure).

mucosectomy, EUS using the thin ultrasound probe is useful for preventing esophageal perforation [22] (*Figure 6*).

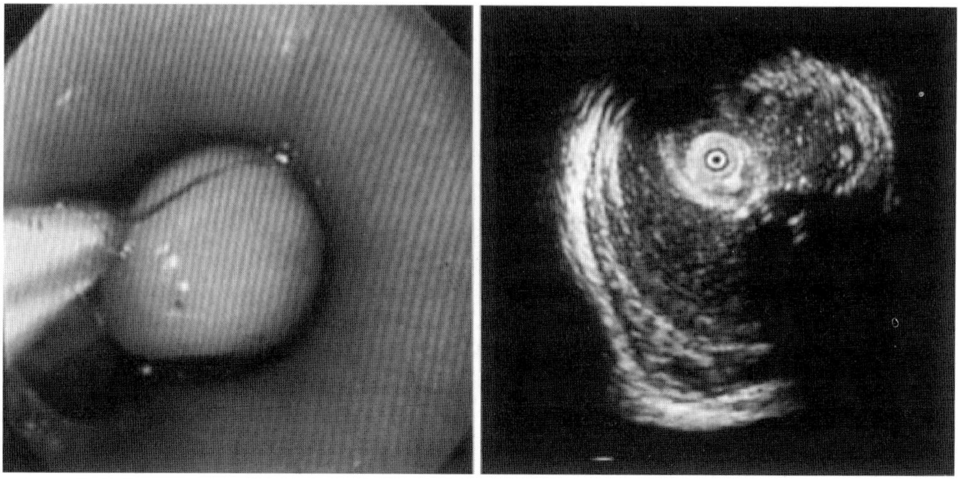

Figure 6. Endosonography during endoscopic resection (cited from [21] with permission). (See page VII for colour figure).

In Japan, outstanding progress in gastrointestinal diagnostics by X-ray and endoscopy has made it possible to treat many early cancers as compared with other countries. Progress in EMR techniques for gastrointestinal mucosa also owes greatly to the advanced diagnostics in Japan. Under these circumstances, progress has been made in the use of EUS as an alternative diagnostic modality to the conventional practice. Although the equipment has improved, EUS is not at present a stand alone diagnostic method, and its significance should be discussed in combination with other image diagnostic methods. In the near future, we believe that EUS will become the standard diagnostic modality for esophageal lesions, as sonogram analyses become clearer, interpretation criteria are established, and examination techniques are improved.

The usefulness of the thin ultrasound probe exists in its ability to obtain clear tomograms of minute changes in the esophageal wall that can not be obtained by X-ray and endoscopy. Its usefulness should not be discussed from the standpoint of its simple usage and accuracy rate for diagnosis. That is to say, EUS by the thin ultrasound probe is most suitable for visualizing various lesions located within the mucosa and submucosa, and takes the position to provide the most objective images for managing superficial carcinoma. Considering this, efforts to attain precise imaging are required for the rapid establishment of the efficacy of EUS by the thin ultrasound probe.

References

1. Murata M. Diagnosis of advancement of superficial esophageal cancer by US and histopathological and clinical prognostic evaluation. Jpn Gastroenterol Surg 1989;22:195-204 (in Japanese with English abstract).
2. Kouzu T, Arima M, Hishikawa E, et al. How detail interpretation is possible for superficial esophageal cancer by EUS. Stomach Intest 1992;27:213-221 (in Japanese with English abstract).
3. Kulling D, Feldman DR, Kay CL, et al. Local staging of esophageal cancer using endoscopic magnetic resonance imaging: prospective comparison with endoscopic ultrasound. Endoscopy 1998;30:745-749.
4. Kawano T. EUS of the esophagus and 20MHz sonogram by Sonoprobe using a transparent overtube. Gastroenterol Endos 1992;34:1237-1251 (in Japanese with English abstract).
5. Kawano T, Ohshima M, Endo M. Endoscopic ultrasonography. Stomach Intest 1995;30:365-374 (in Japanese).
6. Endo M, Yoshino K, Kawano T, et al. Diagnosis of superficial esophageal cancer from the standpoint of preoperative examination. Gastroenterol Surg 1992;15:1741-1747 (in Japanese with English abstract).
7. Hosoi T, Nishizawa M, Omura T, et al. Invasion depth diagnosis of early esophageal cancer by X-ray radiography majoring judgment of m and sm cancer. Stomach Intest 1994;25:1039-1050 (in Japanese with English abstract).
8. Yoshida M, You R, Hirose T, et al. Endoscopic diagnosis of esophageal cancer. Clin Sci 1994;30:658-665 (in Japanese with English abstract).
9. Makuuchi H, Machimura T, Mizutani T, et al. Accuracy of endoscopic diagnosis of invasion depth for superficial esophageal cancer. Stomach Intest 1992;27:175-184 (in Japanese with English abstract).
10. Waxman I, Saitoh Y. Clinical outcome of endoscopic mucosal resection for superficial GI lesions and the role of high-frequency ultrasound probe sonography in an American population. Gastrointest Endosc 2000;52:322-327.
11. Silverstein FE, Martin RW, Kimmey MB, et al. Experimental evaluation of an edoscopic ultrasound probe. In vitro and in vivo canine studies. Gastroenterology 1989;96:1058-1062.
12. Aibe T. Basic and clinical study on the layer structure of the gastrointestinal wall (2) - the layer structure of the esophagus and colon. Gastroenterol Endosc 1984;26:1465-1473 (in Japanese with English abstract).
13. Kimmy MB, Martin RW, Haggitt RC, et al. Histologic correlates of gastrointestinal ulrasound images. Gastroenterology 1989;96:433-441.
14. Inoue H, Nara T, Izumi Y, et al. Contrivance for EUS of the esophagus using the thin probe. Gastroenterol Endosc 1994;36:800-803 (in Japanese with English abstract).
15. Kawano T, Endo M. In cases of endoscopic mucosal resection, should EUS evaluation by a miniature probe be recommended to make the indication more accurate? In : Giuli R, Galmiche JP, Jamieson GC, Scarpignato C, eds. The esophagogastric junction. Paris : John Libbey Eurotext, 1998:1204-1206.
16. Makuuchi H. Endoscopic mucosal resection for early esophageal cancer – indication and techniques. Dig Endosc 1996;8:175-179.
17. Kawano T, Endo M. Step up strategy in the treatment for superficial esophageal cancer. In : Bismuth H, Galmiche JP, Huguier M, Jaeck D, es. The International Gastro-surgical Club. Rome : Monduzzi, 1998:23-26.
18. Kawano T, Endo M. A new multipurpose tube for esophageal endoscopy. Endoscopy 1997;29:526-527.
19. Inoue H, Kawano T, Tani M, et al. Endoscopic mucosal resection using a cap: techniques for use and preventing perforation. Can J Gastroenterol 1999;13:477- 480.
20. Endo M, Yoshino K, Kawano T, et al. Clinicopathologic analysis of lymph node metastasis in surgically resected superficial cancer of the thoracic esophagus. Dis Esophagus 2000;13:125-129.
21. Kawano T, Nagai K, Inoue H, et al. Endoscopic ultrasonography for patients with an esophageal cancer invading to the deep mucosa or superficial submucosa. Stomach Intest 1998;33:969-974 (in Japanese with English abstract).
22. Izumi Y, Inoue H, Kawano T, et al. Endosonography during endoscopic mucosal resection enhance its safety -A new technique-. Surg Endosc 1999;13:358-360.

For the most accurate diagnosis of superficial carcinomas, what is the compared value of ultrasound miniprobe and of the radial scanning echo-endoscope?

N. Marcon (Toronto)

There is confusion as to what is meant by superficial carcinoma. It is carcinoma limited to the mucosa, which does not penetrate below the muscularis mucosa. There may be some difficulty on histological interpretation of endoscopic biopsies in separating high-grade dysplasia (HGD) *versus* more involvement of the lamina propria. Excisional snare biopsies with saline assist would seem to be the only way to tell the depth of invasion, short of esophagectomy. Conventional diagnosis depends on endoscopic recognition and random biopsies as per protocol for dysplasia detection. Can endoscopic ultrasound be of use in diagnosing Barrett's esophagus or searching for the presence of dysplasia or mucosal cancer in an otherwise flat mucosa?

Instrumentation?

There are two ultrasound devices currently used to assess the wall of the esophagus. There is the echo-endoscope with frequencies of 7.5 and 12 MHz and miniprobes, which pass through the accessory channel. The commercially available probes are 12 and 20 MHz and soon to be released 30 MHz. The higher the frequency, the more clarity and detail but with the compromise of lower penetration and therefore only a limited area is examined beyond the wall. The focusing point for the 7.5 scope is 30 millimeters, for the 12 MHz probe 20 millimeters and for the 20 MHz probe 2-3 millimeters. The depth of penetration is also in similar proportions. For the 7.5 it is 40 millimeters and for the 12 it is 30 millimeters and the 20 MHz probe it is a radius of 15 millimeters. The major manufacturer of the radial scanning echo-endoscope is Olympus, older models have diameters between 11 and 13 millimeters and have a rigid end, which is 4-5 centimeters in length. Newer scopes have a diameter of 9.5 millimeters. They function best in the esophagus with a balloon for better interfacing. A disadvantage of these scopes in surveying the esophageal mucosa is, when the balloon is inflated with water, they can compress subtle lesions and the mucosal layers. Probes are able to pass down a conventional endoscope, their diameter is 2.5 millimeters. The presence of air, the enemy of endoscopic ultrasonography (EUS), may be corrected by either filling the esophagus with water, with appropriate positioning of the patient, which can sometimes be anatomically difficult, use probes that have incorporated balloons or fashion homemade balloons (condoms). These can be taped over the end of the mother scope, filled with water and yet are transparent, allowing the mucosa to be seen. A recent editorial suggests that probes give good information of the wall of the esophagus and the nearby mediasternum, equal to echo-endoscopes.

The issues to be resolved are:

- is endoscopic ultrasonography useful in the diagnosis of Barrett's?
- is endoscopic ultrasonography helpful in the detection of dysplasia?

- what is the confidence using EUS in the staging of mucosal carcinoma when considering endoscopic ablation in the operable patient.

There are few published papers and a small number of abstracts that study the ability of EUS to differentiate the mucosal thickness in Barrett's from that of normal squamous.

The assumption to begin with is that Barrett's mucosa is thicker than normal squamous mucosa. Scivastava *et al.* [1] found that the esophageal wall of patients with Barrett's mucosa was slightly thicker than that of controls. However, the difference between the wall thickness in segments of dysplastic and non-dysplastic epithelium did not reach statistical significance. They used a conventional echo-endoscope at both 7.5 and 12 MHz.

A more recent study by Miller's group in Philadelphia [2] used high frequency ultrasound probes of 20 MHz and concluded that high resolution ultrasound probes were able to detect Barrett's esophagus, however they were not successful in being able to identify areas of dysplasia. They studied 17 patients with Barrett's esophagus, of which 3 had dysplasia, and 12 normal control patients. Barrett's esophagus was diagnosed if the second hypoechoic layer was thicker than the first hyperechoic layer of the mucosa. Dysplasia was diagnosed if a focal hypoechoic area was seen within the mucosa. A blinded investigator reviewed all tapes to validate these criteria. All 17 patients with Barrett's epithelium were correctly identified as were 10 out of the 12 controls. They were unable to identify dysplasia in the three patients who had dysplasia. No other groups have been published in this area. A European consensus study downplays the usefulness of using EUS to confirm this feature of Barrett's [3].

What about endosonography and its ability to screen for high-grade dysplasia in Barrett's mucosa?

There have been a few studies looking at this. Kinjo *et al.*, Mayo Clinic [4], looked at 56 patients with Barrett's. They did show that the wall thickness was increased in patients with Barrett's *versus* non-Barrett's, but they did not find any statistical difference in the wall thickness among the different grades of dysplasia. This study used an echo-endoscope of 7.5 and 12 MHz and overall because of both false negatives and false positives this group concluded that EUS is not cost effective for the detection of cancer in Barrett's. Falk *et al.* [5] used an echo-endoscope on 9 patients who had biopsy proven HGD and who were slated for esophagectomy. EUS was able to identify only one out of three cancers found at surgery. It was felt that EUS was not a useful exercise for the screening of dysplasia or cancer in the patient who did not have any endoscopically visible nodularity.

What about the utility of endoscopic ultrasonography in staging?

Staging of disease determines the treatment algorithm. As endoscopic ablative therapy becomes more recognized as a useful alternative to resective surgery, the endoscopist must have a high degree of confidence that with intramucosal cancer, the disease is indeed mucosal and does not extend into the submucosa where there is a 20-30% chance of lymph node involvement. The higher the ultrasound frequency, the better the clarity and resolution in the staging of mucosal disease [6-8]. There is relatively little that has been published. The endoscopist relies more on the fact that the muscularis mucosa or the second hypoechoic layer is intact. If there is evidence of a hypoechoic lesion in the submucosa, using at least current probes, this may be tumor invasion and endoscopic ablation in operable patients would not be appropriate. There is fortunately an extensive bibliography on resective surgery for mucosal disease both squamous and in Barrett's where localization of carcinoma to the mucosa is rarely associated with lymphatic involvement. It is on this premise of an intact muscularis mucosa that the endoscopist has the confidence to proceed with local ablative therapy. For staging of the esophageal wall, endoprobes are better than traditional dedicated echo-endoscopes [6-10].

Conclusion

In the most accurate diagnosis of superficial carcinoma, endoscopic ultrasound has no role but is necessary to determine the staging and localization to decide treatment algorithms, especially endoscopic ablation.

References

1. Scrivastava AK, Vanagunas A, Kamel P, et al. Endoscopic ultrasound in the evaluation of Barrett's esophagus:A preliminary report.Am J Gastroenterol 1994;89:2192-2195.
2. Miller LS, Adrain AL, Ter HC, Cassidy MJ, Schiano TD, Liu JB. High-resolution endoluminal sonography is a sensitive modality for the identification of Barrett's metaplasia. Gastrointest- Endosc- 1997;46(2):147-151.
3. Axon A, Lambert R, Robaszkiewicz M, Rosch T, Sonnenberg A. The Second European Endoscopy Forum (Sintra, Portugal, 17-18 June 1999). Twenty questions on the esophagogastric junction. Is there a place for endosonography in BE? Endoscopy 2000;32:413.
4. Kinjo M, Maringhini A, Wang KK, et al. Is endoscopic ultrasonography (EUS) cost effective to screen for cancer in patients with Barrett's esophagus? Gastrointest Endosc 1994;40:205A.
5. Falk GW, Catalano MF, Sivak MV Jr, et al. Endosonography in the evaluation of patients with Barrett's esophagus and high-grade dysplasia. Gastrointest Endosc 1994;40:207-212.
6. Chak A. How far have we come with ultrasound miniprobes? Endoscopy 1999;31(4):329-332.
7. Menzel J, Hoepffner N, Nottberg H, Schulz C, Senninger N, Domschke W. Preoperative staging of esophageal carcinoma: miniprobe sonography versus conventional endoscopic ultrasound in a prospective histopathology verified study. Endoscopy 1999;31(4):291-297.
8. Murata Y, Suzuki S, Ohta M, Mitsunaga A, Hayashi K, Yoshina K, Ide H. Small ultrasonic probes for determination of the depth of superficial esophageal cancer. Gastrointest Endosc 1996;44:23-28.
9. Hasegawa N, Niwa Y, Arisawa T, Hase S, Goto H, Hayakawa T. Preoperative staging of superficial esophageal carcinoma: comparison of an ultrasound probe and standard endoscopic ultrasonography. Gastrointest Endosc 1996;44:388-393.
10. Yanai H, Yoshida T, Harasa T, Matsumoto Y, Nishiaki M, Shigemitsu T, Tada M, Okita K, Kawano T, Nagasaki S. Endoscopic ultrasonography of superfical cancers using a thin ultrasound probe system equipped with switchable radial and linear scanning modes. Gastrointest Endosc 1996;44:578-582.

What are the results of photodynamic therapy in early esophageal adenocarcinoma?

J. Spénard (Québec)

Esophageal adenocarcinoma is a possible complication of long-standing Barrett's esophagus, and often the 2 conditions coexist in patients with adenocarcinoma. Since patients with Barrett's esophagus are usually under a strict surveillance program, esophageal adenocarcinoma is often detected at an early stage (T_{is}- or T_1- N_0M_0). Treatment options are numerous and include, among other, endoscopic mucosal removal, esophagectomy, and photodynamic therapy (PDT). This review looks at the published results of PDT in the treatment of early esophageal adenocarcinoma.

Methods

Literature was searched by Medline with the key words: photodynamic, esophageal, and cancer. Names of authors who have already published on these topics or related ones were also used as well as the "related articles" function. Abstracts from major gastroenterology meetings from 1995 to Aug 2000 were also revised.

The manuscripts with the following criteria were not considered: PDT and other interventions in the same patients without breakdown of results, PDT with more than one photosensitising agent without breakdown of results, unspecified or multiple stages of esophageal cancer without breakdown of results, cancer of esophagus and other organs in the same publication without breakdown of results for esophagus, squamous cell carcinoma or unspecified type of esophageal cancer. Duplicate reporting or updated reports involving previously published partial results where counted only once. Four authors were contacted by email for additional precisions and three replied in a timely fashion; their publications are included in this survey.

Results

Eleven studies matching the criteria and involving 142 patients were retrieved: 7 full manuscripts and 4 abstracts.

Results are presented in the *Table I*. The overall cure rate, defined as complete removal of adenocarcinoma after one or repeated PDT courses, is 75%. When the results are further broken down by the type of photosensitising agent, 5-aminolevulinic acid (5-ALA) or a porphyrin, the cure rates are 70% and 81% respectively. *A posteriori* exploratory analysis by 2-tailed Fisher test did not show a difference between the 2 agents ($p = 0.1696$).

Table I. Efficacy rates for ablation of early stage adenocarcinoma by photodynamic therapy in the literature.

First author	Treated	Cured	%	Treatment
Sibille [1]	18	16	89%	POR
Mc Caughan [2]	7	6	86%	POR
Gossner [3]	22	17	77%	5-ALA
Gossner [4]	42	34	81%	5-ALA
Tan [5]	12	2	17%	5-ALA
Overholt [6]	13	10	77%	POR
Scotiniotis [7]	12	9	75%	POR
Wolfsen [8]	2	2	100%	POR
Lovat [9]	3	2	67%	mTHPC
Panjehpour [10]	7	7	100%	POR
Corti [11]	4	1	25%	POR
TOTAL	142	106	75%	
95% CI			58.2-91.1%	
5-ALA	76	53	70%	
95% CI			52.4-87.1%	
Porphyrin	63	51	81%	
95%CI			66.1-95.8%	

5-ALA: 5-aminolaevulinic acid; POR: porphyrin derivative; mTHPC: mesotetrahydroxyphenylchlorin; CI: Confidence interval

Conclusions

PDT seems a valid approach for treatment of superficial esophageal adenocarcinoma, often associated with Barrett's esophagus, with an overall success rate of about 76%. A prospective randomized study comparing 5-ALA to porfimer, with an adequate sample size to detect a difference, could provide valuable information.

References

1. Sibille A, Lambert R, Souquet JC, Sabben G, Descos F. Long-term survival after photodynamic therapy for esophageal cancer. Gastroenterology 1995;108:337-344.
2. McCaughan JS Jr, Ellison EC, Guy JT, Hicks WJ, Jones JJ, Laufman LR, May E, Nims TA, Spiridonidis CH, Williams TE. Photodynamic therapy for esophageal malignancy: a prospective twelve-year study. Ann Thorac Surg 1996;62(4):1005-1009.
3. Gossner L, Stolte M, Sroka R, Rick K, May A, Hahn EG, Ell C. Photodynamic ablation of high-grade dysplasia and early cancer in Barrett's esophagus by means of 5-aminolevulinic acid. Gastroenterology 1999;114:448-455.
4. Gossner L, May A, Sroka R, Rabenstein T, Schneider TH, Hahn EG, Stolte M, Ell C. Photodynamic therapy of Barrett's esophagus with high-grade dysplasia and early cancer. Digestive Disease Week, Abstract book, 1998.
5. Tan WC, Fulljames C, Stone N, Dix AJ, Shepherd N, Roberts DJH, Brown SB, Krasner N, Barr H. Photodynamic therapy using 5-aminolaevulinic acid for esophageal adenocarcinoma associated with Barrett's metaplasia. J Photochem Photobiol 1999;53:75-80.
6. Overholt BF, Panjehpour M, Haydek JM. Photodynamic therapy for Barrett's esophagus: follow-up in 100 patients. Gastrointest Endosc 1999;49(1):1-7.
7. Scotiniotis IA, Kochman ML, Sanfilipo N, Hahn S, Rosato E, Ginsberg G. Management of superficial esophageal cancer: outcomes of esophagectomy, photodynamic therapy, or endoscopic mucosal resection. Digestive Disease Week, Abstract book, 2000.

8. Wolfsen HC, Woodward TA. Photodynamic therapy for dysplastic Barrett's esophagus and mucosal esophageal adenocarcinoma: the value of endoscopic ultrasound and results using the bare fiber technique. Digestive Disease Week, Abstract book, 2000.
9. Lovat LB, Whitelaw DE, Spencer GM, Thorpe SM, Mlkvy PP, Buonaccorsi G, Bown SG. Photodynamic therapy for gastrointestinal tumours using mTHPC. Digestive Disease Week, Abstract book, 2000.
10. Panjehpour M, Overholt BF, Haydek JM, Lee SG. Results of photodynamic therapy of ablation of dysplasia and early cancer in Barrett's esophagus and effect of oral steroids on stricture formation. Am J Gastroenterol 2000;95(9):2177-2184.
11. Corti L, Skarlatos J, Boso C, Cardin F, Kosma L, Koukourakis M, Giatromanolaki A, Norberto L, Shaffer M, Beroikas K. Outcome of patients receiving photodynamic therapy for early esophageal cancer. Int J Rad Oncol Biol Phys 2000;47(2):419-424.

What is the compared value of the various techniques of endoscopic mucosal resection for superficial lesions?

W. Mayoral, C. Tombazzi, G. Marino, T.L. Tio (Washington)

Barrett's esophagus is considered a precancerous condition. Patients with Barrett's are estimated to be 30 to 125 times more likely to have adenocarcinoma than the general population [1, 2]. Esophagectomy is the treatment of choice with a curative intent. However, a large number of patients are inoperable, or do not want surgery because of the associated 3-5% mortality even in centers with experience. Despite the lack of large series, endoscopic mucosal resection (EMR) has emerged as an alternative for patients with Barrett's esophagus and high-grade dysplasia (HGD) or carcinoma *in situ*.

Endoscopic mucosal resection techniques

EMR refers to the endoscopic removal of a mucosal lesion using a diathermic snare.

It is advisable to mark the outer margins of a lesion before EMR is performed, specially when a submucosal injection for lifting purposes is going to be performed. Four-point markings are commonly made with the tip of the snare. Three main types of EMR have been described with modalities; *i.e.*:

- resection without injection;
- injection of submucosal saline/methylene blue followed by resection;
- suck-cut using the Inohue cap;
- mucosectomy with snare over the Makuuchi rigid overtube;
- suck-cut with the rubber-band technique;
- injection-cut with the endo-snare.

Inject-and-cut

Deyhle *et al.* [3] described in 1973 submucosal injection with normal saline as a technique for raising sessile polyps in the colon to facilitate their excision. The injected saline separated the lesion in the mucosa/submucosa from the underlying muscularis propria minimizing the risk of perforation. The absence of rising or lifting of the lesion after saline injection, is suggestive that the tumoral lesion is invading or is adherent to the muscularis propria, which is a contraindication for EMR. Hypertonic saline, hypertonic glucose, indigo carmine and ethylene blue have also been used to as submucosal agents; however no difference between these agents has been so far reported.

Lift-and-cut

This technique was described in 1976 by Martin *et al.* [4] using a double-channel endoscope while trying to provide a bleeding-ulcer model. A forceps for lifting was used in one channel, and a snare for resection in the other. But to the authors surprise, submucosa was always present on each tissue sample, so it was reported as alternative for large tissue biopsy. Tada *et al.* [5] described the strip biopsy as an extension of the lift-and-cut technique with double lumen endoscopes in early cancers. They injected 3-5 ml of normal saline submucosally before the lift-and-cut technique was applied. This technique requires the use of a double channel endoscope which may not be widely available. Takechi [6] described an approach using two thin endoscopes placed next to each other; one will be used to lift and the other one to snare. But this technique is awkward and not widely used.

Suck-and-cut

An artificial polypoid lesion from the tumor's mucosa using suction is created. A special EMR Olympus transparent overtube with an outer diameter of 18 mm is used for this purpose. It contains a small accessory channel for insertion of a snare, which exits at the open-circle slit. Inoue *et al.* [7] described the use of the transparent cap adapter in the variceal banding ligator kit (Bard Interventional Products; Tewksbury MA) to perform EMR. Sakai *et al.* [8] in 6 patients with T1N0 early tumors, and Fleischer *et al.* [9] in 5 patients with moderate dysplasia, applied this equipment and technique of variceal band ligation to perform EMR. Recently, Ell *et al.* [10] reported 120 resections in 64 patients with high-grade dysplasia (HGD) or early carcinoma. They used 2 different polypectomy techniques: submucosal injection of diluted epinephrine followed by snare resection, and the suck and ligate" technique. They reported recurrent carcinoma in 14% of patients after a mean follow-up of 12 ± 8 months. In our group here reported, we performed 12 resections using different techniques. The biggest resection we performed was 2.9 cms. Despite the lack of randomized, large studies in the literature, EMR has become an encouraging alternative for patients with Barrett's esophagus and HGD or carcinoma *in situ*. Aggressive anti-acid therapy and close follow-up of this patients is warranted after EMR. The different available techniques for EMR are all effective means. However, prospective studies need to be done to confirm this.

We report 4 of 29 patients with Barrett's adenocarcinoma or HGD, of whom 12 underwent resections.

Patients and methods

From June 1997 and May of 2000, 29 patients with endoscopically and histologically proven Barrett's adenocarcinoma or HGD were referred and evaluated with at Georgetown University Medical Center. All patients underwent endoscopy, endosonography (Olympus UM20, and Pentax linear array echo-endoscope); and catheter ultrasound (20MHz probe) with a therapeutic scope for lesion identified at endoscopy. All patients were sprayed with acetic acid followed by chromoendoscopy (methylene blue or lugol) for adequate identification of mucosal lesions prior to biopsy. Biopsies were obtained from visible lesions and quadrant biopsies were taken every 2 cms of the entire Barrett's segment. Three patients had HGD; 8 patients had T1 lesions; 4 patients had T2 lesions; 9 had T3 lesions and 4 patients had T4 lesions. EMR was performed using the suck and snare technique after submucosal injection had been performed (normal saline and methylene blue).

Results

Of this group, 10 (34%) patients underwent surgery; 10 patients (34%) were not surgical candidates and underwent chemotherapy and radiotherapy; 5 patients were lost to follow-up and 4 patients underwent EMR, which constitute the sample of our study. A total of 12 resections were performed in these 4 patients. The mean age of the patients in the resection group was 67.7 (range 48-80). One patient had HGD and underwent 2 resections; 2 patients had a T1N0Mx lesion and underwent 3 and 4 resections respectively, and 1 patient had a T1bN0Mx lesion and underwent 4 resections. This last patient finally underwent an esophagectomy and gastric pull-up and the pathology specimen was negative for malignant tissue. The other 3 patients are being currently followed-up and have had no malignant tissue at histological evaluation of their biopsies. *Table I* depicts some of the characteristics of these patients. One case of oozing hemorrhage was observed immediately after resection, but the bleeding was controlled after endoscopic hemostasis with epinephrine (1:10.000). Mild transitory epigastric discomfort that ceased spontaneously and did not require additional work-up was present after 3 resections. No perforations or other major complications were encountered. All patients were treated after resection with proton pump inhibitors.

Discussion

EMR refers to the endoscopic removal of a mucosal lesion using a diathermic snare. It was initially described in 1973 by Ottenjann *et al.* [11] in obtaining adequate tissue samples for histopathologic analysis. They originally used a snare for colonic polypectomy to excise large samples in the upper gastrointestinal tract of 11 patients. Deyhle *et al.* [12] in Zurich in 1974 removed a 6 mm-polypoid well-differentiated gastric adenocarcinoma with a polypectomy snare; pathology evaluation revealed only one focus of penetration into the muscularis propia of the tumor resected. However, the operative specimen after the patient went to surgery revealed no residual tumor or lymph node metastasis. In the mid and late 1980's, EMR was popularized by Japanese authors in the treatment of early cancers of the upper gastrointestinal tract. In the 1990's, this therapeutic modality has gained more popularity and acceptance, becoming every day easier and safer.

Table I. Characteristics of patients with endoscopic mucosal resection.

Age/ gender	Diagnosis	TNM	Barrett's location	Stain used	Resection number	Technique	Pathology
48/M	HGD	–	33-37cm	MB	1	Inject and cut	HGD-Cis
					2	Inject and cut	HGD with free margins
73/M	Cis	T1N0Mx	36-39cm	MB	1	Injection-lift-cut	Cis
				MB	2	Injection-lift-cut	Cis
				MB	3	Injection-lift-ut	No evidence of malignancy or dysplasia
80/M	Cis	T1N0Mx	32-36cm	MB	1	Rubber-band suck-cut	Cis
					2	Endo-loop, Inohue cap	Dysplasia-no malignancy
					3	Endo-loop Inohue-cap	No malignancy or dysplasia
73/M	Cis	T1bN0M0	35-39cm	MB	1	Inohue cap	Adenocarcinoma, signet ring features invading muscularis mucosa
					2	Inohue cap*	Adenocarcinoma
					3	Inohue-cap	Adenocarcinoma
					4	Inohue-cap	Dysplasia
					Esophagectomy and gastric pull-up		Negative for malignancy

* Largest resection obtained (2.9 cms); HGD: High-grade dysplasia; Cis: Carcinoma *in situ*

By definition, Barrett's esophagus is the presence of columnar epithelium with intestinal metaplasia in the distal esophagus. The intestinal-type metaplasia with goblet cells is at increased risk for malignant transformation. The choice of therapy depends on the existence and the grade of dysplasia. It is accepted that if dysplasia is absent, the aim of therapy will be the reflux symptoms of the patient. If low-grade dysplasia is present, aggressive anti-acid medical therapy and endoscopic surveillance are recommended. If carcinoma is present, esophagectomy is the standard of care. But in patients with Barrett's esophagus and HGD the management is still controversial because esophagectomy, endoscopic surveillance and endoscopic ablation therapy are acceptable. Endoscopic ablation therapies include:

- thermal ablation (multipolar electrocoagulation), and laser coagulation (contact or non-contact);
- chemical ablation (photodynamic therapy);
- mechanical ablation (EMR).

EMR is a diagnostic and therapeutic modality. The degree of dysplasia in patients with Barrett's esophagus – or the tumor differentiation grade if a superficial cancer is present –, the depth of infiltration, the presence or not of lymphatic compromise or invasion at the tumor-free margins, will determine the definitive

Table II. 1997, TNM-revised classification.

Primary tumor - T -	
TX →	Primary tumor cannot be assessed
T0 →	No evidence of primary tumor
Tis →	Carcinoma *in situ*
T1 →	Tumor invades lamina propria or submucosa
T2 →	Tumor invades muscularis propria
T3 →	Tumor invades adventitia
T4 →	Tumor invades adjacent structures
Regional lymph nodes -N –	
NX →	Regional lymph nods cannot be assessed
N0 →	No regional lymph node metastasis
N1 →	Regional lymph node metastasis
Distant metastasis	
MX →	Distant metastasis cannot be assessed
M0 →	No distant metastasis
M1 →	Distant metastasis
Tumors of the lower thoracic esophagus	
M1a →	Metastasis in celiac lymph nodes
M1b →	Other distant metastasis
Tumors of the mid-thoracic esophagus	
M1a →	Not applicable
M1b →	No regional lymph nodes
Tumors of the upper thoracic esophagus	
M1a →	Metastasis in cervical lymph nodes
M1b →	Other distant metastasis

Table III. Japanese society for esophageal diseases: classification of early cancer.

T1-m1→	Intraepithelial invasion (carcinoma *in situ*)
T1-m2 →	Invasion of the lamina propria mucosae
T1-m3 →	Invasion of the muscularis mucosa
T1-sm1 →	Superficial layer of the submucosa involved
T1-sm2 →	Deeper layer of the submucosa involved

treatment strategy after EMR has been performed. Superficial or "early" cancers by definition involve the mucosal or submucosal layers. According to the TNM-1987 classification, this would correspond to a T1 lesion. But the 1997 TNM-revised classification distinguishes between carcinoma *in situ* (intraepithelial) and T1 stage cancers (invasion into the lamina propia and submucosa) [13]. *Table II* depicts this classification. The differentiation of the infiltration depth is important due to the fact that the risk of lymphatic invasion increases with progression in depth. In tumors limited to the intraepithelial layers, the risk of metastatic spread is non-existent; if the muscularis mucosa is invaded, this risk increases to 10%; if the superficial mucosa is invaded this risk is near 20%; and up to 40% if the submucosa is invaded. The Japanese society for esophageal diseases has a more differentiated classification (*Table III*) and they differentiate between intra-epithelial invasion (T1-m1), infiltration of the lamina propria (T1-m2), and infiltration of the muscularis mucosa (T1-m3).

References

1. Falk GW. Barrett's esophagus. Gastrointest Endosc Clin N Am 1994;4:773-789.
2. Sampliner RE. Practice guidelines on the diagnosis, surveillance, and therapy of Barrett's esophagus. Am J Gastroenterol 1998;93:1028-1032.
3. Deyhle H, Largiader F, Jenny S, et al. A method for endoscopic electroresection of sessile colonic polyps. Endoscopy 1973;5:36-40.
4. Martin TR, Onstad GR, Silvis SE, et al. Lift and cut biopsy technique for submucosal samplings. Gastrointest Endosc 1976;23:29-30.
5. Tada M, Murata M, Murakami F, et al. Development of strip-off biopsy. Gastrointest Endosc 1984;26:833-839.

6. Takechi K, Mihara M, Saito Y, et al. A modified technique for endoscopic mucosal resection of small early gastric carcinomas. Endoscopy 1992;24:215-217.
7. Inohue H, Endo M, Takeshita K, et al. A new simplified tehcnique of endoscopic esophageal mucosal resection suing a cap-fitted panendoscope (EMRC). Surg Endosc 1992;6:215-217.
8. Sakai P, Filho FM, Iryia K, et al. An endoscopic technique for resection of small gastrintestinal carcinomas. Gastrointes Endosc 1996;44:65-68.
9. Fleischer DE, Wang GQ, Dawsey S, et al. Tissue band ligation followed by snare resection (band and snare): a new technique for tissue adquisition in the esophagus. Gastrointest Endosc 1996;44:68-72.
10. Ell, C, May A, Gossner L, et al. Endoscopic mucosl resectin of early cancer and high-grade dysplasia in Barrrett's esophagus. Gastroenterology 2000;118:670-677.
11. Ottenjam R, Lux G, Henke M, et al. Big particle biopsy. Endoscopy 1973;5:139-143.
12. Deyhle P, Sulser H, Sauberli H. Endoscopic snare ectomy of an early gastric cancer: a therapeutic method? Endoscopy 1974;6:195-198.
13. AJCC Cancer Staging Manual (Ed 3). Philadelphia, PA: Lippincott-Raven, 1997.

In early adenocarcinomas, are endoscopic ultrasonography findings of value for the indications of endoscopic mucosal resection?

H. Inoue, K. Nagai, T. Kawano, T. Iwai, M. Endo (Tokyo)

Barrett's epithelium has been highlighted because of its high potential risk of carcinogenesis, compared with normal squamous epithelium. Therefore once intestinalized mucosa is detected in distal tubular esophagus, multiple biopsies and periodical follow-up endoscopy are strongly recommended. When adenocarcinoma or high-grade dysplasia (HGD) is identified, esophagectomy has been recommended as the first choice of treatment.

On the other hand, technique of endoscopic mucosal resection (EMR) has already been established and applied successfully to a large number of squamous cell esophageal carcinomas [1]. EMR is now regarded to be technically feasible and a potentially safe procedure.

In this preliminary study, we applied EMR to resect the short segment Barrett's mucosa or carcinoma on Barrett's mucosa, intending not only to perform a total biopsy, but also a curative resection for Barrett's cancer.

Patients and methods

Four cases underwent EMR, two cases of Barrett's cancer (T1a), and two cases of short segment Barrett's mucosa. As a method for mucosal resection, the EMRT (transparent tube) and EMRC (cap-fitted endoscope) procedures [2, 3] were applied. Technical details of the procedures are equal to the published reports, with 200,000 diluted epinephrine saline solution (10% epinephrine 0.5 ml and normal saline solution 100 ml) injected in the submucosa.

After mucosal resection, proton-pump inhibitors were prescribed for one month, followed by another one month administration of H_2 antagonist in case 2, 3 and 4. Antibiotics were administered intravenously on the first two days, and then continued perorally during 14 days. In all cases endoscopic follow-up with biopsy was carried out each month during the first 3 months and then continued every 6 months.

Results

In 1989, the first case of a T1a cancer on Barrett's esophagus (0-IIa) was successfully treated by EMR. Eleven years later no recurrence was proved. The second case patient with T1a cancer on Barrett's esophagus (0-IIc) underwent EMR. In the two other cases, the short segment Barrett's mucosa was totally resected, leaving almost half circumferential artificial ulcer. Prior to resection of the Barrett's mucosa, more than 20 ml epinephrine-added saline (from 15 to 30 ml, average 22) was submucosally injected in each case. Lifing of Barrett's mucosa was observed in all cases by submucosal injection. In the third and fourth cases, short segment Barrett's mucosa was completely resected by two cauterizations, leaving half circumferential ulcer. In the second case, three cauterizations were necessary to resect the whole Barrett mucosa. No bleeding and no muscle injury were encountered. The whole EMR procedure was carried out within thirty minutes in each case under intravenous anesthesia with diazepam or midazoram. Two hours after the procedure, patients started drinking cold water, and on the following day, normal diet was started. Antibiotics were administered intravanously for two days, followed by peroral administration. Anti-acid drugs were also given according to the protocol.

After EMR, one out of four patients expressed no particular complaint, and the others only mild dull retrosternal pain.

The first endoscopic check-up of artificial ulcer was carried out on the first or second postoperative day. Ulcers were covered by white coat with neither bleeding nor stricture. One month after EMR, they healed with longitudinal linear scar covered by normal squamous epithelium in an acid suppressive environment. During the follow-up period, no residual columnar epithelium or cancer were identified.

Discussion

How to ablate Barrett's epithelium is one of the challenging decisions for the gastroenterologist. Endoscopic ablation, including laser treatment, is now considered to be a generally accepted procedure. Sampliner *et al.* reported on 10 patients with Barrett's esophagus who were treated with one-half circumferential ablation using multipolar electrocoagulation with replacement of the mucosa by a new squamous epithelium under acid suppressive condition [4]. The resected area was successfully recovered by squamous epithelium, but residual intestinal metaplasia (IM) was identified beneath the new squamous epithelium in two patients. In Barham's experience, glandular epithelium underlying the areas of regeneration of squamous epithelium was also observed in 11 of 16 patients (69%). Overholt *et al.* treated 36 patients with dysplasia or early cancer with photodynamic therapy. These lesions were successfully ablated in 29 of 36 patients (81%) and Barrett's epithelium was completely ablated in 10 of 36 (28%). During the follow-up period, one patient developed adenocarcinoma underneath the new squamous epithelium after being treated for HGD [5]. IM on esophagal glandular epithelium, originally situated deep in the submucosal layer, could not be destroyed by mucosal-surface ablation alone, and may still remain beneath the regenerated new squamous epithelium. These reports suggest that superficial epithelial ablation might not be satisfactory for treating Barrett's esophagus.

Compared to those ablation therapies, EMR can directly resect full-thickness mucosa including epithelium, lamina propria, muscularis mucosa and 2/3 of submucosal layer. Esophageal glands are totally involved in the resected specimen, and this fact can strengthen the concept that EMR may be a more appropriate treatment modality for eradication of Barrett's epithelium.

The other major advantage of EMR is the obtention of a specimen which allows for further histopathological evaluation. If cancer and submucosal layer or lymphatic vessels involvement is shown by microscopic observation, additional surgery with lymph-node dissection will be recommended. In our experiences of EMR for 150 cases of squamous cell carcinoma, surgical resection was actually performed in two cases of submucosal cancer.

The first experience of EMR for adenocarcinoma on short segment Barrett's mucosa was reported by the authors in 1990 [2]. This patient is still in life with no evidence of cancer recurrence.

Our experience is still of a limited number of cases, but endoscopic resection of Barrett's mucosa is considered to be a potentially feasible technique. Application of EMR for Barrett's esophagus deserves to be evaluated by further studies.

References

1. Inoue H, Tani M, Nagai K, et al. Treatment of esophageal and gastric tumors. Endoscopy 1999;31:47-55.
2. Inoue H, Endo M. Endoscopic esophageal mucosal resection using a transparent tube. Surg Endosc 1990;4:198-201.
3. Inoue H, Takeshita K, Hori H, et al. Endoscopic mucosal resection with a cap-fitted pan endoscope for esophagus, stomach and colon mucosal lesions. Gastrointest Endosc 1993;39:58-62.
4. Sampliner RE. Practice guidelines on the diagnosis, surveillance, and therapy of Barrett's esophagus. Am J Gastroenterol 1998;93:1028-1032.
5. Overholt BF, Panjehpour M. Barrett's esophagus: photodynamic therapy for ablation of dysplasia, reduction of specialized mucosa, and treatment of superficial esophageal cancer. Gastrointest Endosc 1995;42:64-70.

P. Spinelli (Milan)

Barrett's esophagus is a sequela of chronic injury due to gastroesophageal reflux. It has been established that Barrett's esophagus is a precancerous condition with an increased risk of development of esophageal adenocarcinoma [1]. Patients with specialized columnar epithelium have a 30- to 52-fold increase in developing esophageal cancer. Data on the incidence of malignant transformation range from 1 of 46 to 1 of 441 patients/years [2].

Barrett's patients should undergo regular endoscopic and histologic follow-up in order to detect high-grade dysplasia (HGD) or early adenocarcinoma.

The management of patients with HGD is still debatable. It has been reported that not every patient with this condition will develop adenocarcinoma [3]. On the other hand, 11% to 67% of patients with HGD showed foci of simultaneous adenocarcinoma in the resected specimen [4]. Even an aggressive endoscopic biopsy protocol, cannot differentiate HGD from early invasive adenocarcinoma [5]. Dysplastic areas are scattered in the mucosa and can be easily overlooked.

Esophageal resection has been recommended in patients with HGD, However, even in referral centers, surgery has mortality rates ranging form 3% to 5% in patients with early adenocarcinoma and HGD [6, 7].

Neoplastic progression usually occurs in elderly patients and in this group the risk of esophagectomy is higher. For this reason, until now, surveillance endoscopy was not recommended for patients unfit for surgery. The development of minimally invasive endoscopic therapy of Barrett's esophagus would change the fate of these patients.

Several endoscopic techniques have been developed to ablate the mucosa: Nd:YAG laser, argon plasma coagulator photodynamic therapy (PDT). However, their main disadvantages include the need of multiple sessions and the impossibility to perform an histologic evaluation, with the risk of missing an invasive cancer [8].

Data derived from Japanese literature, focusing on endoscopic mucosal resection (EMR) of early gastric cancers, have shown that patients with type I lesions smaller than 20 mm in diameter, and type I-IIa, IIb, IIc $\leq$ 10 mm have a 5-year survival ranging between 80% and 95% [9].

It has also been reported that the lymph node metastases rate in Barrett's esophagus patients with early adenocarcinoma is 0% and 1% in patients with squamous cell carcinoma of the mucosal type [10].

The aim of this short review is to summarize the current methods of endoscopic ablation in patients with HGD and early adenocarcinoma in Barrett's esophagus.

Thermal ablation

Thermal ablation can be performed by using Nd:YAG laser and potassium titanyl phosphate (KTP) laser. The depth of the necrosis depends on the characteristics of laser. The advantage of laser treatment is the possibility to destroy tissue in a "paint-brush" way, better than thermal contact methods.

KTP laser, with a power density ranging from 12 to 18 Watts, allows the selective destruction of mucosa. This would avoid lesions to the muscularis propria and the onset of iatrogenic stenoses. Gossner *et al.* [11] reported the first clinical experience in 4 patients with HGD and 2 with early adenocarcinoma. The laser treatment was associated with proton pump inhibitor therapy (80 mg omeprazole daily). An average of 2.4 sessions were carried out. A successful response was observed in all patients and no complications occurred. Specialized intestinal metaplasia was detected at histology underneath the normal squamous epithelium. The authors recommend the use of this technique in patients with short dysplastic Barrett's segments.

The number of patients treated with Nd:YAG laser is limited. The results are disappointing as 5 (29%) out of 17 patients with Barrett's esophagus, had residual areas of Barrett's esophagus during the follow-up. This type of laser has also been used to obtain reversal of columnar epithelium in patients without HGD. A recent study showed that only 2 out of 11 patients had remnants of specialized columnar epithelium, after a follow-up of two years [4].

Chemical ablation

PDT involves the administration of a photosensitizer which accumulates in premalignant and malignant tissues. The photoactivation by a laser light produces cytotoxic singlet oxygen that destroys the target tissue. PDT is performed by administrating intravenously an hematoporphyrin derivative (Photofrin®), followed by the exposure to a 630 nm wavelength after 48 hours. Unfortunately, the drug causes skin photosensitivity lasting for 4 to 6 weeks. Complications, like esophageal stenoses, transient dyspnea and chest pain, can occur [12].

The largest series has been reported by Overholt *et al.* [13]. They treated 100 patients with dysplasia in Barrett's esophagus. Among them, 11 had superficial cancer (T1 and T2). In 84 patients Nd:YAG laser was used to ablate residual areas of metaplastic epithelium. A complete reversal of the columnar epithelium was observed in 43% of patients. Ten out of 13 cases of early adenocarcinoma were healed and dysplasia disappeared in 78 patients. In 3 patients a progression of subsquamous specialized columnar epithelium to HGD or cancer occurred after 6, 18 and 22 months after PDT. Stenoses have been reported in 34% of patients and repeated bougienage was necessary.

A different photosensitizer, 5-aminolevulinic acid (5-ALA), has been used. The advantages are represented by its rapid clearance with a reduction of the sun sensitivity and its accumulation in the mucosa. The latter characteristic would avoid the onset of esophageal strictures [14].

Gossner *et al.* [15] used ALA in 32 patients with HGD (10 patients) and superficial cancer (22 patients). Complete regression was obtained in patients with lesions less than 2 mm in thickness. During the follow-up (mean 9.9 months), subsquamous specialized columnar epithelium was detected in two patients. No major complications occurred.

Endoscopic mucosal resection

EMR has gained popularity in the treatment of early cancers of the gastrointestinal tract. The technique has been developed by Japanese endoscopists and its application in the Western countries is not widespread. EMR provides a complete specimen, permitting a more confident diagnosis of the depth and extension of the neoplastic lesion. The ability to gain superior histologic sampling is one of the prime driving forces behind refining EMR. Strip-biopsy or EMR has been refined, but problems still remain. The depth of the resection cannot be tailored properly and a risk of deep thermal injury, causing scarring, remain. Pre-injection with saline avoids penetration of thermal energy transmurally, and reduces major complications [16, 17].

EMR can be performed according three techniques: "lift-and-cut", "suck-and-cut", and with the variceal ligating device which is used to create an artificial polyp.

"Lift-and-cut" consists in injecting a solution into the submucosa, deep to the lesion. The submucosal fluid cushion minimizes thermal damage and facilitates grasping of the targeted tissue. The simultaneous use of a grasping forceps allows a correct placement of the snare around the mucosa. This requires the use of a double-channel instrument which can make the resection cumbersome. In some areas, such as upper lesser curve and the antrum of the stomach, the submucosal injection does not create an adequate bleb and the lesion cannot be snared properly. Recently, the endoscopic resection of gastric and esophageal tumors without submucosal injection has been reported. The resection of gastric cancers was unsuccessful in patients with lesions larger than 20 mm, with submucosal infiltration, in those showing depressed-type cancer greater than 10 mm, and ulcerated tumors [18, 19].

Using an esophageal variceal ligation device similar to that used for varices can perform mucosectomy. An artificial polyp is created and the resection can be performed with a standard polypectomy snare. It has been used for minute gastric cancers (5 mm) with the diameter of the resected mucosa ranging from 10 to 15 mm [20].

Torii *et al.* [21] proposed endoscopic aspiration mucosectomy ("suck-and-cut"). It consists of aspirating a selected area into a plastic cap fixed at the tip of the endoscope and cutting it with a snare fixed outside of the cap. A complete resection was obtained in 81.8% of patients with early gastric cancer. One out of 24 patients had a perforation. To avoid perforation, the authors recommend endoscopic ultrasonography (EUS) after the submucosal injection in order to evaluate the effect of the solution between the wall layers.

Adding a gutter distally and on the inside of the cap has modified the transparent plastic cap. This allows passage of a snare through the biopsy channel and deployment of the snare before the mucosal aspiration. After the resection, aspirating it inside the cap retrieves the specimen. The therapeutic results are satisfactory with a negligible complication rate [22]. Takeshita *et al.* [23] performed EMR in 56 patients with early esophageal cancer, in whom the lesions were less than 20 mm and involved one third of the circumference. No complications were recorded and complete healing was observed one month later.

Recently, Ell *et al.* [24] reported their experience of EMR in patients with early cancer and HGD in Barrett's esophagus. EMR was performed in 61 patients with early adenocarcinoma and 3 with HGD. Thirty-five patients with type I (polypoid) lesions $\leq$ 20 mm in diameter were treated with the polypectomy technique after submucosal injection of diluted epinephrine solution. The remaining 29 patients with types II (a,b,c,) and III (ulcerated) lesions > 20 mm were treated using the variceal ligation device. Complete remission was achieved in 97% of the patients with smaller lesions and in 59% of the remaining patients. Active bleeding immediately after the EMR, occurred in one patient. However, it was controlled endoscopically.

Combination of EMR and PDT is an attractive therapy for Barrett's esophagus patients with macroscopic dysplastic lesions. Preliminary EMR of the dysplastic lesion permits an adequate histologic examination and may facilitate subsequent PDT. PDT is essential in eliminating invisible multiple dysplastic areas and in reducing the risk of local recurrence.Our group [25] has been the first to evaluate this therapy for endoscopically detectable HGD lesions in 4 patients with Barrett's esophagus. EMR was performed by polypectomy snare excision of grossly abnormal tissue. Patients underwent EUS staging prior to EMR. PDT was performed 5 weeks after EMR with porfimer sodium (Photofrin®)

(2mg/kg i.v.) using 630 nm monochromatic light. All patients received 40 mg of omeprazole daily following PDT. The mean Barrett's esophagus length was 9.2 cm (range 8-11 cm). Dysplastic lesions were nodular, with a diameter from 5 to 13 mm. Two patients had two lesions. Combined treatment (EMR + PDT) was initially performed in all patients. The mean follow-up was 15 (range 4-24) months. Large areas of squamous re-epithelialization were detected in all patients. Two patients had macroscopic sessile regrowth of HGD at the resection site, and underwent combination re-treatment. In one patient EMR was not possible and the lesion was destroyed with monopolar electrocoagulation prior to PDT.

In conclusion, the results of EMR in Barrett's patients with HGD and early adenocarcinoma are encouraging. However, further studies involving a larger number of patients, with a long-term follow-up, are mandatory in order to establish the clinical value of the technique.

References

1. Spechler SJ, Goyal RK. Barrett's esophagus. N Engl J Med 1986;315:362-371.
2. Hameeteman W, Tytgat GNJ, Houthoff HJ, van den Tweel JG. Barrett's esophagus: development of dysplasia and adenocarcinoma. Gastroenterology 1989;96:1249-1256.
3. Levine DS, Haggitt RC, Irvine S, et al. Natural history of high-grade dysplasia in Barrett's esophagus. Gastroenterology 1996;110:A550.
4. Van den Boogert J, van Hillegersberg R, Siersema PD, de Bruin RWF, Tilanus HW. Endoscopic ablation therapy for Barrett's esophagus with high-grade dysplasia: a review. Am J Gastroenterol 1999;94:1153-1160.
5. Levine DS, Haggitt RC, Blount PL, et al. An endoscopic biopsy protocol can differentiate high-grade dysplasia from early adenocarcinoma in Barrett's esophagus. Gastroenterology 1993;105:105:40-50.
6. Heitmiller RF, Redmond M, Hamilton SR. Barrett's esophagus with high-grade dyplasia: an indication for prophylactic esophagectomy. Ann Surg 1996;224:66-71.
7. Hölscher AH, Bollschweller E, Schroder W, Gutschow C, Siewert JR. Prognostic differences between early squamous cell and adenocarcinoma of the esophagus. Dis Esophagus 1997;10:179-184.
8. Lim KN, Waring PJ, Saidi R. Therapeutic options in patients with Barrett's esophagus. Dig Dis 1999;17:145-152.
9. Kojima T, Parra-Blanco A, Takahashi H, Fujita R. Outcome of endoscopic mucosal resection for early gastric cancer: review of the Japanese literature. Gastrointest Endosc 1998;48:550-555.
10. Hölscher AH, Bollschweller E, Schneider PM, Siewert JR. Prognosis of early esophageal cancer: comparison between adeno- and squamous cell carcinoma. Cancer 1995;76:178-186.
11. Gossner L, May A, Stolte M, Seitz G, Hahn EG, Ell C. KTP laser destruction of dysplasia and early cancer in columnar-lined Barrett's esophagus. Gastrointest Endosc 1999;49:8-12.
12. Overholt BF, Panjehpour M. Photodynamic therapy in Barrett's esophagus. J Clin Laser Med Surg 1996;14:245-249.
13. Overholt BF, Panjehpour M, Haydek JM. Photodynamic therapy for Barrett's esophagus: follow-up in 100 patients. Gastrointest Endosc 1999;49:1-7.
14. Barr H, Shepherd NA, Dix A, et al. Eradication of high-grade dysplasia in columnar-lined (Barrett's) esophagus by photodynamic therapy with endogenously generated protoporphyrin IX. Lancet 1996;348:584-585.
15. Gossner L, Stolte M, Sroka R, et al. Photodynamic ablation of high-grade dysplasia and early cancer in Barrett's esophagus by means of 5-aminolevulinic acid. Gastroenterology 1998;114:448-455.
16. Karita m, Tada M, Okita K. The successive strip biopsy partial resection technique for large early gastric and colon cancers. Gastrointest Endosc 1992;38:174-178.
17. Shirai M, Nakamura T, Matsuda A, Ito Y, Kobayashi S. Safer colonoscopic polypectomy with local submucosal injection of hypertonic saline-epinephrine solution. Am J Gastroenterol 1994;89:334-338.
18. Iishi H, Tatsuta M, Yano H, Narahara H, Iseki K, Ishiguro S. More effective endoscopic resection with a two-channel colonoscope for carcinoid tumors of the rectum. Dis Colon Rectum 1996;39:1438-1439.
19. Endo M. Endoscopic resection as local treatment of mucosal cancer of the esophagus. Endoscopy 1993;25:672-674.
20. Lee DK, Lee SW, Kwon SO, Jang WI, Shim YH, Cho MY. Endoscopic mucosectomy using an esophageal variceal ligation device for minute gastric cancer. Endoscopy 1996;28:386-389.
21. Torii A, Sakai M, Kajiyama T, Kishimoto H, Kin G, Inoue K, Koizumi T, Ueda S, Okuma M. Endoscopic aspiration mucosectomy as curative endoscopic surgery: analysis of 24 cases of early gastric cancer. Gastrointest Endosc 1995;42:475-479.

22. Tada M, Inoue H, Yabata E, Okabe S, Endo M. Feasibility of the transparent cap-fitted colonoscope for screening and mucosal resection. Dis Colon Rectum 1997;40:618-621.
23. Takeshita K, Tani M, Inoue H, Saeki I, Hayashi S, Honda T, Kando F, Saito N, Endo M. Endoscopic treatment of early esophageal or gastric cancer. Gut 1997;40:123-127.
24. Ell C, May C, Gossner L, et al. Endoscopic mucosal resection of early cancer and high-grade dysplasia in Barrett's esophagus. Gastroenterology 2000;118:670-677.
25. P.Spinelli, M.Conio, A.Mancini, M.Falsitta, F.De Paoli, A.Schicchi. The association of endoscopic mucosal resection and photodynamic therapy in the treatment of nodular dysplastic areas arising in Barrett's esophagus. Gastrointest Endosc 2000;51:A3475.

Is lymphadenectomy necessary for intramucosal carcinoma?

S.R. DeMeester (Los Angeles)

The value of lymphadenectomy in patients with epithelial cancers has been questioned, but it is steadily becoming recognized as an important component of surgical treatment for these patients. As in other epithelial cancers, surgical resection with extended lymphadenectomy can be curative in patients with esophageal carcinoma, even when multiple lymph glands are involved. This indicates that esophageal carcinoma is not a systemic disease in everyone at the time of diagnosis, and that in a subset of patients resection of the primary tumor with lymphadenectomy is appropriate, curative therapy.

Barrett's esophagus, or intestinalized columnar mucosa within the esophagus occurs as a consequence of long-standing gastroesophageal reflux. Barrett's esophagus is premalignant, and Barrett's has been demonstrated to progress to dysplasia and adenocarcinoma. Consequently, it is generally recommended that patients with Barrett's esophagus undergo surveillance endoscopies with biopsies to watch for progression. In those patients found to have progression there is a unique opportunity to intervene and alter the natural history of this disease. The opportunity exists to cure patients unequivocally prior to the development of invasive adenocarcinoma, and prior to the opportunity for lymph node or systemic metastases to occur.

Important issues in regard to intervention include at what point intervention should be recommended, and what intervention represents the best therapy for these patients. Implicit in these two questions are such factors as the rapidity of development of invasive cancer in a patient with Barrett's esophagus, the morbidity and mortality of the proposed intervention, and the quality of life after the intervention. Obviously, an intervention is only worthwhile if the mortality rate of the intervention is less than the mortality rate for untreated patients. The greater the divergence in mortality rates in favor of the intervention, the less important issues such as morbidity and quality of life become. Conversely, as the mortality rate for the intervention approaches that of the untreated patient, the more important quality of life and morbidity rates become.

One of the troubling aspects of Barrett's esophagus with high-grade dysplasia (HGD) is our imprecise understanding of the natural history of this condition. We and others have demonstrated that the majority of patients with HGD will ultimately, either on either additional biopsies or analysis of the resected surgical specimen, be found to have an area of invasive adenocarcinoma [1, 2]. However, in these patients without a visible lesion the likelihood of lymphatic metastases is extremely small. We found that in 10 patients with occult esophageal cancer only a single lymph node out of 370 analyzed by both routine histology and immunohistochemistry contained tumor 51] Likewise, Rice *et al.* found that only 1 of 38 patients (2.6%) with intramucosal esophageal cancer had lymph node metastases [3]. Consequently, the possibility of lymph node metastases exists once the tumor has invaded the lamina propria; however, compared to tumors that penetrate into the submucosa the likelihood of lymph node metastases is small.

Given the low likelihood of lymph node metastases in these patients and the excellent prognosis for surgical cure of their cancer, the focus should be on minimizing morbidity and maximizing quality of life. The esophagus should be removed to ensure that the primary tumor is completely eliminated, but the resection should be done in the least invasive fashion possible. In our experience the least invasive method of esophagectomy is a stripping procedure. This can be done in such a fashion that the vagal nerves are preserved. A limited analysis of nodes along the lesser curve can be performed while the tumor is pathologically examined to determine precisely the depth of invasion. We have found that if lymph node metastases are present in patients with intramucosal tumors they occur along the lesser curve. If the tumor is found to have penetrated into the submucosa the likelihood of lymph node metastases increases to 50%, and a formal lymphadenectomy should be performed to maximize the likelihood of cure for the patient [4]. In patients with an expectation of cure or prolonged survival our preferred method of reconstruction is with an isoperistaltic left colon graft. This is required in patients undergoing vagal-sparing esophagectomy. All anastomoses are performed in the neck. This is particularly important when using a gastric pull-up to prevent the development of Barrett's above the esophagogastric anastomosis long-term.

If the surgeon does not perform a vagal-sparing esophagectomy, there is no reason not to perform an intra-abdominal lymphadenectomy, as it adds little or no morbidity to the procedure. However, postoperative alimentation and quality of life are likely compromised by this approach. Alternative therapies such as photodynamic therapy often leave residual Barrett's, have a high stricture rate, and risk incomplete or inadequate treatment for these early, curable tumors. Consequently, with excellent postoperative quality of life, and low operative morbidity and mortality, vagal-sparing esophagectomy should become the standard treatment for this disease.

References

1. Nigro JJ, et al. Occult esophageal adenocarcinoma: extent of disease and implications for effective therapy. Ann Surg 1999;230:433-440.
2. Ferguson MK, Naunheim KS. Resection for Barrett's mucosa with high-grade dysplasia: implications for prophylactic photodynamic therapy. J Thorac Cardiovasc Surg 1997;114:824-829.
3. Rice TW, Zuccaro G Jr, Adelstein DJ, Rybicki LA, Blackstone EH, Goldblum JR. Esophageal carcinoma: depth of tumor invasion is predictive of regional lymph node status. Ann Thorac Surg 1998;65:787-792.
4. Nigro JJ, et al. Prevalence and location of nodal metastases in distal esophageal adenocarcinoma confined to the wall:implications for therapy. J Thorac Cardiovasc Surg 1999;117(1):16-25.

What is the clinical impact of micrometastases in esophageal adenocarcinoma?

G.C. O'Sullivan, D. Maguire, J.K. Collins, F. Shanahan (Cork)

Despite optimal treatment, including multimodal and radical surgical therapy, most patients with clinically manifest esophagogastric cancer die from metastatic disease within three years of presentation [1]. Their outcome is predetermined by the presence of widespread, occult metastatic cancer cells that have disseminated prior to treatment and are in many patients chemoresistant [2]. In 90% of patients who are subjected to curative excisional surgery for esophageal cancer, analysis of haemopoietic bone marrow reveals metastatic cell dissemination. This asymptomatic clinical state, after optimal locoregional therapy, is known as minimal residual disease and is represented by either isolated or microaggregates of malignant tumor cells which have the potential to establish overt metastases. This explains the frequent early tumor recurrences that occur following radical resection.

Bone marrow micrometastases

Cells derived from esophageal adenocarcinomas retain expression of epithelial cell-specific proteins (cytokeratins and carcinoembryonic antigen) that are not constitutively expressed in bone marrow (derived from the embryonic mesoderm). The finding of such markers in bone marrow indicates the presence of metastatic cells [3]. These cells are usually referred to as micrometastases as they are not otherwise identifiable by conventional microscopy and radiology. Strategies to identify these micrometastases within marrow include morphological detection by immunohistochemical staining (*Figure 1*), antibody-based methods by flow cytometry and gene expression techniques by reverse transcriptase-polymerase-chain reaction. These analytic techniques have been validated with false positive identification in less than 2% of cases [3, 4]. The incidence of false negative analysis is unknown but this may be reduced by concurrent examination for a number of markers and by improved marrow sampling (two or more sites). Currently, analysis of marrow from a resected segment of rib obtained at thoracotomy (prior to manipulation of the tumor) is the "gold standard" for detecting micrometastases in esophageal cancer [2].

Biology of micrometastases

The finding of micrometastases in bone marrow of patients with adenocarcinoma of the esophagus is an independent negative prognostic indicator. The viability and proliferative capacity of micrometastases have been confirmed *in vitro* using combinations of growth factors in the presence of extracellular matrix proteins [3]. In patients with esophageal adenocarcinoma, tumor cell lines may be generated from rib marrow aspirates. These cell lines establish xenografts when transferred to immunodeficient athymic nude mice, confirming tumorogenicity [2].

The finding of bone marrow micrometastases in the preoperative setting does not universally predict poor outcome. Some micrometastatic cells are possibly transitory and are unable to establish at a secondary site or unable to escape destruction by the immune system, or remain in a dormant state. A study of bone marrow from patients with esophageal adenocarcinoma before and six months after "curative" surgery showed that occasional patients were able to clear their marrow of metastatic cells, but persistence of the cells was noted in most and carried a high risk of developing overt metastatic disease within the subsequent months [5]. The majority of these patients with persistent micrometastases developed overt disease on follow-up but a small number of long-term survivors emerged suggesting dormant disease in some. Often in this context recurrent disease is precipitated by systemic events such as infection, surgery, or immunesuppression suggesting loss of biological control by inhibition of immune containment or by stimulation of pro-tumorigenic mechanisms such as angiogenesis or phenotypic aggressiveness. It is likely that the transition from dormancy to progressive disease involves to some degree cellular genetic changes, angiogenic stimulation and immune evasion. Thus, sequential analysis of bone marrow allows a precise diagnosis of dormancy and study of relevant gene expression and determination of the cell cycle and proliferative status of the metastatic cells.

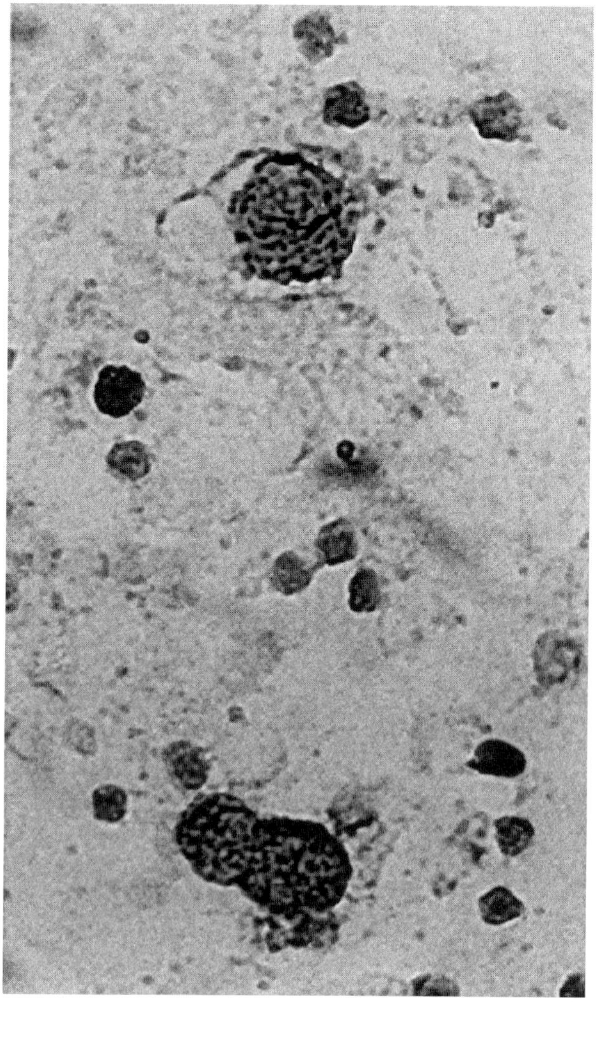

Figure 1. This is an example of tumor cells in a bone marrow aspirate from a patient with esophageal adenocarcinoma. Alkaline phosphatase anti-alkaline phosphatase staining for cytokeratin 18 demonstrates hyperchromatic tumor cells staining positive (red). (See page VIII for colour figure).

Targets for development of effective systemic therapy

Most cells within the primary tumor are terminally differentiated, and do not possess the intrinsic capabilities necessary for dissemination and propagation. Cells that disseminate have the inherent capability to detach from the primary growth, travel through extracellular matrix and basement membrane into the local microvasculature, survive transit in the circulation, and exit by attaching and extravasating through the endothelium at another site [2, 3]. This complex process involves several interdependent steps regulated by cascades of cytokines, chemokines, growth factors and matrix metalloproteinases [3, 6, 7]. The presence of viable micrometastatic deposits in tissues implies dissemination of cancer cells with the facility for independent survival and growth [2]. These are most likely metastatic stem cells and are the appropriate targets for systemic therapy.

Spread of esophagogastric cancer

Traditionally, esophagogastric cancers have been thought to spread sequentially from mucosa to the esophageal wall, to the regional lymph-nodes and lastly systemically. This model has dominated patient care from preoperative staging investigations, to endeavours at disease control. In the absence of overt metastatic disease, by conventional staging investigations, the lymph node status has been used as a "proxy" indicator of systemic spread, but the majority of patients with node-negative cancer also die of metastases. This suggests that haematogenous dissemination may have occurred independent of lymphogenous spread. This has recently been confirmed by the detection of micrometastases in bone marrow samples from resected rib segments of patients with node negative cancers [2]. Metastatic cells in the marrow of these patients were viable, capable of proliferation, grew independently in tissue culture and formed malignant tumors when injected into immunocompromised mice. Thus, both clinical experience and bone marrow analysis suggest that most patients have residual disease after resection of the primary cancer and the regional lymph nodes and that lymph node status alone is not an accurate marker for systemic spread [1, 2].

Implications for neoadjuvant therapy

To date, improvements in survival from multimodal programs have been modest, with most patients succumbing to metastases [8-10]. There is general acceptance that for chemotherapy or chemoradiotherapy to be effective against esophagogastric cancer it must be given in a neoadjuvant setting, before tumor vascularity and patient fitness are compromised by excisional surgery. The choice of chemotherapeutic agents needs to be determined by the responses of both the primary tumor and the sensitivity/resistance of disseminated metastatic cells. In a recent large scale clinical trial of fluoruracil and platinum the clinical response rate of the primary tumor was not reflected in improved survival [11]. That this was due to resistance of minimal residual disease or micrometastases to the chemotherapeutic agents has been confirmed by the finding of viable tumor cells in bone marrow of patients who received similar treatment [2]. The responsiveness to neoadjuvant therapy should be assessed at the level of micrometastases (accessible in bone marrow) rather than by measurements of shrinkage of primary tumors where the terminally differentiated cells may be induced to die whilst the metastatic stem cells are chemo-resistant and remain viable.

Towards the control of minimal residual disease

The control of minimal residual disease is potentially a realisable goal. Repeated access of bone marrow will help define minimal residual disease status, responsiveness to therapy, and provide a source of micrometastases for genetic modification and manufacture of tumor-specific vaccines. Until more specific antitumor drugs are developed, the residual disease burden in most patients can only be controlled by ablation of the primary tumor, and adjuvant biological approaches at general host and metastatic cell level. This will involve the development of means to control the imunosuppressive and angiogenic responses to surgical trauma and infection.

Recent successes in murine models suggest that effective tumor specific vaccines can be developed for even MHC negative cancers without prior antigen isolation [13]. Data from studies utilising dendritic cells that were primed *in vitro* by fusion with tumor cells or by pulsing with RNA or membrane components have also been encouraging. Genetic modification of tumor cells to secrete GMCSF and to express the B7 co-stimulatory molecule, permit undefined tumor antigen presentation by dendritic cells, and tumor control by specific natural killer cells. The clinical application of these vaccines is now feasible with the culture of metastatic cell lines from bone marrow aspirates.

Conclusions

Conventional methods for assessment of tumor load understage patients. Bone marrow micrometastases are viable cells with proliferative and tumorigenic potential. Persistence of micrometastases following "curative" surgery indicates minimal residual disease that also carries a poor prognosis, whereas clearance of marrow micrometastases is associated with a favourable outcome.

Since the outcome of patients with esophagogastric and other cancers is determined by the fate of disseminated micrometases, it is time to direct attention to the study of these cells. This may offer the best hope for development of rational treatments which can be based on biological control mechanisms of dormancy or clearance. Whether specific immune, anti-angiogenic or chemo/radiotherapeutic strategies are adopted, the study of systemic micrometastatic disease in esophageal cancer will be critical to predict and assess clinical responsiveness.

References

1. Bytzer P, Christensen PB, Damkier P, Vinding K, Seersholm N. Adenocarcinoma of esophagus and Barrett's esophagus: a population based study. Am J Gastroenterology 1999;94:86-91.
2. O'Sullivan G, Sheahan D, Clarke A, Stuart R, Walsh T, Kelly J, Kiely MD, Collins JK, Shanahan F. Micrometastases in esophagogastric cancer: high detection rate in resected rib segments. Gastroenterology 1999;116:543-548.
3. Maguire D, O'Sullivan GC, Collins JK, Morgan J, Shanahan F. Bone marrow micrometastases and gastrointestinal cancer detection and significance. Am J Gastroenterol 2000;95:1644-1651.

4. Schlimok G, Funke I, Pantel K, Strobel F, Lindemann F, Witte J, Reithmüller G Micrometastatic tumour cells in bone marrow of patients with gastric cancer: methodological aspects of detection and prognostic significance. Eur J Cancer 1991;27(11):1461-1465.
5. O'Sullivan G, Collins JK, Kelly J, Morgan J, Madden M, Shanahan F Micrometastases: marker of metastatic potential or evidence of residual disease Gut 1997;40:512-515.
6. Banks RE, Gearing AJ, Hemmingway IK, Norfolk DR, Perren TJ, Selby PJ. Circulating intercellular adhesion molecule-1 (ICAM-1), E-selectin and vascular cell adhesion molecule-1 (VCAM-1) in human malignancies Br J Cancer 1993;68:122-124.
7. Gearing AJ, Hemingway K, Pigott R, Hughes J, Rees AJ, Cashman SJ. Soluble forms of vascular adhesion molecules E-selectin, ICAM-1, and VCAM-1: pathological significance Ann NY Acad Sci 1992;667:324-331.
8. Altorki NK, Skinner DB. Occult cervical nodal metastases in esophageal cancer: preliminary results of three field lymphadenectomy. J Thorac Cardiovasc Surg 1997;113:540-544.
9. Walsh TN, Noonan N, Hollywood D, Kelly A, Keeling N, Hennessy TPJ. A comparison of multimodal therapy with surgery for esophageal adenocarcinoma. N Engl J Med 1996;335:462-467.
10. Shanahan F, O'Sullivan GC. Progress in treating esophageal adenocarcinoma Gastroenterology 1997;112:1417-1418.
11. Kelsen DP, Ginsberg R, Pajak TF, Sheahan DG, Gunderson L, Mortimer J, Estes N, Haller DG, Ajani J, Kocha W, Minsky BD, Roth JA. Chemotherapy followed by surgery compared with surgery alone for localised esophageal cancer. N Engl J Med 1998;339:1979-1984.
12. Braun, S, Pantel, K, Muller, P. et al. Cytokeratin positive cells in the bone marrow and survival of patients with stage I II or III breast cancer. N Engl J Med 2000;342:525-533.

What long-term results can be expected from laser ablation in adenocarcinomas?

P. Sharma (Kansas City)

Esophageal adenocarcinoma develops through the metaplasia-carcinoma sequence from Barrett's esophagus without dysplasia → low-grade dysplasia (LGD) → high-grade dysplasia (HGD) → adenocarcinoma. The diagnosis of early adenocarcinoma in patients with Barrett's esophagus needs a curative resection. However, given the high morbidity and mortality rates reported with esophagectomy, and the comorbidities frequently present in these older patients – local endoscopic ablative techniques have been utilized for the eradication of early cancer. Moreover, certain patients may not be deemed fit to undergo surgery after a surgical evaluation or may decline esophagectomy.

ND:YAG laser

Barrett's mucosa, including HGD and early adenocarcinoma, can be destroyed by laser photocoagulation. Thermal energy is delivered to the tissue by means of a fiber inserted through the channel of an endoscope and given the greater depth of injury with laser, one of its potential uses is in patients with early Barrett's adenocarcinoma. Patients with documented Barrett's esophagus and early adenocarcinoma who had either refused surgery or were poor candidates for surgery were offered endoscopic therapy of their tumor with Nd:YAG plus electrocoagulation [1]. The patients were treated with 20 mg of omeprazole twice a day and underwent therapy with Nd:YAG laser and multipolar electrocoagulation

Table I. Laser ablation of Barrett's with and without adenocarcinoma.

Author	Laser	n	Mean f/u (months)	Residual IM
Berenson [6]	Argon	10 patients (40 areas)	N/A	17
Salo [5]	Nd:YAG	11	26	–
Meyer [4]	Nd:YAG	19	3	9
Sharma [1]	Nd:YAG	6	41	3
Barham [2]	KTP	16	3-18	11
Gossner [3]	KTP	10	11	0

n: number of patients; f/u: follow-up; IM: intestinal metaplasia

(MPEC). All 6 patients had a complete initial response to therapy. One patient on chronic immunosuppressive therapy had recurrence of the tumor after a 36 month follow-up. The cancer was eliminated in the remaining 5 patients, with 2 having complete reversal of their Barrett's esophagus as well. The patients were followed up for a mean of 3.4 years (range 9-86 months).

Potassium titanyl phosphate laser

Two published reports have utilized potassium titanyl phosphate (KTP) laser for reversal of Barrett's esophagus. Sixteen patients with long segment Barrett's esophagus were treated with KTP laser and 40 mg of omeprazole [2]. Eleven of 16 patients had intestinal metaplasia (IM) underlying squamous mucosa following treatment, whereas 9 demonstrated squamous mucosa regeneration within previous Barrett's glands.

In the second study on KTP, Gossner *et al.* treated 10 patients with Barrett's esophagus including 4 with LGD, 4 with HGD, and 2 with early adenocarcinoma using KTP laser while the patients were maintained on omeprazole 80 mg/day [3]. Dysplasia was eliminated in all 10 patients who were followed for a mean of 10.6 months. Two of the 10 patients showed IM underlying the normal squamous mucosa and no complications were reported in this pilot study.

References

1. Sharma P, Jaffe PE, Bhattacharyya A, Sampliner RE. Laser and multipolar electrocoagulation ablation of early Barrett's aenocarcinoma: long-term follow-up. Gastrointest Endosc 1999;49:442-446.
2. Barham CP, Jones RL, Biddlestone LR, Hardwick RH, Shepherd NA, Barr H. Photothermal laser ablation of Barrett's esophagus: endoscopic and histological evidence of squamous re-epithelialization. Gut 1997;41:281-284.
3. Gossner L, May A, Stolte M, Seitz G, Hahn E, Ell C. KTP laser destruction of dysplasia and early cancer in columnar-lined Barrett's esophagus. Gastrointest Endosc 1999;49:8-12.
4. Meyer B, Boyer S, Nawau G, et al. Nd:YAG laser combined with omeprazole as a treatment of Barrett's esophagus. Preliminary results of a prospective multicenter study. Endoscopy 1996;38:P03.
5. Salo J, Salminen J, Kiviluoto T, Namoander A, Ramo O, Farkkila M, et al. Treatment of Barrett's esophagus by endoscopic laser ablation and antireflux surgery. Ann Surg 1998;227:40-44.
6. Berenson MM, Johnson TD, Markowitz NR, Buchi KN, Samowitz WS. Restoration of squamous mucosa after ablation of Barrett's esophagus epithelium. Gastroenterology 1993;104:1686-1691.

In Barrett's carcinoma, is incipient invasion of the lamina propria the minimal criteria for performing lymph node clearance?

J.E. Hagen (Los Angeles)

The traditional approach to patients with cancer of the esophagus in most centers has included complete removal of the esophagus, with a formal two-field or three-field lymph node dissection. In the past decade, however, Barrett's surveillance programs in the western world, and screening studies in Asia have led to an increase in the number of patients diagnosed with early stage esophageal cancer. At the same time, a number of alternatives to traditional resection have been described, including non-operative techniques such as endoscopic mucosal resection and mucosal ablation and less invasive resection techniques such as the vagal sparing esophagectomy [1]. These developments have lead some to question the need for the type of aggressive surgical approach that has been used in the past [2]. Before these alternative treatments can be accepted, however, it needs to be determined whether or not they effectively deal with the extent of disease present, so as not to compromise the benefits of early detection by incomplete removal. In theory, mucosal ablation and endoscopic mucosal resection should effectively deal with the primary tumor itself, so long as it is truly confined to the mucosa. However, there remains considerable debate regarding the ability of the various techniques to accomplish complete removal of the mucosa, an issue that is important, but will not be discussed further in this article. An equally important but often overlooked question that arises is whether or not these alternatives to standard resections would be expected to deal effectively with the possibility of lymph node involvement. In the case of mucosal ablation and endoscopic mucosal resection the answer is clearly no. When the treatment focuses only on mucosal therapy, any lymph node involvement would result in inadequate therapy. In the case of more limited resections, such as the vagal sparing esophagectomy, the answer is perhaps yes, if it can be shown that the potentially involved nodes are likely to be limited in number, in close proximity to the primary tumor. Therefore, in order to determine circumstances under which it might be appropriate to apply these more limited therapies, the patterns of lymphatic spread and the frequency of nodal involvement in early esophageal adenocarcinoma must be clearly defined. Furthermore, practical reliable means of selecting patients for these treatment options must be developed.

As we investigate the clinical application of these alternatives to standard resection, we can minimize the number of patients who may suffer the consequences of inadequate treatment, by using the lessons of the past as a guide, including observations about the anatomy of the esophagus, and information about the frequency and location of node involvement in esophageal cancer. We also need to look at our ability to accurately diagnose early cancers preoperatively if these new treatments are to be applied clinically.

Esophageal anatomy

The anatomy of the human esophagus is unique amongst hollow organs in the presence of a rich interconnecting network of lymphatic vessels in the lamina propria and especially in the submucosa. These vessels actually outnumber the capillaries in this area [3]. In contrast, in the stomach and intestine, these lymphatic vessels are first encountered in the submucosa, increasing as one progresses more deeply into the esophageal wall. This observation would suggest that a tumor that breaches the basement membrane to any significant extent may be at risk for dissemination to the regional nodes, and that certainly by the time the tumor has reached the muscularis mucosa and the submucosa, lymph node spread would be expected to be fairly common.

Clinical experience with cancer of the esophagus would support the concept that the rich lymphatic network in the mucosa and submucosa would be expected to result in early lymph node spread in patients with superficial esophageal cancer. Rice *et al.* made this point in a study of 54 patients with cancers confined to the mucosa and submucosa of the esophagus [4]. Of these, 19 were *in situ* cancers, 18 were limited to the mucosa (T1 (m)), and 17 invaded into the submucosa (T1(sm)). Overall, 9.3% had positive nodes, with 5.6% of the tumors confined to the mucosa alone having lymph node involvement, compared to positive nodes in 23.5% of the T1-submucosal tumors. As the anatomic studies would predict, lymph node involvement can occur early in cancer of the esophagus.

This initial publication included patients with both squamous cell cancer and adenocarcinoma. In a subsequent publication, looking only at patients with adenocarcinoma, the same group reported 65 T1 tumors, 38 of which were T1(m), and 27 of which were T1(sm) [5]. Overall, 10.8% of the T1 tumors had involved nodes. In this series, 2.6% of the T1(m) tumors had involved nodes, compared to a frequency of node involvement of 22.2% in the T1(sm) group, a difference that was statistically significant.

Our own experience with adenocarcinoma confined to the esophageal wall [6] has been similar. We studied 37 patients, 15 with T1(m) tumors and 12 with T1(sm) tumors (*Table I*). We found a similar 7% prevalence of involved nodes in the intramucosal group, but the frequency of involved nodes in the T1-submucosal group was higher, 50% in our series. The reported high prevalence of lymph node involvement in superficial esophageal adenocarcinoma has led us to the conclusion that invasion of the lamina propria is an important indicator of the possibility of lymph node involvement, which would indicate that a lymph node dissection is advisable.

Table I. Prevalence of lymph node involvement and number of involved nodes in patients undergoing en bloc esophagectomy

Tumor depth	Prevalence of involved nodes	Nb of involved nodes (median, range)
Intramucosal	1/15 (7%)[1]	0 (0-1)
Submucosal	6/12 (50%)[1]	0.5 (0-9)[2]
Intramuscular	8/10(80%)[1]	1.0 (0-6)[2]

1. χ^2 = 14.05, p = 0.00089
2. p < 0.01 *versus* intramucosal group

Role of endoscopic ultrasound

It could be argued that the very low prevalence of node involvement in tumors confined to the mucosa alone does not justify the performance of a lymph node dissection. This may be true if the incidence of node involvement is closer to the 2.2% that Rice *et al.* have reported, but as the frequency of involved nodes approaches 10%, as in our recent series, elimination of a node dissection becomes less defensible. However, from a clinical practice perspective, this may not be an important issue when one considers the difficulty we have in identifying tumors that are limited to the mucosa with presently available techniques.

At present, the best available means of staging esophageal cancer is by endoscopic ultrasound (EUS). *Table II* summarizes the recent series that report on the accuracy of EUS in patients with superficial esophageal cancer. Overall, the accuracy with which we can assess the T status is somewhere between 60 and 92%. However, a closer look at these series reveals that the accuracy of assessment of T status depends heavily on the patient group studied. Groups such as Vickers *et al.* [7] that report the highest accuracy rates tend to have very small numbers of T1 tumors. In contrast, Salminen *et al.* [8] report an accuracy of EUS of only 66%, in their series that included 22% T1 tumors. It would appear that the near-field effect of conventional ultrasound, and the distortion caused by the balloon limit the identification of tumors confined to the mucosa. Even with higher frequency probes that are commonly used in Asia but rarely reported in other parts of the world, the accuracy of assessment of T1 tumors is only about 80% (80.7%) [9]. This is similar to the results reported in superficial gastric cancer, where the accuracy of high frequency ultrasound is only 70%. Clearly if high frequency ultrasound is not used, (and perhaps even if it is), it would appear that EUS cannot reliably tell if the tumor is confined to the mucosa.

Table II. Literature review on the accuracy of endoscopic ultrasound in early esophageal cancer.

Author	Nb of patients	Accuracy	Nb of T1 tumors
Rice (1991)	28	59%	N/S
Peters (1994)	42	85%	5 (12%)
Salminen (1999)	32	65.6%	7 (22%)
Vickers (1998)	50	92%	1 (2%)

Importance of a visible lesion

Since as many as one half of the patients with T1(sm) tumors have involved nodes, and since we cannot at present reliably differentiate between these patients and those with T1(m) disease with EUS, it would appear advisable to recommend surgical resection with lymph node dissection in all patients with early esophageal cancer. However, when a patient presents for Barrett's surveillance and a biopsy shows high-grade dysplasia (HGD) or intramucosal cancer in the absence of a grossly evident tumor mass, the need for a formal lymph node dissection continues to be questioned. The occasional occurrence of serious morbidity (or even mortality) following resection, when the final pathology report shows only dysplasia, prompts consideration of less invasive treatment options. Although EUS has not proven sufficiently reliable to identify candidates in whom it might be safe to eliminate a node dissection in such patients, a recent study from our institution [10] would suggest that a practical approach to this problem might be possible. This approach is based on the appearance of the esophagus at endoscopy as a guide to therapy.

We reviewed our experience with surgical resections performed in patients with endoscopically occult cancers. These patients presented for Barrett's surveillance endoscopy in which a biopsy showed either HGD, or intramucosal cancer. A total of 37 patients were studied. We found that the presence of a visible area of ulceration or nodularity in the Barrett's mucosa was a predictor a more advanced tumor, as well as an indicator of the likelihood of node involvement. In the presence of a visible lesion, 75% of the tumors invaded the submucosa or beyond. In contrast, 88% of the patients with no visible abnormalities in the Barrett's mucosa had tumors that were confined to the lamina propria (*Figure 1*).

The likelihood of node involvement also correlated with the presence or absence of a visible lesion (*Figure 2*). In the presence of a visible lesion, over half of the patients had at least one involved node, compared to a single patient in the group without a visible lesion.

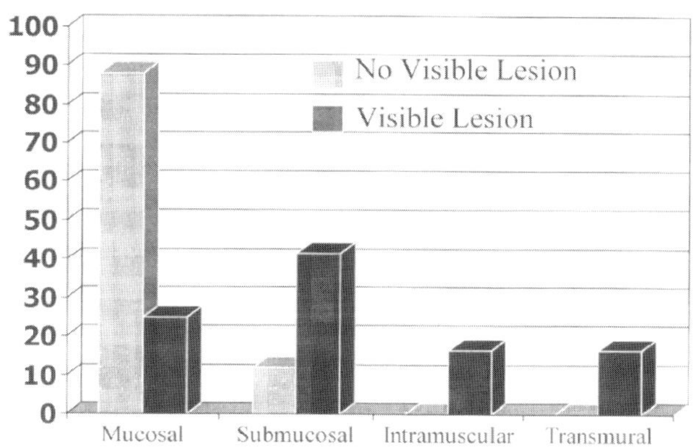

Figure 1. Depth of tumor invasion in patients with and without endoscopically visible lesions on surveillance endoscopy.

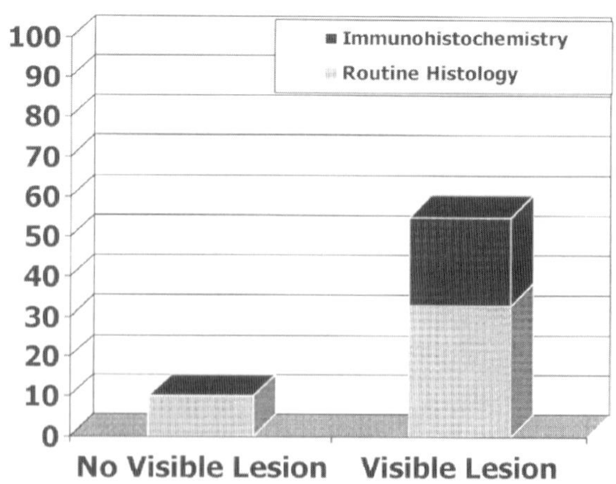

Figure 2. Prevalence of lymph node involvement in patients with and without endoscopically visible lesions on surveillance endoscopy.

These data would suggest that the presence or absence of a visible lesion might be the best way to identify candidates for limited treatment. Until we can develop better methods of identifying tumors that are truly confined to the mucosa, with advancements in imaging techniques, we may be best to learn form the Japanese experience with squamous cell cancer, and use morphology at endoscopy rather than imaging studies to identify these patients.

References

1. Akiyama H, Tsurumaru M, Ono Y, Udagawa H, Kajiyama Y. Esophagectomy without thoracotomy with vagal preservation. J Am Coll Surg 1994;178(1):83-85.
2. Sampliner RE, Jaffe P. Malignant degeneration of Barrett's esophagus: the role of laser ablation and photodynamic therapy. Dis Esophagus 1995;8:104-108.
3. Liebermann-Meffert D, Duranceau A, Zuidema GD, Orringer MB. Anatomy of the esophagus. In: Shakelford's surgery of the alimentary tract, 4th ed. Philadelphia: WB Saunders, 1996:3-21.
4. Sabik JF, Rice TW, Goldblum JR, Koka A, Kirby TJ, Medendorp SV, Adelstein DJ. Superficial esophageal carcinoma. Ann Thorac Surg 1995;60(4):896-901.
5. Rice TW, Zuccaro G Jr, Adelstein DJ, Rybicki LA, Blackstone EH, Goldblum JR. Esophageal carcinoma:depth of tumor invasion is predictive of regional lymph node status. Ann Thorac Surg 1998;65:787-792.
6. Nigro JJ, Hagen JA, DeMeester TR, DeMeester SR, Peters JH, Oberg S, Theisen J, Kiyabu M, Crookes PF, Bremner CG. Prevalence and location of nodal metastases in distal esophageal adenocarcinoma confined to the wall: implications for therapy. J Thorac Cardiovasc Surg 1999;117(1):16-25.
7. Vickers J, Alderson D. Esophageal cancer staging using endoscopic ultrasonography. Br J Surg 1998;85:994-998.
8. Salminen JT, Farkkila MA, Ramo OJ, Toikkanen V, Simpanen J, Nuutinen H, Salo JA. Endoscopic ultrasonography in the preoperative staging of adenocarcinoma of the distal esophagus and esophagogastric junction. Scand J Gastroenterol 1999;34(12):1178-1182.
9. Fukuda M, Hirata K, Natori H. Endoscopic ultrasonography of the esophagus. World J Surg 2000;24(2):216-226.
10. Nigro JJ, Hagen JA, DeMeester TR, DeMeester SR, Theisen J, Peters JH, Kiyabu M. Occult esophageal adenocarcinoma:extent of disease and implications for effective therapy. Ann Surg 1999;230(3):433-440.

What is the rate of nodal invasion in small primary lesions?

A.H. Hölscher, W. Schröder (Cologne)

Small primary adenocarcinomas of the esophagus are classified as early esophageal cancer which is defined as a tumor limited to the mucosa (pT1a) or submucosa (pT1b) [1]. The distinction between mucosal and submucosal carcinoma is of pathological and prognostic relevance since the majority of lymphatic channels is located in the submucosal but not the mucosal layer [2]. The difference in lymphatic drainage has an impact on the frequency of nodal metastases. This is the reason that different therapeutic strategies have been emerged for these malignant entities. Whereas pT1a carcinomas can be treated by local endoscopic resection pT1b carcinomas require a resection with lymphadenectomy [3].

The question of this article was to assess the exact percentage of lymph node metastases in pT1a and pT1b tumors of esophageal adenocarcinoma.

A review of the present literature shows that almost all studies investigating early adenocarcinoma of Barrett's esophagus have been undertaken in Western countries. In contrast to this, authors from Japan demonstrate greater experience concerning early squamous cell carcinoma of the esophagus which is not the topic of this review. A total of 6 series published between 1991 and 1999 were analyzed, of which the main results are summarized in *Table I* [3-8]. This includes the authors own experience with 41 cases of early adenocarcinoma of Barrett's esophagus [3].

This rather small number of studies is due to the fact that other authors do not differentiate between pT1a and pT1b category but classify carcinomas only according to the UICC stage [9-12]. In addition, the rate of nodal metastases related to the different pT categories is not quoted in other series [9-12].

Results

A total of 145 patients with early adenocarcinoma of Barrett's esophagus were analyzed. The median follow-up of these patients ranged from 1.7 to 5.5. years. Fifty nine patients were classified to have a pT1a carcinoma, in 86 patients the diagnosis of a pT1b carcinoma was made. None of the patients with a mucosal carcinoma (pT1a) had metastasis to locoregional lymph nodes. In 16 of 86 patients (18.6%) with submucosal carcinoma lymph node metastases were demonstrated (range: 0-44.4%). Except for one series of Menke *et al.* [5] the 5 year survival rate of patients with a pT1a carcinoma was 100%. The 5 year survival for patients with a pT1b carcinoma ranged from 36% to 85%. The difference in survival between patients with mucosal and submucosal infiltration was not significant in any study, most likely due to the small number of patients included.

In our own series of 41 patients, the average number of removed lymph nodes was 23 (range: 10-48). Nineteen percent of the removed lymph nodes were infiltrated in the 5 pN1 carcinomas of the submucosal type.

Table I.

Author	Year	Patients	Follow-up		Mucosa			Submucosa			Significance
		n	Median years	Range years	pT1a n	pN1 n	Survival 5-year	pT1b n	pN1 n	Survival 5-year	p
Streitz [4]	1991	22	–	–	4	0	100%	18	8	53-85%	–
Menke [5]	1992	12	1,7	0,1-9	2	0	76%	10	0	47%	NS
Pera [6]	1992	16	2,8	0,2-9,6	9	0	100%	7	1	36%	–
Paraf [7]	1995	21	4,3	1,8-11,3	9	0	–	12	1	–	–
Hölscher [3]	1997	41	5,5	0,7-12,9	10	0	100%	31	5	79%	NS
Nigro [8]	1999	33	3,6	0,3-9,8	25	0	–	8	1	–	–
Total		145			59	0 (0%)	76-100%	86	16 (19%)	36-85%	

Discussion

In several studies it could be clearly demonstrated that lymph node metastases are a strong prognostic factor for survival in patients with Barrett's carcinoma [10, 13, 14]. The most significant variation in long-term survival is found between pT1 and pT2 tumors caused by an increase in lymph node metastases [8, 14]. Therefore, early detection substantially increases the chances for cure by diminishing the risk of lymph node involvement.

This review clearly demonstrates that mucosal adenocarcinoma of the esophagus is not associated with locoregional lymph node metastases whereas submucosal cancer has a substantial risk of almost 20% to have metastatic lymph nodes. These findings are in contrast to early squamous cell carcinoma of the esophagus for which Japanese authors report nodal metastases in up to 6,5% of patients with mucosal cancer and up to 50% of patients with submucosal cancer (survey in [15]). These different rates of nodal metastasis explain the poorer survival rates for patients with early squamous cell carcinoma [15].

Since nodal metastases are not present in mucosal cancer of esophageal adenocarcinoma it appears consequent to treat those carcinomas by local resection, for example by endoscopic mucosal stripping. However, before these alternative therapies can be widely accepted, the preoperative diagnostic imaging, in particular the endoscopic ultrasound has to be able to safely differentiate between pT1a and pT1b carcinomas in order not to compromise the benefit of early detection by incomplete removal. Local endoscopic resection of the mucosal adenocarcinoma is also limited by the multicentricity which is seen in up to 15% of tumors [3].

A complete removal (R0) by a standardized surgical resection is associated with an excellent prognosis of mucosal Barrett's carcinoma and should be the gold standard for evaluation of other less invasive treatment options. Because of the relevant rate of nodal metastases the submucosal carcinoma of the Barrett's esophagus remains the domain of a subtotal esophagectomy with at least 2-field lymphadenectomy and contributes to a 5-year survival of almost 80% [15].

References

1. Hermanek P, Hutter RVP, Sobin LH, Wagner G, Wittekind C. UICC TNM classification of malignant tumors, 4th ed. Berlin: Springer, 1998:71-80.
2. Patti MG, Gantert W, Way LW. Surgery of the esophagus. Anatomy and Physiology. Surg Clin North Am 1997;77(5):959-970.
3. Hölscher AH, Bollschweiler E, Schneidert PM, Siewert JR. Early adenocarcinoma in Barrett's esophagus. Br J Surg 1997; 84:1470-1473.
4. Streitz JM, Ellis FH, Gibb SP, Balogh K, Watkins E. Adenocarcinoma of the Barrett's esophagus – a clinicipathologic study of 65 cases. Ann Surg 1991;213(2):122-125.
5. Menke-Pluymers MBE, Schoute NW, Mulder AH, Hop WCJ, van Blankenstein M, Tilanus HW. Outcome of surgical treatment of adenocarcinoma in Barrett's esophagus. Gut 1992;33:1454-1458.
6. Pera M, Trastek VF, Carpenter HA, Allen MS, Deschamps C, Pairolero P. Barrett's esophagus with high-grade dysplasia: an indication for esophagectomy? Ann Thorac Surg 1992;54:199-204.
7. Paraf F, Flejou JF, Pignon JP, Potet F. Surgical pathology of adenocarcinoma arising in Barrett's esophagus – analysis of 67 cases. Am J Pathol 1995;19(2):183-191.
8. Nigro JJ, Hagen JA, DeMeester TR, DeMeester SR, Theisen J, Peters JH, Kiyabu M. Occult esophageal adenocarcinoma. Extent of disease and implications for effective therapy. Ann Surg 1999; 230(3):433-440.
9. Collard JM, Romagnoli R, Hermans BP, Malaise J. Radical esophageal resection for adenocarcinoma arising in Barrett's esophagus. Am J Surg 1997;174:307-311.

10. Lerut T, Coosemans W, van Raemdonck D, Dillemans B, de Leyn P, Marnette JM, Geboes K. Surgical treatment of Barrett's carcinoma; correlations between morphologic findings and prognosis. J Thorac Cardiovasc Surg 1994;107:1059-1066.
11. Peters JH, Clark GWB, Ireland AP, Chandrasoma TP, Smyrk TC, DeMeester TR. Outcome of adenocarcinoma arising in Barrett's esophagus in endoscopically surveyed and nonsurveyed patients. J Thorac Cardiovasc Surg 1994;108:813-822.
12. Levine DS, Haggitt RC, Blount PL, Rabinovitch PS, Rusch VW, Reid BJ. An endoscopic biopsy protocol can differentiate high-grade dysplasia from early adenocarcinoma in Barrett's esophagus. Gastroenterology 1993; 105:40-50.
13. Hölscher AH, Bollschweiler E, Bumm R, Bartels H, Höfler H, Siewert JR. Prognostic factors of resected adenocarcinoma of the esophagus. Surgery 1995;118:845-855.
14. Hölscher AH, Becker K, Höfler H, Fink U, Siewert JR. Plattenepithel-Frühcarcinom des esophagus. Multizentrität, Metastasierungsmuster und Prognose. Chirurg 1996; 67:357-361.
15. Hölscher AH, Bollschweiler E, Schröder W, Gutschow C, Siewert JR. Prognostic difference between early squamous-cell and adenocarcinoma of the esophagus. Dis Esophagus 1997;10:17-184.

Can unnecessary surgery be avoided by endoscopic ultrasound guided fine needle aspiration?

M. Giovannini (Marseille)

Endoscopic ultrasound (EUS) is now widely used for the assessment of locoregional involvement of adenocarcinoma of the esophagus and the esophagogastric junction. It allows accurate assessment of wall involvement in 85% of cases and lymph node involvement in 75% of cases. But the EUS specificity to distinguish malignant from inflammatory lymph nodes is low, no more than 50%. A correct staging is mandatory before treatment. According to the UICC classification, distant lymph nodes are considered as metastasis and surgery is not recommended. The main problem is the EUS specificity to distinguish malignant and benign lymph nodes. EUS lymph node imaging has poor specificity, but as the therapeutic decision depends on the lymph node staging, it is essential to have an histologic characterisation of the lymph nodes. Recent series published about EUS guided biopsy show that, with this new technique, a specificity of 95% to differentiate malignant and inflammatory lymph nodes can be expected [1].

In our Institution, we have performed a prospective study on the impact of EUS guided lymph node biopsy in patients with esophageal adenocarcinoma [2].

From January 1994 to January 1998, 77 patients (52 men and 25 women) with a mean age of 66 years (range: 42-76 years) underwent EUS for the local staging of an adenocarcinoma of the esophagus before treatment. In all patients pretreatment work-up included gastrointestinal fiberoscopy, thoracic CT scan and abdominal ultrasonography. All patients were considered as operable and CT scan didn't show local contraindication to surgery.

EUS was performed using an echoendoscope with a curved array transducer (FG32UA-FG 36-X, Pentax). Wall involvement was staged according to the EUS TN classification and lymph nodes were considered as metastases if 3 of the following 4 criteria were observed: round shape, hypoechogenic, well-defined borders, and diameter greater than 1 cm. However, when the lymph node was located in a distant area (aortico-cava, superior mediastinal and cervical) EUS guided biopsy was performed even if the EUS malignancy criteria were not observed.

The puncture is realized at the end of the examination, the patient being in left lateral decubitus. A neuroleptanalgesia is generally necessary. The technique of puncture is the following:

- positioning of the lesion on the way of exit of the needle;
- withdrawal of the stylet, then introduction of the needle in the tumor. The visualization of the echo-tip of the needle allows to verify its good positioning in the lesion;
- aspiration with a 20 ml syringe associated with back and forth movements of the needle in the tumor.

One to three passages are generally necessary to obtain a microbiopsy. It is currently possible to obtain microfragments of tissue in approximately 90% of cases with the needle of Vilmann-Hancke (22 gauges and 12 cm length. Microbiopsies are obtained as follows:

- the totality of the specimen contained inside the needle is collected with the reintroduction of the stylet;
- this microcore is then put in the formalin-adelhyde, then included in paraffin.

Contrarily to American teams, we do not administer systematically an injection of antibiotic following the biopsy. At the end of the examination, it is necessary to watch over the patient during at least three hours. The EUS guided biopsy can, in the majority of cases, be performed ambulatory. The main limits to the technique are size of the lesion lesser than 5 mm, the depth of the lesion, as compared to the probe, greater than 6-7 cm, and a trouble of blood coagulation (TP < 60%, platelets < 80,000/mm^3).

Ten over 77 patients (13%) underwent EUS - lymph node a guided biopsy. Patient tolerance was excellent and the insertion of the needle into the lesion was always successful. The mean size of the lymph nodes was 8.6 mm (range: 6-11 mm). The mean number of needle passages was 1,3 (range: 1-2). The diagnosis of malignant lymph nodes was obtain on microhistology and cytology in 6 cases, on microhistology alone in 3 cases and on cytology alone in 1 case. These 10 patients were treated by concomitant chemo-radiation therapy.

EUS guided biopsy of lymph nodes resulted in a change in the stage of the tumor in 10/77 cases, these tumors with distant lymph node involvement being considered as metastatic according the UICC classification.

References

1. Wieserma M, Vilmann P, Giovannini M, Chang KJ. Endosonography-guided fine needle aspiration biopsy: diagnostic accuracy and complication assessment. Gastroenterology 1997;112;1087-1095.
2. Giovannini M, Monges G, Seitz JF, Moutardier V, Bernardini D, Thomas P, Houvenaeghel G, Delpero JR, Giudicelli R, Fuentes P. Distant lymph node metastases in esophageal cancer: impact of endoscopic ultrasound guided biopsy. Endoscopy 1999;31:795-801.

What are the means of esophagogastric resection and reconstruction for Barrett's adenocarcinoma?

R. Romagnoli, C. Gutschow, J.-M. Collard (Brussels)

Barrett's adenocarcinoma arises either in the esophageal tube or on the gastroesophageal junction (GEJ) [1]. Numerous surgical techniques are available for the resection of this peculiar neoplasm and subsequent gastric and/or esophageal replacement.

Resection

Parameters that direct the choice of the surgical procedure with respect to extent of both esophageal and gastric resections are the following:

- the exact location of the tumor [2] (*i.e.* in the esophageal tube or on the GEJ) as assessed by preoperative endoscopic and radiologic examinations of the upper gastrointestinal tract and intraoperative findings;
- the length of the metaplastic area, which must be encompassed to prevent subsequent development of a second neoplastic lesion from a residual dysplastic focus [3, 4];
- the existence of a short esophagus (fixed hiatal hernia – HH) or not (no HH or a HH reducible to the abdomen in the erect position). For instance, esophageal shortening was found in 20 among 55 consecutive patients (36%) operated on in our institution for Barrett's adenocarcinoma or high-grade dysplasia [4].

Figure 1 shows a personal classification of different neoplastic processes that may arise in an esophageal metaplastic area into 5 different types according to these three criteria [4]:

- type I: short esophagus, tumor extending over the GEJ;
- type II: short esophagus, tumor not involving the GEJ;
- type III: normal length esophagus, tumor extending over the GEJ, > 3 cm metaplastic area;
- type IV: normal length esophagus, tumor not involving the GEJ, > 3 cm metaplastic area;
- type V: normal length esophagus, tumor centered on the GEJ, < 3 cm metaplastic area.

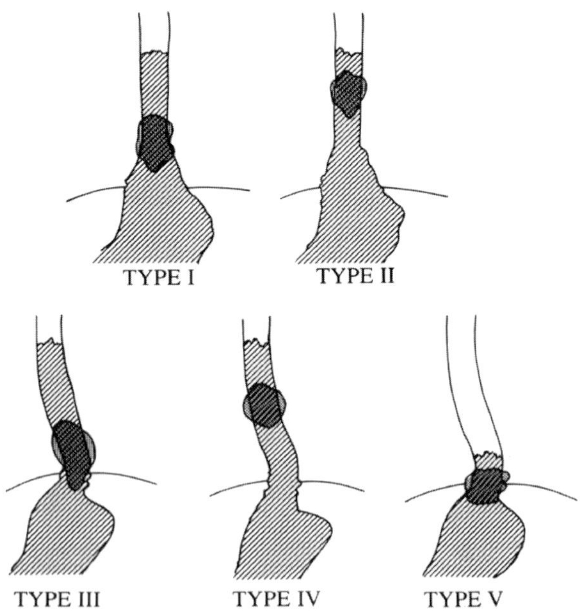

Figure 1. Classification of Barrett's adenocarcinomas according to the existence of a short esophagus or not, location of the tumor, and length of the metaplastic area.

Actually, each individual anatomical situation deserves a specific resective technique, to be chosen among the following:

- subtotal esophagectomy without any gastric resection: this technique addresses type II and IV tumors that are located in the esophageal tube at a rather long distance away from the GEJ;
- subtotal esophagectomy with resection of both lesser curvature and subcardial area of the stomach: this technique is indicated in those tumors involving a fixed intrathoracic GEJ (type I) or in those esophageal tube tumors extending over an intra-abdominal GEJ but arising in a long esophageal metaplastic area (type III);
- subtotal esophagectomy with proximal two-third or total gastrectomy: this technique may be used for the resection of tumors centered on the GEJ and extending to both the esophageal tube and the proximal stomach (types I and III);
- distal esophagectomy with proximal one-third or total gastrectomy: this technique is indicated in those tumors that are centered on an intra-abdominal GEJ and arising in a short Barrett's segment (type V). In this regard, a study [5] comparing various types of gastrectomy for cancer of the GEJ showed that extended total gastrectomy including splenectomy and celiac lymph node dissection resulted in a significantly higher survival rate than proximal gastrectomy. In addition, the latter carried a significantly higher risk for local neoplastic recurrence than the former;
- distal esophagectomy with no gastric resection: the exceedingly low prevalence of lymph node metastasis in intramucosal Barrett's neoplasic lesions [6, 7] together with the wish for reducing side-effects of the classic esophagogastric resections including bilateral vagotomy have led to the development of so-called vagus-sparing esophagectomy techniques. A first technique consists of the stripping of the esophageal tube [7] according to a principle applied previously by Akiyama *et al.* to early squamous neoplastic lesions [8]. More recently, a vagus-sparing technique of distal esophagectomy with subsequent interposition of a 15 cm jejunal loop between the esophageal remnant and the intact stomach has been described [9] and applied to patients operated on for an early neoplastic lesion arising in a short Barrett's segment. Potential advantages of vagal-sparing over conventional techniques of esophagectomy in terms of postoperative alimentary comfort and quality of life are obvious. As the normally-innervated stomach is left in place, postoperative symptoms in relation to gastric denervation such as diarrhea, early postprandial fullness and "slow digestion" are less likely.

However, recent observations from experienced Eastern [10] and Western [11, 12] teams quantify at about 30% the likelihood of upper mediastinal lymph node involvement from an adenocarcinoma of the lower esophagus and GEJ. Even though a benefice in terms of survival and cure has not been reported yet, this finding might justify the performance of a subtotal esophagectomy with so-called 3-field lymph node dissection in every patient operated on for Barrett's adenocarcinoma.

Reconstruction

Digestive continuity after resection of Barrett's adenocarcinoma can be re-established using one of three organs: the jejunum, the colon, or the stomach (*Table I*).

Table I. Re-establishment of digestive continuity according to types of esophageal and/or gastric resection for Barrett's adenocarcinoma.

Resection	Reconstruction
Distal esophagectomy with total gastrectomy	60 cm Roux-en-Y or jejunal loop interposition
Distal esophagectomy without any gastric gastric resection	15 cm jejunal loop interposition
Subtotal esophagectomy with proximal two-third or total gastrectomy	Colon transplant
Vagal-sparing subtotal esophagectomy without any gastric resection	Colon transplant
Distal esophagectomy with proximal one-third gastrectomy	Distal two thirds of the stomach
Subtotal esophagectomy with resection of both lesser curve and subcardial area of the stomach	Greater curvature tube
Subtotal esophagectomy without any gastric resection	Whole stomach

Jejunum

The jejunum is the reconstruction organ of choice after combined distal esophagectomy and total gastrectomy. The most common techniques of jejunal preparation are the Roux-en-Y loop [13] and the jejunal interposition [14, 15]. When distal esophagectomy is performed without any gastric resection [9], a 15-cm jejunal segment according to Merendino technique[16] can be interposed between the esophageal stump and the whole stomach.

Main advantage of esophageal replacement with the jejunum lies on the existence of a residual motor activity within the jejunal wall, even after vagotomy [17]. However, fundamental studies [18, 19] of the electrical or mechanical activity of the jejunal loop have evidenced a number of motor abnormalities that may account for the stasis of jejunal juice in the lumen of the loop and for its reflux into the proximal organ. In this respect, protection of the remaining esophageal segment against the harmful effects of pathologic jejuno-esophageal reflux after total gastrectomy requires the construction of a very long (> 60 cm) jejunal loop [20].

Colon

For a long period over the 20th century, the colon transplant has been the esophageal substitute of choice after subtotal esophagectomy because of the great length of the colic segment. As shown by DeMeester *et al.* [21], more than 80% of patients get satisfactory alimentary comfort with a colic graft, which has been ascribed to the presence of residual contractions in the colic wall [22] and the maintenance of the whole gastric reservoir.

Nowadays, however, colon interposition has been abandoned for the stomach by many surgical teams. Disadvantages of the colon in comparison with the stomach [23] are:

- the need for three to four anastomoses with the colon instead of only one with the stomach;
- the potential for contamination of the operative field by colon contents;
- unfavorable congenital variations in the mesocolic vasculature or the presence of severe atheromatous lesions in supplying arteries, both conditions predisposing to graft necrosis;

- the risk (up to 33%) for subsequent reoperations to manage late technical complications such as kinking of the colon segment above the diaphragm or anastomotic stricture [24].

In this setting, residual indications of the colon transplant after esophageal resection for Barrett's adenocarcinoma are the following:

- subtotal esophagectomy combined with total or proximal two-third gastrectomy;
- vagal-sparing subtotal esophagectomy without any gastric resection;
- history of previous gastric resection;
- salvage procedure following inadvertent injury to the basal pedicle of a gastric transplant;
- re-establishment of digestive continuity after postoperative necrosis of a gastric transplant [25].

Stomach

After distal esophagectomy and proximal one-third gastrectomy, the residual gastric pouch can be used to re-establish digestive continuity with construction of a low intrathoracic esophagogastric anastomosis [26]. However, this kind of operation has been abandoned by many surgical teams because it may induce severe postoperative gastroesophageal reflux symptoms and lesions. Indeed, a 24 hour pH-monitoring study comparing patients having a lower mediastinal esophagogastric anastomosis with those having an upper mediastinal anastomosis [27] indicates that although gastric acid secretion was identical in the two groups, esophageal exposure to acid in patients with a low anastomosis was much longer than that in patients with an anastomosis at the apex of the chest.

After subtotal esophagectomy, the stomach has proved to be an excellent esophageal substitute because of its extraordinary plasticity and stretchability and the richness of its submucosal vascular network. The stomach can be used either in its entirety [28] or as a greater curvature tube [29, 30]. Principles of these two techniques of gastric tailoring can be summarized as follows:

- whole stomach with denudation of the lesser curvature [28]: the lesser curvature is denuded by division of the terminal rami of both right and left gastric vessels flush with the gastric wall from the gastric angle up to the GEJ; potentially involved lymph nodes [31] within the lesser omentum are separated from the gastric wall while the right side of the stomach is unfolded; the esophagus is then separated from the stomach by application of a single cartridge of a linear stapler on the GEJ;
- greater curvature tube with resection of the lesser curvature [29, 30]: stapling resection of the proximal three fourths of the lesser curvature is started by division of the lesser omentum 4 to 5 cm proximal to the pylorus for the application of a linear stapler on the gastric wall; the distal segment of the first cartridge is applied at an angle of 60 degrees to the right border of the stomach; the next cartridges are applied in totality parallel to and 20 mm away from the free edge of the lesser curvature up to the left side of the GEJ.

Main advantages of the whole stomach transplant over the greater curvature tube are the following:

- lower risk of postoperative technical complications [32]: anastomotic stenoses and fistulas are siginificantly less frequent with the whole stomach transplant than with a greater curvature tube; this may be explained by a better blood supply to the anastomotic site in the fundus with the whole stomach technique, since this supply mainly comes from vessels that are located within the wall of the lesser curvature rather than from the vascular arcade of the greater curvature. Recently, the use of an original technique of cervical esophagogastrostomy in which a large posterior communication between the two lumina is created by stapling [33] has been shown to create a large-bore anastomosis, so that most of the patients are able to swallow large pieces of meat or bread at early follow-up;

- better alimentary comfort [32]: in comparison with patients having a greater curvature tube, patients having their whole stomach as an esophageal substitute take fewer meals and snacks per day, complain less frequently of a sensation of early fullness at or just after meal, and are able to consume more calories at a test meal. Better alimentary comfort of patients having a whole stomach transplant in comparison with those having a greater curvature tube may be explained by the maintenance of the entire gastric volumetric capacity [32] on the one hand and better spontaneous recovery of the gastric contractility with time [34, 35] on the other. In fact, contrary to the classic opinion, the denervated stomach as an esophageal substitute is a contractile organ that recovers more and more motor activity over the years [36]. Better motor recovery within the wall of the whole stomach is likely related to the maintenance of the vagus-dependent command ganglia within the lesser curvature [37]. Moreover, the spontaneous motor recovery process within the gastric wall after extrinsic denervation can be enhanced [38] by postoperative administration of erythromycin (750 mg daily for a minimum 6-month period), a prokinetic drug that acts as a motilin-receptor agonist [39]. In some patients, enhancement of gastric contractility may even persist after discontinuation of the drug [38].

The main drawback of the gastric transplant technique consists of a progressive normalization of the intraluminal pH profile with time that probably reflects progressive re-increase in acid production [40]. This phenomenon obviously alters alimentary comfort, so that > 3 years after the operation, one third of patients complain of severe cervical heartburn with endoscopic esophagitis, and in some of them, intestinal metaplasia may even develop in the cervical esophageal remnant [40-42]. Prevention of such a metaplastic transformation by chronic intake of a proton pump inhibitor is unlikely [43]. In contrast, construction of a fundoplication around the cervical anastomosis has been shown to create a high-pressure zone that can oppose gastroesophageal reflux [44]. Such a long-term deterioration of the alimentary comfort questions the use of the stomach as esophageal replacement in dysplastic and early neoplastic diseases of the esophagus.

As for exposure of the denervated gastric transplant to bile, it is lengthened significantly in comparison with healthy subjects when the patient assumes the supine position during the night [45]. However, pathologic gastric exposure to bile tends to normalize if both a gastric drainage procedure such as a pyloroplasty or a pyloromyotomy is added and erythromycin is given at early follow-up [46]. Here again, the effect of erythromycin may persist after discontinuation of the drug [46].

In conclusion, esophagogastric resection and subsequent restoration of digestive continuity calls for numerous surgical techniques, each of which has to be used with eclecticism according to both anatomical and histological characteristics of the neoplastic disease, patient's general condition and past surgical history, and potential chances of long-term survival and cure [47].

References

1. Hamilton SR, Smith RRL, Cameron JL. Prevalence and characteristics of Barrett esophagus in patients with adenocarcinoma of the esophagus or esophagogastric junction. Hum Pathol 1988;19:942-948.
2. Siewert JR, Holscher AH, Becker K, Gossner W. Cardia cancer: attempt at a therapeutically relevant classification. Chirurgie 1987;58:25-32.
3. Berenson MM, Riddell RH, Skinner DB, Freston JW. Malignant transformation of esophageal columnar epithelium. Cancer 1978;41:554-561.
4. Collard JM, Romagnoli R, Hermans BP, Malaise J. Radical esophageal resection for adenocarcinoma arising in Barrett's esophagus. Am J Surg 1997;174:307-311.
5. Papachristou DN, Fortner JG. Adenocarcinoma of the gastric cardia. The choice of gastrectomy. Ann Surg 1980;192:58-64.
6. Hölscher AH, Bollschweiler S, Schneider PM, Siewert JR. Early adenocarcinoma in Barrett's esophagus. Br J Surg 1997;84:1470-1473.
7. Nigro JJ, Hagen JA, DeMeester TR, et al. Occult esophageal adenocarcinoma: extent of disease and implications for effective therapy. Ann Surg 1999;230:433-440.
8. Akiyama H, Tsurumaku, M, Kawamura T, Ono Y. Esophageal stripping with preservation of the vagus nerve. Int Surg 1982;67:125-128.
9. Salo JA, Sihvo EI, Salminen JT, Toikkanen VK, Isolauri JO. Vagal-preserving esophageal resection. 6th World Congress of OESO, Paris, September 1-6, 2000, Book of abstracts, 87.
10. Kinoshita Y, Udagawa H, Tsutsumi K, et al. Lymph node dissection for cancer of the gastroesophageal junction. 6th World Congress of OESO, Paris, September 1-6, 2000, Book of abstracts, 126.
11. Altorki NK, Skinner DB. Occult cervical nodal metastasis in esophageal cancer: preliminary results of three-field lymphadenectomy. J Thorac Cardiovasc Surg 1997;113:540-544.
12. Lerut T, Coosemans W, De Leyn P, et al. Reflections on three field lymphadenectomy in carcinoma of the esophagus and gastroesophageal junction. Hepatogastroenterology 1999;46:717-725.
13. Allison PR, Tavares Da Silva L. The Roux loop. Br J Surg 1953;41:173-180.
14. Henley FA. Gastrectomy with replacement. Br J Surg 1952;40:118-123.
15. Longmire WP, Beal JM. Construction of a substitute gastric reservoir following total gastrectomy. Am Surg 1952;135:673-676.
16. Merendino KA, Thomas GE. The jejunal interposition operation for substitution of the esophagogastric sphincter. Surgery 1958;44:1112-1115.
17. Nishihira T, OE H, Sugawara K, et al. Reconstruction of the thoracic esophagus with jejunal pedicled segments for cancer of the thoracic esophagus. Dis Esophagus 1995;8:30-39.
18. Vantrappen G, Coremans G, Janssens J, et al. Inversion of the slow-wave frequency gradient in symptomatic patients with Roux-en-Y anastomoses. Gastroenterology 1991;101:1282-1288.
19. Woodward A, Sillin LF, Bortoff A. Migrating myoelectric complex and jejunal slow-wave propagation after Roux gastrectomy in dogs. Dig Dis Sci 1993;38:1073-1078.
20. Collard JM, Romagnoli R. Roux-en-Y jejunal loop and bile reflux. Am J Surg 2000;179:298-303.
21. Demeester TR, Johansson KE, Franze I, et al. Indications, surgical technique, and long-term functional results of colon interposition or by-pass. Ann Surg 1988;208:460-474.
22. Benages A, Moreno-Osset E, Paris F, et al. Motor activity after colon replacement of the esophagus. J Thorac Cardiovasc Surg 1981;82:335-340.
23. Collard JM, Otte JB, Kestens PJ. Reconstruction after esophagectomy. In: Steichen FM, Welter R, eds. Minimally invasive surgery and new technology. St Louis: Quality Medical Publishing, 1994:629-633.
24. Jeyasingham K, Lerut T, Belsey RHR. Functional and mechanical sequelae of colon interposition for benign disease. Eur J Cardiothorac Surg 1999;15:327-331.
25. Obertop H, Bosscha K, de Graaf PW. Mediastinitis from anastomotic disruption after esophageal resection and reconstruction for cancer: results of salvage surgery. Dis Esophagus 1994;7:184-187.
26. Sweet RH. Surgical management of carcinoma of the midthoracic esophagus. Preliminary report. N Engl J Med 1945;233:1-7.
27. Domergue J, Veyrac M, Huin-Yan S, et al. pH monitoring for 24 hours of gastroesophageal reflux and gastric function after intrathoracic gastroplasty after esophagectomy. Surg Gynecol Obstet 1990;171:107-110.
28. Collard JM, Otte JB, Jamart J, Reynaert M, Kestens PJ. An original technique for lengthening the stomach as an esophageal substitute after esophagectomy. Preliminary results. Dis Esophagus 1989;2:171-174.
29. Akiyama H, Miyazono H, Tsurumaru M, Hashimoto C, Kawamura T. Use of the stomach as an esophageal substitute. Ann Surg 1978;188:606-610.
30. Gignoux M, Segol P, Ollivier JM, Bricard H. L'œsophagoplastie cervicale dans le traitement du cancer de l'œsophage. Lyon Chir 1978;74:262-264.
31. Akiyama H, Tsurumaru M, Kawamura T, Ono Y. Principles of surgical treatment for carcinoma of the esophagus: analysis of lymph node involvement. Ann Surg 1981;194:438-446.

32. Collard JM, Tinton N, Malaise J, Romagnoli R, Otte JB, Kestens PJ. Esophageal replacement: gastric tube or whole stomach? Ann Thorac Surg 1995;60:261-267.
33. Collard JM, Romagnoli R, Goncette L, Otte JB, Kestens PJ. Terminalized semimechanical side-to-side suture technique for cervical esophagogastrostomy. Ann Thorac Surg 1988;65:814-817.
34. Collard JM, Romagnoli R, Otte JB, Kestens PJ. The denervated stomach as an esophageal substitute is a contractile organ. Ann Surg 1998;227:33-39.
35. Collard JM, Romagnoli R. Human stomach has a recordable mechanical activity at a rate of about three cycles/minute. Eur J Surg 2001;167:188-194.
36. Andrews PLR, Bingham S. Adaptation of the mechanisms controlling gastric motility following chronic vagotomy in the ferret. Exp Physiol 1990;75:811-825.
37. Schemann M, Grundy D. Electrophysiological identification of vagally-innervated enteric neurons in guinea pig stomach. Am J Physiol 1992;263:G709-718.
38. Collard JM, Romagnoli R, Otte JB, Kestens PJ. Erythromycin enhances early postoperative contractility of the denervated whole stomach as an esophageal substitute. Ann Surg 1999;229:337-343.
39. Peeters T, Matthijs G, Depoortere I, Cachet T, Hoogmartens J, Van Trappen G. Erythromycin is a motilin receptor agonist. Am J Physiol 1989;257:G470-474.
40. Gutschow C, Collard JM, Romagnoli R, Salizzoni M, Hölscher AH. Denervated stomach as an esophageal substitute recovers intraluminal acidity with time. Ann Surg 2001;233:509-514.
41. Lindhal H, Rintala R,Sariola H, Louhimo I. Cervical Barrett's esophagus: a common complication of gastric tube reconstruction. J Pediat Surg 1990;25:446-448.
42. Derocha JR, Ceconello I, Zilberstein B, et al. Barrett's esophagus in the esophageal stump after subtotal esophagectomy with cervical esophagogastroplasty. Rev Hosp Clin Fac Med Sao Paulo 1992;46:69-70.
43. Wetscher GJ, Profanter C, Gadenstätter M, Perdikis G, Glaser K, Hinder RA. Medical treatment of gastroesophageal reflux disease does not prevent the development of Barrett's metaplasia and poor esophageal body motility. Langenbecks Arch Surg 1997;382:95-99.
44. Okada N, Kuriyama T, Umemoto H, et al. Esophageal surgery: a procedure for posterior invagination esophagogastrostomy in one-stage without positional change. Ann Surg 1974;179:27-34.
45. Romagnoli R, Bechi P, Salizzoni M, Collard JM. Combined 24-hour pH and bile monitoring of the denervated whole stomach as an esophageal substitute. Hepatogastroenterology 1999;46:86-91.
46. Gutschow C, Collard JM, Govaerts B, et al. Effect of vagotomy, posture, gastric drainage, and erythromycin therapy on bile exposure of the stomach as esophageal replacement. Submitted for publication.
47. Collard JM, Otte JB, Fiasse R, et al. Skeletonizing en-bloc esophagectomy for cancer. Ann Surg 2001;234:25-32.

What is the most efficient current multimodality therapy to be applied?

T.N. Walsh (Dublin)

At least 50% of esophageal cancers have overt metastases at presentation and the majority of the rest will die despite apparent curative surgery, suggesting occult systemic metastases [1]. The need for adjuvant systemic therapy is not disputed, just the most effective protocol. There are few randomized trials of multimodal therapy for adenocarcinoma and none comparing regimens. Information from non-randomized studies and squamous carcinoma must be interpreted with caution as the two tumors differ in aetiology, distributions, stage at presentation and survival for each stage. The response rate and outcome following response also differs [2] but there is no evidence to suggest that a regimen effective for one will not benefit the other.

Realistically the best regimen can only improve outcome by single or low double percentage figured as with breast and colon cancer. Large trials are needed to prove such differences significant. Most trials on esophageal cancer are underpowered. Hence, in one an increase in survival from 15% to 32% is not statistically significant [3]. Because of the paucity of adenocarcinoma data this paper examines some randomized trials of squamous carcinoma as well as non-randomized trials of esophageal adenocarcinoma for evidence of efficacy.

What works for squamous cell carcinoma? Evidence from randomized trials

Chemotherapy

The most promising agents studied are 5-fluorouracil (5-FU), cisplatin, mitomycin and paclitaxel. Single agent therapy is more effective than combination therapy.

Preoperative chemotherapy

Early randomized trials with smaller numbers comparing preoperative chemotherapy with surgery alone found no benefit for chemotherapy with considerable toxicity [4, 5]. Recent larger trials have been more optimistic. Law *et al.* [6] reported on 147 patients with esophageal cancer randomized to preoperative cisplatin and 5-FU or surgery alone. Median survival figures (16.8 *versus* 13 months) were not statistically different. The Medical Research Council [7] randomized 802 patients with operable squamous and adenocarcinoma to two cycles of cisplatin and 5-FU or surgery alone. Median survivals of 17.6 *versus* 13.6 months were statistically significantly different. The Rotterdam Esophageal Tumour Study Group [8] randomized 148 patients with operable squamous cancer to preoperative cisplatin and etoposide or surgery alone. Early results indicate an enhanced median survival of 18.7 months *versus* 11 months. Thus, differences in survival become significant in larger trials.

Postoperative chemotherapy

Pouliquen *et al.* [9] found no benefit for postoperative chemotherapy with low-dose 5-FU and cisplatin. Recently Ando *et al.* [10] presented preliminary data on a randomized trial of postoperative cisplatin (80 mg/m^2) and 5-FU (800 mg/m^2 x 5 days) *versus* surgery alone in 242 patients who underwent transthoracic esophagectomy with lymphadenectomy. Five-year disease free survival was 58% *versus* 46% favouring postoperative chemotherapy. Overall survival was similar but a trend favoured therapy in the node-positive subgroup.

Pre- and postoperative chemotherapy

Roth *et al.* [11] compared preoperative and postoperative cisplatin, vindesine and bleomycin with surgery alone in 36 patients and found no survival difference between the limbs. Saltz and Kelsen [12] randomized patients to receive pre- and postoperative cisplatin, vinblastin and bleomycin or surgery alone and again found no survival advantage. More recently Kelsen *et al.* [13] reported on 467 patients with operable squamous or adenocarcinoma of the esophagus randomized to 3 cycles of preoperative cisplatin and

5-FU followed by 2 cycles postoperatively. Median and 3-year survival figures were similar.

Radiotherapy

Preoperative radiotherapy

Seven randomized trials have compared preoperative radiotherapy with surgery for squamous cell carcinoma, of which six have found no survival advantage for neoadjuvant radiotherapy [14-19]. Only one describe a survival advantage for preoperative radiotherapy [5] but patients receiving preoperative chemotherapy and radiotherapy were pooled with those who had radiotherapy only.

Postoperative radiotherapy

Three trials comparing postoperative radiotherapy with surgery alone found no survival advantage for adjuvant radiotherapy, which was associated with significant morbidity. Following curative resection Zieren *et al.* [20] randomized 68 patients to 55.8 Gy radiotherapy or surgery alone, a French group [21] randomized 221 patients to 45-55 Gy postoperative radiotherapy or surgery and Fok *et al.* [22] randomized 60 patients to 49 Gy radiotherapy or surgery alone. None found an advantage and one [21] found a significantly disadvantage for postoperative therapy.

Chemoradiotherapy

Chemoradiotherapy versus radiotherapy

Four randomized trials compared radiotherapy and chemotherapy with radiotherapy alone. Araujo *et al.* [23] reported no difference in outcome in 59 patients with squamous carcinoma randomized to 5-FU, mitomycin C and bleomycin and radiotherapy or radiotherapy alone. Roussel *et al.* [24] reported no survival advantage in 144 patients with advanced carcinoma randomized to methotrexate and 56 Gy radiotherapy over radiotherapy alone. Sischy *et al.* [25] treated 135 patients with 5-FU and mitomycin C and 40 Gy radiotherapy or radiotherapy alone. The median survival for the multimodality group was significantly longer at 14 months than 9 months for radiotherapy alone. Herskovic *et al.* [26] randomized 121 potentially curable patients to 64 Gy radiation alone or 50 Gy concurrent with two courses of cisplatin and 5-FU. Long-term follow-up confirms a 3-year survival of 30% *versus* 0% favouring multimodal therapy [27]. These trials support concurrent chemotherapy and radiotherapy over radiotherapy alone.

Chemoradiotherapy plus surgery versus surgery

Five randomized trials have compared preoperative chemotherapy and radiotherapy with surgery alone for squamous cancer and one trial pooled adenocarcinoma (75%) and squamous cancer. Half used consecutive, the rest concurrent chemoradiotherapy. Nygaard *et al.* [5] randomized 186 patients into four subgroups, two of which were to receive sequential chemotherapy and radiotherapy or surgery alone. They found a survival advantage for neoadjuvant radiotherapy over surgery alone but no further advantage for added chemotherapy. LePrise *et al.* [28] reported no survival advantage in 86 patients randomized to receive sequential preoperative chemotherapy (5-FU and cisplatin) and low dose radiotherapy (20 Gy) over surgery alone. Bosset *et al.* [29] reported on the EORTC trial of 282 patients randomized to sequential 37 Gy together with single-agent cisplatin chemotherapy. Disease-free survival was 40% *versus* 28% favouring multimodal therapy but there was no overall survival difference (36% *versus* 34%) at 3 years. Apinop *et al.* [30] reported on 69 patients with squamous cell carcinoma randomized to preoperative concurrent CRT with two cycles of cisplatin and 5-FU plus 40 Gy radiotherapy. The difference in survival of 10 months *versus* 7 months was not significant. Urba *et al.* [3] randomized 100 patients with squamous or adenocarcinoma (70%) to concurrent cisplatin, vinblastin and 5-FU plus 45 Gy radiotherapy or surgery only. There was a trend in 3 years survival of 15% *versus* 32% favouring multimodal therapy (p = 0.07) not reaching significance. Walsh *et al.* [31] randomized 98 patients with squamous cell carcinoma of the esophagus to preoperative concurrent cisplatin and 5-FU and 40 Gy radiotherapy or surgery alone. Survival at 3 years was 32% for the multimodal limb and 16% for surgery alone while the 5-year survival was 36% *versus* 11% for surgery. In summary, trials support a trend or significant difference especially for concurrent and multi-agent treatment.

What works for adenocarcinoma? Evidence from non-randomized trials

Preoperative chemotherapy

The only trials on preoperative chemotherapy have been single arm and uncontrolled [32, 33] showing some promise but poorly tolerated.

Pre- and postoperative chemotherapy

Ajani *et al.* [34] reported a median survival of 24 months in 35 patients with resectable adenocarcinoma treated with preoperative and postoperative etoposide, cisplatin and 5-FU. In a further trial they treated 26 potentially resectable patients with preoperative etoposide, doxorubicin, cisplatin and GM-CSF and a further three postoperative doses to responding patients [35]. They concluded that less toxic and more effective regimens were required.

Combined chemotherapy and radiotherapy

Chemotherapy and radiotherapy without surgery

Coia *et al.* [36], in an uncontrolled study, treated 20 patients with adenocarcinoma with combined 5-FU, mitomycin and radiation therapy. The median relapse-free survival was 10 months and the median survival was 15 months.

Hoff *et al.* [37] treated 39 patients with adenocarcinoma with two cycles of cisplatin, 5-FU, etoposide, leucovorin and 30 Gy radiation therapy followed by resection [40]. A complete response to preoperative therapy was seen in 19%. Actuarial survival at 12, and 24 months was 72 and 51%. Stewart *et al.* [38] reported an uncontrolled trial of cisplatin, 5-FU and leucovorin, and concomitant 30 Gy radiation in 24 patients with adenocarcinoma. The median survival was more than 26 months. Wolfe *et al.* [2] used preoperative multi-agent chemotherapy and radiotherapy in 93 patients with adenocarcinoma. The 5-year survival amongst resected patients was 25%. Twenty percent of those resected had a sterilised specimen with a 5-year survival of 60%. Urba *et al.* [39] reported on 5-FU as single agent therapy with 49 Gy radiotherapy followed by transhiatal esophagectomy in 24 patients. The median survival was only 11 months. Naunheim *et al.* [40] treated 28 patients preoperatively with two courses of cisplatin and 5-FU and 30 or 36 Gy radiation. Seventeen percent had a complete response. Actuarial survival at 2, and 3 years was 28 and 20% respectively. Algan *et al.* [41] compared high-dose chemoradiation with high-dose chemoradiation followed by esophagectomy in a study of patients with potentially resectable adenocarcinoma and found no survival advantage for esophagectomy after treatment. Keller *et al.* [42] studied 46 patients with stage I or II adenocarcinoma of the esophagus or gastroesophageal junction treated with concomitant 60 Gy radiation and 5-FU and mitomycin (10 mg/m^2 bolus). Overall median survival was 16.6 months and 2-year survival 27%.

What works for adenocarcinoma? Evidence from randomized trials

There are no randomized trials on chemotherapy *versus* surgery or radiotherapy *versus* surgery. Neither are there randomized trials comparing different agents. Urba *et al.* pooled adenocarcinoma (75%) with squamous cell carcinoma and found a survival trend favouring multimodal therapy as reported above. Walsh *et al.* [43] reported the only randomized trial comparing preoperative 5-FU and cisplatin and 40 Gy radiotherapy with surgery alone in 113 patients. Chemotherapy consisted of two cycle of. Radiation therapy was given over 15 days, the first five concurrent with the first course of chemotherapy. The median survival based on intention to treat, was 17 *versus* 12 months favoring multimodality therapy ($p = 0.003$). The actual five-year survival rates were 34% and 2% respectively. Multimodal treatment was superior to surgery alone for resectable adenocarcinoma.

Summary

Preoperative but not postoperative chemotherapy has shown promise in large randomized trials. Neither preoperative nor postoperative radiotherapy has proven efficacy. Concurrent combined treatment given preoperatively using multiple agents has shown a complete pathological response of 20-30% for adenocarcinoma with a survival advantage over surgery alone. Refinements of current agents may add a few percentage points of difference. For a radical difference new strategies are needed.

References

1. O'Sullivan GC, Sheehan D, Clarke A, et al. Micrometastases in esophagogastric cancer: high detection rate in resected rib segments. Gastroenterology 1999;116 (3):543-548.
2. Wolfe WG, Vaughn AL, Seigler HF, et al. Survival of patients with carcinoma of the esophagus treated with combined-modality therapy. J Thorac Cardiovas Surg 1993;105:749-755.
3. Urba S, Orringer M, Turris A, et al. A randomized trial comparing surgery to preoperative concomitant chemoradiation plus surgery in patients with resectable esophageal cancer: updated analysis. Proc ASCO 1997;16:227a.
4. Schlag PM. Randomized trial preoperative chemotherapy for squamous cell cancer Arch Surg 1992;127:1446-1450.
5. Nygaard K, Hagen S, Hansen HS, et al. Pre-operative radiotherapy prolongs survival in operable esophageal carcinoma: a randomized, muilticenter study of pre-operative radiotherapy and chemotherapy. World J Surg 1992;16:1104-1110.
6. Law SY, Fok M, Chow S, et al. Preoperative chemotherapy versus surgical therapy alone for squamous cell carcinoma of the esophagus. A prospective randomized trial. J Thorac Cardiovasc Surg 1997;114:210-217.
7. Medical Research Council. MRC/UKCCCR Upper GI Tract Cancer National Meeting, London, UK. 10th Feburary 2000.
8. Kok TC, Lanschot JV, Siersema PD, et al. Neoadjuvant chemotherapy in operable esophageal squamous cell cancer:final report of a phase III multicentre randomized controlled trial. Proc Am Soc Clin Oncol 1997;16:277a.
9. Pouliquen X, Levard H, Hay JM, et al. 5-Fluouracil and cisplatin therapy after palliative surgical resection of squamous cell carcinoma of the esophagus. A multicenter randomized trial. French Association for Surgical Research. Ann Surg 1996;223:127-133.
10. Ando N, Iizuka T, Ide H, et al. A randomized trial of surgery alone vs surgery plus postoperative chemotherapy with cisplatin and 5-fluorouracil for localized squamous carcinoma of the thoracic esophagus: the Japan Clinical Oncology Group Study (JCOG 9204). Presented at ASCO, Atlanta, 1999.
11. Roth JA, Pass HI, Flanagan MM, et al. Randomized clinical trial of preoperative and postoperative adjuvant chemotherapy with cisplatin, vindesine and bleomycin for carcinoma of the esophagus. J Thorac Cardiovasc Surg 1988;96:242-246.
12. Saltz L, Kelsen D. Combined modality therapy in the treatment of loco-regional esophageal cancer. Ann Oncol 1992;3:793-799.
13. Kelsen DP, Ginsberg R, Pajak TF, et al. Chemotherapy followed by surgery compared with surgery alone for localised esophageal cancer. N Eng J Med 1998;114:210-217.
14. Arnott SJ, Duncan W, Kerr GR, et al. Low dose preoperative radiotherapy for carcinoma of the esophagus: results of a randomized clinical trial. Radiother Oncol 1992;24:108-113.
15. Gignoux M, Roussel A, Paillot B, et al. The value of preoperative radiotherapy in esophageal cancer: results of a study of the EORTC. World J Surg 1987;11:426-432.
16. Launois B, Delarue D, Campion JP, Kerbaol M. Preoperative radiotherapy for carcinoma of the esophagus. Surg Gynaecol Obst 1981;153:690-692.
17. Huang GJ, Gu XZ. Experience with combined preoperative irradiation and surgery for squamous-cell carcinoma of the esophagus. In: Wagner G, Zhang YH, eds. Cancer of the liver, esophagus and nasopharynx. New York: Springer-Verlag, 1987:134.
18. Mie W, Xian-Zhi G, Wiebo Y, et al. Randomized clinical trial on the combination of preoperative irradiation and surgery in the treatment of esophageal carcinoma: a report of 206 patients. Int J Radiat Oncol Biol Phys 1989;16:325-330.
19. Husemann B. Preoperative radiotherapy or chemotherapy. In: Giuli R, ed. Cancer of the esophagus in 1984. Paris: Maloine, 1984:55-58.
20. Zieren HU, Müller JM, Jacobi CA, et al. Adjuvant postoperative radiation therapy after curative resection of squamous cell carcinoma of the thoracic esophagus: a prospective randomized study. World J Surg 1995;19:444-449.
21. The French University Association for Surgical Research. Postoperative radiation therapy does not increase survival after curative resection for squamous cell carcinoma of the middle and lower esophagus as shown by a multicenter controlled trial. Surg Gynaecol Obst 1991;173:123-130.
22. Fok M, Sham J, Choy D, et al. Postoperative radiotherapy for carcinoma of the esophagus: a prospective randomized controlled trial. Surgery 1993;113:138-147.
23. Araujo CM, Souhami L, Gil RA, et al. A randomized trial comparing radiation therapy versus concomitant radiation therapy and chemotherapy in carcinoma of the thoracic esophagus. Cancer 1991;67:2258-2261.
24. Roussel A, Bleiberg H, Dalesio O, et al. Palliative therapy of inoperable esophageal cancer with radiotherapy and methotrexate: final results of a controlled clinical trial. Int J Radiat Oncol Biol Phys 1988;16:67-72.
25. Sischy B, Ryan L, Haller D, et al. Interim report of EST 1282 phase III protocol for the evaluation of combined modalities in the treatment of patients with carcinoma of the esophagus, stage I and II. Proc Am Soc Clin Oncol 1990;9:105.
26. Herskovic A, Martz K, Al-Sharaf M, et al. Combined chemotherapy and alone in patients with cancer of the esophagus. N Engl J Med 1992, 326:24;1593-1598.
27. Cooper JS, Guo MD, Herskovic A, et al. Chemoradiotherapy of locally advanced esophageal cancer. JAMA 1999;281:1623-1627.

28. LePrise E, Etienne P, Meunier B, et al. A randomized study of chemotherapy, radiation therapy and surgery versus surgery for localised squamous cell carcinoma of the esophagus. Cancer 1994;74:1779-1784.
29. Bosset JF, Gignoux M, Triboulet JP, et al. Chemoradiotherapy followed by surgery compared with surgery alone in squamous cell cancer of the esophagus. N Engl J Med 1997;337:161-167.
30. Apinop C, Puttisak P, Preecha N. A prospective study of combined therapy in esophageal cancer. Hepatogastroenterology 1994;41:391-393.
31. Walsh TN, McDonnell CO, Mulligan E, et al. Multimodal therapy versus surgery alone for squamous cell carcinoma of the esophagus:a prospective randomized trial. Gastroenterology 2000;11:A1008.
32. Kies MS, Rosen ST, Tsang TK, et al. Cisplatin and 5-fluorouracil in the primary management of squamous esophageal cancer. Cancer 1987;60:2156-2160.
33. Adelstein DJ, Rice TW, Boyce GA, et al. Adenocarcinoma of the esophagus and gastroesophageal junction. Clinical and pathologic assessment of response to induction chemotherapy. Am J Clin Oncol 1994;17:14-18.
34. Ajani JA, Roth JA, Ryan B, et al. Evaluation of pre- and post-operative chemotherapy for resectable adenocarcinoma of the esophagus. J Clin Oncol 1990;8:1231-1234.
35. Ajani JA, Roth JA, Ryan MB, et al. Intensive preoperative chemotherapy with colony-stimulating factor for resectable adenocarcinoma of the esophagus or gastroesophageal junction. J Clin Oncol 1993;11:22-28.
36. Coia LR, Paul AR, Engstrom PF. Combined radiation and chemotherapy as primary management of adenocarcinoma of the esophagus and gastroesophageal junction. Cancer 1988;61:643-649.
37. Hoff SJ, Stewart JR, Sawyers JL, et al. Preliminary results with neoadjuvant therapy and resection for esophageal carcinoma. Ann Thorac Surg 1993;56:282-286.
38. Stewart JR, Hoff SJ, Johnson DH, et al. Improved survival with neoadjuvant therapy and resection for adenocarcinoma of the esophagus. Ann Surg 1993;218:571-576.
39. Urba SG, Orringer MB, Perez-Tamayo C, et al. Concurrent preoperative chemotherapy and radiation therapy in localized esophageal adenocarcinoma. Cancer 1992;69:285-291.
40. Naunheim KS, Petruska PJ, Roy TS, et al. Multimodality therapy for adenocarcinoma of the esophagus. Ann Thoracic Surg 1995;59:1085-1090.
41. Algan O, Coia LR, Keller SM, et al. Management of adenocarcinoma of the esophagus with chemoradiation alone or chemoradiation followed by esophagectomy: results of sequential nonrandomized phase II studies. Int J Radiat Oncol Biol Phys 1995;32:753-761.
42. Keller SM, RyanLM, Coia LR, et al. High dose chemoradiotherapy followed by esophagectomy for adenocarcinoma of the esophagus and gastroesophageal junction. Cancer 1998;83:1908-1916.
43. Walsh TN, Noonan N, Hollywood D, et al. A comparison of multimodal therapy and surgery for esophageal adenocarcinoma. N Engl J Med 1996;335:462-467.

Following resection, can DNA ploidy be considered as a prognostic factor?

B.P.L. Wijnhoven, H.W. Tilanus (Rotterdam)

Transformation from a normal to a malignant cell may be associated with changes in total DNA content or ploidy. A normal cell has a chromosome number of 2N, for which the term diploid is applied. A cell with numerical aberrations is designated as aneuploid. Barrett's dysplasia and esophageal adenocarcinomas are characterized by chromosomal instability leading to aneuploidy. It is suggested that chromosome instability, tetraploidization, and asymmetrical chromosome segregation during cell division are the result of dysfunctioning human mitotic checkpoint genes. But also genes with multiple functions that normally exert active checks on the cell cycle processes including apoptosis and chromosome stability, *e.g.* p53 and k-ras genes, can be deregulated.

Table I.

First author	Aneuploid tumors/ tumors analyzed (%)	Pathological characteristics of the tumor that correlate with DNA ploidy	Factors predicting survival	
			univariate	multivariate analysis
Finley *et al.*	61/75 (81)	pN tumor stage	Tumor grade, pT, pN, ploidy	Tumor grade, pT, pN
Nakamura *et al.*	69/80 (86)	pN	pT, pN, pM, ploidy	pT, pM, ploidy (N0/R0 patients)
Sarbia *et al.*	59/65 (61)	Ming's classification*	pT, pN, pR, tumor grade, Lauren and Ming's classification, size of tumor	No data
Schneeberger *et al.*	61/75 (81)	pN, tumor stage	pT, pN, tumor grade (overall surv.) ploidy (dis. free survival)	pT, pN, tumor grade
Bittinger *et al.*	25/50 (50)	Tumor grade, pN	Ploidy, pT, pN, pM, stage, pR, lymphangio-invasiveness	Ploidy, pT, pM (R0 patients)
Flejou *et al.*	16/23 (80)	pT, pN	No statistical analysis	No statistical analysis
Khan *et al.*	24/30 (80)	No correlation	No correlation	No data
Gleeson *et al.*	16/20 (80)	No correlation	No data	No data

* Expansive *versus* infiltrative carcinomas

By using flow cytometry, it is possible to provide objective information about the ploidy status of the tumor with reference to cells with a normal diploid amount of DNA. It has been shown that the evolution from normal esophagus to premalignant Barrett's metaplasia is frequently associated with abnormal DNA content and increased G2/M fraction (4N) of the metaplastic cells. Moreover, abnormal DNA content shows a correlation with the histologic diagnosis of dysplasia and carcinoma. Flow cytometry also detects a subset of patients whose biopsies are histologically indefinite or negative for dysplasia and carcinoma, but who have DNA content abnormalities similar to those otherwise seen only in dysplasia and carcinoma. Therefore, this technique (in combination with histology) may be of use in screening patients with Barrett's esophagus for early signs of malignant change. As their precursor lesion, Barrett's adenocarcinomas often demonstrate aneuploidy. Several studies have consistently documented high levels of DNA aneuploidy, typically ranging from 50-85% [1-6].

What is the relationship between DNA ploidy and pathological characteristics of the tumor?

Most studies report that aneuploid tumors are significantly associated with infiltration of the wall of the esophagus (pT-stage), increased lymph node metastases (pN) and/or advanced stage of disease [2, 3, 5, 6]. Only two studies could not establish a significant relationship between DNA ploidy and pathology.

What is the relationship between DNA ploidy and survival in patients after resection for esophageal adenocarcinoma?

DNA ploidy can predict overall survival or disease free survival after resection, but only two studies identified DNA ploidy as an independent predictor of survival: in patients with Barrett's adenocarcinoma after curative resection (R0) [3], and in lymph node-negative (N0), R0-resected patients [6]. Bittinger *et al.* found that DNA ploidy is the strongest predictor of survival (and not pTNM stage): patients with diploid or tetraploid tumors had a significantly better prognosis with a 3-year survival rate of 35% in contrast to 8% for aneuploid tumors. Furthermore, within the pT2 and pT3 tumors, DNA ploidy allowed additional prognostic information [3].

In conclusion, current data from the literature demonstrate that aneuploidy in esophageal adenocarcinomas reflects the numerous chromosomal aberrations and this correlates well with the aggressiveness of the tumor. Aneuploid tumors are generally more likely to have positive lymph nodes, which is usually one of the most important prognostic variable in predicting disease free and overall survival. Considering the information obtained from pathological examination of the esophagogastric specimen, the addition of tumor ploidy can alert the clinician to high-risk groups, namely those with increased incidence of lymph node metastases, recurrence, and poorer survival. However, further studies on a larger series of patients with adenocarcinomas of the esophagus will be necessary for verification of these results. One of the great advantages of flow cytometric analysis of DNA ploidy is that it can be reliable on routine, paraffin-embedded tissues and pre-operative mucosal biopsies, thereby enabling assessment of prognosis at the time of cancer diagnosis. However, their clinical relevance for therapeutic decision making (*e.g.* extent of surgical resection, indication for neo-adjuvant radiotherapy or chemotherapy) remains to be demonstrated.

References

1. Gleeson CM, Sloan JM, McManus DT, Maxwell P, Arthur K, McGuigan JA, Ritchie AJ, Russel SHE. Comparison of p53 and DNA content abnormalities in adenocarcinoma of the esophagus and gastric cardia. Br J Cancer 1998;77:277-286.
2. Finley RJ, Inculet RI. The results of esophagogastrectomy without thoracotomy for adenocarcinoma of the esophagogastric junction. Ann Surg 1989;210:535-542.
3. Bittinger T, Dutkowski P, Kirkpatrick CJ, Junginger T. Prognostic significance of tumor ploidy and histomorphological parameters in adenocarcinoma of Barrett's esophagus. Dig Surg 1999;16:180-185.
4. Sarbia M, Molsberger G, Willers R, Horstmann O, Schroders C, Porschen R, Gabbert HE. The prognostic significance of DNA ploidy in adenocarcinomas of the esophagogastric junction. J Cancer Res Clin Oncol 1996;122:186-188.
5. Schneeberger AL, Finley RJ, Troster M, Lohmann R, Keeney M, Inculet R. The prognostic significance of tumor ploidy and pathology in adenocarcinoma of the esophagogastric junction. Cancer 1990;65:1206-1210.
6. Nakamura T, Nekarda H, Hoelscher AH, Bollschweiler E, Harbec N, Becker K, Siewert JR. Prognostic value of DNA ploidy and c-erbB-2 oncoprotein overexpression in adenocarcinoma of Barrett's esophagus. Cancer 1994;73:1785-1794.
7. Flejou JF, Doublet B, Potet F, Metayer J, Hemet J. Etude de l'AND-ploïdie dans les adénocarcinomes sur endobrachyoesophage. Ann Pathol 1990;10:161-165.
8. Khan M, Bui HX, del Rosario A, Abdulla M, Ballouk F, Sim YJ, Ross JS. Role of DNA content determination by image analysis in confirmation of dysplasia in Barrett's esophagus. Mod Pathol 1994;7:169-174.

What is the compared value of tumor stage and lymph node invasion in cancers of the cardia?

H. Udagawa, Y. Kinoshita, M. Ueno, K. Tsutsumi, T. Nakamura, T. Iidsuka, H. Akiyama (Tokyo)

Cancer of the gastric cardia poses many problems for surgeons because of its unique location. In Western countries, cancer of the cardia is attracting attention because its incidence is thought to be rapidly increasing. In this study, we retrospectively reviewed our data on this disease to clarify the significance of the T and N categories of the TNM system with respect to prognosis and preoperative decision-making.

Material and methods

The subjects were 68 consecutive patients with adenocarcinoma of the cardia (Siewert type II [1]) who underwent surgical resection at Toranomon Hospital from 1990 to 1999 without preoperative adjuvant treatment. The relationship between the pT, pN, or pM categories and survival was investigated. The actual locations of lymph node metastasis were investigated in a special group of patients and the pattern of recurrence was also investigated.

Results

The relationship between the pT and pN (including pM1-lym, pM1 due to extra-regional lymph node involvement) categories is shown in *Table I*, and the metastasis rates to various lymph node groups are listed in *Table II*. Disease-specific survival curves stratified by pT and pN status are shown in *Figures 1 and 2*, respectively, Also, disease-specific survival curves stratified by the number of metastatic lymph nodes (regional and extraregional) are shown in *Figure 3*. The clinical features of three pM1-lym patients who survived more than 2 years are described in *Table III*. Recurrence was experienced by 11 patients. Among these 11 patients, hematogenous metastasis was found in 9 patients, lymph node metastasis in 3, and peritoneal dissemination in 2. Among the 3 patients with lymph node recurrence, 2 developed cervical lymph node metastasis and 2 had abdominal paraaortic node recurrence.

Table I. Relationship between pT and pN.

	pN[2]					
pT	0	1	2	3	Total	pN4[1]
1a	8	0	0	0	8	0
1b	12	2	0	0	14	0
2	9	15(1)	4(2)	0	28	3
3	3	8(1)	4(2)	1(1)	16	4
4	1	0	1	0	2	0
Total	33	25	9	1	68	0

1. pM1-lym (pM1 due to extra-regional lymph node involvement) is expressed here and in *Figure 2* as pN4
2. Numbers in parentheses show the number of pN4 patients

Table II. Rate of metastasis to different lymph node groups.

Lymph node group[1]	Number of n+ patients	% in the 68 subjects
Cervical	1	1.5
Upper mediastinal	0	0
Middle mediastinal	0	0
Lower mediastinal	4	5.9
Paracardiac-left gastric a. (1,2,3,7)	34	50.0
Around celiac a. (8,9,11,20)	13	19.1
Short gastric a.-left. gastroepiploic a. (4s)	2	2.9
Right gastroepiploic a. & infrapyloric (4d,6)	0	0
Suprapyloric (5)	1	1.5
Splenic hilum (10)	1	1.5
Extra-regional nodes in the abdomen (16,19)	4	5.9

1. Numbers in parentheses show the lymph node group numbers in the Japanese Classification of Gastric Carcinoma [3]

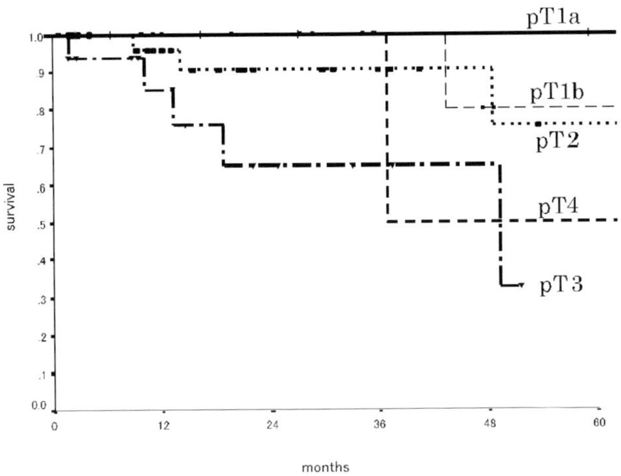

Figure 1. Disease-specific survival curves stratified by pT.

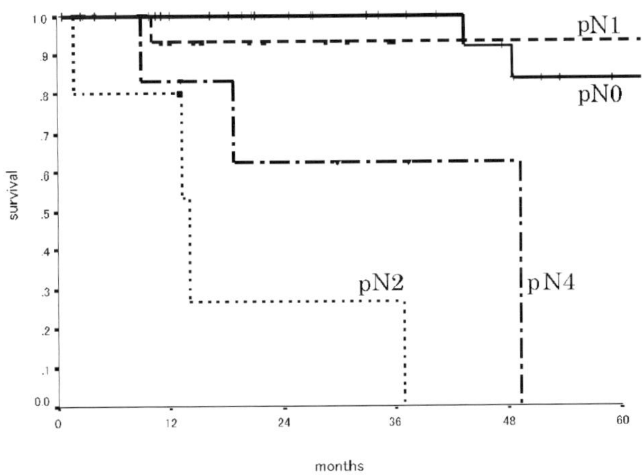

Figure 2. Disease-specific survival curves stratified by pN (Refer to comment 1. of *Table I*).

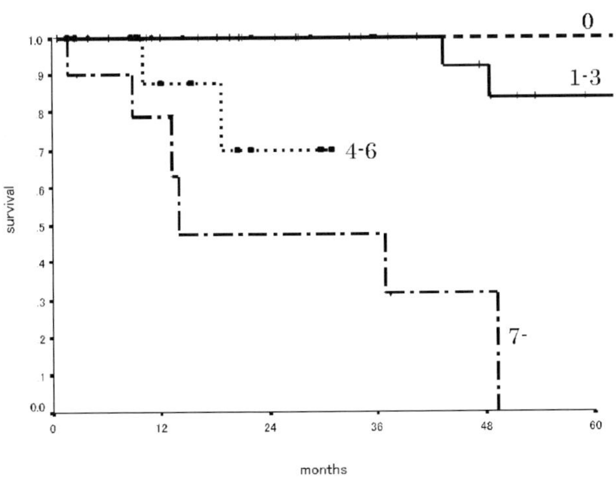

Figure 3. Disease-specific survival curves stratified by the number of metastatic lymph nodes regardless of regional or extraregional development.

Table III. Clinical features of patients who survived for more than 2 years with TNM extraregional lymph node metastasis.

Age	Sex	Tumor length (cm)	Approach	Nb of positive nodes	pT	Site of M1 nodes	Months after operation	Prognosis
49	M	5	LTA[1]	9	3	LM[2]	49.3	Dead of lung metastasis
41	M	8	LTA[1]	13	3	PA[3]	37.4	Alive without metastasis
58	M	4	LTA[1]	6	2	C[4], LM[2]	29.8	Alive without metastasis

1. Left thoracoabdominal approach
2. Lower mediastinal node
3. Abdominal paraaortic node
4. Cervical node

Discussion

As shown in *Table I*, pT1a tumors, which are limited to the mucosa (epithelium, lamina propria mucosae, and muscularis mucosae), were not associated with lymph node metastasis in our series. Although the number of cases is too small to conclude that T1a tumors are never associated with lymph node metastases (a large-scale study has given different results), limited procedures such as endoscopic mucosal resection (EMR) or laparoscopic local resection have a good chance of achieving a cure. T1b tumors, which invade the submucosa, have about a 15% risk of lymph node involvement, but it is limited to the regional lymph nodes of the TNM system and the number of metastatic nodes is relatively small. This means that a good prognosis can be expected after complete removal of the primary tumor and thorough dissection of the regional nodes. Once a tumor invades the proper muscle layer (T2), the number of metastatic nodes increases and the extraregional lymph node involvement may also occur. At the same time, no metastasis was seen to the infra-pyloric nodes or the right gastroepiploic nodes (*Table II*), implying that even when extraregional node involvement occurs, proximal gastrectomy is still possible for Siewert type II tumors.

As shown in *Figures 1 and 2*, pT and pN are both meaningful prognostic factors. When pM1-lym is categorized as pN4 and considered together with pN0~pN3 (*Figure 2*), an interesting inversion of the survival curves between pN2 and pN4 occurs. When survival curves are drawn according to a simpler grading of the number of metastatic nodes, this shows a better correlation with the prognosis (*Figure 3*). This tells us that even when a patient has a few extraregional lymph node metastases, a fair prognosis can still be achieved if such nodes are completely cleared (*Table III*). Accordingly, the total number of metastatic lymph nodes is a better prognostic indicator than a crude regional *versus* extraregional classification.

Although pT and pN are correlated with each other, as shown in *Table I*, they essentially express different aspects of tumor spread. It should be noted that pT1a has an absolutely good prognosis, while pN0 does not. Also, complete cure is very difficult in pN2-3 patients with 7 or more lymph nodes involved, while pT4 patients have a much higher chance of cure. The lesson from this is that efforts to remove the primary tumor (pT) and lymph node metastases (pN) are equally important, and a good result is only possible when both are achieved. In this sense, preoperative staging is extremely important to determine the proper approach and the extent of lymph node dissection. However, preoperative diagnosis of lymph node metastasis is not completely accurate. Therefore, we decide the approach and the extent of lymph node dissection according to the cT category and the tumor location [2].

As a general rule for cT1b or deeper tumors, we perform upper median laparotomy and abdominal lymphadenectomy when the tumor is limited to the stomach, and adopt a left thoracoabdominal approach for the clearance of lower mediastinal nodes when the tumor invades the abdominal esophagus. When the upper margin of the tumor is located in the thoracic esophagus, we perform right thoracotomy to allow complete mediastinal lymph node clearance. We think that the low rate of lymph node recurrence supports the validity of our criteria for selection of the surgical approach.

References

1. Siewert JR, Stein HJ. Carcinoma of the cardia: carcinoma of the gastroesophageal junction; classification, pathology, and extent of resection. Dis Esophagus 1996;9:173-182.
2. Udagawa H, Tsutsumi K, Kinoshita Y, Nakamura T, Ueno M, Kajiyama Y, Tsurumaru M. Therapeutic strategy for adenocarcinoma in Barrett's esophagus: a study based on a comparison with squamous cell carcinoma. J Japan Surg Soc 1999;100(3):261-264
3. Japanese Gastric Cancer Association. Japanese Classification of Gastric Carcinoma,13th ed. Tokyo: Kanehara, 1999:7-9.

What information can be expected from immunohistochemistry in the evaluation of late survival of patients with esophageal adenocarcinoma?

B.P.L. Wijnhoven, H.W. Tilanus (Rotterdam)

Factors that are relevant to prognosis should be considered in the treatment of adenocarcinoma of the esophagus to allow for the identification of patients who may benefit from esophageal resection in terms of survival. Factors relevant to prognosis that are based on the histologic assessment of the resected esophagus are known. Nevertheless there is variability and heterogeneity among tumor stages, and none of the available staging criteria accurately reflects the prognosis of an individual patient.

Since the rise of the molecular biology, many researchers studied the relationship between the immunohistochemical detection of new tumor markers (usually oncogene or tumor suppressor gene products) and clinicopathological features of the tumor. Besides the current TNM staging system, there are some promising markers that might stratify patients with esophageal adenocarcinoma into short and long-term survivors. Since immunohistochemistry has now become a routine technique in most laboratories, this has widened the door for application of new tumor markers in clinical practice. However, immunohistochemistry is still rather time-consuming and expensive compared to haematoxylin and eosin staining. Secondly, the prognostic significance of many tumor markers has not been proven to be superior above the current used prognostic variables based on histology such as tumor grade, number of positive lymph nodes, distant metastases or lymphangio invasiveness.

Usually in a retrospective fashion, the level of expression of oncogene and tumor suppressor gene products (as deermined by immunohistochemistry) is correlated with pathological characteristics of the tumor, stage of disease and overall or disease free survival. One of the best-studied molecular alteration in the Barrett esophageal adenocarcinoma sequence is the p53 gene alteration, that has been demonstrated in 40-80% of the tumors and appear to occur relatively early. Retrospective studies have linked p53 immunoreactivity, which reflects p53 protein dysfunction, with a poorer prognosis [1]. However, others report that mutational analysis is a better determinant of p53 function than immunohistochemistry [2]. Survival of patients with p53 mutations was significantly lower than that of patients without mutations: overall survival 21.6 months *versus* 40 months) and disease free survival (14.1 months *versus* 38 months) [3]. Other tumor markers studied are genes/proteins involved in cell proliferation and apoptosis (*e.g.* PCNA, Ki-67, Fas/APO-1) [4], cell cycle genes (*e.g.* retinoblastoma, cyclin D1, p21, p27) [5], genes involved in signal transduction (*e.g.* EGFR, TGF, c-erbB2 and VEGF) [6] and cell-cell adhesion molecules (*e.g.* E-cadherin-catenin complex and CD44 family) [7]. Some studies report additional prognostic value of a tumor marker besides the current TNM classification based on histology. However, a possible independent prognostic value in the evaluation of survival in patients after resection for esophageal adenocarcinoma can not be demonstrated or has not been studied.

New sensitive immunohistochemical assays that employ monoclonal antibodies directed against epithelial or tumor-associated marker proteins, can detect single isolated epithelial tumor cells in mesenchymal secondary organs (*e.g.* bone marrow and lymph nodes). Applying immunohistochemistry to the reanalysis of lymph nodes classified as "tumor free" by routine histopathological examination reveals considerable rates of early lymphatic dissemination in patients with resectable primary esophageal adenocarcinoma: 50% of patients with no nodal involvement on routine histopathological examination, were judged nodal positive after immunohistochemistry [8]. The presence of these tumor cells is an independent prognostic factor in terms of relapse free survival. Remarkably, all patients who were found to be free of nodal tumor involvement by both histopathological and immunohistochemical analysis survived the median observation period of 22 months without recurrence [8]. However, there is no correlation between the presence of micrometastatic cancer cells in bone marrow obtained from the rib or iliac crest and TNM status, nor was there a difference in the prevalence of micrometastases in rib marrow between patients who received neoadjuvant chemotherapy and patients who underwent surgery alone [8, 9]. In other tumor types, the presence of micrometastatic tumor cells in bone marrow are a marker of poor prognosis. For esophageal adenocarcinoma this needs a more extensive study.

In conclusion, immunocytochemical assays should become acceptable for international tumor staging classifications. However, future studies need a careful statistical evaluation of the data with multivariate analysis in order to prove independent prognostic significance of the new tumor markers. Combined analysis with expression of several markers in the same tumor specimen may even more accurately identify subgroups with poor or good prognosis. However, protein expression as determined by immunohistochemistry does not always reflect protein function. Therefore, genetic analysis might be a more sensitive predictor of tumor aggressiveness as has been shown for the p53 tumor suppressor gene. Ideally, one should be informed about the biological behavior of the tumor before surgery is applied. Pre-operative mucosal biopsies or cytological brushes can enable assessment of prognosis at the time of cancer diagnosis and might aid in therapeutic decision making (*e.g.* extent of surgical resection, indication for neo-adjuvant radiotherapy or chemotherapy). Finally, immunohistochemical assessment of lymph nodes can be used to refine the staging system for esophageal adenocarcinoma and help identify patients who will be short or long term survivors and/or not be cured by surgery alone. However, further research into this interesting field is necessary before translation into the clinical setting can be made.

References

1. Casson A, Kerkvliet N, O'Malley F. Prognostic value of p53 protein in esophageal adenocarcinoma. J Surg Oncol 1995;60:5-11.
2. Ireland AP, Clark GWB, DeMeester TR. The significance of p53 in clinical practice. Ann Surg 1997;225:17-30.
3. Ribeiro U, Finkelstein SD, Safatle-Ribeiro AV, Landreneau RJ, Clarke MR, Bakker A, Swalsky PA, Gooding WE, Posner MC. P53 sequence analysis predicts treatment response and outcome of patients with esophageal adenocarcinoma. Cancer 1998;83:7-18.
4. Yasunaga M, Tabira Y, Kondo K, Okuma T, Kitamura N. The prognostic significance of cell cycle markers in esophageal cancer after neoadjuvant therapy. Dis Esophagus 1999;12:120-127.
5. Kuwahara M, Hirai T, Yoshida K, Yamashita Y, Hihara J, Inoue H, Toge T. P53, p21 (Waf1/Cip1) and cyclin D1 protein expression and prognosis in esophageal cancer. Dis Esophagus 1999;12:116-119.
6. Yacoub L, Goldman H, Odze R. Transforming growth factor-α, epidermal growth factor receptor, and MiB-1 expression in Barrett's associated neoplasia: correlation with prognosis. Mod Pathol 1997;10:105-112.
7. Krishnadath KK, Tilanus HW, van Blankenstein M, Hop WCJ, Kremers ED, Dinjens WNM, Bosman FT. Reduced expression of the E-cadherin-catenin complex in esophageal adenocarcinoma correlates with poor prognosis. J Pathol 1997;182:331-338.
8. Izbicki JR, Hosch SB, Pichlmeier U, Rehders A, Busch C, Niendorf A, Passlick B, Broelsch CE, Pantel K. prognostic value of immunohistochemically identifiable tumor cells in lymph nodes of patients with completely resected esophageal cancer. New Engl J Med 1997;337:1188-1194.
9. O'Sullivan, GC, Sheehan D, Clarke A, Stuart R, Kelly J, Kiely B, Walsh T, Collins JK, Shanahan FLJ. Micrometastases in esophagogastric cancer: high detection rate in resected rib segments. Gastroenterology 1999;116:543-548.

Should Barrett's esophagus be treated at all?

S.J. Sontag (Hines)

The management of Barrett's esophagus is controversial. Current surveillance recommendations for patients with documented Barrett's esophagus are predicated on the hope that Barrett's cancer either can be prevented or can be detected early enough so that therapy prevents death from the cancer. The frequency of surveillance endoscopies needed to accomplish this goal is not known. Frequency intervals vary from every 3 months for Barrett's with high-grade dysplasia (HGD) to every 3-5 years for Barrett's without dysplasia. Thus, if the goal of treatment is early detection of esophageal cancer, it is imperative to know something about the natural history of the disease.

It is generally accepted that the development of Barrett's cancer follows a dysplasia-carcinoma sequence: intestinal metaplasia (IM) without dysplasia progresses to IM with low-grade dysplasia (LGD) to IM with HGD to cancer [1]. The factors that encourage or discourage the leap to cancer remain unidentified. A few facts, however, are generally accepted:

- the vast majority of patients with Barrett's esophagus are rather healthy, and thus remain undiagnosed;
- the vast majority of patients with Barrett's cancer come to endoscopy when it is too late.

Based on our 20-year Hines VA database, the prevalence and incidence of Barrett's esophagus and Barrett's cancer as follows

• Prevalence:
- 15% of all adults with gastroesophageal reflux (GER) symptoms have Barrett's esophagus;
- 0.7% of all adults with GER symptoms will have Barrett's cancer at first endoscopy.

• Incidence:
- 2% of all Barrett's esophagus patients will develop Barrett's cancer during a mean of 7 years (0.3% per year);

- 15% of all Barrett's HGD patients will develop Barrett's cancer during a mean of 7 years (2.2% per year).

Based on national statistics, the importance of esophageal cancer as the percentage of all cancers, the percentage of all cancer deaths and the esophageal cancer death rate can be placed into perspective

• *Figure 1a* shows that esophageal cancer is uncommon.
Esophageal cancer in 1998 represented only 1% of all new cancers [1].
- # of new esophageal cancers: 12,200
- total # of cancers: 1,220,000
- percentage: 1%

• *Figure 1b* shows that esophageal cancer in 1998 represented only 2% of all cancer deaths [1].
- # of esophageal cancer deaths: 11,800
- total # of cancer deaths: 578,200
- percentage: 2%

• *Figure 1c* shows the percentage of patients with esophageal cancer that died.
- 97% of esophageal cancer patients died (11,800 of 12,200)
- 3% did not die (400 of 12,200)

From these statistics, it appears that only a small minority of patients with Barrett's esophagus will go on to develop HGD and eventually cancer. Indeed, only 12,200 new cases of esophageal cancer are diagnosed each year, and about half of those are squamous cell carcinomas. Thus, about 6,000 cases of Barrett's cancer occur each year, and almost all are diagnosed when it is too late.

It seems, therefore, that if any major decrease in the mortality of Barrett's cancer is to be achieved, it will be brought about only by the large-scale identification of patients with Barrett's esophagus who do not yet have cancer. At the present time, such identification could occur only by massive screening of individuals at high risk for Barrett's and cancer.

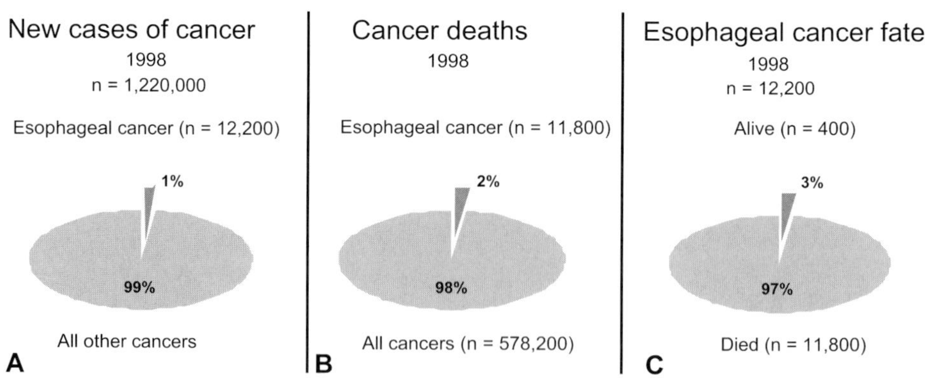

Figure 1. A. In 1998, esophageal cancer represented only 1% of all new cancers in the US. **B.** In 1998, esophageal cancer represented only 2% of all cancer deaths in the US. **C.** In 1998, 97% of patients diagnosed with esophageal cancer died.

Such individuals are otherwise healthy, although heartburn symptoms may make them easily identifiable. Indeed, a recent study from Sweden showed that the presence of heartburn, regurgitation or both at least one time per week increases the risk of esophageal cancer 8-fold [2]. If the symptoms are frequent, severe and of 20 years duration, the cancer risk increases 44-fold. In order to substantially reduce the esophageal cancer death rate, this group would need to be targeted for early endoscopic examination. Anything short of a full-blown attack on this group with symptomatic GER will necessarily fail to achieve that goal. On the other hand, a full-blown attack on this group would require massive investment of time and energy by currently available endoscopists.

Figure 2 is a decade-old poll demonstrating that 44% of adult Americans have heartburn at least once monthly and 18% take indigestion medication at least twice a week [3]. These numbers indicate that 18 million – at minimum – adult Americans would need screening endoscopy to detect Barrett's esophagus, so that they could be enrolled in a surveillance program of additional endoscopies.

Figure 3 compares the incidence of esophageal cancer and colon cancer in the United States. Colon cancer occurs 13 times as often as Barrett's cancer, raising the important question of whether we should divert our resources to the other end of the intestine. Indeed, every 90-minutes in the United States, one individual dies from esophageal cancer, while 13 die from colon cancer.

Given the high prevalence of symptomatic GER in the general population, the low prevalence of Barrett's esophagus in the symptomatic GER population, the very low Barrett's esophagus diagnosis rate in the total Barrett's population, the minuscule incidence of cancer in the Barrett's population, and the dismal survival rate of patients with Barrett's cancer, it is unlikely that a major decrease in mortality from Barrett's cancer will occur in the near future. There is, however, a possibility that a completely different form of therapy may have an impact in the morbidity and mortality of esophageal cancer.

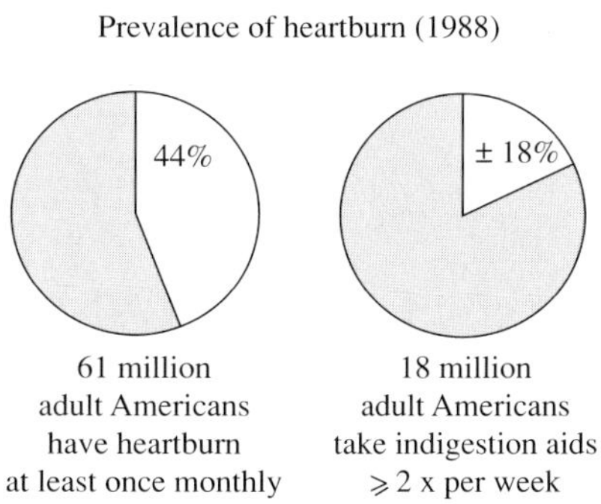

Figure 2. Gallop survey showing that 44% of adult Americans have heartburn at least once monthly and 18% take indigestion medication at least twice a week.

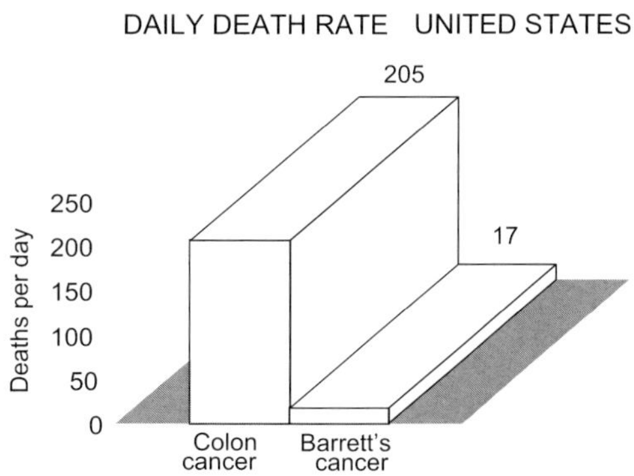

Figure 3. The incidences of esophageal cancer and colon cancer.

A different approach

If we must question the wisdom of spending a hunk of our resources on a disease in which 97% of its victims are "goners" from the time of first diagnosis, and less than 3% are potentially treatable or curable, then perhaps we might find some hope in the concept of chemoprevention. Although still untested and unproven, chemoprevention – in the form of COX-2 inhibitors – are now being studied for the prevention and regression of colon polyps and the prevention and regression of Barrett's esophageal dysplasia.

Chemoprevention

The theoretical goal of cancer chemoprevention is to inhibit or reverse pre-invasive carcinogenesis before the development of clinical cancer. The goals of current clinical studies are to demonstrate regression of existing neoplasia, prevention of recurrent neoplasia, and prevention of first-time neoplasia. The genetic targets for chemoprevention are genetic damage and genetic defects. If chemoprevention, whether through COX-2 inhibitors or some other agents, eventually proves to be a reliable discipline in the reversal of dysplasia or the prevention of the ultimate dysplasia – cancer – its eventual impact would depend completely on how the medical community responded to the following question: *"If physicians – and their patients with Barrett's esophagus – could be relatively certain that they would not develop cancer – regardless of the current grade of dysplasia – would the medical community accept in lieu of repeated endoscopies and surgical resection a lifetime daily dose of a chemopreventive agent, such as a COX-2 inhibitor?"*

References

1. Cancer Statistics. CA. A cancer journal for physicians. Am Cancer Soc 1998;48:6-30.
2. Lagergren J, Bergstrom R, Lindgren A, et al. Symptomatic gastroesophageal reflux as a risk factor for esophageal adenocarcinoma. N Engl J Med 1999;340:825-831.
3. Gallup Survey. Heartburn across America. Princeton, NJ: Gallup Orgainzation, 1988:Mar 24.

AUTHORS INDEX

SUBJECT INDEX

Treatments

Medical treatments

Surgical treatments

Ablation therapy

Screening and surveillance

Regression

Adenocarcinomas

Achevé d'imprimer par Corlet, Imprimeur, S.A. - 14110 Condé-sur-Noireau
N° d'Imprimeur : 72580 - Dépôt légal : août 2003 - *Imprimé en France*